NERVOUS CONTROL OF BLOOD VESSELS

The Autonomic Nervous System

A series of books discussing all aspects of the autonomic nervous system. Edited by Geoffrey Burnstock, Department of Anatomy and Developmental Biology, University College of London, UK.

Volume 1
Autonomic Neuroeffector Mechanisms
edited by *G. Burnstock* and *C.H.V. Hoyle*

Volume 2
Development, Regeneration and Plasticity
of the Autonomic Nervous System
edited by *I.A. Hendry* and *C.E. Hill*

Volume 3
Nervous Control of the Urogenital System
edited by *C.A. Maggi*

Volume 4
Comparative Physiology and Evolution of
the Autonomic Nervous System
edited by *S. Nilsson* and *S. Holmgren*

Volume 5
Disorders of the Autonomic Nervous System
edited by *D. Robertson* and *I. Biaggioni*

Volume 6
Autonomic Ganglia
edited by *E.M McLachlan*

Volume 7
Autonomic Control of the Respiratory
System
edited by *P. Barnes*

Volume 8
Nervous Control of Blood Vessels
edited by *T. Bennett* and *S.M. Gardiner*

Additional Volumes in Preparation

Nervous Control of the Heart
J.T. Shepherd and *S.F. Vatner*

Autonomic – Endocrine Interactions
K. Unsicker

Central Control of Autonomic Function
D. Jordan

Nervous Control of the Eye
G. Burnstock and *A.M. Sillito*

Autonomic Innervation of the Skin
I.L. Gibbins and *J.L. Morris*

Nervous Control of the Gastrointestinal Tract
M. Costa

This book is part of a series. The publisher will accept continuation orders which may be cancelled at any time and which provide for automatic billing and shipping of each title in the series upon publication. Please write for details.

NERVOUS CONTROL OF BLOOD VESSELS

Edited by

Terence Bennett

and

Sheila M. Gardiner

*Department of Physiology
and Pharmacology
University of Nottingham Medical School
Nottingham
UK*

harwood academic publishers

**Australia • Canada • China • France • Germany • India • Japan
Luxembourg • Malaysia • The Netherlands • Russia • Singapore
Switzerland • Thailand • United Kingdom**

Emmaplein 5
1075 AW Amsterdam
The Netherlands

British Library Cataloguing in Publication Data

Nervous control of blood vessels. — (The autonomic
    nervous system; v. 8)
    1. Blood-vessels   2. Autonomic nervous system   3. Vascular
    smooth muscle
    I. Series   II. Bennett, Terence   III. Gardiner, Sheila M.
    612.8'49

ISBN 3-7186-5139-4

Contents

Preface to the Series — Historical and Conceptual Perspective of The Autonomic Nervous System Book Series

The pioneering studies of Gaskell (1886), Bayliss and Starling (1899), and Langley and Anderson (*see* Langley, 1921) formed the basis of the earlier and, to a large extent, current concepts of the structure and function of the autonomic nervous system; the major division of the autonomic nervous system into sympathetic, parasympathetic and enteric subdivisions still holds. The pharmacology of autonomic neuroeffector transmission was dominated by the brilliant studies of Elliott (1905), Loewi (1921), von Euler and Gaddum (1931), and Dale (1935), and for over 50 years the idea of antagonistic parasympathetic cholinergic and sympathetic adrenergic control of most organs in visceral and cardiovascular systems formed the working basis of all studies. However, major advances have been made since the early 1960s that make it necessary to revise our thinking about the mechanisms of autonomic transmission, and that have significant implications for our understanding of diseases involving the autonomic nervous system and their treatment. These advances include:

(1) Recognition that the autonomic neuromuscular junction is not a 'synapse' in the usual sense of the term where there is a fixed junction with both pre- and postjunctional specialization, but rather that transmitter is released from mobile varicosities in extensive terminal branching fibres at variable distances from effector cells or bundles of smooth muscle cells which are in electrical contact with each other and which have a diffuse distribution of receptors (*see* Hillarp, 1959; Burnstock, 1986a).

(2) The discovery of non-adrenergic, non-cholinergic nerves and the later recognition of a multiplicity of neurotransmitter substances in autonomic nerves, including monoamines, purines, amino acids, a variety of different peptides and nitric oxide (Burnstock *et al.*, 1964; Burnstock, 1986b; Rand, 1992; Milner and Burnstock, 1995; Lincoln *et al.*, 1995; Zhang and Snyder, 1995).

(3) The concept of neuromodulation, where locally released agents can alter neurotransmission either by prejunctional modulation of the amount of transmitter released or by postjunctional modulation of the time-course or intensity of action of the transmitter (Marrazzi, 1939; Brown and Gillespie, 1957; Vizi, 1979; Fuder and Muscholl, 1995).

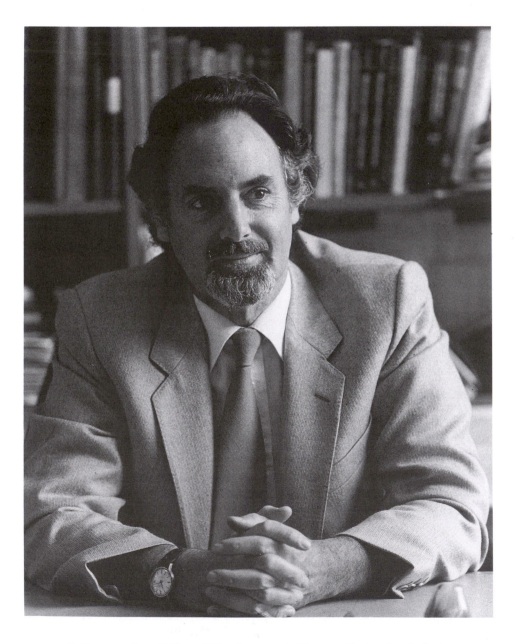

G. Burnstock — Editor of The Autonomic Nervous System Book Series

(4) The concept of cotransmission that proposes that most, if not all, nerves release more than one transmitter (Burnstock, 1976; Hökfelt, Fuxe and Pernow, 1986; Burnstock, 1990a; Burnstock and Ralevic, 1996) and the important follow-up of this concept, termed 'chemical coding', in which the combinations of neurotransmitters contained in individual neurones are established, and whose projections and central connections are identified (Furness and Costa, 1987).

(5) Recognition of the importance of 'sensory-motor' nerve regulation of activity in many organs, including gut, lungs, heart and ganglia, as well as in many blood vessels (Maggi, 1991; Burnstock, 1993), although the concept of antidromic impulses in sensory nerve collaterals forming part of 'axon reflex' vasodilatation of skin vessels was described many years ago (Lewis, 1927).

(6) Recognition that many intrinsic ganglia (e.g., those in the heart, airways and bladder) contain integrative circuits that are capable of sustaining and modulating sophisticated local activities (Saffrey et al., 1992; Ardell, 1994). Although the ability of the enteric nervous system to sustain local reflex activity independent of the central nervous system has been recognized for many years (Kosterlitz, 1968), it has been generally assumed that the intrinsic ganglia in peripheral organs consist of parasympathetic neurones that provided simple nicotinic relay stations.

(7) The major subclasses of receptors to acetylcholine and noradrenaline have been recognized for many years (Dale, 1914; Ahlquist, 1948), but in recent years it has become evident that there is an astonishing variety of receptor subtypes for autonomic transmitters (*see Pharmacol. Rev.*, **46**, 1994). Their molecular properties and transduction mechanisms are being characterized. These advances offer the possibility of more selective drug therapy.

(8) Recognition of the plasticity of the autonomic nervous system, not only in the changes that occur during development and aging, but also in the changes in expression of transmitter and receptors that occur in fully mature adults under the influence of hormones and growth factors following trauma and surgery, and in a variety of disease situations (Burnstock, 1990b; Saffrey and Burnstock, 1994).

(9) Advances in the understanding of 'vasomotor' centres in the central nervous system. For example, the traditional concept of control being exerted by discrete centres such as the vasomotor centre (Bayliss, 1923) has been supplanted by the belief that control involves the action of longitudinally arranged parallel pathways involving the forebrain, brain stem and spinal cord (Loewy and Spyer, 1990; Jänig and Häbler, 1995).

In addition to these major new concepts concerning autonomic function, the discovery by Furchgott that substances released from endothelial cells play an important role in addition to autonomic nerves, in local control of blood flow, has made a significant impact on our analysis and understanding of cardiovascular function (Furchgott and Zawadski, 1980; Burnstock and Ralevic, 1994). The later identification of nitric oxide as the major endothelium-derived relaxing factor (Palmer et al., 1988; *see* Moncada et al., 1991) (confirming the independent suggestion by Ignarro and by Furchgott) and endothelin as an endothelium-derived constricting factor (Yanagisawa *et al.*, 1988; *see* Rubanyi and Polokoff, 1994) have also had a major impact in this area.

In broad terms, these new concepts shift the earlier emphasis on central control mechanisms towards greater consideration of the sophisticated local peripheral control mechanisms.

Although these new concepts should have a profound influence on our considerations of the autonomic control of cardiovascular, urogenital, gastrointestinal and reproductive systems and other organs like the skin and eye in both normal and disease situations, few of the current textbooks take them into account. This is largely because revision of our understanding of all these different specialised areas in one volume by one author is a near impossibility. Thus, this Book Series of 14 volumes is designed to try to overcome this dilemma by dealing in depth with each major area in separate volumes and by calling upon the knowledge and expertise of leading figures in the field. Volume 1, deals with the basic mechanisms of *Autonomic Neuroeffector Mechanisms* which sets the stage for later volumes devoted to autonomic nervous control of particular organ systems, including *Heart, Blood Vessels, Respiratory System, Urogenital Organs, Gastrointestinal Tract, Eye* and *Skin.* Another group of volumes will deal with *Central Nervous Control of Autonomic Function, Autonomic Ganglia, Autonomic–Endocrine Interactions, Development, Regeneration and Plasticity* and *Comparative Physiology and Evolution of the Autonomic Nervous System.*

Abnormal as well as normal mechanisms will be covered to a variable extent in all these volumes depending on the topic and the particular wishes of the Volume Editor, but one volume edited by Robertson and Biaggioni, 1995, has been specifically devoted to *Disorders of the Autonomic Nervous System* (*see* also Bannister and Mathias, 1992).

A general philosophy followed in the design of this book series has been to encourage individual expression by Volume Editors and Chapter Contributors in the presentation of the separate topics within the general framework of the series. This was demanded by the different ways that the various fields have developed historically and the differing styles of the individuals who have made the most impact in each area. Hopefully, this deliberate lack of uniformity will add to, rather than detract from, the appeal of these books.

G. Burnstock

Series Editor

REFERENCES

Ahlquist, R.P. (1948). A study of the adrenotropic receptors. *Am. J. Physiol.*, **153**, 586–600.

Ardell, J.L. (1994). Structure and function of mammalian intrinsic cardiac neurons. In: *Neurocardiology.* (Eds.) Armour, J.A. and Ardell, J.L. pp. 95–114. Oxford University Press: Oxford.

Bannister, R. and Mathias, C.J. (Eds.) (1992). *Autonomic Failure.* Third Edition. Oxford University Press: Oxford.

Bayliss, W.B. (1923). *The Vasomotor System.* Longman: London.

Bayliss, W.M. and Starling, E.H. (1899). The movements and innervation of the small intestine. *J. Physiol. (Lond.)*, **24**, 99–143.

Brown, G.L. and Gillespie, J.S. (1957). The output of sympathetic transmitter from the spleen of a cat. *J. Physiol. (Lond.)*, **138**, 81–102.

Burnstock, G. (1976). Do some nerve cells release more than one transmitter? *Neuroscience*, **1**, 239–248.

Burnstock, G. (1986a). Autonomic neuromuscular junctions: Current developments and future directions. *J. Anat.*, **146**, 1–30.

Burnstock, G. (1986b). The non-adrenergic non-cholinergic nervous system. *Arch. Int. Pharmacodyn. Ther.*, **280** (suppl.), 1–15.

Burnstock, G. (1990a). Co-Transmission. The Fifth Heymans Lecture - Ghent, February 17, 1990. *Arch. Int. Pharmacodyn. Ther.*, **304**, 7–33.

Burnstock, G. (1990b). Changes in expression of autonomic nerves in aging and disease. *J. Auton. Nerv. Syst.*, **30**, 525–534.

Burnstock, G. (1993). Introduction: Changing face of autonomic and sensory nerves in the circulation. In: *Vascular Innervation and Receptor Mechanisms: New Perspectives*. (Eds.) by L. Edvinsson and R. Uddman, pp. 1–22. Academic Press Inc: San Diego.

Burnstock, G., Campbell, G., Bennett, M. and Holman, M.E. (1964). Innervation of the guinea-pig taenia coli: Are there intrinsic inhibitory nerves which are distinct from sympathetic nerves? *Int. J. Neuropharmacol.*, **3**, 163–166.

Burnstock, G. and Ralevic, V. (1994). New insights into the local regulation of blood flow by perivascular nerves and endothelium. *Br. J. Plast. Surg.*, **47**, 527–543.

Burnstock, G. and Ralevic, V. (1996). Cotransmission. In: *The Pharmacology of Smooth Muscle*. (Eds.) Garland, C.J. and Angus, J. Oxford University Press: Oxford.

Dale, H. (1914). The action of certain esters and ethers of choline and their reaction to muscarine. *J. Pharmacol. Exp. Ther.*, **6**, 147–190.

Dale, H. (1935). Pharmacology and nerve endings. *Proc. Roy. Soc. Med.*, **28**, 319–332.

Elliott, T.R. (1905). The action of adrenalin. *J. Physiol. (Lond.)*, **32**, 401–467.

Fuder, H. and Muscholl, E. (1995). Heteroceptor-mediated modulation of noradrenaline and acetylcholine release from peripheral nerves. *Rev. Physiol. Biochem. Physiol.*, **126**, 265–412.

Furchgott, R.F. and Zawadski, J.V. (1980). The obligatory role of endothelial cells in the relaxation of arterial smooth muscle by acetylcholine. *Nature*, **288**, 373–376.

Furness, J.B. and Costa, M. (1987). *The Enteric Nervous System*. Churchill Livingstone: Edinburgh.

Gaskell, W.H. (1886). On the structure, distribution and function of the nerves which innervate the visceral and vascular systems. *J. Physiol. (Lond.)*, **7**, 1–80.

Hillarp, N.-Å. (1959). The construction and functional organisation of the autonomic innervation apparatus. *Acta Physiol. Scand.*, **46** (suppl. 157), 1–38.

Hökfelt, T., Fuxe, K. and Pernow, B. (Eds.) (1986). Coexistence of neuronal messengers: A new principle in chemical transmission. In *Progress in Brain Research*, vol. 68, Elsevier: Amsterdam.

Jänig, W. and Häbler, H.-J. (1995). Visceral-Autonomic Integration. In: *Visceral Pain, Progress in Pain Research and Management*, (Ed.) Gebhart, G.F. Vol. 5, 311–348. IASP Press: Seattle.

Kosterlitz, H.W. (1968). The alimentary canal. In *Handbook of Physiology*, vol. IV, (Ed.) C.F. Code, pp. 2147–2172. American Physiological Society: Washington, DC.

Langley, J.N. (1921). *The Autonomic Nervous System*, part 1. W. Heffer: Cambridge.

Lewis, T. (1927). *The Blood Vessels of the Human Skin and Their Responses*. London: Shaw & Sons.

Lincoln, J., Hoyle, C.H.V. and Burnstock, G. (1995). Transmission: Nitric oxide. In: *The Autonomic Nervous System, Vol. 1* (reprinted): *Autonomic Neuroeffector Mechanisms*. (Eds.) Burnstock, G. and Hoyle, C.H.V. pp. 509–539. Harwood Academic Publishers: The Netherlands.

Loewi, O. (1921). Über humorale Übertrangbarkeit der Herznervenwirkung. XI. Mitteilung. *Pflügers Arch. Gesamte Physiol.*, **189**, 239–242.

Loewy, A.D. and Spyer, K.M. (1990). *Central Regulations of Autonomic Functions*. Oxford University Press: New York.

Maggi, C.A. (1991). The pharmacology of the efferent function on sensory nerves. *J. Auton. Pharmacol.*, **11**, 173–208.

Marrazzi, A.S. (1939). Electrical studies on the pharmacology of autonomic synapses. II. The action of a sympathomimetic drug (epinephrine) on sympathetic ganglia. *J. Pharmacol. Exp. Ther.*, **65**, 395–404.

Milner, P. and Burnstock, G. (1995). Neurotransmitters in the autonomic nervous system. In: *Handbook of Autonomic Nervous Dysfunction*. (Ed.) Korczyn, A.D. pp. 5–32. Marcel Dekker: New York.

Moncada, S., Palmer, R.M.J. and Higgs, E.A. (1991). Nitric oxide: Physiology, pathophysiology, and pharmacology. *Pharmacol. Rev.*, **43**, 109–142.

Palmer, R.M.J., Rees, D.D., Ashton, D.S. and Moncada, S. (1988). Arginine is the physiological precursor for the formation of nitric oxide in endothelium-dependent relaxation. *Biochem. Biophys. Res. Commun.*, **153**, 1251–1256.

Rand, M.J. (1992). Nitrergic transmission: nitric oxide as a mediator of non-adrenergic, non-cholinergic neuroeffector transmission. *Clin. Exp. Pharmacol. Physiol.*, **19**, 147–169.

Rubanyi, G.M. and Polokoff, M.A. (1994). Endothelins: Molecular biology, biochemistry, pharmacology, physiology, and pathophysiology. *Pharmacol. Rev.*, **46**, 328–415.

Saffrey, M.J. and Burnstock, G. (1994). Growth factors and the development and plasticity of the enteric nervous system. *J. Auton. Nerv. Syst.*, **49**, 183–196.

Saffrey, M.J., Hassall, C.J.S., Allen, T.G.J. and Burnstock, G. (1992). Ganglia within the gut, heart, urinary bladder and airways: studies in tissue culture. *Int. Rev. Cytol.*, **136**, 93–144.

Vizi, E.S. (1979). Prejunctional modulation of neurochemical transmission. *Prog. Neurobiol.*, **12**, 181–290.

von Euler, U.S. and Gaddum, J.H. (1931). An unidentified depressor substance in certain tissue extracts. *J. Physiol.*, **72**, 74–87.

Yanagisawa, M., Kurihara, H., Kimura, S., Tomobe, Y., Kobayashi, M., Mitsui, Y., Yazaki, Y., Goto, K. and Masaki, T. (1988). A novel potent vasoconstrictor peptide produced by vascular endothelial cells. *Nature*, **332**, 411–415.

Zhang, J. and Snyder, S.H. (1995). Nitric oxide in the nervous system. *Annu. Rev. Pharmacol. Toxicol.*, **35**, 213–233.

Preface

When invited to edit this volume on Nervous Control of Blood Vessels for the series The Autonomic Nervous System, we took a very broad look at the topic and then invited contributions from experts in the field, as judged by our reading of the literature. A particular advantage of this approach is that it allowed each of the contributors free rein within the area of their interest, and this has, we believe, resulted in a series of fresh commentaries with some inevitable, but valuable, overlap.

It was our intention to have coverage of all aspects of the control of blood vessels, including endothelial function, afferent and efferent innervation and the associated chemical messengers, together with integrated accounts of the control of the vasculature of all the major organ systems. We consider this objective has been met in the present volume which complements recent publications on related topics (e.g. Edvinsson and Uddman, 1993; Burnstock and Ralevic, 1994).

Even within the time-frame over which this book was conceived and produced, our understanding of the complexity of cardiovascular control mechanisms has developed apace. Much recent work has focused on molecular biological and cellular events, particularly related to the physiology and pathophysiology of endothelial, vascular smooth muscle, and myocardial cells. However, as pointed out elsewhere (Folkow, 1994, 1995; Böttiger, 1995; Lenfant, 1995), the ultimate challenge is to bring all this information together in a way that allows proper understanding of integrative cardiovascular control *in vivo*. We believe consideration of vascular mechanisms at the level of the organ system, as here, taking into account the 'new' biology, is an important move towards this final objective. However, it is unlikely that a full understanding of the complexity of *in vivo* vascular control mechanisms will ever be achieved without increased efforts being made to obtain detailed haemodynamic data in the absence of the confounding effects of anaesthetic agents. In this regard it is notable how few laboratories have taken advantage of those technological advances which allow, for example, on-line monitoring of regional haemodynamics in conscious unrestrained animals. In our experience, such an approach can provide valuable information about the influence of endothelial dilator and constrictor factors, neurotransmitters, neuropeptides, and novel therapeutic agents on haemodynamics (e.g. Gardiner and Bennett, 1988; Gardiner *et al.*, 1988, 1989, 1990, 1994). A criticism that may be levelled at this approach concerns the complexity of the system being studied, as evidenced by the number of variables monitored. However, confining measurement to systemic arterial blood pressure alone, for example, is a spurious simplification, since all those variables not monitored will be changing nonetheless. So, we look forward to the day when cutting-edge molecular biology

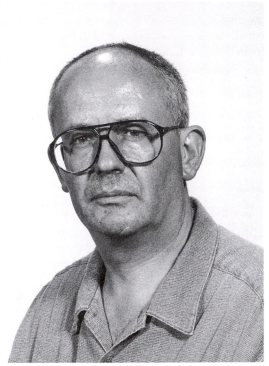

Terence Bennett

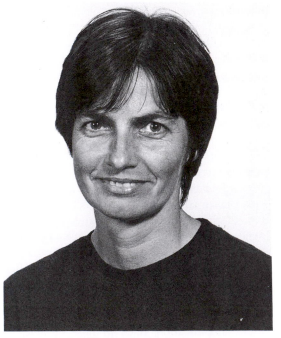

Sheila M. Gardiner

is brought into conjunction with state-of-the-art cardiovascular monitoring, to achieve a fuller understanding of all the nuances of the control of blood vessels. We hope this volume will tempt researchers in that direction.

REFERENCES

Böttiger, L.E. (1995). Integrative biology (physiology) — a necessity! *J. Int. Med.*, **237**, 345–347.

Burnstock, G. and Ralevic, V. (1994). New insights into the local regulation of blood flow by perivascular nerves and endothelium. *Br. J. Plast. Surg.*, **47**, 527–543.

Edvinsson, L. and Uddman, R. (1993). Vascular innervation and receptor mechanisms. *Academic Press, Inc.* San Diego.

Folkow, B. (1994). Increasing importance of integrative physiology in the era of molecular biology. *NIPS*, **9**, 93–95.

Folkow, B. (1995). Integration of hypertension research in the era of molecular biology: G.W. Pickering Memorial Lecture (Dublin 1994). *J. Hypertens.*, **13**, 5–18.

Gardiner, S.M. and Bennett, T. (1988). Regional haemodynamic responses to adrenoceptor antagonism in conscious rats. *Am. J. Physiol.*, **255**, H813–H824.

Gardiner, S.M., Compton, A.M. and Bennett, T. (1988). Regional haemodynamic effects of depressor neuropeptides in conscious, Long Evans and Brattleboro rats. *Br. J. Pharmacol.*, **95**, 197–208.

Gardiner, S.M., Compton, A.M. and Bennett, T. (1989). Regional haemodynamic effects of human α- and β-calcitonin gene-related peptide in conscious Wistar rats. *Br. J. Pharmacol.*, **98**, 1225–1232.

Gardiner, S.M., Compton, A.M., Kemp, P.A. and Bennett, T. (1990). Regional and cardiac haemodynamic responses to glyceryl trinitrate, acetylcholine, bradykinin and endothelin-1 in conscious rats: effects of N^G-nitro-L-arginine methyl ester. *Br. J. Pharmacol.*, **101**, 632–639.

Gardiner, S.M., Kemp, P.A., March, J.E., Bennett, T., Davenport, A.P. and Edvinsson, L. (1994). Effects of an ET_1-receptor antagonist, FR139317, on regional haemodynamic responses to endothelin-1 and [Ala^{11,15}]Ac-endothelin-1 (6–21) in conscious rats. *Br. J. Pharmacol.*, **112**, 477–486.

Lenfant, C. (1995). Integrative physiology: remember the big picture. *Circulation*, **91**, 1901.

Contributors

Bell, Christopher
Physiology Department
The University of Dublin
Trinity College
Dublin 2
Republic of Ireland

Bennett, Terence
Department of Physiology and
    Pharmacology
University of Nottingham
    Medical School
Queen's Medical Centre
Nottingham NG7 2UH
UK

Brain, Susan D.
Pharmacology Group
Biomedical Sciences Division
King's College London
Manresa Road
London SW3 6LX
UK

Breslow, Michael J.
Department of Anesthesiology/
    Critical Care Medicine
The Johns Hopkins Medical
    Institutions
600 North Wolfe Street
Meyer 299A
Baltimore, MD 21287-7294
USA

Burnstock, Geoffrey
Department of Anatomy and Developmental
    Biology and Centre for Neuroscience
University College London
Gower Street, London WC1E 6BT
UK

Busija, David W.
Physiology and Pharmacology
Bowman Gray School of Medicine
    of Wake Forest University
Medical Center Boulevard
Winston-Salem, NC 27157
USA

Chaudhuri, K. Ray
Cardiovascular Medicine Unit
Department of Medicine
St Mary's Hospital Medical School
Praed Street, London W2 1NY
UK

Dey, Malay
Department of Physiology
West Virginia University
Health Sciences Center South
Morgantown, WV 26506
USA

Dunn, William R.
Department of Physiology and Pharmacology
University of Nottingham Medical School
Queen's Medical Centre
Nottingham NG7 2UH
UK

Edvinsson, Lars
Department of Internal Medicine
University Hospital of Lund
S-221 85 Lund
Sweden

Franco-Cereceda, Anders
Department of Thoracic Surgery
Karolinska Hospital
S-171-76 Stockholm
Sweden

Frayn, K.N.
Oxford Lipid Metabolism Group
Radcliffe Infirmary
Oxford OX2 6HE
UK

Gardiner, Sheila M.
Department of Physiology and
   Pharmacology
University of Nottingham
   Medical School
Queen's Medical Centre
Nottingham NG7 2UH
UK

Gulbenkian, Sergio
Department of Cell Biology
Gulbenkian Institute of Science
2781 Oeiras
Portugal

Gutterman, David D.
Department of Internal Medicine
University of Iowa College of Medicine
Iowa City, IA 52242
USA

Hall, John E.
Department of Physiology and Biophysics
University of Mississippi Medical Center
2500 North State Street
Jackson, MS 39216-4505
USA

Hanley, Daniel F.
Department of Anesthesiology/
   Critical Care Medicine
The Johns Hopkins Medical Institutions
600 North Wolfe Street
Meyer 299A
Baltimore, MD 21287-7294
USA

Hedge, George A.
Department of Physiology
West Virginia University
Health Sciences Center South
Morgantown, WV 26506
USA

Hjemdahl, Paul
Department of Clinical Pharmacology
Karolinska Hospital
PO Box 60 500
S-171 76 Stockholm
Sweden

Huffman, Linda J.
Department of Physiology
West Virginia University
Health Sciences Center South
Morgantown, WV 26506
USA

Jansen-Olesen, Inger
Department of Experimental Research
University of Lund
Malmö General Hospital
S-214 01 Malmö
Sweden

Kahan, Thomas
Division of Internal Medicine
Karolinska Institute
Danderyd Hospital
S-182 88 Danderyd
Sweden

Lautt, W. Wayne
Department of Pharmacology and
  Therapeutics
Faculty of Medicine
University of Manitoba
Winnipeg, Manitoba
Canada R3E 0W3

Lohmeier, Thomas E.
Department of Physiology and
  Biophysics
University of Mississippi Medical Center
2500 North State Street
Jackson, MS 39216-4505
USA

Macdonald, I.A.
Department of Physiology and
  Pharmacology
University of Nottingham Medical School
Queen's Medical Centre
Nottingham NG7 2UH
UK

Mathias, Christopher J.
Cardiovascular Medicine Unit
Department of Medicine
St Mary's Hospital Medical School
Praed Street
London W2 1NY
UK

Michalkiewicz, Mieczyslaw
Department of Physiology
West Virginia University
Health Sciences Center South
Morgantown, WV 26506
USA

Mizelle, H. Leland
Department of Physiology and Biophysics
University of Mississippi Medical Center
2500 North State Street
Jackson, MS 39216-4505
USA

Ralevic, V.
Department of Anatomy and Developmental
  Biology and Centre for Neuroscience
University College London
Gower Street
London WC1E 6BT
UK

Schnoll, Danna
Department of Internal Medicine
University of Iowa College of Medicine
Iowa City, IA 52242
USA

Thomaides, Thomas
Cardiovascular Medicine Unit
Department of Medicine
St Mary's Hospital Medical School
Praed Street
London W2 1NY
UK

Traystman, Richard J.
Department of Anesthesiology/
  Critical Care Medicine
The Johns Hopkins Medical Institutions
600 North Wolfe Street
Meyer 299A
Baltimore, MD 21287-7294
USA

Uddman, Rolf
Department of Otorhinolaryngology
University of Lund
Malmö General Hospital
S-214 01 Malmö
Sweden

Van Vliet, Bruce N.
Division of Basic Medical Sciences
Faculty of Medicine
The Health Sciences Centre
Memorial University of Newfoundland
St John's, Newfoundland
Canada A1B 3V6

Wilson, David
Department of Anesthesiology/
    Critical Care Medicine
The Johns Hopkins Medical Institutions
600 North Wolfe Street
Meyer 299A
Baltimore, MD 21287-7294
USA

Wilson, V.G.
Department of Physiology and Pharmacology
University of Nottingham Medical School
Queen's Medical Centre
Nottingham NG7 2UH
UK

1 Noradrenergic Neurotransmission in Blood Vessels

V.G. Wilson and W.R. Dunn

Department of Physiology and Pharmacology,
University of Nottingham Medical School,
Queen's Medical Centre, Nottingham, UK

Noradrenaline is the principal neurotransmitter released upon sympathetic nerve stimulation at the vascular neuroeffector junction. Evidence to support this statement has accumulated since the beginning of the century, fulfilling the four criteria, (anatomical, biochemical, physiological and pharmacological), necessary to define a substance as a neurotransmitter. In more recent times, practical information about the role of noradrenaline at the vascular neuroeffector junction has been obtained using selective adrenoceptor antagonists. Recent attempts at further subdividing adrenoceptors, using molecular biological techniques, have yet to be translated into a functional role for these adrenoceptor subtypes at the vascular neuroeffector junction. This is partly the consequence of the relatively poor selectivity displayed by antagonists for the proposed subtypes, and also of the experimental systems studied.

Noradrenaline can modulate neurotransmitter release by interacting with prejunctional adrenoceptors; β_2-adrenoceptor stimulation enhances transmitter release while α_2-adrenoceptor stimulation reduces transmitter output. More recently, electrophysiological techniques have demonstrated that this modulation of transmitter release does not occur locally, but at some distant site (lateral modulation). On the postjunctional membrane, the most common consequence of noradrenaline release from nerves is vasoconstriction, an effect mediated via α-adrenoceptors. The concept that α_1-adrenoceptors are solely responsible for mediating noradrenergic neurovascular contraction is no longer tenable. Recent evidence from studies of large arteries and veins, and more importantly small resistance arteries, indicates that noradrenaline released from nerves produces vasoconstriction by acting on postjunctional α_2-adrenoceptors. Neither receptor subtype is mutually exclusive however, and in many cases, postjunctional α_1- and α_2-adrenoceptors coexist and interact in a positive, synergistic manner. Discrimination of the relative importance of pre- and postjunctional mechanisms for noradrenaline at the neurovascular junction has proved difficult. However, evidence is accumulating that the postjunctional interaction between α_2-adrenoceptors, with either α_1-adrenoceptors or humoral agents such as angiotensin II, is of greater importance than prejunctional regulation of transmitter release, in determining the end-organ response. Activation of the sympathetic nervous system can also produce distinct regional vascular effects, as evidenced by the predominance of β_2-adrenoceptor-mediated vasodilatation in some vascular beds.

The importance of noradrenaline as a neurotransmitter at the vascular neuroeffector junction is reflected in the action of many antihypertensive drugs. α_1-adrenoceptor antagonists have been used clinically for many years, while the potential for an α_2-adrenoceptor antagonist, which discriminates between pre- and postjunctional α_2-adrenoceptors, awaits realisation. In addition, many of the clinically useful effects of ACE inhibitors are a consequence of interference with noradrenergic neurotransmission in blood vessels.

KEY WORDS: noradrenaline; α_1-adrenoceptors; α_2-adrenoceptors; β_2-adrenoceptors; prejunctional modulation; postjunctional facilitation; blood pressure.

INTRODUCTION

The role of noradrenaline as a sympathetic neurotransmitter to control the calibre of blood vessels has long been established. Indeed, the development of antihypertensive drugs which interfere with the function of noradrenaline attests to its pivotal role in the nervous control of blood pressure. In comparison to the cotransmitters, ATP and neuropeptide Y, there is a wealth of information on almost every aspect of this topic which, in itself, can create problems for the reviewer. For example, during the last seven years there have been major reviews on the pharmacological characteristics of the receptors through which noradrenaline produces its biological effects (McGrath, Brown and Wilson, 1989; Lomasney *et al.*, 1991), the regulation of transmitter release from the vascular neuroeffector junction (Starke, 1987) and the electrophysiological aspects of sympathetic neurotransmission (Hirst and Edwards, 1989; Brock and Cunnane, 1991). Most of these reviews have focused on the findings obtained with one or two major techniques and this has provided detailed insights into factors contributing to, or directly involved in, noradrenergic transmission in blood vessels. There are, however, few reviews that have attempted to cross the artificial boundaries created by different technical approaches and confront the real challenge of 'integrative physiology' (Noble and Boyd, 1993).

In attempting to provide an overview of vascular noradrenergic transmission, we have considered studies that have employed a wide range of experimental techniques — from the use of the polymerase chain reaction to identify the messenger RNA for α-adrenoceptor subtype(s) on vascular smooth muscle, to the determination of blood pressure in man — often in combination with selective pharmacological tools. It has been necessary, however, to focus on aspects of noradrenergic transmission that bridge the gap between the individual varicosity and the whole animal; factors regulating the release of noradrenaline and those that influence the end-organ response. Thus, we have used information relating to α_2-adrenoceptors, which reside on both sides of the neuroeffector junction, as a cornerstone for much of our discussion to assess the relative importance of pre- and postjunctional events. This integrative approach has also allowed us to reevaluate the action of antihypertensive agents known to affect noradrenergic transmission, and highlight potential targets for the future.

METHODOLOGICAL CONSIDERATIONS

In 1981 Gainer and Brownstein modified Dale's original proposal and suggested that there are four criteria, each reflecting a different methodological approach, that should (ideally) be fulfilled before considering a particular substance as a neurotransmitter.

(1) Anatomical   The presence of the substance in the appropriate amounts in presynaptic processes.

(2) Biochemical   Recovery of the compound from the perfusate of an innervated structure during periods of nerve stimulation, but not (or in greatly reduced amounts) in the absence of stimulation. In addition, the presence and operation of enzymes that synthesize the substance in the presynaptic neurons and processes, and remove or inactivate the substance should be demonstrable at the synapse.

(3) Physiological   Ionophoretic application of the substance to the synapse in appropriate amounts mimics the natural response.

(4) Pharmacological   Drugs that affect the different enzymatic or biophysical steps have predictable effects on synthesis, storage, release, action, inactivation and reuptake of the substance.

In practice, however, findings from a single experimental approach have often been employed to advocate that a particular substance is a neurotransmitter. This was certainly true for early observations on sympathetic neurotransmission.

The first suggestion that noradrenaline, rather than adrenaline, functioned as the principal neurotransmitter in the mammalian sympathetic nervous system was speculatively made 60 years ago by Bacq (1934). This hypothesis was suggested in an attempt to simplify the sympathin E/sympathin I model for adrenaline as a sympathetic neurotransmitter (Cannon and Rosenblueth, 1937), and to accommodate the finding that the 'sympathin' released by the liver during excitation of the nerves running along the hepatic artery, was more active than adrenaline on the sensitized nictitating membrane (α-adrenoceptor effect) than on the non-pregnant uterus (β-adrenoceptor effect). As Bacq (1975) explained many years later, a variety of factors conspired to delay the incontrovertible proof from von Euler (1946). Principal amongst these were the dependence upon bioassay, rather than direct chemical means for the determination of 'activity', coupled with the fact that pharmacopoeal standard l-adrenaline (extracted from bovine adrenals) was contaminated with l-noradrenaline. In the intervening 48 years since von Euler's seminal publication, the application of an ever-increasing range of techniques and pharmacological tools has ensured that the evidence for noradrenergic, sympathetic neurotransmission in the vasculature has continued unabated.

The introduction of a histochemical method for the detection of noradrenaline (Falck, Thieme and Torp, 1962) provided evidence that in the majority of blood vessels sympathetic nerve terminals formed a dense network which was largely confined to the adventitia-media border (see: Bevan, Bevan and Duckles, 1980). This technique also had the distinct advantage of providing evidence for the presence of noradrenaline in resistance arteries which, at the time, were too small for routine isometric tension recordings and failed to release noradrenaline in a sufficient quantity to allow biochemical detection, i.e., detection of noradrenaline release had been restricted to large conduit arteries or entire vascular beds. The further development of immunohistochemical methods for the detection of biosynthetic enzymes in intact nerves and subcellular fractionation techniques, most notably for dopamine-β-hydroxylase (DBH), provided evidence for the existence of the appropriate biosynthetic pathways in nerves for the production of noradrenaline (Chubb, De Potter and De Sehaepdryver, 1970; Pickel, Joh and Reis, 1976). Histochemical evidence alone, however, is insufficient to prove that noradrenaline is the most important sympathetic neurotransmitter in any given blood vessel. Such methods have also provided evidence for the presence of neuropeptide Y and other peptides in sympathetic nerves innervating vascular preparations, which are released upon activation (see Morris and Gibbins, 1991; Franco-Cereceda this volume). Therefore, other methods are required to determine which substance(s) is responsible for the neurogenic response.

An approach to this problem, which also satisfies one of the above criteria for a neurotransmitter, is to compare the response to the putative neurotransmitter with the neurogenic response. This approach, again, however, is not without complications when used in isolation. For example, in the case of noradrenaline, the existence of α- and β-adrenoceptors on vascular smooth muscle and their different locations, can lead to anomalies between the effects of application of exogenous noradrenaline and activation of sympathetic nerves. This point is illustrated by the observations of Pegram, Bevan and Bevan (1976), who demonstrated that electrical field stimulation of the rabbit facial vein produced sustained vasodilatation, yet noradrenaline produced only small, poorly sustained dilator responses. This anomaly was resolved however, since after α-adrenoceptor blockade, the response to exogenous noradrenaline mimicked that to nerve stimulation. It would appear that the β-adrenoceptor and α-adrenoceptors in this preparation are located intra- and extrajunctional, respectively.

While each of the above techniques have their advantages and disadvantages, in practice the participation of noradrenaline in neurogenic responses of blood vessels is usually made solely on the basis of the effect of receptor antagonists. In some instances, this has been wisely coupled with an anatomical approach, using either the Falck technique or glyoxylic acid staining (see Bevan, Bevan and Duckles, 1980). It is important to recognize, however, that the use of antagonists also has its limitations, and that the drug used to identify a receptor participating in neurogenic responses, and by implication the neurotransmitter, should ideally be employed within a concentration-range devoid of other pharmacological effects. This may be of particular importance for co-transmission in blood vessels, where there is a possibility that the non-adrenergic component of neurogenic responses might be suppressed, or enhanced, by an adrenoceptor antagonist, thereby giving a false view of the contribution of noradrenaline to a given response. It is noteworthy that the Burn-Rand Cholinergic Link Hypothesis for adrenergic neurotransmission was largely rejected on the basis that the cholinergic modifying drugs employed were of questionable specificity (Ferry, 1966). Examples of some of the principal drugs employed in the study of adrenergic neurotransmission, and some of their additional actions, are shown in Table 1.1.

For the most part, however, the use of adrenoceptor antagonists has been successful in identifying noradrenaline as the main sympathetic neurotransmitter responsible for regulating vascular smooth muscle. This probably reflects the fact that non-specific depressant effects of adrenoceptor antagonists have been encountered in relatively few preparations (see Table 1.1), and because of the minor role of 5-HT as a sympathetic neurotransmitter in peripheral blood vessels.

TABLE 1.1

The pharmacological agents used to identify and study noradrenergic neurotransmission

Drugs	Principal action	Limitations and additional actions	References
Phenoxy-benzamine	Irreversible α-adrenoceptor antagonists (1 nM–1 μM)	Inhibition of neuronal and extraneuronal uptake (>1 μM) Inhibition of H_1, muscarinic and 5-$HT_{(2)}$ receptors (10 nM–1 μM)	Furchgott (1972)
Phentolamine	Competitive α-adrenoceptor antagonist (10 nM–3 μM)	Inhibition of 5-$HT_{(2)}$ receptors (0.3 μM) and 5-HT_1-like receptors (1 μM) Inhibition of cromkalin-sensitive K^+ channels (10 μM) Non-specific depression of excitation-contraction coupling (10 μM) In vivo α-adrenoceptor activity in the rabbit, but not in the dog Activation of non-adrenoceptor, imidazoline receptors regulating transmitter release from noradrenergic neurones (> 1 μM)	Limberger et al. (1989) Wilson, Brown and McGrath (1991) McPherson and Angus (1989) Holman and Suprenant (1980) Bell (1988) Göthert and Molderings (1991)
Prazosin	Selective α_1-adrenoceptor antagonist	Variable affinity at α_1-adrenoceptors (pA_2—11-8) — very potent (1 nM–0.3 μM) in the rat, but less pronounced in other species Relatively high affinity for α_{2B}-adrenoceptor subtype (pA_2—6.5) Exocytotic action on noradrenergic vesicles (1 μM) Non-specific depression of excitation-contraction coupling (> 3 μM)	Wilson, Brown and McGrath (1991) Wilson, Brown and McGrath (1991) Davey (1987) Holman and Suprenant (1980)
Rauwolscine and Yohimbine	Selective α_2-adrenoceptor antagonists (10 nM–3 μM)	Recognition 5-HT_1-like receptors (0.1 μM) Activation of 5-HT_1-like receptors Facilitation of α_1-adrenoceptor-mediated contractions	De Vos et al. (1991) Shimamoto et al. (1993) Guan, Chen and Sun (1991)

TABLE 1.1
Continued.

Drugs	Principal action	Limitations and additional actions	References
Idazoxan	Selective α_2-adrenoceptor antagonist (10 nM–1 μM)	Activation of α_1-adrenoceptors Activation of prejunctional α_2-adrenoceptors Activation of prejunctional non-adrenoceptor-imidazoline binding sites	van der Graaf *et al.* (1992) Limberger and Starke (1983) Göthert and Molderings (1991)
Propranolol	β-adrenoceptor antagonist	Local anaesthetic effect (30 μM) α-adrenoceptor agonism (pA$_2$—5)	Furchgott (1972) Ashbrook *et al.* (1980)
α-β-methylene ATP	Desensitization of P$_{2X}$ purinoceptors	Potentiation of adrenergic responses due to concomitant membrane depolarization	Neild and Kotecha (1986) Nagao and Szuki (1988)

The literature pertinent to the identity of the neurotransmitter responsible for the motor response of the rabbit isolated basilar artery, illustrates the need to integrate findings gleaned from different experimental approaches to establish that a particular substance is a neurotransmitter. It indicates at the very least the functional importance of data obtained with selective concentrations of receptor antagonists. For example, glyoxylic acid staining for noradrenaline (Lee, Su and Bevan, 1976) and immunohistochemical staining for 5-HT (Saito and Lee, 1987) revealed the presence of a network of fluorescence for each biogenic amine typical of a nerve plexus. Following surgical denervation (proximal to the cervical ganglion) the fluorescence for both amines disappeared, as did the motor response. Further support for the involvement of noradrenaline was provided by the finding that the adrenergic neuron blockers guanethidine and bretylium, and reserpine-pretreatment abolished the motor response (Lee, Su and Bevan, 1976). On the other hand, the use of a biochemical technique, direct measurement of 5-HT metabolites by HPLC following nerve stimulation, indicated that 5-HT was released from sympathetic nerves and was, therefore, a potential transmitter (Edvinsson *et al.*, 1984). Indeed a role for 5-HT, rather than noradrenaline, as a neurotransmitter contributing to the motor response, was provided by the findings that neurogenic contractions were resistant to α-adrenoceptor antagonists (Lee, Su and Bevan, 1976; Saito and Lee, 1987), but were partially reduced by the 5-HT receptor antagonists ketanserin and methergoline (Edvinsson *et al.*, 1984). Thus, although noradrenaline and 5-HT are contained in, and released from, sympathetic nerves innervating the rabbit basilar artery, the available evidence only provides support for 5-HT as a potential transmitter. The identity of the transmitter responsible for the non-α-adrenoceptor, non-5-HT$_2$, receptor component of the neurogenic contraction awaits the development of specific receptor antagonists capable of reducing the response.

Most studies of sympathetic neurovascular transmission have used relatively large blood vessels that, for the most part, do not make a significant contribution to arterial resistance. Two recent technological advances indicate that detection of transmitter release and neurogenic responses in small, resistance vessels may now be possible. Stjärne and coworkers (Mermet, Gonon and Stjärne, 1990; Msghina *et al.*, 1992; Bao, Gonon and Stjärne, 1993) have developed a voltammetric technique which they have used for on-line detection of noradrenaline 'clearance', from perivascular, sympathetic nerves of the rat tail artery. This method overcomes the problem of detecting [^{3}H]-transmitter release from isolated blood vessels, which often requires unphysiological, stimulation parameters and the inclusion of an uptake inhibitor in the bathing medium to increase the likelihood of detection of the amine (Starke *et al.*, 1974; Starke, Borowski and Endo, 1975a; Starke, Endo and Taube, 1975b) and can, potentially be applied to examining transmitter release from arteriolar blood vessels. Secondly, the Halpern-pressure myograph allows resistance blood vessels, as small as 100 μm in diameter, to be examined under conditions similar to those experienced *in vivo*. This technique involves cannulation and subsequent pressurization of small arteries, with responses detected as a change in diameter rather than isometric force. Under these conditions, the vessel develops calcium-dependent myogenic tone which appears to render the preparation more sensitive to constrictor influences (Dunn, Wellman and Bevan, 1994). This is dramatically demonstrated in Figure 1.1 which shows that segments of the rabbit isolated middle cerebral artery mounted on a Halpern-pressure myograph are 1000-fold

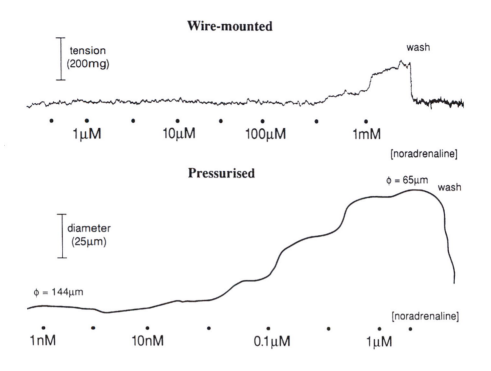

Figure 1.1   Comparison of responses to noradrenaline of the rabbit isolated middle cerebral artery, set up in either an isometric 'wire' myograph (top) or a Halpern pressure myograph (bottom). The readers attention is drawn to the threshold concentration of noradrenaline for vasoactivity; 1 mM for wires cf. 10 nM for pressurised arteries (Dunn and Bevan, unpublished observations).

more sensitive to noradrenaline, than when examined under isometric conditions (an effect mediated by α_1-adrenoceptors; Dunn and Bevan, unpublished observations). This increase in sensitivity also has implications for studies examining neurogenic response in isolated blood vessels.

Using a conventional isometric 'wire' myograph, van Riper and Bevan (1991) have shown that the motor response of the rabbit isolated middle cerebral artery is sensitive to α-adrenoceptor antagonists only after desensitization of NPY receptors. In view of the differential sensitivity of responses to exogenous noradrenaline when this preparation is mounted on a Halpern-pressure myograph, it seems likely that a similar effect will be observed for the motor response, thereby allowing demonstration of neurotransmission via α_1-adrenoceptors in cerebral arteries. This may help to explain the finding that prazosin inhibited sympathetically-mediated reduction in cerebral blood flow in the anaesthetized rabbit (Busija, 1985). Finally, it is noteworthy that the development of myogenic tone in resistance vessels mounted on a Halpern-pressure myograph will also permit examination of neurogenic vasodilation (see Han, Naes and Westfall, 1990; Kawasaki *et al.*, 1990), without recourse to pre-constriction of vessels with a spasmogen.

The above account has emphasized the primacy of the end-organ response, and the appropriate use of receptor antagonists, when determining the involvement of noradrenaline in neurogenic responses. However, before considering the experimental evidence implicating noradrenaline as a neurotransmitter in blood vessels, it is necessary to consider the pharmacological characteristics of adrenoceptors.

PHARMACOLOGICAL CHARACTERISTICS OF ADRENOCEPTORS

Preliminary evidence for the existence of adrenoceptor subtypes was apparent as early as the beginning of this century when Dale (1906) demonstrated, in pithed cats, that pressor responses to adrenaline could be blocked by ergot alkaloids unmasking a depressor response to the agonist. It was not until 1948 however, that Ahlquist demonstrated that a series of catecholamines had two distinct orders of potency when tested in a wide variety of preparations, one for excitatory events, which he termed α- and one for mainly inhibitory events which he termed β (Ahlquist, 1948). Confirmation of the existence of α- and β-subtypes of adrenoceptors was confirmed by the development of selective β-adrenoceptor antagonists a decade later (Powell and Slater, 1958; Black and Stephenson, 1962; Black *et al.*, 1964).

CLASSIFICATION OF β-ADRENOCEPTOR

In contrast to the subclassification of α-adrenoceptors, the information obtained from molecular, functional and radioligand binding studies converge relatively clearly, to provide evidence for the existence of three β-adrenoceptors (Michel, Philipp and Brodde, 1992). The initial subdivision of β-adrenoceptors into β_1- and β_2-subtypes was made on the basis of differences in the rank order of potency of a series of catecholamines, for a variety of β-adrenoceptor-mediated responses (Lands *et al.*, 1967). The seminal observation of this group was, that while adrenaline was equipotent with noradrenaline on the β-adrenoceptors controlling cardiac stimulation, fatty acid metabolism and gastrointestinal smooth muscle relaxation (β_1), it was much more effective than noradrenaline at mediating bronchodilatation, vasodilatation and inhibition of uterine contractions (β_2). The potential for the development of compounds to selectively modulate the β receptors, principally in the heart (β_1) and in bronchial smooth muscle (β_2) meant this subclassification received considerable interest from the pharmaceutical industry. This permitted the consolidation of this classification with the development of selective β_1-adrenoceptor antagonists such as practolol (Dunlop and Shanks, 1968), atenolol (Barret *et al.*, 1973) and more recently CGP 20,712A (Dooley, Bittiger and Reymann, 1986), and the development of selective β_2-agonists such as salbutamol (Brittain *et al.*, 1968) and antagonists such as butoxamine (Burns and Lemberger, 1965) and ICI 118,551 (Bilski *et al.*, 1993). Pharmacological evidence for the existence of a third β-adrenoceptor has amassed since the initial subdivision into β_1- and β_2. β-mediated responses have been noted to be 'atypical' in a number of preparations within the gastrointestinal tract (Bristow, Sherrod and Green, 1970) and in skeletal muscle (Challis *et al.*, 1988) and adipocytes (Harms, Zaagsma and De Vente, 1977), since they are relatively resistant to the actions of β_1- and β_2-antagonists. A number of agonists, such as BRL 28410 and BRL 37344, have also been developed and shown to specifically stimulate 'atypical' β-adrenoceptors in similar preparations (Arch *et al.*, 1984; Challis *et al.*, 1988; McLaughlin and MacDonald, 1990). This has led to the proposal that 'atypical' β receptors should be termed β_3-adrenoceptors (Tan and Curtis-Prior, 1983; Arch, 1989). Furthermore, a novel β_3-adrenoceptor has recently been cloned which expresses similar pharmacology to that obtained in functional studies (Emorine *et al.*, 1989). Interestingly, it has recently been reported that BRL 37344 increases blood flow to skin and fat, in conscious dogs, in the presence of combined $\beta_{1/2}$ blockade (with propranolol), suggesting a role for 'β_3-adrenoceptors' in mediating peripheral vasodilatation (Shen, Zhang and Vatner, 1994). The development of a selective antagonist for this 'atypical' (β_3-) receptor will finally confirm classification and may help clarify some anomalies reported for 'atypical' β-adrenoceptors in the heart in comparison with other preparations (Kaumann, 1989).

CLASSIFICATION OF α-ADRENOCEPTORS

The pharmacological subdivision of α-adrenoceptors awaited the realisation that nor-adrenaline was able to limit its own release from sympathetic nerves via prejunctional α-adrenoceptors in a negative feedback system. The first evidence which indicated this mechanism came from the experiments of Brown and Gillespie (1956, 1957) who observed that dibenamine, an irreversible α-adrenoceptor antagonist, increased the amount of noradrenaline appearing in venous blood from the cat spleen following nerve stimulation. However, this observation was complicated by the fact that dibenamine blocked the end-organ response. It was therefore not until the observations of Langer *et al.* (1971) and Starke (1972), who demonstrated increased transmitter overflow, produced by α-adrenoceptor antagonists, in tissues where the end-organ response was mediated via β-adrenoceptors (and hence the end-organ response was also increased) that this view gained promi-nence. Differences between pre- and postjunctional α-adrenoceptors were subsequently demonstrated by examining agonist and antagonist potencies at increasing transmitter output, or in blocking the concomitant contractions produced by nerve stimulation. Of particular importance at the time were the agonists, clonidine and phenylephrine, which appeared to preferentially activate pre- and postjunctional α-adrenoceptors, respectively, and the antagonists yohimbine and phenoxybenzamine, which preferentially inhibited pre and postjunctional α-adrenoceptors respectively (Dubocovich and Langer, 1974; Starke, Borowski and Endo, 1975a; Starke, Endo and Taube, 1975b).

The original split into α- and β-adrenoceptors explained why "α-blockers" such as ergotamine failed to block sympathetic responses in some tissues such as the heart (since they were mainly β-adrenoceptor-mediated). The new division (pre-/postjunctional) allowed the resolution of the old "yohimbine paradox", i.e., yohimbine and a few other agents now known to be α_2-adrenoceptor antagonists, could block responses to adrenaline but not responses to sympathetic nerve stimulation (since they increased transmitter output and this offset postjunctional blockade) (Bacq, 1935). Although there were attempts to classify α-adrenoceptor subtypes based upon location, α_1- for 'postjunctional' sites and α_2- for 'prejunctional' sites (e.g., Langer, 1974), a pharmacological basis for this subdivision was subsequently proposed by several workers following numerous reports of differences between agonist and antagonist selectivity profiles in various systems (Starke, 1977; Vizi, 1977; Westfall, 1977).

During the late 1970s, work with the aminoquinazoline derivative, prazosin, and the yohimbine diastereoisomers, rauwolscine and corynanthine, consolidated this classification scheme and provided tools that were to prove crucial in the demonstration of postjunctional α_2-adrenoceptors on vascular smooth muscle. First, Cambridge, Davey and Massingham (1977) demonstrated that prazosin, in marked contrast to yohimbine, possessed a 1000-fold greater affinity for postjunctional (α_1-) adrenoceptors in the rabbit main pulmonary artery. Secondly, Weitzell, Tanaka and Starke (1979) showed that rauwolscine possessed 100-fold greater affinity for prejunctional (α_2-) adrenoceptors than corynanthine, while at the postjunctional site corynanthine was 5–10 fold more potent than rauwolscine. These isomers have the advantage of possessing similar physicochemical properties, which ensures that the potency ratio at each subtype is not affected by the diffusional characteristics of the receptor biophase, and, as such, provides an alternative basis for discriminating between α_1- and α_2-adrenoceptor. This is now particularly important since there is evidence that prazosin can discriminate between subtypes of α_2-adrenoceptors (see below). Finally, Drew and Whiting (1979) demonstrated that pressor responses (mediated by a postjunctional α-adrenoceptor) to noradrenaline in the pithed rat and anaesthetized cat were less sensitive to prazosin than similar responses to phenylephrine, suggesting the presence of postjunctional α-adrenoceptors with pharmacological characteristics comparable to those on sympathetic nerves. Confirmation that these postjunctional receptors were of the α_2-adrenoceptor subclass was provided by the observation that the prazosin-resistant pressor response to adrenaline in the pithed rat was sensitive to yohimbine (Flavahan and McGrath, 1980).

These findings prompted Starke (1981) to propose that α_1-adrenoceptor mediated responses would be sensitive to low concentrations of prazosin, and that corynanthine would be more potent than rauwolscine, while α_2-adrenoceptor mediated responses would be preferentially antagonised by rauwolscine, and be insensitive to corynanthine and prazosin. McGrath (1982), recognising that rauwolscine, like yohimbine, also inhibited responses to 5-HT, suggested that any putative α_2-adrenoceptor response which was sensitive to rauwolscine or yohimbine should also be resistant to a 5-HT receptor blocker.

The pharmacological basis for this subclassification has proved extremely valuable, not only for examining noradrenergic neurotransmission in blood vessels and defining the roles of pre- and postjunctional α-adrenoceptors, but also for the development of more subtype-selective antagonists. An example of a selective α_1-adrenoceptor antagonist is the phenethylamine derivative YM-12617, which possesses a degree of selectivity comparable to that of prazosin (Honda, Nakagawa and Terai, 1987). Examples of selective α_2-adrenoceptors antagonists, comparable to rauwolscine, but devoid of activity at 5-HT receptors, include the imidazoline derivative idazoxan (Doxey et al., 1984), and the berbane derivatives, CH-38083 (Vizi et al., 1986) and RS-15385-197 (MacKinnon et al., 1992).

The motivation to subdivide adrenoceptors into α- and β-subtypes and to subsequently subdivide the α subtype into α_1- and α_2-adrenoceptors arose from a need to explain irregularities in the quantitative interactions between agonist and antagonist drugs, either in different tissues or within the same preparation. Neither of these subdivisions was embraced wholeheartedly when first proposed, requiring rigorous examination (and a period of several years) to overcome prevailing opinion. However, the combination of the synthesis of a range of structurally-dissimilar, subtype-selective antagonists and the development of new methodological approaches, e.g., radioligand binding, biochemical examination of receptor function, and gene sequencing of receptor protein with expression in cultured cell lines, has generated a wealth of information on α_1 and α_2-adrenoceptors consistent with further fragmentation of α-adrenoceptors. Such studies have far outpaced work on the pharmacological characteristics of noradrenergic neurotransmission in blood vessels. Although much of the work in this area still revolves around the relatively simple definition provided above, we feel it appropriate to discuss the recent evidence that neither α_1- nor α_2-adrenoceptors on blood vessels consist of a homogeneous population of receptors.

Classification of α_1-adrenoceptors

At the time of writing, cloning studies have revealed the existence of at least four subtypes of α_1-adrenoceptors (A, B, C and D subtypes) which have a different sequence of amino acids (Lomasney *et al.*, 1991; Perez, Paiscik and Graham, 1991). Using polymerase chain reaction analysis, Ping and Faber (1993) have recently reported that smooth muscle cells from the rat thoracic aorta and vena cava possess mRNA for both α_{1A}- and α_{1B}-adrenoceptors, and that the adventitia possesses the mRNA for the α_{1A}-subtype. The essentially qualitative nature of the technique unfortunately did not permit any analysis of the relative abundance of the receptor 'message'. Given the known heterogeneity of vascular smooth muscle (McGrath, Brown and Wilson, 1989), the results of similar analysis in sympathetically-innervated arteries and veins are eagerly awaited.

Presently, much of our knowledge on the heterogeneity of α_1-adrenoceptors relies upon the pharmacological characteristics exhibited in radioligand binding studies, biochemical studies or functional (contraction-based) experiments and, therefore, is dependent upon the properties of the agents employed and the system under examination. Two different classification schemes, α_{1A}- and α_{1B}- (Han, Abel and Minneman, 1987; Minneman, 1988), and α_{1H}-, α_{1L}- and α_{1N}- (Murumatsu, Kigoshi and Oshita, 1990a; Murumatsu *et al.*, 1990b) have been proposed, and their relative merits have been discussed in detail elsewhere (see: Wilson, Brown and McGrath, 1991). However, some of the key antagonists at these putative receptor subtypes are given in Table 1.2. Prazosin describes fundamental differences between the two schemes, failing to discriminate between the $\alpha_{1A/B}$-subtypes, but exhibiting different potencies at $\alpha_{1H/L/N}$-subtypes. On the other hand, the alkylating agent, chlorethylclonidine, is able to inactivate α_{1B}- and α_{1H}-subtypes, but is relatively inactive at the other α_1-adrenoceptor subtypes. The competitive antagonist, WB-4101, preferentially inhibits the α_{1A}-subtype compared to the α_{1B}-subtype, but exhibits a range of potencies at the $\alpha_{1H/L/N}$-adrenoceptors. These points are used to illustrate that none of the antagonists presently available exhibit subtype-selectivity comparable to that possessed by prazosin and rauwolscine for α_1- and α_2-adrenoceptors, respectively.

TABLE 1.2

The effect of selected α-adrenoceptor antagonists at putative subtypes of α_1-adrenoceptors

	α_{1A}	α_{1B}	α_{1H}	α_{1L}	α_{1N}	References
Prazosin	high[4,12] (9.3–9.4)	high[4,12] (9.4–9.6)	high[1,5,6,13] (9.6–10.0)	low[1,5,13] (7.9–8.6)	low[5,6] (8.2–8.3)	1) Murumatsu, Ohmura and Oshita (1989)
WB 4101	high?[2,3,4,7,8] (8.4–9.5)	low?[2,3,4,7,8] (7.3–8.9)	low[6] (8.1)	?	high[6] (9.0)	2) Suzuki et al. (1990)
CEC	resistant[11,14]	sensitive[11,14] (10–100 μM, 10–20 mins)	sensitive[1]	resistant[6]	resistant[5,6]	3) Satoh, Kojima and Takayangi (1993)
5-MeU	high[2,3,4,7,8] (7.8–9.4)	low[2,3,4,7,8] (5.1–7.4)	?	?	?	4) Aboud, Shafii and Docherty (1993)
HV 723	?	?	low[5,6] (8.5–8.7)	low[1,6] (8.5)	high[5,6] (9.4)	5) Murumatsu (1991)
SLZ 49	sensitive[9] (0.1 μM, 30 mins)	resistant	?	?	?	6) Murumatsu et al. (1990b)

7) Michel, Loury and Whiting (1990)
8) Hoyer et al. (1990)
9) Piascik et al. (1988)
10) Piascik et al. (1991)
11) Han, Abel and Minneman (1987)
12) Morrow and Creese (1986)
13) Flavahan and Vanhoutte (1986b)
14) Minneman (1988)

Values shown are the pK_i determined from radioligand binding studies or pA_2 values from functional studies.

Despite these problems, the most convincing pharmacological evidence for the existence of α_1-adrenoceptor subtypes on vascular smooth muscle has been obtained from radioligand binding studies using the thoracic aorta from rats and rabbits. In 1983, Awad, Payne and Deth, demonstrated specific binding of [^{3}H]prazosin in membrane preparations from the rabbit aorta. Functional studies demonstrated that contractile responses were antagonised by prazosin but not yohimbine, leading them to conclude that contractions were mediated by a homogeneous population of α_1-adrenoceptors. However, Piascik *et al.* (1988), following on from observations that noradrenaline and another α-agonist, metaraminol, could displace [^{3}H]prazosin from two sites (Babich *et al.*, 1987), subsequently demonstrated that prazosin bound to a high and a low affinity site ($\alpha_{1L/1H}$?) which were affected differentially by a chemically reactive alkylating analogue of prazosin, SZL-49. Further support for the presence of two α_1-adrenoceptors in the rabbit aorta has been provided by several other studies. First, Murumatsu *et al.* (1990b) observed that [^{3}H]-prazosin recognized two distinct sites, one of which was sensitive to chlorethylclonidine (the α_{1H}?). Secondly, Tsujimoto *et al.* (1989), Suzuki *et al.* (1990) and Satoh, Kojima and Takayanagi (1992) demonstrated that chlorethylclonidine inactivated only a proportion of α_1-adrenoceptors in the rabbit aorta, but these authors elected to use the $\alpha_{1A/B}$ subclassification to describe their results. Thirdly, the α_{1A}-adrenoceptor selective antagonist, WB4101, displaced [^{3}H]prazosin from two binding sites on rat aortic membranes with affinities consistent with those found in non-vascular preparations (Piascik *et al.*, 1991). Thus, although two pharmacologically distinct α_1-adrenoceptors have been detected in aortic membranes, supporting the observations of Ping and Faber (1993), there is no antagonist which permits unequivocal identification of the subtypes involved (see Table 1.2). This problem is further compounded in functional experiments where the characteristics of the system under examination is an additional factor.

First, there is evidence in some tissues that chlorethylclonidine (rat aorta) and SLZ-49 (rat and rabbit aorta) alkylate α-adrenoceptors in a novel manner, and this confers upon them properties in functional systems not normally associated with irreversible antagonists (Tian, Gupta and Deth, 1990; Paiscik *et al.*, 1991). Unlike phenoxybenzamine, both agents produced a rightward displacement of the noradrenaline concentration-response curve which was **not** associated with a reduction in the maximum response. Although this could be taken as evidence that the α_1-adrenoceptor subtype remaining after treatment with either chlorethylclonidine or SLZ-49 is sufficiently well coupled to mediate a full contractile response, the pharmacological characteristics of the remaining response implied the involvement of a non-α-adrenoceptor, because the response was resistant to prazosin, WB-4101, and even phenoxybenzamine (Oriowo and Bevan, 1990; Tian, Gupta and Deth, 1990; Piascik *et al.*, 1991). Since under normal conditions responses to noradrenaline in both tissues are clearly mediated by α-adrenoceptors, e.g., Oriowo and Bevan (1990) demonstrated that phenoxybenzamine can abolish responses to noradrenaline, it would seem logical to presume that chlorethylclonidine and SLZ-49 are able to selectively prevent phenoxybenzamine (and prazosin and WB-4101) access to its normal binding site. Interestingly, while preventing antagonist attachment to the receptor (irreversibly), SZL-49 and chlorethylclonidine appeared to behave as competitive antagonists with respect to the response to noradrenaline, because there was no reduction in the maximum response. This concept deviates from traditional receptor theory, but clearly indicates that more information

TABLE 1.3

The effect of selected α-adrenoceptor antagonists at putative subtypes of α_2-adrenoceptors

	α_{2A}	α_{2B}	α_{2C}	α_{2D}
Rauwolscine	(9.0–9.4)	(8.9–9.4)	(9.7–10.4)	(8.3–8.5)
Prazosin	(5.6–6.5)	(7.4–7.6)	(7.1–7.8)	(6.8–7.0)
WB 4101	8.9	8.1	9.6	8.1
ARC 239	(6.0–6.8)	(8.0–8.7)	(7.4–7.9)	(6.4–6.8)
BAM 1303	(7.9–8.6)	(7.3–7.6)	(8.7–9.4)	(7.1–7.3)
SKF 104078	(7.0–7.5)	(7.1–7.3)	(7.2–7.4)	(6.4–6.7)
Oxymetazoline	(8.7–9.1)	(6.6–7.2)	(7.2–7.4)	(7.9–8.8)
Corynanthine	6.9	7.0	7.6	6.1
cell	HT-29 cell	NG108-15 cells	OK cells	bovine pineal or rat
(or tissue) type		or rat lung		sublingual gland

Values shown are the pK_i determined from radioligand binding studies from the following references (and references therein). Bylund and Ray-Prenger (1989), Michel, Loury and Whiting (1989), Simonneaux, Ebadi and Bylund (1991), Gleason and Hieble (1992).

is required on the precise mechanism of action of these 'atypical' irreversible antagonists. The explanation forwarded by Piascik *et al.* (1991) to describe their observations was that the α_1-adrenoceptor subtypes interacted in such a way that attachment of either chlorethylclonidine or SLZ-49, altered the binding characteristics of the other receptor subtype. Were this to be true, the usefulness of these agents for examining neurogenic responses in blood vessels is questionable.

Secondly, many blood vessels possess prejunctional α_2-adrenoceptors that regulate transmitter release, and postjunctional α_2-adrenoceptors which mediate contraction (see later), and the presence of these receptors further reduces the value of WB-4101 and the chlorethylclonidine for examining neurogenic responses. For example, WB-4101, the "selective" α_{1A}-receptor antagonist (pA_2 value 9.2; Table 1.2) also possesses high affinity at α_2-adrenoceptor binding sites (pK_i as high as 9, Table 1.3), while its selectivity between α_{1A}- and α_{1B} receptors is relatively modest (~10-fold) (see above discussion and Wilson, Brown and McGrath, 1991 for further details). These findings support earlier functional experiments questioning the α_1-/α_2-selectivity of WB-4101 (Massingham *et al.*, 1981). Furthermore, chlorethylclonidine has been reported to be an irreversible agonist at prejunctional α_2-adrenoceptors in the rat vas deferens (Bultmann and Starke, 1993), postjunctional α_1-adrenoceptors in the rat aorta (LeClerc *et al.*, 1980; Oriowo and Bevan, 1990) and postjunctional α_2-adrenoceptors in the dog saphenous vein (Nunes and Guimaraes, 1993).

Thus, although the above agents have supported findings from cloning studies that α_1-adrenoceptors are not a homogeneous group, the irreversible action of SLZ-49 and chlorethylclonidine, and the failure of chlorethylclonidine and WB-4101 to discriminate between α_1- and α_2-adrenoceptors, effectively limits our ability to probe the contribution of subtypes of α_1-adrenoceptors to neurogenic responses in blood vessels.

Classification of α_2-adrenoceptors

On the basis of radioligand binding and molecular cloning studies in many tissues, four subtypes of α_2-adrenoceptors (A, B, C and D) have been proposed (Nahorski, Barnett and

Cheung, 1985; Bylund, 1985, 1988; Michel, Loury and Whiting, 1989; Blaxall *et al.*, 1991; Bylund *et al.*, 1991; Lomasney *et al.*, 1991; Simonneaux, Ebadi and Bylund, 1991; Bylund, 1992). To date, polymerase chain reaction analysis has only been performed on the rat aorta and vena cava, and this has revealed the presence of mRNA for α_{2A}- and α_{2B}-adrenoceptors, respectively (Ping and Faber, 1993). The surprising feature of these findings is that as yet there is no evidence for α_2-adrenoceptor-mediated contractions in the aorta (McGrath, Brown and Wilson, 1989). There are two possible explanations for the discrepancy between the PCR analysis (molecular biology) and contraction-based (functional) approaches. Either the α_2-adrenoceptors have a non-contractile function in this tissue or, the value of the former technique has been overestimated, were PCR analysis to detect receptors present in such small numbers, that they have no measurable physiological effect.

Unlike the subclassification scheme for α_1-adrenoceptors, pharmacological differences between α_2-adrenoceptors have been exclusively based upon the use of competitive antagonists (Table 1.3). In the majority of functional studies examining the α_2-autoreceptor, such as those in rabbit and human cortex (Limberger, Spath and Starke, 1991; Raiteri *et al.*, 1992), guinea-pig urethra (Alberts, 1992), rat vas deferens (Connaughton and Docherty, 1990) and presynaptic cholinergic and sympathetic fibres of the guinea-pig submucosal plexus (Shen, Barajas-Lopez and Surprenant, 1990), the authors have concluded that α_{2A}-adrenoceptors mediate autoinhibition, largely based upon the insensitivity of responses to prazosin and ARC-239. In contrast, presynaptic modulation in rat atrium and rabbit iris display sensitivity to prazosin and ARC-239 thereby implicating α_{2B}-receptors (Connaughton and Docherty, 1990; Fuder and Selbach, 1993). More recently, α_{2D}-adrenoceptors have been proposed to be functionally important in the submaxillary gland (Limberger, Trendelenburg and Starke, 1992). With respect to vascular smooth muscle, we have recently demonstrated that α_2-adrenoceptor binding sites on vascular smooth muscle cells of the porcine thoracic aorta and marginal ear vein belong to the prazosin-insensitive, $\alpha_{2A/D}$-subclass, and mediate contractions in both preparations, which are also resistant to prazosin (Blaylock and Wilson, 1993; Wright, Blaylock and Wilson, unpublished observations).

In the majority of instances, however, the functional correlates of the four α_2-adrenoceptor binding sites are poorly defined and attempts at classifying α_2-adrenoceptor-mediated responses must be treated with extreme caution. This is evident since the selectivity of agents for the proposed α_2-adrenoceptor subtypes is frequently modest. Furthermore, as shown in Tables 1.2 and 1.3, many of the agents currently employed to distinguish between α_2-adrenoceptor binding sites (e.g., prazosin and WB-4101) are also potent antagonists at α_1-adrenoceptors. This has important implications for attempts to identify neurogenic α_2-adrenoceptor responses *in vitro*, particularly as there is extensive data to indicate that vascular α_1- and α_2-adrenoceptor mediate responses of the same functional polarity (in contrast to α- and β-adrenoceptors) with the potential to interact. Some examples which highlight the complications produced by interactions between α_1- and α_2-adrenoceptors for receptor characterisation are outlined below.

In the tail artery from the normotensive rat, responses to noradrenaline are mediated via α_1-adrenoceptors (prazosin-sensitive, rauwolscine-resistant) under standard experimental conditions. However in the presence of tone, induced with either vasopressin, 5-HT or endothelin, a sizeable component of the response to noradrenaline becomes prazosin-resistant, rauwolscine-sensitive (α_2-mediated) (Templeton *et al.*, 1989; MacLean and McGrath, 1990). This quiescent adrenoceptor population has been shown to have sufficient influence to produce discrepancies in the potency of selective antagonists against various agonists (Rajanayagam and Medgett, 1987). Secondly, in the rabbit saphenous artery, a very dramatic demonstration of synergistic interactions with α_2-adrenoceptors could be shown with tachyphylactic concentrations of angiotensin II (Dunn, McGrath and Wilson, 1989). In the absence of angiotensin II, the 'selective' α_2-adrenoceptor agonist, UK-14304, produced contractions which were sensitive to low concentrations of prazosin. In the presence of this peptide however, the threshold sensitivity to UK-14304 was increased 300-fold and this 'unmasked' response was prazosin-resistant, rauwolscine-sensitive (α_2-adrenoceptor-mediated). Similar observations were made using low (barely contractile) concentrations of the relatively selective α_1-adrenoceptor agonist, phenylephrine, demonstrating a direct synergistic interaction between α_1- and α_2-adrenoceptors (Dunn, McGrath and Wilson, 1991a). Furthermore, although angiotensin II had no effect on the potency of noradrenaline *per se*, a prazosin-resistant component, not evident in the absence of angiotensin II, was uncovered (Dunn *et al.*, 1991a). Finally in the rabbit saphenous vein, contractile responses to noradrenaline are sensitive to low concentrations of both prazosin and rauwolscine. However, following exposure to either angiotensin II or the calcium channel facilitator Bay K 8644, responses become more resistant to prazosin (Dunn *et al.*, 1991c). Examined under standard experimental conditions, quantitative studies in these three preparations would have given the false impression of the presence of only one subtype (α_1) or of an adrenoceptor displaying characteristics differing from the classical α_1-α_2 subdivision (see McGrath *et al.*, 1991). Figure 1.2 shows a schematic representation of the interaction between postjunctional α_1- and α_2-adrenoceptors and how angiotensin II, for example, can allow functional expression of postjunctional α_2-adrenoceptors.

The study of Smith, Connaughton and Docherty (1992), on the pharmacological characteristics of α-adrenoceptors mediating contractions to noradrenaline in the human isolated saphenous vein, illustrates the potential for confusion when a preparation possesses postjunctional α_1- and α_2-adrenoceptors. These workers examined a range of selective α_1- and α_2-adrenoceptor antagonists against noradrenaline-induced contractions in the human saphenous vein, and compared their effect with the inhibitory constants obtained against α_{2A}- and α_{2B}-adrenoceptor binding sites on human platelet and rat kidney membranes, respectively. Parallel rightward displacement of the noradrenaline concentration-response curve was produced by all antagonists, when employed over a limited 3-fold concentration range, and the estimated dissociation constants correlated better with the α_{2B}-adrenoceptor binding site. The finding that the selective α_1-adrenoceptor antagonists prazosin and ARC-239 were more potent than expected at α_{2A}-adrenoceptors, was particularly important in arriving at the above conclusion. However, since the estimated dissociation constants for the selective α_2-adrenoceptor antagonists, BDF-8933 and CH-38083, were **less** than the inhibition constants at either α_{2A}- or α_{2B}-adrenoceptor binding sites (by a factor of 10), one possible explanation is that the saphenous vein possesses both α_1- and α_2-adrenoceptors. This is precisely the conclusion arrived at by Roberts *et al.* (1992), who observed that low concentrations of prazosin (10 nM) and rauwolscine (10 nM) produced an approximate 10-fold rightward displacement of the noradrenaline concentration response curve in the

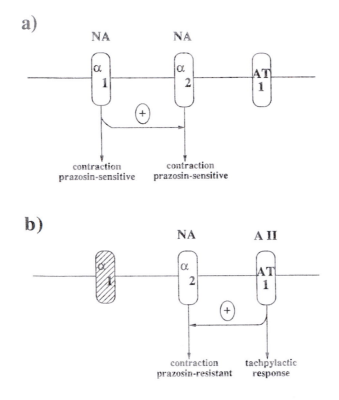

Figure 1.2 Diagrammatic representation of the positive interaction between postjunctional α_1- and α_2-adrenoceptors which renders responses to noradrenaline mediated via α_2-adrenoceptors sensitive to prazosin in some blood vessels, e.g., the rabbit isolated distal saphenous artery (Dunn, McGrath and Wilson, 1991a).

(a) Under normal conditions noradrenaline mediates contractile responses via postjunctional α_1-adrenoceptors. In addition stimulation of α_1-adrenoceptors has a positive influence on the expression of functional responses to noradrenaline mediated via postjunctional α_2-adrenoceptors. The dependency of α_2-adrenoceptor-mediated responses on α_1-adrenoceptor activation however, renders responses mediated via this subtype sensitive to α_1-adrenoceptor antagonists, such as prazosin.

(b) If the function of α_1-adrenoceptors is removed, the positive influence required for α_2-adrenoceptor functional expression can be provided by tachyphylactic concentrations of angiotensin II. Under this circumstance responses to noradrenaline mediated via postjunctional α_2-adrenoceptors are resistant to blockade by prazosin.

human isolated saphenous vein. Furthermore, since the presence of angiotensin II reduced the sensitivity of UK-14304 induced contractions to prazosin, the α_2-adrenoceptor is of the A/D (prazosin-resistant) rather than the B/C (prazosin-sensitive) subtype.

These studies also underline the fact that, since prazosin is still central to any functional study aiming to distinguish between vascular α_1 and α_2-adrenoceptors, it is unlikely that attempts to differentiate between the prazosin-sensitive (B/C) and the prazosin-insensitive (A/D) vascular α_2-adrenoceptor will be successful. As indicated by investigations on non-vascular tissues, identification of the α_2-adrenoceptor subtype implicated in a given functional response often requires in excess of seven antagonists.

In summary, α_1- and α_2-adrenoceptors have each been divided into four putative subgroups, while β-adrenoceptors appear to exist as three subtypes. At present, it is not known how many of these subtypes are located at the vascular neuroeffector junction, or even on vascular smooth muscle. Neither the pharmacological tools nor the molecular biological techniques available allow for convincing demonstration of the functional importance of any of the putative subtypes. The problem is made all the more difficult by the ability of the receptor subtypes to interact to produce the biological response. For the remainder of this chapter we will limit much of our discussion on the role of adrenoceptors within the vascular neuroeffector junction to the β_2-, α_1- and α_2- subtypes. The role of specific subgroups of these receptors will only be considered when studies have been conducted in an appropriately rigorous manner, or when observations with a 'selective' compound produced interesting observations.

PREJUNCTIONAL ADRENOCEPTOR MODULATION OF NORADRENALINE RELEASE FROM SYMPATHETIC FIBRES

As indicated in Figure 1.3 the prejunctional membranes of individual varicosities on sympathetic fibre are endowed with both α_2- and β_2-adrenoceptors which, when activated by noradrenaline, have the potential to modify further transmitter release. We will attempt to assess the relative importance of each receptor system, but focus mainly upon the α_2-adrenoceptors, since these have received more attention.

PREJUNCTIONAL β_2-ADRENOCEPTORS

Evidence for facilitatory prejunctional β_2-adrenoceptors on sympathetic nerve terminals has long been recognized (Langer, 1981; Kawasaki, Cline and Su, 1984) but, compared to inhibitory α_2-adrenoceptors, has received little attention. Part of the problem has been that demonstration of the facilitatory effect of β_2-adrenoceptor activation *in vitro* often requires prior disruption of autoinhibitory feedback by α_2-adrenoceptors (Johnston and Majewski, 1986; Costa and Majewski, 1988), and this has been interpreted as indicating that it is of minor importance. Also, β-adrenoceptor antagonists do not reduce transmitter output from vascular preparations examined *in vitro*. However, several observations appear to indicate that noradrenaline may not be the endogenous activator of prejunctional β-adrenoceptors, and necessitates revision of its physiological importance.

First, Borkowski *et al.* (1989) demonstrated that adrenaline enhanced neurogenic responses in the dog mesenteric artery (without affecting responses to exogenous noradrenaline). This facilitation was unaffected by the selective β_1-adrenoceptor antagonist atenolol, but was sensitive to the non-selective β-adrenoceptor antagonist, timolol, indicating the involvement of β_2-adrenoceptors. Secondly, Remie *et al.* (1988) reported that the β_2-adrenoceptor agonist, fenoterol, produced a 3-fold increase in plasma noradrenaline in freely moving rats, even in the absence of α_2-adrenoceptor blockade. Finally, Scheurink *et al.* (1989) demonstrated that the 4-fold elevation of plasma noradrenaline in exercising rats was greatly reduced following adrenodemedullation or administration of the selective β_2-adrenoceptor antagonist, ICI-118551. These latter findings appear to indicate that

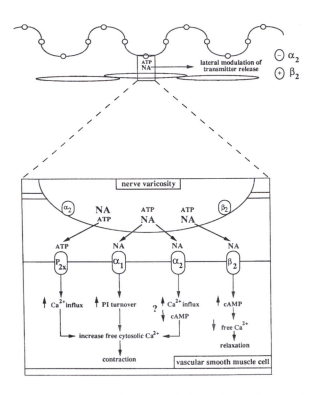

Figure 1.3 Overall schematic of a post-ganglionic sympathetic axon innervating a blood vessel. The small beads represent an individual varicosity — the site of release of the neurotransmitters. The expanded diagram of an individual varicosity shows that vascular neurotransmission may involve the release of a least two transmitters (noradrenaline and ATP) and activation of several receptors (α_1-, α_2- and β-adrenoceptors and P_{2x} purinoceptors). The coupling mechanism through which postjunctional responses are produced are also shown (details of which can be found in McGrath, Brown and Wilson, 1989, 1991). Prejunctional regulation of noradrenaline released by α_2-adrenoceptors and β_2-adrenoceptors, monitored by the magnitude of the excitatory junctional potential associated with activation of P_{2x} purinoceptors, is thought to occur at varicosities distant from the site of release — lateral modulation (Brook and Cunnane, 1991b; Stjärne et al., 1993). Please note that in order to simplify the diagram the sympathetic neurotransmitter neuropeptide Y (Franco-Cereceda, this volume) has not been included.

facilitatory β_2-adrenoceptors are activated by adrenaline derived from the adrenal gland. However, the physiological consequence of the elevated plasma noradrenaline is not clear, since both experimental manipulations also interfere with the direct effects of adrenaline on the vasculature.

PREJUNCTIONAL α_2-ADRENOCEPTORS

Local or lateral modulation of transmitter release?

There is a wealth of evidence to indicate that when noradrenaline is released from sympathetic fibres innervating blood vessels, it is capable of reducing further release by activating prejunctional α_2-adrenoceptors — the so-called autoinhibitory feedback mechanism

(Gillespie, 1980; Starke, 1987). As explained earlier (Classification of adrenoceptors), this concept developed from the observations that α_2-adrenoceptor antagonists increase noradrenaline release from sympathetic nerves, by interrupting the negative feedback mechanism, and that α_2-adrenoceptor agonists reduced transmitter release, by mimicking the endogenous ligand. Additional supports for this mechanism came from the general observations that α_2-adrenoceptor antagonists failed to influence transmitter release to a limited number of pulses, presumably because the intrajunctional concentration of noradrenaline was too low to further modify transmitter release, while, under the same conditions, synthetic α_2-adrenoceptor agonists were effective (for the same reason). This negative feedback mechanism has, until recently, been presumed to operate at the level of each individual varicosity in such a manner as to ensure pulse-by-pulse regulation of noradrenaline release and, therefore, vascular calibre. This model of sympathetic neurotransmission requires that a high percentage of varicosities release transmitter following each nerve action potential, thereby allowing noradrenaline to accumulate and exert a local effect.

The majority of the above studies have involved either measurement of $[^3H]$-noradrenaline overflow or indirect assessment of transmitter release by monitoring the excitatory junction potential (ejp) produced by the sympathetic cotransmitter ATP (see Figure 1.3), and represent findings from a large population, rather than for an individual varicosity. The recent development of focally applied extracellular suction electrodes has allowed recording of excitatory junction currents (ejc) from individual varicosities in the guinea-pig vas deferens (Brock and Cunnane, 1987) and the rat tail artery (Astrand and Stjärne, 1989; Stjärne et al., 1993), and findings from these studies challenge the above view that transmitter release is modulated on a pulse-by-pulse basis. First, transmitter release from a given varicosity has been shown to be intermittent, with a probability of 0.01, thus making it unlikely that noradrenaline can build up to sufficient levels to reduce subsequent release from the same site. Secondly, during a long train of stimuli there is actually a transient **increase** in the likelihood that transmitter release will occur from the same or closely related release site. Both of these findings support earlier electrophysiological studies that questioned the existence of local regulation of transmitter release (Blakeley, Cunnane and Petersen, 1982). It should be noted, however, that since the postjunctional event is thought to be mediated by ATP, but prejunctional modulation involves noradrenaline, the above interpretation depends upon the release of both substances being affected similarly, i.e., there is no differential modulation of transmitter release. There are a number of observations which challenge this view (Forsyth and Pollock, 1988).

In spite of the difficulty encountered in observing prejunctional feedback at the level of an individual varicosity, synthetic α_2-adrenoceptor agonists, when added **outside** the extracellular recording electrode, have been shown to reduce the ejcs **inside** the recording electrode (Stjärne et al., 1993). These findings have been interpreted as evidence that the effect of activation of prejunctional α_2-adrenoceptors is not exclusively local, but can spread along the nerve terminal — so-called lateral modulation of transmitter release (Brock and Cunnane, 1991a, b; Stjärne et al., 1993) (see Figure 1.3). The precise mechanism involved is not known, but Stjärne and coworkers (1993) have proposed a chaotic model whereby an additional factor, integral to the probability of transmitter release, is inhibited by α_2-adrenoceptor activation. Brock and Cunnane (1991b), on the other hand, have been more cautious and suggested that 'the terminal network of sympathetic fibres has a complex three-dimensional branching anatomical arrangement the function of which is not fully appreciated'.

If the concept of lateral inhibition of transmitter release applies to noradrenaline, then it is likely that both ATP and neuropeptide Y, also released from sympathetic fibres innervating blood vessels (Morris and Gibbins, 1991; Franco-Cereceda, this volume), will influence prejunctional events in a similar fashion. In the opinion of the authors, this radical revision of factors regulating transmitter release has implications for assessing the relative importance of pre- and postjunctional factors influencing the end-organ response in vascular smooth muscle.

Pharmacological characterization of prejunctional α_2-adrenoceptors

As indicated earlier (Subclassification of α-adrenoceptors) the application of radioligand binding and molecular biological techniques has suggested that there may be as many as four different subtypes of α_2-adrenoceptors. Two different pharmacological approaches have been used to determine which of these subtypes reside on noradrenergic neurones in the periphery and, although only a limited number of studies have been conducted, it is clear that the choice of method will have a bearing on the accuracy with which antagonist potency can be determined.

The first method, identical to that originally employed by Starke and coworkers (1974, 1975a), involves an assessment of antagonist potency at enhancing transmitter ($[^3H]$-noradrenaline) release by 30% above control values. This method relies upon the pre-existing autoinhibition of transmitter release, and has been used to suggest that prejunctional α_2-adrenoceptors in the rat vas deferens may be of the α_{2A}-subclass, while those in the rat atrium belong to the α_{2B}-subclass (Connaughton and Docherty, 1990). One major disadvantage of this approach however, is that the true maximum effect of the antagonist cannot be determined, and this reduces confidence in values of antagonist potency obtained from the attainment of a fixed response. The second method involves careful selection of stimulation parameters to either minimize or eliminate autoinhibition, as assessed by the absence of the release-enhancing effect of antagonists. Under these conditions, it is possible to use selective α_2-adrenoceptor agonists to generate a concentration-related inhibition of stimulated transmitter release, and then to repeat this in the presence of various concentrations of an antagonist. This method has the advantage of allowing accurate determination of agonist potency, and the antagonist dissociation constant. Using this approach, prejunctional α_2-adrenoceptors in the rat kidney (Schwartz and Malik, 1992; Bohmann, Schollmeyer and Rump, 1993) and the rat submaxillary gland (Limberger, Trendelenburg and Starke, 1992) have been classified as belonging to the α_{2D}-subclass, while those on the rat atrium (Limberger, Trendelenburg and Starke, 1992) were considered to be different from both the α_{2B}- and α_{2D}. A particularly important feature of the above studies is that they have all been conducted in the rat, thereby eliminating species differences in the same receptors as a complicating factor (see McGrath, Brown and Wilson, 1989).

The more rigorous approach permitted by the second method also allowed Limberger, Trendelenburg and Starke (1992) to eliminate the possibility that inhibitory prejunctional α_1-adrenoceptors (see Starke, 1987) or inhibitory prejunctional imidazoline receptors (Göthert and Molderings, 1991; Molderings, Hentrich and Göthert 1991; Fuder and Schwarz 1993), contributed to the effect of UK-14304. The existence of prejunctional inhibitory imidazoline receptors on postganglionic sympathetic fibres accounts for a previously reported difference between the α_2-adrenoceptor antagonists rauwolscine (a non-imidazoline) and BDF-6143 (an imidazoline derivative) in their ability to enhance [^{3}H]-noradrenaline release in the rabbit pulmonary artery (Docherty *et al.*, 1982). The possibility exists that these prejunctional non-adrenoceptors may be activated by endogenous agmatine (decarboxylated arginine), a candidate for the previously described 'clonidine-displacing substance' (Li *et al.*, 1994).

To date, there have been no detailed studies of the pharmacological characteristics of prejunctional α_2-adrenoceptors in isolated blood vessels, presumably because the amount of transmitter released in the absence of autoinhibition is too low. In the future it may be possible to adapt the on-line voltammetric method for the detection of noradrenaline (Mermet, Gonon and Stjärne, 1990) to allow measurement of transmitter release in the absence of autoinhibition. This will be particularly important for the development of antagonists with the potential to discriminate between pre- and postjunctional α_2-adrenoceptors.

Physiological aspects of prejunctional α_2-adrenoceptor regulation of
transmitter release at the vascular neuroeffector junction

There are numerous studies showing that disruption of autoinhibition at the vascular neuroeffector junction causes increased transmitter release from isolated blood vessels, and this appears to account for the 4-fold increase in plasma noradrenaline produced by yohimbine in freely moving rats (Remie and Zaagma, 1986). However, the functional consequence of this effect is most easily observed when the postjunctional response does not involve α-adrenoceptors. For example, Morris and Gibbins (1991) demonstrated that phentolamine increased the motor response in the guinea-pig thoracic inferior vena cava, a response which appears to be mediated by NPY. Similarly, von Kügelgen and Starke (1985), Murumatsu, Ohmura and Oshita (1989) and Bulloch and Starke (1990) noted that α_2-adrenoceptor antagonists increased the motor response in blood vessels (rabbit and dog mesenteric arteries) where the dominant component of the response is purinergic. A particularly dramatic demonstration of the effect of prejunctional regulation by noradrenaline of postjunctional responses was reported by Yamamoto, Cline and Takasaki (1988). These authors observed that the neurogenic pressor response in the perfused rat mesenteric bed was practically abolished by 30 nM prazosin. However, the use of higher concentrations of prazosin (to 1 μM) was associated with the appearance of a response that was sensitive to α, β-methylene ATP. Thus, it would appear that under normal conditions the motor response is entirely noradrenergic, being mediated by α_1-adrenoceptors, but that high concentrations of prazosin remove autoinhibitory feedback control of ATP release by blocking prejunctional α_2-adrenoceptors, and this is manifest as a pressor response. These observations support earlier findings that prazosin can increase noradrenaline release from sympathetic nerve endings (Cavero *et al.*, 1979), and emphasizes that even for this antagonist, usually considered the most selective α_1-adrenoceptor ligand, care must be exercised in the choice of concentration for experiments designed to assess the contribution of α_1-adrenoceptors in a physiological response (see Table 1.1).

In view of the relative ease with which the autoinhibitory feedback can be demonstrated by α_2-adrenoceptor antagonists, it is somewhat surprising that there are relatively few reports illustrating that selective α_2-adrenoceptor agonists can inhibit motor responses in isolated blood vessels (see Table 1.6 below). Part of the problem may be that contractile responses are only obtained with stimulation parameters that also activate autoinhibitory feedback by noradrenaline. However, Su (1980) showed that, even in the rabbit isolated mesenteric artery, where activation of prejunctional α_2-adrenoceptors reduces [^{3}H]-noradrenaline release, the postjunctional response (purinergic) was enhanced by α_2-adrenoceptor agonists. Qualitatively similar results have also been reported in perfused cat spleen (Dubocovich, Langer and Massingham, 1980) and canine isolated saphenous vein (Senaratne, Jakakody and Kappagoda, 1987). One possible explanation for the discrepancy between pre- and postjunctional actions of α-adrenoceptor agonists is that postjunctional facilitation of contractile responses overcomes the consequence of prejunctional inhibition of transmitter release. The general implications of these observations, in terms of the relative importance of pre- and postjunctional mechanisms at the vascular neuroeffector junction, will be addressed later.

α_2-adrenoceptor modulation of noradrenaline release from sympathetic nerves has also been observed in human pulmonary artery (Hentrich, Göthert and Greschuchna, 1986), gall bladder artery (Kaposci et al., 1987) and saphenous vein (Roberts et al., 1992) and the widespread distribution of these receptors appears to account for the ability of yohimbine (Goldberg, Hollister and Robertson, 1983; Grossman et al., 1993) and idazoxan (Brown et al., 1985) to elevate plasma noradrenaline in man. Interestingly, both antagonists produced a small elevation of blood pressure. This suggests that the functional consequence of disruption of autoinhibitory feedback in man is increased activation of postjunctional non-α_2-adrenoceptors. However, since both of these compounds can cross the blood-brain barrier, the possibility exists that the transient hypertension is a result of inhibition of central α_2-adrenoceptors rather than a functional consequence of disruption of autoinhibitory feedback at the vascular neuroeffector junction. In support of this mechanism of actions, Szemeredi et al. (1989) have reported that the selective α_2-adrenoceptor antagonist, L-659,066, elevated plasma noradrenaline and produced a transient **decrease** in blood pressure. Since this compound does not cross the blood-brain barrier (Clineschmidt et al., 1988), it would appear that, at least in rats, disruption of autoinhibitory feedback alone is not sufficient to elevate blood pressure. Moreover, the transient reduction in blood pressure would appear to indicate that postjunctional α_2-adrenoceptors make a significant contribution to peripheral resistance in conscious animals. A similar haemodynamic study with L-659,066 in man is clearly warranted!

In summary, the application of biochemical, electrophysiological and pharmacological approaches to the study of noradrenergic transmission at the sympathetic neuroeffector junction has provided detailed insights into the prejunctional factors regulating transmitter release, and also an indication of their functional importance. Demonstration of the physiological role of facilitatory β_2-adrenoceptors is easier *in vivo*, and these observations suggest that adrenaline, rather than noradrenaline, is the endogenous activator. It is unclear, however, whether the action of adrenaline is a 'hormonal' effect or the result of prior uptake into sympathetic nerves and subsequent release with noradrenaline at the vascular neuroeffector junction. On the other hand, the role of inhibitory α_2-adrenoceptors in regulating transmitter release can be demonstrated *in vitro* and *in vivo*, which suggests that it is activated by noradrenaline. In many peripheral tissues the receptors appear to be of the α_{2D}-subclass although there is evidence, most notably in the atrium, that other subtypes may be involved. Finally, the elegant work of Brock and Cunnane, and Stjärne's group has challenged the concept of local regulation of transmitter release by prejunctional adrenoceptors, and places the site of modulation some distance from the site of release. We endorse the view of Brock and Cunnane (1991b) that microanatomical examination of the three dimensional structure of sympathetic innervation may provide an explanation for lateral modulation of transmitter release.

THE ROLE OF POSTJUNCTIONAL ADRENOCEPTORS AT THE VASCULAR NEUROEFFECTOR JUNCTION

In considering the role of postjunctional adrenoceptors in neurogenic modulation of vascular smooth muscle, we will mainly focus upon the evidence for the involvement of α_2-, β_2- and non-α-, non-β (γ) adrenoceptors. Since the role of postjunctional α_1-adrenoceptor in neurogenic contractions is well established, and has been thoroughly addressed elsewhere (Davey, 1989; McGrath, Brown and Wilson, 1989; Morris and Gibbins, 1991), we will limit our discussion of the involvement of this subtype to recent attempts to further characterize the pharmacological characteristics of the receptor involved.

α_1-ADRENOCEPTOR-MEDIATED RESPONSES

In 1991 Murumatsu found that the irreversible antagonist, chlorethylclonidine, abolished neurogenic contractions in the dog carotid artery, but only reduced responses in the dog mesenteric artery and rabbit carotid artery by 30–40%. In addition prazosin exhibited a 3 to 10-fold greater potency in the dog carotid artery, compared to the dog mesenteric artery and rabbit carotid artery, leading the authors to suggest that the α_{1H}-subtype mediated the responses in the dog carotid artery, but that a combination of α_{1H}- and α_{1N}-adrenoceptors was responsible for responses in the other two vessels. In another study, Sulpizio and Hieble (1991) examined the pharmacological characteristics of electrically-evoked responses to 2 Hz stimulation for 2 min in the rat tail artery. The phasic and tonic components of the neurogenic contractions were similarly affected by 5-methylurapidil (putative α_{1A}-antagonist), chlorethylclonidine (putative α_{1B}-adrenoceptor antagonist) and prazosin (non-selective $\alpha_{1A/B}$-adrenoceptor antagonist; see Table 1.2). The authors concluded that only a single α_1-adrenoceptor, possessing the pharmacological characteristics of the A and B subtypes, was implicated in neurogenic responses in this tissue. It is noteworthy that, while both studies employed chlorethylclonidine to discriminate between putative subtypes, and adopted procedures to eliminate the involvement of α_2-adrenoceptors and purinoceptors, each arrived at different conclusions. This emphasizes that progress in this area is critically dependent upon the availability of pharmacological tools that possess high selectivity for the putative α_1-adrenoceptor subtype.

Another potential problem with the pharmacological characterization of transient neurogenic contractions, is also highlighted in the study of Sulpizio and Hieble (1991). The putative α_{1A}-adrenoceptor antagonist, WB-4101, which was slightly more potent than prazosin, selectively inhibited the phasic component of the neurogenic contractions. Although this might be taken as evidence for further receptor heterogeneity, we believe that this is a function of potent antagonists at α_1-adrenoceptors on arterial smooth muscle in the rat. For example, low concentrations of prazosin have been reported to produce an insurmountable inhibition of the phasic response to noradrenaline in the aorta (Downing, Wilson and Wilson, 1983), perfused mesenteric bed (Downing, Wilson and Wilson, 1985) and the perfused tail (Templeton et al., 1989), but a competitive inhibition of the tonic (sustained) component of contractions. Significantly, qualitatively similar observations have also been reported for WB-4101 (Downing, Wilson and Wilson, 1983) and YM-12617 (McGrath and Wilson, 1987). Since both are potent antagonists, structurally unrelated to prazosin, it seems likely that this property is a function of α_1-adrenoceptor blockade per se, rather than an ability to discriminate between receptor subtypes.

α_2-ADRENOCEPTOR-MEDIATED RESPONSES

Following the demonstration of postjunctional α_2-adrenoceptors on vascular smooth muscle (see classification of α-adrenoceptors), several groups noted that α_1-adrenoceptor antagonists were potent inhibitors of sympathetically-mediated pressor responses in the pithed rat (Docherty and McGrath, 1980; Yamaguchi and Kopin, 1980; Wilffert, Timmermans and Van Zwieten, 1982) and the canine hindlimb (Langer, Massingham and Shepperson, 1980). This prompted suggestions that postjunctional α_1-adrenoceptors were innervated, whereas α_2-adrenoceptors were extrajunctional and responded to circulating catecholamines (McGrath, 1982). This view was supported by findings in numerous isolated blood vessels at the time, e.g., rabbit pulmonary artery (Cambridge, Davey and Massingham, 1977), rabbit thoracic aorta (Docherty and Starke, 1982) rat tail artery (Medgett and Langer, 1984), perfused rat mesenteric bed (Yamamoto, Cline and Takasaki, 1988) and perfused cat spleen (Massingham et al., 1981), where prazosin was a potent inhibitor of neurogenic constriction, and also by the observations that stimulation of the adrenal medulla in pithed rats produced a response which was more sensitive to α_2-adrenoceptor antagonists than equivalent sized nerve-mediated responses (Flavahan et al., 1985). While this situation may still apply in some vascular beds (Willette, Hieble and Sauermilch, 1991), it is now clear that this generalisation does not hold. Indeed, it seems that in most instances where postjunctional α_2-adrenoceptors can be demonstrated responding to exogenous noradrenaline, they will also respond to nerve-released noradrenaline, when examined under the appropriate experimental conditions. We will first discuss the regional distribution of postjunctional α_2-adrenoceptors on vascular smooth muscle, and then consider the evidence that these receptors contribute to sympathetically-mediated responses.

Location of α_2-adrenoceptors

Postjunctional α_2-adrenoceptors were first detected in large cutaneous veins. De Mey and Vanhoutte (1981) demonstrated that contractions of the canine saphenous vein and femoral vein to noradrenaline were inhibited (in a non-competitive manner) by prazosin and yohimbine, which suggested the presence of a heterogeneous population of α-adrenoceptors. Unequivocal demonstration of α_2-adrenoceptors in the canine saphenous vein awaited the work of Constantine, Lebel and Archer (1982), who showed that responses to noradrenaline were resistant to prazosin but sensitive to yohimbine (following inactivation of α_1-adrenoceptors by phenoxybenzamine). Functional α_2-adrenoceptors were subsequently demonstrated in a number of other venous preparations from different species and vascular beds, such as the canine spleen (Hieble and Woodward, 1984) and mesentery (Kou, Ibengwe and Suzuki, 1984), guinea-pig kidney (Makita, 1983), rabbit ear vein (Daly, McGrath and Wilson, 1988c) and the saphenous veins from rats, rabbits and humans respectively (Alabaster, Keir and Peters, 1985; Cheung, 1985; Docherty and Hyland, 1985; Daly, McGrath and Wilson, 1988b; Daly et al., 1988d; Akers et al., 1991). In most cases (with the possible exception of the rabbit ear vein) responses to noradrenaline are antagonised potently by both yohimbine and prazosin, which suggests that postjunctional α_2-adrenoceptors co-exist with a population of postjunctional α_1-adrenoceptors. It should also be noted that not all venous preparations possess functional α_2-adrenoceptors, e.g., rabbit renal vein (Daly, McGrath and Wilson, 1988a).

In contrast, with the exception of feline cerebral (Skarby, Andersson and Edvinsson, 1983) and human digital arteries (Stevens and Moulds, 1985), there was very little evidence for functional α_2-adrenoceptors on large arteries. Contractile responses to noradrenaline were invariably sensitive to low concentrations of prazosin, and resistant to α_2-adrenoceptor blockers, even where there was radioligand binding evidence for α_2-adrenoceptors on arterial smooth muscle (Weiss, Webb and Smith, 1983; Shi, Kwan and Daniel, 1989). This can be partly explained by the density of α_2-adrenoceptor expression on vascular smooth muscle (Shi, Kwan and Daniel, 1989; Wright et al., 1994).

A more subtle factor accounting for the difficulty in demonstrating postjunctional α_2-adrenoceptor mediated responses in vitro appears to be the lack of humoral agents normally present in the whole animal. For example, Schumman and Lues (1983) demonstrated that responses to BHT-920 were potently antagonised by prazosin in the rabbit saphenous vein. However, in the presence of angiotensin II, responses became resistant to prazosin and therefore more classically α_2-adrenoceptor-mediated. Similar observations have been made with noradrenaline in this preparation (Dunn et al., 1991c), and an even more dramatic demonstration of the interaction between angiotensin II and α_2-adrenoceptors has been reported in the equivalent arterial preparation (Dunn, McGrath and Wilson, 1989, 1991a). Furthermore, the presence of tissue stimulants has been shown to be a prerequisite for the clear demonstration of α_2-adrenoceptors in a number of other isolated arterial and venous preparations (Sulpizio and Hieble, 1987; Furuta, 1988; Shi, Kwan and Daniel, 1989; Templeton et al., 1989). A schematic representation of the dependence of postjunctional α_2-adrenoceptors on a humoral agent is shown in Figure 1.2.

Thus, the density of α_2-adrenoceptor on vascular smooth muscle and also the experimental conditions employed are important determinants of the functional expression of α_2-adrenoceptors on large blood vessels. In addition, it is now clear that another factor which accounts for the difficulty detecting these responses in vitro is their preferential location on resistance vessels. This is supported by the recent finding of an inverse correlation between human arterial vessel diameter and the magnitude of the α_2-adrenoceptor mediated response observed (Nielsen et al., 1989). Furthermore, a greater dominance of α_2-adrenoceptor-mediated responses was observed in decreasing branches of the arteriolar tree in the blood-perfused cremaster vasculature of the rat (Faber, 1988). Postjunctional α_2-adrenoceptors have also been shown to be present in human resistance arteries isolated from the omentum, colon, pericardial fat and skeletal muscle (Nielsen, Mortensen and Mulvany, 1990, 1991a), and in porcine and human mesenteric resistance arteries (Nielsen *et al.*, 1991b). These observations support a role for α_2-adrenoceptors in the resistance vasculature, although it is not an exclusive role either between or within species, since responses in rat and rabbit mesenteric resistance arteries and in bovine retinal small arteries are mediated solely via postjunctional α_1-adrenoceptors (Nielsen and Nyborg, 1988; Nielsen *et al.*, 1991b).

The above studies illustrate that postjunctional α_2-adrenoceptors are widely distributed throughout the cardiovascular system, although the density of expression appears to be greater in veins, particularly cutaneous veins, and resistance vessels. The arteriolar location of α_2-adrenoceptors ensures that they are ideally-placed to influence peripheral resistance and, therefore, blood pressure. Evidence presented below suggests they are also located within the vascular neuroeffector junction and respond to noradrenaline released from sympathetic neurons.

Innervated α-adrenoceptors

Table 1.4 details the *in vivo* and *in vitro* evidence that activation of sympathetic nerves causes α_2-adrenoceptor vasoconstriction in a wide number of vascular beds, and Figure 1.3 gives a diagrammatic representation of 'innervated' α_2-adrenoceptors. In the majority of these preparations there is evidence that α_1-adrenoceptors are also activated, which increases the potential for synergistic interaction between the two receptors (see Figure 1.2). It should be noted that our assessment of the relative contribution of α_1- and α_2-adrenoceptors to the evoked response is, at best, semiquantitative, and does not take into account the different stimulation parameters employed in each study. There is evidence both for preferential activation of α_2-adrenoceptors by the nerves in some preparations and also that, in others, responses via this receptor are dependent upon prior neuronal activation of α_1-adrenoceptors. For example, Bao, Gonon and Stjärne (1993) reported that single pulse stimulation of the tail artery often caused a small contraction which was sensitive to yohimbine, but resistant to prazosin. In contrast, stimulation with several pulses produced larger contractions which were sensitive to prazosin. These observations suggest that α_2-adrenoceptors are 'intrajunctional' while α_1-adrenoceptors are located further away from the site of release, and helps to explain earlier reports that neurogenic contractions in this preparation (with longer trains of pulses) were 'exquisitely sensitive' to prazosin (Medgett and Langer, 1984). At present it is not known which of the two responses are physiologically more important. On the other hand, MacDonald *et al.* (1992) reported that neurogenic contractions in the rabbit isolated saphenous vein can be resolved into a fast and slow component, mediated by α_1- and α_2-adrenoceptors, respectively, but that the slower (rauwolscine-sensitive) component was also reduced by prazosin. This suggests that neuronal activation of α_2-adrenoceptors, like that by exogenous noradrenaline (Daly, McGrath and Wilson, 1988b), is critically dependent upon the level of α_1-adrenoceptor-mediated contraction.

The parallel between studies with exogenous noradrenaline and neuronally released noradrenaline are further highlighted by observations in the rabbit isolated saphenous artery; a preparation in which angiotensin II plays a permissive role for the expression of

TABLE 1.4

Examples of preparations responding to sympathetic nerve stimulation via postjunctional
α_2-adrenoceptors

Preparation	Method	Relative contribution to response to nerve stimulation		Reference
		α_1	α_2	
rat				
tail artery	*in vitro*	+	+++	Bao, Gonon and Stjärne (1993)
		+++	+	Rajanayagam, Medgett and Rand (1990)
cremaster muscle	*in vivo*			
(large arterioles)		+++++	–	Ohyanagi, Faber and Nishigaki (1991)
(small arterioles)		–	+++++	
saphenous vein	*in vitro*	–	+++++	Cheung (1985)
rabbit				
saphenous artery	*in vitro*	+++++	–*	Dunn, McGrath and Wilson (1991)
saphenous vein	*in vitro*	+++++	+*	MacDonald *et al.* (1992)
plantaris vein	*in vitro*	+++++	+	see Figure 5
knee circulation	*in vivo*	–	+++++	Najafipour and Ferrell (1993)
feline				
cutaneous bed	*in vivo*	+	+++	Koss, Kawari and Ito (1991)
hindlimb bed	*in vivo*	+++	+	Gardiner and Peters (1982)
pulmonary bed	*in vivo*	+++	+	Hyman, Lippton and Kadowitz (1990)
canine				
mesenteric vein	*in vitro*	+	+++	Kou, Ibengwe and Suzuki (1984)
saphenous vein	*in vitro*	+++	+++	Flavahan *et al.* (1984)
hindlimb	*in vivo*	+++	+++	Gardiner and Peters (1982)
coronary bed	*in vivo*	+++	+++	Woodman (1987)
skeletal muscle	*in vivo*	+	+++	Kubes *et al.* (1992)
human				
digital blood flow	*in vivo*	–	+++	Coffman and Cohen (1988)
digital artery	*in vitro*	+++	+++	Stevens and Moulds (1985)
metatarsal vein	*in vitro*	+++++	+++++	Stevens and Moulds (1985)
saphenous vein	*in vitro*	+	+++	Docherty and Hyland (1985)
subcutaneous fat	*in vitro*	+++	+++	Stephens *et al.* (1992)

* indicates that nerve-mediated α_2-adrenoceptors are demonstrated only under appropriate experimental conditions.

functional α_2-adrenoceptors to either noradrenaline or selective α_2-adrenoceptor agonists (Dunn, McGrath and Wilson, 1989, 1991b, Figure 1.2). In this preparation, nerve-mediated responses (following desensitization of purinoceptors) can be virtually eliminated by prazosin under normal experimental conditions. In the presence of angiotensin II however, part of the response becomes resistant to prazosin but susceptible to rauwolscine, and hence, by definition, is mediated via postjunctional α_2-adrenoceptors (McGrath, Brown and Wilson, 1989). Other experimental manipulations that have been reported to increase the magnitude of the α_2-adrenoceptor (rauwolscine-sensitive) component of neurogenic contractions in isolated blood vessels include inhibition of nitric oxide synthase (Gordon *et al.*, 1992; MacLean *et al.*, 1993), and inhibition of neuronal uptake (MacDonald *et al.*, 1992). The latter effect may be a consequence of either higher concentrations of noradrenaline within the neuroeffector junction, or the recruitment of 'extrajunctional' α_2-adrenoceptors.

Finally, a major problem in attempting to resolve the importance of α_2-adrenoceptors for nerve-mediated responses is that the available antagonists do not readily discriminate between pre- and postjunctional α_2-adrenoceptors. Thus, rauwolscine, for example, will inhibit α_2-mediated autoregulation of transmitter release, which will increase the non-α_2-adrenoceptor responses and cause underestimation of the consequence of postjunctional inhibition. It is hoped that the development of compounds which are selective for postjunctional α_2-adrenoceptor will make this analysis simpler (Ruffolo *et al.*, 1987; Hieble *et al.*, 1991, 1992).

Taken together it is clear that the role of postjunctional α_2-adrenoceptors in sympathetic neurotransmission in blood vessels has been greatly underestimated. It seems likely that greater recognition of the experimental factors that influence detection of neurogenic vasoconstriction via α_2-adrenoceptors will ultimately lead to a greater appreciation of the physiological function of this particular receptor subtype. Neuronally-activated α_2-adrenoceptors are present on arterioles and cutaneous vessels, which may confer upon them a role in the control of blood pressure and also thermoregulation. In support of the latter possibility, Flavahan and Vanhoutte (1986a) have demonstrated that neurogenic contractions of the canine saphenous vein are enhanced by cooling and that this appears to involve both α_2-adrenoceptors and purinoceptors. Also, Redfern and Clague (1991) have reported that selective α_2-adrenoceptor antagonists, but not prazosin, increase tail skin temperature in conscious rats. Although no evidence was presented to indicate that this was produced by inhibition of sympathetically-activated α_2-adrenoceptors on the rat tail, such a mechanism remains a possibility. The role of postjunctional α_2-adrenoceptors in the control of blood pressure will be discussed later.

β-ADRENOCEPTOR-MEDIATED RESPONSES

Although the principal effect of increased sympathetic nerve activity on vascular smooth muscle is to produce vasoconstriction via α-adrenoceptors, there is evidence in a number of blood vessels and vascular beds, e.g., cutaneous veins (Pegram, Bevan and Bevan, 1976), and the adipose circulation (Frayn and McDonald, this volume), that this can lead to β_2-adrenoceptor-mediated vasodilatation (Figure 1.3). In the former study it was demonstrated that electrical field stimulation of rabbit isolated facial vein produced a relaxation which was converted to vasoconstriction following β-adrenoceptor blockade (Pegram, Bevan and Bevan, 1976). Qualitatively similar observations have also been reported in human facial veins (Mellander *et al.*, 1982) and the cat submaxillary gland (Bloom, Edwards and Garrett, 1987). In the case of the latter preparation, however, α-adrenoceptor-mediated vasoconstriction is the dominant response since β-adrenoceptor-mediated vasodilatation is only observed after α-adrenoceptor blockade.

β-adrenoceptor-mediated neurogenic vasodilatation has also been noted in the hindlimb of the rat (Berecek and Brody, 1982) and the dog (Diana *et al.*, 1990). In both of these studies the method of neuronal activation was different from that generally employed and, more interestingly, the evidence suggests that adrenal-derived adrenaline is responsible for the neurogenic response. The latter point is of great importance since adrenoceptor antagonists do not discriminate between adrenaline and noradrenaline. Both groups have therefore, adopted a number of approaches to implicate adrenaline. Since these essentially physiological manipulations suggest that adrenaline may have a far greater role in neurogenic responses than previously recognized, they are worth considering in greater detail.

Berecek and Brody (1982) noted that electrical activation of the anteroventral region of the third ventricle (AV3V) in anaesthetized rats caused renal and mesenteric vaso-constriction and hindlimb vasodilatation, the latter effect being sensitive to propranolol. Following adrenal demedullation, repeated stimulation of the AV3V region caused a progressive diminution of the response in each vascular bed. Subsequent infusion of adrenaline restored the hindlimb vasodilatation to AV3V stimulation, but this effect was prevented by prior infusion of the neuronal uptake inhibitor desipramine. Thus, the hindlimb vasodilatation produced in adrenal demedullated rats appears to be the result of β-adrenoceptor activation by neuronally-released adrenaline which is of plasma origin. Support for a physiological/pathophysiological role for this mechanism was provided by the observation that hindlimb vasodilatation to AV3V stimulation was greater in stressed rats. These workers also demonstrated that renal and mesenteric vasoconstriction to AV3V stimulation were impaired in adrenal demedullated rats, an effect restored by infusion of adrenaline, which raises the possibility that adrenaline also contributes to neurogenic vasoconstriction *in vivo*. In an equally elegant study, Diana *et al.* (1990) demonstrated that nicotine-induced hindlimb vasodilatation in the dog also involves adrenal-derived adrenaline activating β-adrenoceptors following release from nerves. In this study, nicotine-induced vasodilatation was found to be dependent upon functional nerves (hexamethonium and denervation abolished the responses) and sensitive to adrenalectomy and desipramine (indicating release of adrenal-derived catecholamines and uptake into nerves, respectively) and also sensitive to adrenoceptor blockade. Although we have interpreted the above findings in terms of adrenaline being responsible for the neurogenic β-adrenoceptor vasodilatation, the possibility exists that this effect is an indirect one via facilitatory prejunctional β_2-adrenoceptors, particularly as adrenal-derived adrenaline may be responsible for a 4-fold increase in plasma noradrenaline in exercising rats (Scheurink *et al.*, 1989). However, an indication that activation of postjunctional β-adrenoceptors may be the dominant mechanism is illustrated by an *in vitro* study by Guimaraes and Paiva (1981). Following a 60 min exposure of isolated segments of the canine saphenous vein to adrenaline, the electrically-evoked and tyramine-induced response in pre-constricted (and α-adrenoceptor blocked) preparations consisted of a β-adrenoceptor-mediated relaxation. This contrasts sharply with preparations pre-loaded with noradrenaline, which failed to produce a β-adrenoceptor-mediated vasodilatation under similar conditions.

Thus, activation of sympathetic nerves on blood vessels can result in β-adrenoceptor vasodilatation in a few vascular beds. In addition, there is evidence that adrenaline released from nerves may be directly responsible for postjunctional responses in the vasculature. However, since this adrenaline appears to be of adrenal origin, it does not function as a true neurotransmitter, i.e., it is not synthesized in the neurons from which it is released. In spite of this, further studies on the potential physiological role of adrenaline as a sympathetic 'neurotransmitter' in blood vessels are clearly warranted.

NON-α NON-β-ADRENOCEPTOR NEUROGENIC RESPONSES

In 1980, Hirst and Neild reported that ionophoretic application of high concentrations of noradrenaline, to certain regions of small arterioles, produced an electrophysiological response similar to that evoked by activation of perivascular nerves (excitatory junctional potential), and mechanical responses which were not blocked by α-adrenoceptor antagonists. They termed these receptors γ-adrenoceptors and subsequently suggested that they were closely associated with sympathetic varicosities and hence were of likely importance in mediating the response to nerve stimulation in small arterioles (Hirst and Neild, 1981a). Although there was considerable evidence that α-adrenoceptors were responsible for mediating the end-organ response in many vascular tissues, they argued that these receptors were essentially 'extrajunctional' and that α-adrenoceptor blockers, such as prazosin (Hirst and Neild, 1981b; Hirst, De Gleria and van Helden, 1985) and phentolamine (Holman and Suprenant, 1980), possessed non-specific effects on vascular smooth muscle or interfered with the propagation of muscle action membrane potentials.

Further support for the presence of a non-α-, non-β-adrenoceptor action of noradrenaline on vascular smooth muscle has come from several other studies. First, Laher, Khayal and Bevan (1986) demonstrated that high concentrations of noradrenaline (>100 μM) produced contractions in several arteries from the rabbit via a low affinity "extraceptor" which (like the γ receptor) is relatively resistant to α-adrenoceptor antagonists. Secondly, Benham and Tsien (1988) demonstrated that noradrenaline-induced (>30 μM) stimulation of voltage-operated calcium channels in the rabbit ear artery was resistant to α- and β-adrenoceptor antagonists. Finally, Edwards et al. (1989) noted that following irreversible inactivation of α-adrenoceptors and β-adrenoceptor blockade in the rat middle cerebral artery, changes in membrane potential to high concentrations of noradrenaline ($>$ 1 mM) were only observed in segments known to stain positive for catecholamine-containing nerves. This latter observation further supports the idea of a close association between the distribution of γ-adrenoceptors and sympathetic innervation, which raises the possibility that the latter exerts a trophic effect on the former. If correct, then it might be expected that in vitro chemical sympathectomy with 6-hydroxydopamine would not affect the distribution of γ-adrenoceptors, while in vivo treatment (over a longer period), with the same agents, might eventually cause a loss of both the sympathetic innervation and γ-adrenoceptors.

As the proponents of the the γ-adrenoceptor hypothesis readily concede (Hirst and Edwards, 1989), progress has been slow due to the lack of a selective antagonist. Also, the increasing interest in the role of 'co-transmitters' (particularly purines) in mediating sympathetic vasoconstriction, along with the increasing availability of putative selective antagonist, has provided an alternative explanation for non-α-adrenoceptor neurogenic vasoconstriction. Agents such as α, β-methylene ATP and suramin are able to inhibit the excitatory junctional potential to sympathetic nerve stimulation in large arteries (Bao, Gonon and Stjärne, 1993; Sneddon and Burnstock, 1984) and in small mesenteric arterioles (Angus, Broughton and Mulvany, 1988), and the associated α-adrenoceptor-resistant mechanical response. A more detailed discussion of the role of ATP in sympathetic neurotransmission is given elsewhere (Morris and Gibbins, 1991; Franco-Cereceda, this volume).

It remains to be seen whether there are examples of blood vessels, other than veins (Cheung, 1985; Hirst and Jobling, 1989), where noradrenaline is proven to be the sole mediator of responses to sympathetic nerve stimulation, yet electrical and mechanical responses are resistant to α-adrenoceptor antagonists. This is of particular importance in small resistance arteries where direct evidence that noradrenaline is released during sympathetic nerve stimulation is lacking (see Mulvany and Aalkjaer, 1990). This appears unlikely however, in view of the fact that the majority of responses to sympathetic nerve stimulation in small resistance arteries are susceptible to α-adrenoceptor antagonists (Angus, Broughton and Mulvany, 1988; Parkinson et al., 1992) either alone or in combination with purinoceptor antagonists. In addition, responses to sympathetic nerve stimulation in pithed rats can be blocked completely with the combination of α-adrenoceptor antagonists and α, β-methylene ATP (Bulloch and McGrath, 1988; Dalziel et al., 1990).

Although the weight of evidence is strongly in favour of the involvement of ATP as a cotransmitter at the vascular neuroeffector junction, as discussed by Hirst and Edwards (1889), much depends upon the 'intrajunctional' concentration of the transmitters achieved during nerve stimulation. If the concentration of noradrenaline is very high (albeit very briefly), then it remains possible that the catecholamine may facilitate purinergic mechanism by affecting voltage-operated calcium channels by a non-α-, non-β-adrenoceptor mechanism (see Benham and Tsien, 1988). Since such an effect of noradrenaline may be critically dependent upon resting membrane potential, it would be sensible to examine this possibility in resistance vessels using a Halpern pressure myograph. This technique allows for the development of pressure-induced myogenic tone, which is associated with a reduction in membrane potential (Harder, Gilbert and Lombard, 1987) towards that encountered in vivo (Neild and Keef, 1985).

ANTIHYPERTENSIVE DRUGS, NORADRENALINE AND THE VASCULAR NEUROEFFECTOR JUNCTION

The histochemical, biochemical, physiological and pharmacological evidence for noradrenaline as a neurotransmitter at the vascular neuroeffector junction is overwhelming, and its importance is reflected in the action of some of the drugs currently used to treat various cardiovascular disorders. Principal among these clinically important conditions is essential hypertension. We will discuss three groups of drugs in relation to their use (or potential use) as therapeutic agents in the treatment of hypertension, and present some data which challenges conventional views on their mechanism of action.

α_1-ADRENOCEPTOR ANTAGONISTS

The aminoquinazoline derivatives, prazosin (Davey, 1987), doxazosin (Davey, 1989) and terazosin (Kyncl, 1986) lower blood pressure without causing reflex tachycardia and have been successfully employed as antihypertensive drugs. Each agent possesses >100-fold higher potency at α_1-adrenoceptors than at α_2-adrenoceptors and, their ability to inhibit postjunctional α_1-adrenoceptors at the lung vascular neuroeffector junction without affecting autoinhibitory control of transmitter release, has been considered the basis of their antihypertensive action. For example, prazosin (Elliot et al., 1981) and doxazosin (Vincent et al., 1983) produced a 2–3 fold rightward displacement of phenylephrine pressor responses in man and a significant reduction in blood pressure. However, a recently introduced α_1-selective antagonist, abanoquil (a quinoline derivative), which has been reported to selectively block myocardial α-adrenoceptors, inhibited phenylephrine-induced pressor responses without affecting blood pressure (Schafers *et al.*, 1991; Tham *et al.*, 1992). These findings suggest that inhibition of vascular α_1-adrenoceptors, as indicated by responses to exogenous phenylephrine, may not be sufficient to account for the therapeutic efficacy of aminoquinazoline derivatives in the treatment of essential hypertension. There are two possible explanations.

First, abanoquil may distinguish between subtypes of vascular α_1-adrenoceptors, and fail to affect those directly involved in sympathetic neurotransmission. Interestingly, abanoquil has been reported to selectively inhibit α_{1A}-adrenoceptors (Wenham and Marshall, 1992), a property shared with SLZ-49, a prazosin analogue, which is also able to inhibit pressor responses to phenylephrine in the rat) without affecting blood pressure (Piascik *et al.*, 1989). Thus, a comparison of the potency of prazosin and abanoquil against α_1-adrenoceptor-mediated responses to electrical field stimulation and noradrenaline in isolated blood vessels would indicate whether the difference between the two agents is at the level of the vasculature. Another possibility is that prazosin has a non-vascular action which accounts for the lack of reflex tachycardia associated with the fall in blood pressure. There are several reports from studies on anaesthetized animals, that prazosin, and other antihypertensive α_1-adrenoceptor antagonists, are able to inhibit sympathetic outflow by an effect on central α_1-adrenoceptors (Ramage, 1984, 1986; Yoshioka *et al.*, 1990). Significantly, in conscious dogs, abanoquil was found to produce significant α_1-adrenoceptor blockade without affecting either blood pressure or baroreflex function (Spiers, Harron and Wilson, 1991), while SLZ-49 was reported to cause tachycardia in conscious rats, which offsets the reduction in total peripheral resistance (Piascik, Kusiak and Barron, 1990b). These findings suggest that the central effect of prazosin may be more important in the antihypertensive action than previously recognized.

α_2-ADRENOCEPTOR ANTAGONISTS

As previously indicated, the potential contribution of postjunctional α_2-adrenoceptors to sympathetic vasoconstriction has only recently been fully appreciated. The potential involvement of postjunctional α_2-adrenoceptors in the control of blood pressure has prompted attempts at developing antagonists which can distinguish between pre- and postjunctional α_2-adrenoceptors (these would allow postjunctional blockade without causing prejunctional facilitation).

Potentially, the most useful of these compounds are the benzazepine-based antagonist SKF104078 and a related analogue SKF104856 (Ruffolo *et al.*, 1987; Hieble *et al.*, 1991, 1992). Both compounds were developed from an earlier compound, SKF86446, which selectively inhibited α_2-adrenoceptors and lowered blood pressure in both DOCA-salt and spontaneously-hypertensive rat models (Roesler *et al.*, 1986). In addition, SKF86466 was found to produce a transient increase in heart rate which was attributed to blockade of prejunctional α_2-adrenoceptors in the heart. An analysis of the actions of SKF104078 and SKF104856 suggests that they possess considerably greater potency for postjunctional α_2-adrenoceptors than prejunctional α_2-adrenoceptors and, therefore, are less likely to produce a significant elevation of heart rate (Ruffolo *et al.*, 1987; Hieble *et al.*, 1992; Roberts *et al.*, 1992). Although two groups have been unable to discriminate between pre- and postjunctional effects of SKF104078 in functional studies, demonstrating actions at both sites with similar potencies (Connaughton *et al.*, 1988; Connaughton and Docherty, 1990; Shen, Barajas-Lopez and Surprenant, 1990), observations by Akers *et al.* (1991) indicate that this may be a function of the agonist employed. SKF104078 was found to differentiate between responses mediated by two agonists, B-HT-920 and xylazine, acting on the same (yohimbine-sensitive) prejunctional α_2-adrenoceptor. The significance of these findings, particularly in relation to the current subclassification is not clear, but may be reconciled if further experimental evidence establish that prejunctional α_2-adrenoceptor subtypes are not homogeneous. It is noteworthy that in radioligand binding studies, SKF104078 has been shown to possess high affinity for the $\alpha_{2A/B/C}$ subtypes, but relatively low affinity for α_{2D} adrenoceptors (Michel, Loury and Whiting, 1989, 1990; Simonneaux, Ebadi and Bylund, 1991). As indicated earlier (Classification of adrenoceptors), there is increasing evidence that the α_{2D}-subtype may exist on postganglionic nerve endings in many tissues.

Experimental observations with SKF104078 and SKF104856 are further complicated by their inability to distinguish between postjunctional α_1- and α_2-adrenoceptors (Ruffolo *et al.*, 1987; Akers *et al.*, 1991; Hieble *et al.*, 1992), but this may enhance the ability of these drugs to inhibit sympathetic, α-adrenoceptor-mediated vasoconstriction and also to lower blood pressure when administered intravenously in conscious hypertensive dogs (Hieble *et al.*, 1991, 1992). In addition to the treatment of hypertension, perhaps in conjunction with another antihypertensive agent, selective inhibitors of postjunctional α_2-adrenoceptors may offer clinical benefit in treating congestive heart failure and also Raynaud's disease. Finally, if these drugs prove successful in these conditions this would support our contention that sympathetic tone in many vascular beds is partly dependent upon activation of postjunctional α_2-adrenoceptors.

ANGIOTENSIN-CONVERTING ENZYME INHIBITORS

Angiotensin-converting enzyme (ACE) inhibitors were originally developed to treat high renin hypertension, but have been found to be equally effective against hypertension associated with low or normal-renin states, and also in anephric patients. This has led to the suggestion that these drugs do not act simply by normalizing the levels of angiotensin II, but by interfering with the facilitatory input of angiotensin II on other influences on blood pressure. One such interaction, which has received considerable attention, is that with the sympathetic nervous system (see Squire and Reid, 1993).

An interaction between angiotensin II and the sympathetic nervous system was first implicated by the observations that hindquarter pressor responses to angiotensin II in anaesthetized dog were reduced following sympathectomy or pretreatment with reserpine (Zimmerman, 1962; Baum, 1963). These results suggested that part of the pressor response to angiotensin II was mediated via the sympathetic nervous system. Confirmation of such an action was forthcoming in studies which detailed enhanced responses, in the presence of angiotensin II, to procedures which caused the release of noradrenaline from nerves (McCubbin and Page, 1963), or to direct sympathetic nerve stimulation in the guinea-pig vas deferens and cat spleen (Bennelini, Della Bella and Gandini, 1964). This facilitatory action for angiotensin II has subsequently been described in a number of vascular preparations from a range of species (e.g., Panisset and Bourdois, 1968; Nicholas, 1970; Johnson, Marshall and Needleman, 1974), and can be mimicked with tetradecapeptide renin substrate and angiotensin I, highlighting a possible role for angiotensin II produced at a local tissue level (Malik and Najletti, 1976; Boke and Malik, 1983).

As summarized by Dzau (1988), there is convincing biochemical and pharmacological evidence indicating the presence of a local renin-angiotensin system associated with blood vessels. The physiological importance of this system, particularly in relation to its interaction with the sympathetic nervous system, has been highlighted by Wong, Reilly and Timmermans (1989). A monoclonal antibody to angiotensin II (KAA8) failed to influence the pressor response to either noradrenaline or sympathetic nerve stimulation in the pithed rat, but completely inhibited the pressor responses to exogenous angiotensin II (by effectively removing the peptide from the circulation). In contrast, the angiotensin converting enzyme inhibitor, captopril, was found to attenuate the response to noradrenaline and sympathetic nerve stimulation. In another study (Wong, Reilly and Timmermans, 1990), the angiotensin receptor antagonist, DuP 753 (losartan), was shown to reduce blood pressure in conscious spontaneously hypertensive rats (SHR), but this effect was not mimicked by KAA8. The explanation advanced in both studies was that KAA8, being a large immunoglobulin, failed to gain access to the (non-circulatory) site of angiotensin II production and, therefore, was unable to reduce the facilitatory effect of this peptide on the sympathetic nervous system. As discussed by Squire and Reid (1993), there are two mechanisms that could account for the effect of locally produced angiotensin II at the vascular neuroeffector junction: facilitation of noradrenaline release via a prejunctional mechanism, or a postjunctional (post-receptor) mechanism.

Evidence for prejunctional facilitation of sympathetic neurotransmission

Direct evidence that angiotensin II can increase noradrenaline release from the vascular neuroeffector junction has been obtained in the rabbit pulmonary artery (Costa and Majewski, 1988), human pulmonary and saphenous arteries (Molderings *et al.*, 1988) and the pithed rabbit (Majewski *et al.*, 1984). On the other hand, indirect evidence for a prejunctional action has been based upon the finding that angiotensin II can increase responses to sympathetic neurotransmission without a correspondingly similar augmentation of response to exogenous noradrenaline (Hughes and Roth, 1971; Zimmerman, 1979; Webb *et al.*, 1988). It should be noted, however, that the increment in transmitter output is much smaller than that produced by α_2-adrenoceptor antagonists (see Costa and Majewski, 1988), and that the indirect assessment of prejunctional facilitation presumes that the noradrenaline is the only transmitter contributing to the motor response. As indicated elsewhere (Morris and Gibbins, 1991; Franco-Cereceda, this volume) this is clearly not the case.

Several recent studies highlight further complexities in the interaction between angiotensin II and noradrenergic mechanisms at the level of the vascular neuroeffector junction. First, Kawasaki, Cline and Su (1984) noted that β-adrenoceptor-mediated enhancement of pressor responses to sympathetic nerve stimulation in the rat perfused mesenteric bed was reduced by captopril, saralasin and β-adrenoceptor antagonists. The explanation advanced was that the interaction could be due to the involvement of angiotensin II in β-adrenoceptor-mediated enhancement of transmitter release. This was subsequently demonstrated by Göthert and colleagues, who detected a captopril-sensitive component of the β-adrenoceptor-mediated increase in noradrenaline output in human pulmonary artery, human saphenous vein and rat vena cava (Göthert and Kollecker, 1986; Molderings *et al.*, 1988). Finally, direct evidence that vascular β-adrenoceptors can stimulate local production of angiotensin was provided by Nakamura, Jackson and Inagami (1986). These results provide further evidence for an important role of local tissue production of angiotensin II, and the possibility that circulating catecholamines, particularly adrenaline, could potentiate their own contractile effects on vascular smooth muscle, by stimulating the production of angiotensin II. It should be noted, however, that Li and Zimmerman (1991) reported that β-adrenoceptor-mediated increase in vascular production of angiotensin II in the rabbit is dependent upon the presence of the kidney. This raises the question whether the vascular renin-angiotensin system can be viewed as a true paracrine hormonal system.

The precise location of the β-adrenoceptor-mediated stimulation of angiotensin II production *in vitro* is not known. However, messenger RNA (mRNA) for angiotensinogen, the substrate for renin, has been detected in both adipocytes and fibroblasts within the adventitial layer of blood vessels and also in perivascular fat (Campbell and Habener, 1987; Cassis, Lynch and Peach, 1988a; Cassis, Saye and Peach, 1988b). Interestingly, the levels of angiotensinogen mRNA in 3T3-L1 cells, a pre-adipocyte cell line, is increased following exposure to dexamethasone and the phosphodiesterase inhibitor IBMX (Saye *et al.*, 1989). This indicates that processes capable of elevating cyclic AMP (such as β-adrenoceptor activation) may have the potential to activate the local renin-angiotensin system by increasing angiotensinogen production. Although it is generally acknowledged that renin is the rate-limiting step in the production of circulating angiotensin II, it has been suggested that the local provision of angiotensinogen may be equally important for the operation of the vascular renin-angiotensin system (Frederich *et al.*, 1992).

A dramatic demonstration of the potential influence of perivascular adipose tissue on vascular smooth muscle has been reported by Soltis and Cassis (1991). Electrical field stimulation of the rat thoracic aorta produced small, tetrodotoxin-sensitive, phentolamine-sensitive contractions when the perivascular fat was left on the blood vessel segment. Significantly, prior exposure to saralasin also caused a 50% reduction in the neurogenic response. No response to electrical field stimulation was observed following removal of the adipose tissue; an observation consistent with the known lack of sympathetic innervation in the rat aorta. Thus, neurogenic contractions of the rat aorta appears to be due to noradrenaline generated in surrounding perivascular fat; a component of which may be due to locally generated angiotensin II increasing transmitter release from sympathetic nerves innervating adipose tissues. A diagrammatic representation of the prejunctional effect of adipocyte-generated angiotensin II is shown in Figure 1.4. It is equally possible, however, that perivascular angiotensin II contributed to neurogenic responses by a postjunctional mechanism, and the importance of such an action will now be considered.

Evidence for postjunctional facilitation of sympathetic neurotransmission

Potentiation of noradrenaline-induced responses has been observed in many vascular preparations, and has been proposed as a basis for enhancing sympathetic neurotransmission.

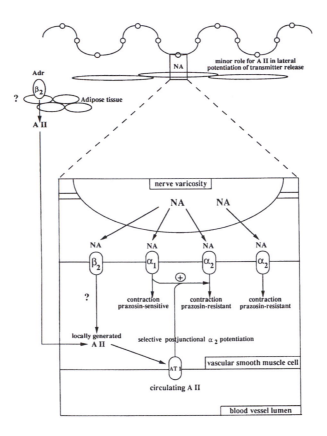

Figure 1.4 Schematic highlighting the involvement of α-adrenoceptor subtypes in mediating responses to sympathetic nerve stimulation at the vascular neuroeffector junction, and the influence of angiotensin II thereon. Neuronally-released noradrenaline can evoke responses via both α_1- and α_2-adrenoceptors (identified by selective antagonists, see Table 4), but in some preparations α_2-adrenoceptor-mediated responses are not observed (α_2-adrenoceptor antagonists fail to affect responses) because they are dependent upon neurogenic activation of α_1-adrenoceptors, e.g., rabbit isolated saphenous artery (Dunn, McGrath and Wilson, 1991b); a positive interaction between α_1- and α_2-adrenoceptors confers prazosin-sensitivity on the adrenergic response. The presence of 'innervated' α_2-adrenoceptors (rauwolscine-sensitive) is revealed by the presence of angiotensin II, which appears to selectively interact with postjunctional α_2-adrenoceptors and replaces the positive input of α_1-adrenoceptors, thereby rendering the responses resistant to prazosin. *In vivo*, the possibility exists that locally-generated angiotensin, perhaps via β-adrenoceptor-activation on adipocytes or fibroblasts, may selectively enhance neurogenic responses via α_2-adrenoceptors. There is also the potential for angiotensin II to enhance transmitter release, which would non-selectively increase responses via α_1- and α_2-adrenoceptors.

For example, angiotensin II has been shown to increase responses to noradrenaline in the perfused rat caudal artery (Nicholas, 1970), rabbit femoral artery (Purdy and Weber, 1988), rabbit saphenous vein (Dunn *et al.*, 1991c) rat, canine and feline mesenteric blood vessels (Panisset and Bourdois, 1968; Malik and Nasjletti, 1976; Chiba and Tsukada, 1986), human digital arteries (Moulds and Worland, 1980), and rabbit aorta (Day and Moore, 1976).

In addition, a number of ACE inhibitors, and the angiotensin II receptor antagonist saralasin, have been demonstrated to reduce responses to both sympathetic nerve stimulation and to exogenous noradrenaline, or α-adrenoceptor agonists in pithed animals, presumably by preventing endogenous angiotensin II formation. (Antonaccio and Kerwin, 1981; Clough et al., 1982; Hatton and Clough, 1982; De Jonge et al., 1983; Grant and McGrath, 1988). Two recent reports have implicated small resistance arterioles as the site for this interaction, since ACE inhibition antagonised α-adrenoceptor mediated increases in total peripheral resistance without influencing corresponding changes in cardiac output (Kaufman and Vollmer, 1985; MacLean and Hiley, 1988).

These studies indicate that in some vascular beds the facilitatory effect of local angiotensin II on sympathetic neurotransmission may involve both pre- and postjunctional mechanisms. We believe, however, that whenever postjunctional facilitation of noradrenaline-induced contractions can be demonstrated, this will be the principal factor influencing the end-organ response. This point is illustrated by examining the effect of agonists known to inhibit transmitter release at the autonomic neuroeffector junction in vascular and non-vascular preparations (Tables 1.5 and 1.6).

Activation of NPY receptors, α_2-adrenoceptors and opioid receptors on cholinergic fibres innervating guinea-pig bronchial and gastrointestinal smooth muscle produces a reduction in the motor response. None of the agonists had a postjunctional action — as judged by the lack of effect against exogenous acetylcholine (Table 1.5). On vascular smooth muscle (Table 1.6), however, the effect of these agonists on the motor response is not strictly related to effects on transmitter release. This is particularly evident for NPY, where enhancement of neurogenic responses is observed in spite of its ability to reduce transmitter output. Thus, the overall effect of NPY on sympathetic neurotransmission is determined by the existence of postjunctional facilitatory mechanisms. In the case of opioid receptors, which have no postjunctional effects on vascular smooth muscle, the motor response is reduced as a result of prejunctional inhibition of transmitter release. If this argument also applies to the effect of angiotensin II at the vascular neuroeffector junction, then we might expect postjunctional facilitation to be the dominant process influencing the magnitude of the motor response. The results shown in Figure 1.5 support this suggestion.

In the rabbit isolated plantaris vein contractions to electrical field stimulation involves activation of both α_1- (prazosin-sensitive), and α_2-adrenoceptors (rauwolscine-sensitive) by noradrenaline. The residual non-α-adrenoceptor component is sensitive to α, β-methylene ATP and is, therefore, purinergic. However, angiotensin II selectively potentiates responses via α_2-adrenoceptors, i.e., those in the absence of rauwolscine. Since neuronally-released noradrenaline is able to activate both α_1- and α_2-adrenoceptors, the selective facilitation by angiotensin II of neurogenic α_2-adrenoceptor venoconstriction is primarily a postjunctional phenomenon. Qualitatively similar observations have also been made in an arterial preparation, the rabbit saphenous artery (Dunn, McGrath and Wilson, 1991b), where the postjunctional effect of angiotensin II is of sufficient magnitude to uncover neurogenic α_2-adrenoceptors not even observed under control conditions. The significance of these findings is further underlined by the report that angiotensin III, an active metabolite of angiotensin II, enhanced neurogenic responses in the rat perfused mesenteric bed without altering transmitter output (Kawasaki et al., 1988).

TABLE 1.5

The effect of opioid agonists, α_2-adrenoceptor agonists and neuropeptide Y against responses to electrical field stimulation and exogenous agonists in bronchial and gastrointestinal smooth muscle

Receptor	Motor Response	Exogenous agonist	Preparation	Reference
Opioid	↓	↔	Guinea-pig bronchioles	Belvisi, Stretton and Barnes (1990)
α_2	↓	↔	Guinea-pig bronchioles	Grundström, Andersson and Wikberg (1984)
Neuropeptide Y	↓	↔	Guinea-pig bronchioles	Grundemar et al. (1990)
Opioid	↓	↔	Guinea-pig isolated ileum	Kosterlitz and Waterfield (1975)
α_2	↓	↔	Guinea-pig isolated ileum	Kosterlitz, Lydon and Watt (1970)
Neuropeptide Y	↓	↔	Guinea-pig isolated ileum	Takaki and Nakayama (1991)

↓ represents decrease, ↔ represents no change.

TABLE 1.6

Comparison of the effect of activation of opioid receptors, α_2-adrenoceptors and neuropeptide Y receptors at the vascular neuroeffector junction

	Motor responses	Transmitter release	Exogenous agonist	Reference
(1) Opioid receptors				
Rabbit ear artery	↓	↓	n.d.	Illes et al. (1985)
	↓	↓	n.d.	Budai and Duckles (1988)
Rat tail artery	↓	↓	n.d.	Illes et al. (1987a)
Rabbit mesenteric artery	↓	↓	n.d.	Illes, Ramme and Busse (1987b)
Pithed rabbit	↓	↓	n.d.	Szabo et al. (1986)
(2) α_2-adrenoceptors				
Rabbit pulmonary artery	↓	↓	n.d.	Starke, Endo and Taube (1975b)
Rabbit saphenous artery	↓	n.d.	n.d.	MacDonald et al. (1992)
Rabbit ear artery	↓	n.d.	n.d.	Budai and Duckles (1989)
	n.d.	↓	n.d.	Limberger and Starke (1983)
Rabbit mesenteric artery	↑	↓	n.d.	Su (1980)
Canine saphenous vein	↑	↓	n.d.	Senaratne et al. (1987)
(3) Neuropeptide Y receptors				
Rabbit ear artery	↑	↓	↑	Wong-Dusting and Rand (1988)
	↑	n.d.	n.d.	Budai, Vu and Duckles (1989)
	↑	n.d.	↑	Saville, Maynard and Burnstock (1990)
Rat tail artery	↑	↔	↑	Vu, Budai and Duckles (1989)
Rat femoral artery	↑	↓	↑	Pernow, Saria and Lundberg (1986)
Rat portal vein	↑	↓	↑	Dahlöf et al. (1985)
	↑	↓	↑	Pernow, Saria and Lundberg (1986)

↑ represents increase, ↓ represents decrease, ↔ represents no change, n.d. represents not determined.

Finally, the ability of angiotensin II to selectively potentiate neurogenic responses mediated by α_2-adrenoceptors may represent an important compensatory mechanism following α_1-adrenoceptor blockade by prazosin. Waeber, Nussberger and Brunner (1983) and Goering and Zimmerman (1986) have reported that the administration of either saralasin,

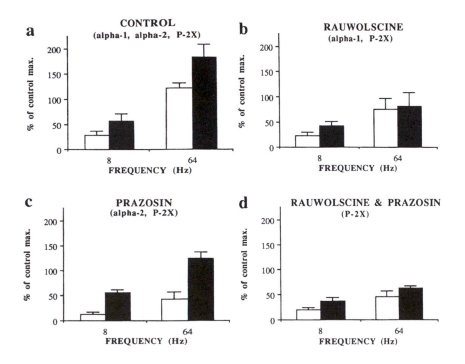

Figure 1.5   The effect of 30 nM angiotensin II (solid bars) on the motor response of the rabbit isolated plantaris vein to 8 and 64 Hz field stimulation (1 sec duration, 0.1 msec pulse width, supramaximal voltage) in the presence of (a) saline, (b) 1 μM rauwolscine, (c) 0.1 μM prazosin and (d) a combination of 1 μM rauwolscine and 0.1 μM prazosin. The contractions were abolished by 0.3 μM tetrodotoxin and, therefore were presumed to be neuronal in origin. Response in the absence of angiotensin II (but in the presence of the antagonists) are represented by (open bars). 30 nM angiotensin II produced a large, transient contraction which returned to baseline with 15 minutes. All responses have been expressed as a percentage of the maximum response prior to exposure to the α-adrenoceptor antagonist(s) and shown as the mean $\pm$ s.e. mean of 6 observations. The readers attention is drawn to the fact that angiotensin II facilitation of nerve responses, only occurs when α_2-adrenoceptors are functionally present (a and c). In the presence of either rauwolscine (not α_2-) or prazosin and rauwolsine (not α_1- nor α_2-), the remaining response is not potentiated. This indicates that any prejunctional enhancement of transmitter release by angiotensin II is not sufficient to produce an increase in the contractile response (Unpublished data, Daly, McGrath and Wilson).

or the ACE inhibitor, enalapril, produced a large reduction in the blood pressure of prazosin-treated conscious rats, while Brown and Dickerson (1991) observed a synergistic interaction between enalapril and doxazosin in man. The potential clinical importance of an interaction between α_2-adrenoceptors and angiotensin II is underlined by studies on human isolated saphenous vein, where angiotensin II reduced the potency of prazosin against noradrenaline-induced contractions (Roberts et al., 1992). Clearly, studies with selective α_2-adrenoceptor antagonists (which do not affect prejunctional α_2-adrenoceptors, e.g., SKF104856), are required to assess the potential for angiotensin II to facilitate α_2-adrenoceptors in vivo.

CONCLUSION

In this chapter we have outlined the experimental evidence indicating a role for noradrenaline as a sympathetic neurotransmitter at the vascular neuroeffector junction. Information from a number of experimental approaches has converged to provide unequivocal evidence that noradrenaline is synthesized and stored in nerves, and released upon sympathetic stimulation. Practical information about the role of noradrenaline at the vascular neuroeffector junction can be obtained with the use of selective antagonists, if sufficient consideration is given both to the concentration of drug used, and the experimental design.

Once released from the nerves, noradrenaline produces its effects by interacting with a variety of adrenoceptor subtypes. Recent developments, using molecular biological and radioligand binding techniques, have indicated that there are multiple subtypes of both α_1- and α_2-adrenoceptors. Advances with this technology have far outstripped functional studies. Unfortunately, the nature of the agents currently available for study do not allow an easy assessment of the role of these subtypes at the neuroeffector junction. It is hoped that more subtype-specific antagonists will be developed to allow clarification. However, since α-adrenoceptor subtypes mediate responses of the same functional polarity, and with the possibility of synergistic interactions between subtypes, caution will still be warranted in interpreting experimental results. This is highlighted by observations with postjunctional α_1- and α_2-adrenoceptors on vascular smooth muscle, where synergistic interactions between the subtypes have been partly responsible for underestimating the role of postjunctional α_2-adrenoceptors in mediating responses to nerve stimulation. It also seems likely that the postjunctional interaction of α_2-adrenoceptors, with either α_1-adrenoceptors or angiotensin II receptors, is of greater importance than pre-junctional regulation of transmitter release in determining the end-organ response. In appreciation of the importance of 'innervated' postjunctional α_2-adrenoceptors and their preferential location on arteriolar smooth muscle, the development of α_2-adrenoceptor antagonists, which can discriminate between pre- and postjunctional α_2-adrenoceptors without affecting α_1-adrenoceptors, is eagerly awaited.

To date, the majority of *in vitro* studies examining vascular neuroeffector mechanisms have been carried out using large (conduit) blood vessels under non-physiological conditions. Two recent technological advances offer an opportunity to examine pre- and postjunctional events under more physiological conditions with vessels that make a significant contribution to total peripheral resistance. First, it is apparent that prejunctional adrenoceptors have the capacity to modulate the release of neurotransmitters. Recent developments, using electrophysiological techniques however, have challenged our understanding of how such modulation occurs. This has led to the realisation that transmitter release from a given varicosity is intermittent and that modulation of transmitter release does not occur locally, but at some distant site (lateral modulation). The development of electrochemical techniques for on-line detection of noradrenaline release, should also allow determination of the physiological role of prejunctional α_2- and β_2-adrenoceptors at regulating transmitter release, using stimulation paradigms that mimic those encountered *in vivo*; intermittent firing of neurons at high frequency (Sjöblom-Widfeldt and Nilsson, 1990; Hardebo, 1992). This will preclude the necessity of using long, non-physiological trains of pulses to detect [3H]-noradrenaline overflow. It will also allow discrimination of the functional importance of pre- and postjunctional facilitatory mechanisms of humoral agents, such as angiotensin II, in various pathological states, e.g., hypertension and diabetes. Secondly, the Halpern pressure-perfusion myograph will allow analysis of small arteries in a situation which closely resembles that found *in vivo*. In view of the pronounced differences in responses to exogenous noradrenaline found with this system compared to isometric techniques (see Figure 1.1 and Dunn, Wellman and Bevan, 1994), there are compelling reasons that this approach should be adopted to assess the role of sympathetic neurotransmission in resistance arteries from different vascular beds. We believe this integrated approach will significantly contribute to our understanding of the physiological processes that regulate resistance blood vessels and, therefore, the control of blood pressure.

REFERENCES

Aboud, R., Shafii, M. and Docherty, J.R. (1993). Investigation of the subtypes of α_1-adrenoceptor mediating contractions of rat aorta, vas deferens and spleen. *British Journal of Pharmacology*, **109**, 80–87.

Ahlquist, R.P. (1948). A study of adrenotropic receptors. *American Journal of Physiology*, **153**, 586–600.

Akers, I., Coates, J., Drew, G.M. and Sullivan, A.T. (1991). α_2-Adrenoceptor blocking profile of SKF104078: further evidence for receptor subtypes. *British Journal of Pharmacology*, **102**, 943–949.

Alabaster, V., Keir, R.F. and Peters, C.J. (1985). Comparison of activity of α-adrenoceptor agonists and antagonists in dog and rabbit saphenous vein. *Naunyn Schmiedeberg's Archives of Pharmacology*, **330**, 33–36.

Alberts, P. (1992). Subtype classification of the presynaptic α-adrenoceptors which regulate [^{3}H]-noradrenaline secretion in guinea-pig isolated urethra. *British Journal of Pharmacology*, **105**, 142–146.

Angus, J.A., Broughton, A. and Mulvany, M.J. (1988). Role of α-adrenoceptors in constrictor responses of rat, guinea-pig and rabbit small arteries to neural activation. *Journal of Physiology*, **403**, 495–510.

Antonaccio, M.J. and Kerwin, L. (1981). Pre- and postjunctional inhibition of vascular sympathetic function by captopril in SHR. *Hypertension*, **3**, (Suppl. 1), 154–162.

Arch, J.R.S. (1989). The brown adipocyte β-adrenoceptor. *Proceedings of the Nutrition Society*, **48**, 215–233.

Arch, J.R.S., Ainsworth, A.T., Cawthorne M.A., Piercy, V., Sennit, M.V., Thody, V.E., *et al.* (1984). Atypical β-adrenoceptors on brown adipocytes as target for anti-obesity drugs. *Nature*, **309**, 163–165.

Ashbrook, D.W., Purdy, R.E., Hurlbett, D.E., Rains, L.A., Reidy, J.P. and Stratford, R.E. (1980). A novel response to propranolol: contractile response in the rabbit isolated ear artery. *Life Sciences*, **26**, 155–163.

Astrand, P. and Stjärne, L. (1989). On the secretory activity of single varicosities in the sympathetic nerves innervating the rat tail artery. *Journal of Physiology*, **409**, 207–220.

Awad, R., Payne, R. and Deth, R.C. (1983). α adrenergic receptor subtype associated with receptor binding, Ca^{++} influx, Ca^{++} release and contractile events in the rabbit aorta. *Journal of Pharmacology and Experimental Therapeutics*, **227**, 60–67.

Babich, M., Pedigo, N.W., Butler, B.T. and Piscik, M.T. (1987). Heterogeneity of α_1 receptors associated with vascular smooth muscle: evidence from functional and ligand binding studies. *Life Sciences*, **41**, 663–673.

Bacq, Z.M. (1934). La pharmacologie due systeme nerveux autonome, et particulierement du sympathique, d'apres la theorie neurohumorale. *Annales de Physiologie*, **10**, 467.

Bacq, Z.M. (1935). Recherches sur la physiologie et al pharmacologie du systeme nerveux autonome. *Archives of Internationales Pharmacodynamics and Therapies*, **52**, 471–492.

Bacq, Z.M. (1975). *Chemical Transmission of Nerve Impulse: a Historical Survey*. Pergammon Press: Oxford, New York, Toronto, Sydney, Braunschweig.

Bao, J.-X., Gonon, F. and Stjärne, L. (1993). Frequency- and train length-dependent variation in the roles of postjunctional α_1- and α_2-adrenoceptors for the field stimulation-induced neurogenic contraction of rat tail artery. *Naunyn Schmiedeberg's Archives of Pharmacology*, **347**, 601–616.

Barret, A.M., Carter, J., Fitzgerald, J.D., Hull, R. and Le Count, D. (1973). A new type of cardioselective adrenoceptor blocking drug. *British Journal of Pharmacology*, **48**, 340P.

Baum, T. (1963). Vascular reactivity of reserpine-pretreated dogs. *Journal of Pharmacology and Experimental Therapeutics*, **141**, 30–35.

Bell, C. (1988). Phentolamine lacks α_2-adrenoceptor agonist activity in anaesthetized dogs. *British Journal of Pharmacology*, **93**, 37–341.

Belvisi, M.G., Stretton, C.D. and Barnes, P.J. (1990). Modulation of cholinergic neurotransmission in guinea-pig airways by opioids. *British Journal of Pharmacology*, **100**, 131–137.

Benham, C.D. and Tsien, R.W. (1988). Noradrenaline modulation of calcium channels in single smooth muscle cells from rabbit ear artery. *Journal of Physiology*, **404**, 767–784.

Bennelini, G., Della Bella, D. and Gandini, A. (1964). Angiotensin and peripheral sympathetic nerve activity. *British Journal of Pharmacology*, **22**, 211–219.

Berecek, K.H. and Brody, M.J. (1982). Evidence for a neurotransmitter role for epinephrine derived from the adrenal medulla. *American Journal of Physiology*, **242**, H539–H601.

Bevan, J.A., Bevan, R.D. and Duckles, S.P. (1980). Adrenergic regulation of vascular smooth muscle. In *American Physiological Society Handbook, Section 2, The Cardiovascular System, 2. Vascular Smooth Muscle*. Eds. D.F. Bohr, A.P. Somlyo and H.V. Sparks, pp. 515–566, American Physiological Society, Bethesda.

Bilski, A., Halliday, S.E., Fitzgerald, J.D. and Wale, J. (1983). The pharmacology of the β_2-selective adrenoceptor antagonist ICI 118,551. *Journal of Cardiovascular Pharmacology*, **5**, 430–437.

Black, J.W. and Stephenson, J.S. (1962). Pharmacology of a new adrenergic β-receptor blocking compound (nethalide). *Lancet*, **II**, 311–314.

Black, J.W., Crowther, A.F., Shanks, R.G., Smith, L. and Dornhorst, A.C. (1964). A new adrenergic β-receptor antagonist. *Lancet*, **I**, 1080–1081.

Blakeley, A.H., Cunnane, T.C. and Petersen, S.A. (1982). Local regulation of transmitter release from rodent sympathetic nerve terminals. *Journal of Physiology*, **325**, 93–109.

Blaxall, H.S., Murphy, T.J., Baker, J.C., Ray, C. and Bylund, D.B. (1991). Characterization of the α_{2C} adrenergic receptor subtype in the opposum kidney and in the OK cell line. *Journal of Pharmacology and Experimental Therapeutics*, **259**, 323–329.

Blaylock, N.A. and Wilson, V.G. (1993). Evidence for functional α_2-adrenoceptors-mediated contractions in the porcine isolated thoracic aorta but not in the splenic artery. *British Journal of Pharmacology*, **109**, 35P.

Bloom, S.R., Edwards, A.V. and Garrett, J.R. (1987). Effects of stimulating the sympathetic innervation in burst on the submandibular vascular and secretory function in cats. *Journal of Physiology*, **393**, 91–106.

Bohmann, C., Schollmeyer, P. and Rump, L.C. (1993). α_2-Autoreceptor subclassification in rat isolated kidney by use of short trains of electrical stimulation. *British Journal of Pharmacology*, **108**, 262–268.

Boke, T. and Malik, K.U. (1983). Enhancement of locally generated angiotensin II of the adrenergic transmitter in the isolated rat kidney. *Journal of Pharmacology and Experimental Therapeutics*, **226**, 900–907.

Borkowski, K.R., Kwan, C.Y. and Daniel, E.E. (1989). Epinephrine facilitates neurogenic responses in isolated segments of dog mesenteric arteries. *Journal of Cardiovascular Pharmacology*, **13**, 760–766.

Bristow, M., Sherrod, T.R. and Green, R.D. (1970). Analysis of receptor drug interactions in isolated rabbit atrium, aorta, stomach and trachea. *Journal of Pharmacology and Experimental Therapeutics*, **171**, 52–61.

Brittain, R.T., Farmer, J.B., Jack, D., Martin, L.E. and Simpson, W.T. (1968). α-((t-butylamino)-methyl)-4-hydroxy-m-xy-lene-α^1-α^3-diol (AH 3365): A selective β-adrenergic stimulant. *Nature*, **219**, 862–863.

Brock, J.A. and Cunnane, T.C. (1987). Relationship between the nerve action potential and transmitter release from sympathetic postganglionic nerve terminals. *Nature*, **326**, 605–607.

Brock, J.A. and Cunnane, T.C. (1991a). Electrophysiology of neuroeffector transmission in smooth muscle. In *Autonomic Neuroeffector Mechanisms*. Eds. G. Burnstock and C.H.V. Hoyle, pp. 121–215. Chur, Switzerland, Harwood Academic Publishers.

Brock, J.A. and Cunnane, T.C. (1991b). Local application of drugs to sympathetic nerve terminals: an electrophysiological analysis of the role of prejunctional α-adrenoceptors in the guinea-pig vas deferens. *British Journal of Pharmacology*, **102**, 595–600.

Brown, G.L. and Gillespie, J.S. (1956). Output of sympathin from the spleen. *Nature*, **178**, 980.

Brown, G.L. and Gillespie, J.S. (1957). The output of sympathetic transmitter from the spleen of the cat. *Journal of Physiology*, **138**, 81–102.

Brown, M.J. and Dickerson, J.E.C. (1991). Synergism between α_1-adrenoceptor blockade and angiotensin-converting enzyme inhibition in essential hypertension. *Journal of Hypertension*, **9**, (Suppl. 6) S362–S363.

Brown, M.J., Struthers, A.D., Di Silvio, L., Yeo, T., Ghatei, M. and Buriin, J.M. (1985). Metabolic and haemodynamic effects of α_2-adrenoceptor stimulation and antagonism in man. *Clinical Sciences*, **68**, (Suppl. 10), 137s–139s.

Budai, D. and Duckles, S.P. (1988). Influence of stimulation train length on opioid-induced inhibition of norepinephrine release in the rabbit ear artery. *European Journal of Pharmacology*, **139**, 61–66.

Budai, D. and Duckles, S.P. (1989). Opioid-induced prejunctional inhibition of vasoconstriction in the rabbit ear artery: α_2-adrenoceptor activation and external calcium. *Journal of Pharmacology and Experimental Therapeutics*, **251**, 497–501.

Budai, D., Vu, H.Q. and Duckles, S.P. (1989). Endothelium removal does not affect potentiation by neuropeptide Y in rabbit ear artery. *European Journal of Pharmacology*, **168**, 97–100.

Bulloch, J.M. and McGrath, J.C. (1988). Blockade of vasopressor and vas deferens responses by α, β-methylene ATP in the pithed rat. *British Journal of Pharmacology*, **94**, 103–109.

Bulloch, J.M. and Starke, K. (1990). Presynaptic α_2-autoinhibition in a vascular neuroeffector junction where ATP and noradrenaline act as cotransmitters. *British Journal of Pharmacology*, **99**, 279–284.

Bultmann, R. and Starke, K. (1993). Chlorethylclonidine: an irreversible agonist at prejunctional α_2-adrenoceptors in rat vas deferens. *British Journal of Pharmacology*, **108**, 336–341.

Burns, J.J. and Lemberger, L. (1965). N-tertiary-butylmethoxamine, a specific antagonist of the metabolic actions of epinephrine. *Federation Proceedings*, **24**, 298.

Busija, D.W. (1985). Role of prostaglandins in modulating sympathetic vasoconstriction in the cerebral circulation in anaesthetized rabbits. *Journal of Cerebral Blood Flow and Metabolism*, **5**, 17–25.

Bylund, D.B. (1985). Heterogeneity of α_2-adrenergic receptors. *Pharmacology, Biochemistry and Behaviour*, **22**, 835–843.

Bylund, D.B. (1988). Subtypes of α_2-adrenoceptors: Pharmacological and molecular biological evidence converge. *Trends in Pharmacological Sciences*, **9**, 356–361.

Bylund, D.B. (1992). Subtypes of α_1- and α_2-adrenergic receptors. *FASEB Journal*, **6**, 832–839.

Bylund, D.B. and Ray-Prenger, C. (1989). α_{2A} and α_{2B} adrenergic receptor subtypes: Attenuation of cyclic AMP production in cell lines containing only one receptor subtype. *Journal of Pharmacology and Experimental Therapeutics*, **251**, 640–644.

Bylund, D.B., Blaxall, H.S., Murphy, T.J. and Simonneaux, V. (1991). Pharmacological evidence for α_{2C}- and α_{2D}-adrenergic receptor subtypes. In *Adrenoceptors: Structure, Mechanisms, Function — Advances in Pharmacological Science*. Edited by E. Szabadi and C.M. Bradshaw, pp. 27–36, Basel: Birkhauser Verlag.

Cambridge, D., Davey, M.J. and Massingham, R. (1977). Prazosin a selective antagonist of postsynaptic α-adrenoceptors. *British Journal of Pharmacology*, **58**, 325–346.

Campbell, D.J. and Habener, J. (1987). Cellular localization of angiotensinogen gene expression in brown adipose tissue and mesentery: quantification of messenger ribonucleic acid abundance using hybridization *in situ*. *Endocrinology*, **121**, 1616–1626.

Cannon, W.B. and Rosenblueth, A. (1937). *Autonomic Neuroeffector Systems*. New York, The Macmillan Company.

Cassis, L.A., Lynch, K.R. and Peach, M.J. (1988a). Localization of angiotensinogen messenger RNA in rat aorta. *Circulation Research*, **62**, 1259–1262.

Cassis, L.A., Saye, J.A. and Peach, M.J. (1988b). Location and regulation of rat angiotensinogen messenger RNA. *Hypertension*, **11**, 591–596.

Cavero, I., Dennis, T., Lefevre-Bog, F., Perrot, P., Roach, A.G. and Scatton, B. (1979). Effects of clonidine, prazosin and phentolamine on heart rate and coronary sinus catecholamines concentration during cardioaccelerator nerve stimulation in spinal dogs. *British Journal of Pharmacology*, **67**, 283–292.

Challis, R.A.J., Leighton, B., Wilson, S., Thorby, P.L. and Arch, J.R.S. (1988). An investigation of the β-adrenoceptor that mediates metabolic responses to the novel agent BRL 28410 in rat soleus muscle. *Biochemical Pharmacology*, **37**, 847–850.

Cheung, D.W. (1985). An electrophysiological study of α-adrenoceptor mediated excitation-contraction coupling in the smooth muscle cells of the rat saphenous vein. *British Journal of Pharmacology*, **84**, 265–271.

Chiba, S. and Tsukada, M. (1986). Potentiating effect of angiotensin II on norepinephrine-induced vasoconstriction in isolated and perfused dog mesenteric arteries. *Japanese Journal of Pharmacology*, **42**, 141–144.

Chubb, I.W., De Potter, W.P. and De Schaepdryver, A.F. (1970). Evidence for two types of noradrenergic storage particles in dog spleen. *Nature*, **228**, 1203–1204.

Clineschmidt, B.V., Pettibone, D.J., Lotti, V.J., Hucker, H.B., Sweeney, B.M., Reiss, D.R., *et al.* (1988). A peripherally acting α_2-adrenoceptor antagonist: L-659,066. *Journal of Pharmacology and Experimental Therapeutics*, **245**, 32–40.

Clough, D.P., Collis, M.G., Conway, J., Hatton, R. and Keddie, J.R. (1982). Interaction of angiotensin converting enzyme inhibitors with the function of the sympathetic nervous system. *American Journal Cardiology*, **49**, 1410–1414.

Coffman, J.D. and Cohen, R.A. (1988). Role of α-adrenoceptor subtypes mediating sympathetic vasoconstriction in human digits. *European Journal of Clinical Investigation*, **18**, 309–313.

Connaughton, S. and Docherty, J.R. (1990). Functional evidence for heterogeneity of peripheral prejunctional α_2-adrenoceptors. *British Journal of Pharmacology*, **101**, 285–290.

Connaughton, S., Moore, D., Sugrue, M. and Docherty, J.R. (1988). Evidence that SKF104078 does not distinguish between pre- and postjunctional α_2-adrenoceptors. *Naunyn Schmiedeberg's Archives of Pharmacology*, **338**, 379–382.

Constantine, J.W., Lebel, W. and Archer, R. (1982). Functional postsynaptic α_2- but not α_1-adrenoceptors in dog saphenous vein exposed to phenoxybenzamine. *European Journal of Pharmacology*, **85**, 325–329.

Costa, M. and Majewski, H. (1988). Facilitation of noradrenaline release from sympathetic nerves through activation of ACTH receptors, β-adrenoceptors and angiotensin II. *British Journal of Pharmacology*, **95**, 993–1001.

Dahlöf, C., Dahlöf, P., Tatemoto, K. and Lundeberg, J.M. (1985). Neuropeptide Y (NPY) reduces field stimulation-evoked release of noradrenaline and enhances force of contraction in the rat portal vein. *Naunyn Schmiedeberg's Archives of Pharmacology*, **328**, 327–330.

Dale, H.H. (1906). On some physiological actions of ergot. *Journal of Physiology*, **34**, 163–206.

Daly, C.J., McGrath, J.C. and Wilson, V.G. (1988a). An examination of the postjunctional α-adrenoceptor subtypes for (–)-noradrenaline in several isolated blood vessels from the rabbit. *British Journal of Pharmacology*, **95**, 473–484.

Daly, C.J., McGrath, J.C. and Wilson, V.G. (1988b). Pharmacological analysis of postjunctional α-adrenoceptors mediating contractions to (–)-noradrenaline in the rabbit isolated saphenous vein can be explained by inter-acting responses to simultaneous activation of α_1- and α_2-adrenoceptors. *British Journal of Pharmacology*, **95**, 485–500.

Daly, C.J., McGrath, J.C. and Wilson, V.G. (1988c). Evidence that the postjunctional α-adrenoceptor mediating contraction of the smooth muscle of the rabbit isolated ear vein is predominantly α_2-. *British Journal of Pharmacology*, **94**, 1085–1090.

Daly, C.J., Dunn, W.R., McGrath, J.C. and Wilson, V.G. (1988d). An attempt at selective protection from phenoxybenzamine of postjunctional α-adrenoceptor subtypes mediating contractions to (–)-noradrenaline in the rabbit isolated saphenous vein. *British Journal of Pharmacology*, **95**, 501–511.

Dalziel, H.H., Gray, G.A., Drummond, R.M., Furman, B.L. and Sneddon, P. (1990). Investigation of the selectivity of α, β-methylene ATP in inhibiting vascular responses *in vivo* and *in vitro*. *British Journal of Pharmacology*, **99**, 820–824.

Davey, M.J. (1987). Mechanism of α blockade for blood pressure control. *American Journal of Cardiology*, **59**, 18G–28G.

Davey, M.J. (1989). Pharmacologic basis for the use of doxazosin in the treatment of essential hypertension. *American Journal of Medicine*, **87**, (Suppl. 2A), 36S–44S.

Day, M.D. and Moore, A.F. (1976). Interaction of angiotensin II with noradrenaline and other spasmogens on rabbit isolated aortic strips. *Archives of Internationales Pharmacodynamie and Therapies*, **219**, 29–44.

De Jonge, A., Knape, J.Th.A., van Meel, J.C.A., Kalkman, H.O., Wilffert, B., Thoolen, M.J.M.C., *et al.* (1983). Effect of captopril on sympathetic neurotransmission in pithed normotensive rats. *European Journal of Pharmacology*, **88**, 231–240.

De Mey, J. and Vanhoutte, P.M. (1981). Uneven distribution of postjunctional α_1 and α_2-like adrenoceptors in canine arterial and venous smooth muscle. *Circulation Research*, **48**, 875–884.

De Vos, H., Cserwiec, E., De Backer, J.P., De Potter, W. and Vauquelin, G. (1991). [^{3}H]-Rauwolscine behaves as an agonist for the 5-HT$_1$-like receptors in human frontal cortex membranes. *European Journal of Pharmacology (Molecular Pharmacology)*, **207**, 1–8.

Diana, J.N., Qian, S., Heesch, C.M., Barron, K.W. and Chien, C.-Y. (1990). Nicotine-induced skeletal muscle vasodilatation is mediated by release of epinephrine from nerve terminals. *American Journal of Physiology*, **259**, H1718–H1729.

Docherty, J.R. and Hyland, L. (1985). Evidence for neuroeffector transmission through postjunctional α_2-adrenoceptors in human saphenous vein. *British Journal of Pharmacology*, **84**, 573–576.

Docherty, J.R. and McGrath, J.C. (1980). A comparison of pre- and postjunctional potencies of several α-adrenoceptor agonists in the cardiovascular system, vas deferens and anococcygeus of the rat. *Naunyn Schmiedeberg's Archives of Pharmacology*, **312**, 107–116.

Docherty, J.R. and Starke, K. (1982). An examination of pre- and postsynaptic α-adrenoceptors involved in neuroeffector mechanisms in rabbit aorta and portal vein. *British Journal of Pharmacology*, **76**, 327–335.

Docherty, J.R., Göthert, M., Diekhöfer, C. and Starke, K. (1982). Effects of 4-chloro-2-(2-imidazolin-2-ylamino)-isoindoline hydrochloride (BE 6143) at pre- and postsynaptic α-adrenoceptors in rabbit aorta and pulmonary artery. *Drug Research*, **32**, 1534–1540.

Dooley, D.J., Bittiger, H. and Reymann, N.C. (1986). CGP20712A: A useful tool for quantitating β_1- and β_2-adrenoceptors. *European Journal of Pharmacology*, **130**, 137–139.

Downing, O.A., Wilson, K.A. and Wilson, V.G. (1983). Non-competitive antagonism of the α-adrenoceptor mediated fast component of contractions of the rat aorta by doxazosin and prazosin. *British Journal of Pharmacology*, **80**, 315–322.

Downing, O.A., Wilson, K.A. and Wilson, V.G. (1985). Perfusion with Ca^{2+} solution potentiates prazosin blockade of noradrenaline-induced pressor responses in the mesenteric bed of the rat. *Journal of Autonomic Pharmacology*, **5**, 295–299.

Doxey, J.C., Roach, A.G. and Strachan, D.A. and Virdee, N.K. (1984). Selectivity and potency of 2-alkyl analogue of the α-adrenoceptor antagonist idazoxan (RX-781094) in peripheral systems. *British Journal of Phamacology*, **83**, 713–722.

Drew, G.M. and Whiting, S.B. (1979). Evidence for two distinct types of postsynaptic α-adrenoceptors in vascular smooth muscle *in vivo*. *British Journal of Pharmacology*, **67**, 207–215.

Dubocovich, M.L. and Langer, S.Z. (1974). Negative feedback regulation of noradrenaline release by nerve stimulation in the perfused cats' spleen: differences in potency of phenoxybenzamine in blocking pre- and postsynaptic adrenergic receptors. *Journal of Physiology*, **237**, 505–519.

Dubocovich, M.L., Langer, S.Z. and Massingham, R. (1980). Lack of correlation between presynaptic inhibition of noradrenaline release and end-organ response during nerve stimulation. *British Journal of Pharmacology*, **69**, 81–90.

Dunlop, D. and Shanks, R.G. (1968). Selective blockade of adrenoceptive β-receptors in the heart. *British Journal of Pharmacology*, **32**, 201–218.

Dunn, W.R., McGrath, J.C. and Wilson, V.G. (1989). Postjunctional α_2-adrenoceptors in the rabbit isolated distal saphenous artery — a permissive role for angiotensin II? *British Journal of Pharmacology*, **96**, 259–261.

Dunn, W.R., McGrath, J.C. and Wilson, V.G. (1991a). Postjunctional α-adrenoceptors in rabbit isolated distal saphenous artery: indirect sensitivity to prazosin of responses to noradrenaline mediated via postjunctional α_2-adrenoceptors. *British Journal of Pharmacology*, **103**, 1484–1492.

Dunn, W.R., McGrath, J.C. and Wilson, V.G. (1991b). Influence of angiotensin II on the α-adrenoceptors involved in mediating the response to sympathetic nerve stimulation in the rabbit isolated distal saphenous artery. *British Journal of Pharmacology*, **102**, 10–12.

Dunn, W.R., Wellman, G.C. and Bevan, J.A. (1994). Enhanced resistance artery sensitivity to agonists under isobaric compared to isometric conditions. *American Journal of Physiology*, **266**, H147–H155.

Dunn, W.R., Daly, C.J., McGrath, J.C. and Wilson, V.G. (1991c). A comparison of the actions of angiotensin II and Bay K 8644 on responses to noradrenaline mediated via postjunctional α_1- and α_2-adrenoceptors in rabbit isolated blood vessels. *British Journal of Pharmacology*, **103**, 1475–1483.

Dzau, V.J. (1988). Circulating versus local renin-angiotensin system in cardiovascular homeostasis. *Circulation*, **77**, (Suppl. 1), I4–I14.

Edvinsson, L., Birath, E., Uddman, R., Lee, J.-F., Duverger, D., MacKenzie, E.T., *et al.* (1984). Indoleaminergic mechanisms in brain vessels; Localization, concentration, uptake and *in vitro* responses for 5-hydroxytryptamine. *Acta Physiologica Scandanavica*, **121**, 291–299.

Edwards, F.R., Hards, D., Hirst, G.D.S. and Silverberg, M.D. (1989). Noradrenaline (γ) and ATP responses of innervated and non-innervated rat cerebral arteries. *British Journal of Pharmacology*, **96**, 785–789.

Elliot, H.L., McLean, K., Summer, D.J., Meredith, P.A. and Reid, J.L. (1981). Immediate cardiovascular responses to oral prazosin — effects of concurrent β-blockers. *Clinical Pharmacology and Therapeutics*, **29**, 303–309.

Emorine, L.J., Marullo, S., Briend-Sutren, M.-M., Patey, G., Tate, K., Delavier-Klutcho, C., *et al.* (1989). Molecular characterization of the human β_3-adrenergic receptor. *Science*, **245**, 1118–1121.

Faber, J.E. (1988). *In situ* analysis of α-adrenoceptors on arteriolar and venular smooth muscle in rat skeletal muscle microcirculation. *Circulation Research*, **62**, 37–50.

Falck, B., Thieme, G. and Torp, A. (1962). Fluorescence of catecholamines and related compounds condensed with formaldehyde. *Journal of Histochemistry and Cytochemistry*, **10**, 348–354.

Ferry, C.B. (1966). Cholinergic link hypothesis in adrenergic neuroeffector transmission. *Physiological Reviews*, **46**, 420–456.

Flavahan, N.A. and McGrath, J.C. (1980). Blockade by yohimbine of prazosin-resistant pressor effects of adrenaline in the pithed rat. *British Journal of Pharmacology*, **69**, 355–357.

Flavahan, N.A., Rimele, T.J., Cooke, J.P. and Vanhoutte, P.M. (1984). Characterization of postjunctional α_1- and α_2-adrenoceptors activated by exogenous or nerve-released norepinephrine in the canine saphenous vein. *Journal of Pharmacology and Experimental Therapeutics*, **230**, 699–705.

Flavahan, N.A., Grant, T.L., Greig, T. and McGrath, J.C. (1985). Analysis of the α-adrenoceptor-mediated and other components in the sympathetic vasopressor responses of the pithed rat. *British Journal of Pharmacology*, **86**, 265–274.

Flavahan, N.A. and Vanhoutte, P.M. (1986a). The effect of cooling on α_1- and α_2-adrenergic responses in canine saphenous vein and femoral veins. *Journal of Pharmacology and Experimental Therapeutics*, **238**, 139–147.

Flavahan, N.A. and Vanhoutte, P.M. (1986b). α_1-adrenoceptor subclassification in vascular smooth muscle. *Trends in Pharmacological Sciences*, **7**, 347–349.

Forsyth, F.M. and Pollock, D. (1988). Clonidine and morphine increase [^{3}H]-noradrenaline overflow in mouse vas deferens. *British Journal of Pharmacology*, **93**, 35–44.

Franco-Cereceda, A. this volume.

Frayn, K. and MacDonald, I.A. this volume.

Frederich, R.C., Kahn, B.B., Peach, M.J. and Flier, J.S. (1992). Tissue specific nutritional regulation of angiotensinogen in adipose tissue. *Hypertension*, **19**, 339–344.

Fuder, H. and Selbach, M. (1993). Characterization of sensory neurotransmission and its inhibition via α_{2B}-adrenoceptors and via non α_2-receptors in rabbit iris. *Naunyn Schmiedeberg's Archives of Pharmacology*, **347**, 394–401.

Fuder, H. and Schwarz, P. (1993). Desensitization of inhibitory prejunctional α_2-adrenoceptors and putative imidazolin receptors on rabbit heart sympathetic nerves. *Naunyn Schmiedeberg's Archives of Pharmacology*, **348**, 127–133.

Furchgott, R.F. (1972). The classification of adrenoceptors (adrenergic receptors). An evaluation from the standpoint of receptor theory. In *Handbook of Experimental Pharmacology*, Vol 33, Catecholamines, Eds. H. Blaschko and E. Muscholl, pp. 283–335, Berlin: Springer-Verlag.

Furuta, T. (1988). Precontraction-induced contractile response of isolated canine portal vein to α_2-adrenoceptor agonists. *Naunyn Schmiedeberg's Archives of Pharmacology*, **337**, 525–530.

Gainer, H. and Brownstein, M.J. (1981). Neuropeptides. In *Basic Neurochemistry*, Eds., G. Siegel, R. Albers, B. Agranoff and J. Katzman, pp. 161–182. Boston: Little Brown.

Gardiner, J.C. and Peters, C.J. (1982). Postsynaptic α_1- and α_2-adrenoceptor involvement in the vascular responses to neuronally released and exogenous noradrenaline in the hindlimb of the dog and cat. *European Journal of Pharmacology*, **84**, 189–198.

Gillespie, J.S. (1980). Presynaptic receptors in the autonomic nervous system. In *Handbook of Experimental Pharmacology*, Vol 54: Adrenergic activators and inactivators. Ed. L. Sezekeres. Part 1, pp. 352–425. Berlin: Springer-Verlag.

Gleason, M.M. and Hieble, J.P. (1992). The α_2-adrenoceptors of the human retinoblastoma cell line (Y79) may represent an additional example of the α_{2C}-adrenoceptor. *British Journal of Pharmacology*, **107**, 222–225.

Goering, J. and Zimmerman, B. (1986). Analysis of adrenoceptor blockade and hypotension elicited by urapidil and prazosin in conscious rat. *Journal of Pharmacology and Experimental Therapeutics*, **237**, 553–557.

Gordon, J.F., Baird, M., Daly, C.J. and McGrath, J.C. (1992). Endogenous nitric oxide modulates sympathetic neuroeffector transmission in the rabbit isolated lateral saphenous vein. *Journal of Cardiovascular Pharmacology*, **20**, (Suppl. 12), S68–S71.

Göthert, M. and Kollecker, P. (1986). Subendothelial β-adrenoceptors in rat vena cava: Facilitation of noradrenaline release via local stimulation of angiotensin II synthesis. *Naunyn Schmiedeberg's Archives of Pharmacology*, **334**, 156–165.

Göthert, M. and Molderings, G.J. (1991). Involvement of presynaptic imidazoline receptors in the α_2-adrenoceptor independent inhibition of noradrenaline release by imidazoline derivatives. *Naunyn Schmiedeberg's Archives of Pharmacology*, **343**, 271–282.

Goldberg, M.R., Hollister, A.S. and Robertson, D. (1983). Influence of yohimbine on blood pressure, autonomic reflexes and plasma catecholamines in humans. *Hypertension*, **5**, 772–778.

Grant, T.L. and McGarth, J.C. (1988). Interactions between angiotensin II and α-adrenoceptor agonists mediating pressor responses in the pithed rat. *British Journal of Pharmacology*, **95**, 1229–1240.

Grossman, E., Rosenthal, T., Pleleg, E., Holmes, C. and Goldberg, D.S. (1993). Oral yohimbine increases blood pressure and sympathetic nervous overflow in hypertensive patients. *Journal of Cardiovascular Pharmacology*, **22**, 22–26.

Grundemar, L., Grundström, N., Johansson, I.G.M., Andersson, R.G.G. and Hakansan, R. (1990). Suppression by neuropeptide Y of capsaicin-sensitive sensory nerve-mediated contraction in guinea-pig airways. *British Journal of Pharmacology*, **99**, 473–476.

Grundström, N., Andersson, G.G. and Wikberg, J.E.S. (1984). Inhibition of the excitatory non-adrenergic, non-cholinergic neurotransmission in the guinea-pig tracheo-bronchial tree mediated by α_2-adrenoceptors. *Acta Pharmacologica et Toxicologica*, **54**, 8–14.

Guan, Y.-Y., Chen, K.-M. and Sun, J.-J. (1991). α_1-adrenoceptors mediate the responses to B-HT-920 and rauwolscine in dog mesenteric artery after partial depolarization by KCl. *European Journal of Pharmacology*, **200**, 283–287.

Guimaraes, S. and Paiva, M.Q. (1981). Two different biophases for adrenaline released by electrical stimulation or tyramine from sympathetic nerve endings of the dog saphenous vein. *Naunyn Schmiedeberg's Archives of Pharmacology*, **316**, 200–204.

Han, C., Abel, P.W. and Minneman, K.P. (1987). Heterogeneity of α_1-adrenergic receptors revealed by chlorethylclonidine. *Molecular Pharmacology*, **32**, 505–510.

Han, S.-P., Naes, L. and Westfall, T.C. (1990). Calcitonin-gene related peptide is the endogenous mediator of noradrenergic-non-cholinergic vasodilation in rat mesentery. *Journal of Pharmacology and Experimental Therapeutics*, **255**, 423–428.

Hardebo, J.E. (1992). Influence of pulse pattern on noradrenaline release from sympathetic nerves in cerebral and some peripheral vessels. *Acta Physiologica Scandanavica*, **144**, 333–339.

Harder, D.R., Gilbert, R. and Lombard, J.H. (1987). Vascular muscle cell depolarization and activation in renal arteries on elevation of transmural pressure. *American Journal of Physiology*, **253**, F778–F781.

Harms, H.H., Zaagsma, J. and De Vente, J. (1977). Differentiation of β-adrenoceptors in the right atrium, diaphragm and adipose tissue of the rat, using stereoisomers of propranolol, alprenolol, nifenalol and practolol. *Life Sciences*, **21**, 123–128.

Hatton, R. and Clough, D.P. (1982). Captopril interferes with neurogenic vasoconstriction in the pithed rat by angiotenin-dependent mechanisms. *Journal of Cardiovascular Pharmacology*, **4**, 116–123.

Hentrich, F., Göthert, M. and Greschuchna, D. (1986). Noradrenaline release in the human pulmonary artery is modulated by presynaptic α_2-adrenoceptors. *Journal of Cardiovascular Pharmacology*, **8**, 539–544.

Hieble, J.P. and Woodward, D.F. (1984). Different characteristics of postjunctional α-adrenoceptors on arterial and venous smooth muscle. *Naunyn Schmiedeberg's Archives of Pharmacology*, **328**, 44–50.

Hieble, J.P., Nichols, A.J., Fredrickson, T.A., DePalma, P.D., Ruffolo, R.R.Jr. and Brooks, D.P. (1992). Cardiovascular actions of a new selective postjunctional α-adrenoceptor antagonist, SKF104856, in normotensive and hypertensive dogs. *British Journal of Pharmacology*, **105**, 992–996.

Hieble, J.P., Sulpizio, A.C., Edwards, R., Chapman, H., Young, P., Roberts, S.P., *et al.* (1991). Additional evidence for functional subclassification of α_2-adrenoceptors based on a new selective antagonist, SKF104856. *Journal of Pharmacology and Experimental Therapeutics*, **259**, 643–652.

Hirst, G.D.S. and Edwards, F.R. (1989). Sympathetic neuroeffector transmission in arteries and arterioles. *Physiological Reviews*, **69**, 546–604.

Hirst, G.D.S. and Jobling, P. (1989). The distribution of γ-adrenoceptors in mesenteric arteries and veins of the guinea-pig. *British Journal of Pharmacology*, **96**, 993–999.

Hirst, G.D.S. and Neild, T.O. (1980). Evidence for two populations of excitatory receptors for noradrenaline on arteriolar smooth muscle. *Nature*, **283**, 767–768.

Hirst, G.D.S. and Neild, T.O. (1981a). Localization of specialised noradrenaline receptors at neuromuscular junctions on arterioles of the guinea-pig. *Journal of Physiology*, **313**, 343–350.

Hirst, G.D.S. and Neild, T.O. (1981b). On the mechanism of action of prazosin at sympathetic nerve-muscle junction of the guinea-pig. *British Journal of Pharmacology*, **74**, 189P.

Hirst, G.D.S., De Gleria, S. and van Helden, D.F. (1985). Neuromuscular transmission in arterioles. *Experientia*, **41**, 874–879.

Holman, M.E. and Suprenant, A.M. (1980). An electrophysiological analysis of the effects of noradrenaline and α-adrenoceptor antagonists on neuromuscular arteries. *British Journal of Pharmacology*, **71**, 651–661.

Honda, Y., Nakagawa, C. and Terai, M. (1987). Further studies on (+)-YM-12617, a potent and selective α_1-adrenoceptor antagonist and its individual optical isomers. *Naunyn Schmiedeberg's Archives of Pharmacology*, **336**, 295–302.

Hoyer, D., Jones, C.R., Ford, W. and Palacios, J.M. (1990). Subtypes of α_1-adrenoceptors in hippocampus of pigs, guinea-pigs, calves and humans: regional differences. *European Journal of Pharmacology (Molecular Biology)*, **188**, 9–16.

Hughes, J. and Roth, R.H. (1971). Evidence that angiotensin enhances transmitter release during sympathetic nerve stimulation. *British Journal of Pharmacology*, **41**, 239–255.

Hyman, A.L., Lippton, H.L. and Kadowitz, P.J. (1990). Analysis of pulmonary vascular responses in cats to sympathetic nerve stimulation under elevated tone conditions: Evidence that neuronally released norepinephrine acts on α_1-, α_2-, and β_2-adrenoceptors. *Circulation Research*, **67**, 862–870.

Illes, P., Pfeiffer, N., von Kügelgen, I. and Starke, K. (1985). Presynaptic opioid receptor subtypes in the rabbit ear artery. *Journal of Pharmacology and Experimental Therapeutics*, **232**, 526–533.

Illes, P., Betterman, R., Brod, I. and Bucher, B. (1987a). β-Endorphin-sensitive opioid receptors in the rat tail artery. *Naunyn Schmiedeberg's Archives of Pharmacology*, **335**, 420–427.

Illes, P., Ramme, D. and Busse, R. (1987b). Photoelectric measurement of neurogenic vasoconstriction of the rabbit mesenteric artery reveals the presence of presynaptic opioid receptor δ-receptors. *Naunyn Schmiedeberg's Archives of Pharmacology*, **335**, 701–704.

Johnson, E.M. Jr., Marshall, G.R. and Needleman, P. (1974). Modification of responses to sympathetic nerve stimulation by the renin-angiotensin system in rats. *British Journal of Pharmacology*, **51**, 541–547.

Johnston, H. and Majewski, H. (1986). Prejunctional β-adrenoceptors in rabbit pulmonary artery and mouse atria: effect of α-adrenoceptor blockade and phosphodiesterase inhibition. *British Journal of Pharmacology*, **87**, 533–562.

Kaposci, J., Zimanyi, I., Farsang, C. and Vizi, E.S. (1987). Presynaptic α_2-adrenoceptors exclusively sensitive to agonists of phenethylamine structure on sympathetic nerves of the human gall bladder artery. *Neuroscience*, **4**, 413–418.

Kaufman, L.J. and Vollmer, R.R. (1985). Endogenous angiotensin II facilitates sympathetically mediated haemodynamic responses in pithed rats. *Journal of Pharmacology and Experimental Therapeutics*, **235**, 128–134.

Kaumann, A.J. (1989). Is there a third heart β-adrenoceptor? *Trends in Pharmacological Sciences*, **10**, 316–320.

Kawasaki, H., Cline, W.H. and Su. C. (1984). Involvement of vascular renin-angiotensin system in β-adrenergic receptor-mediated facilitation of vascular neurotransmission in spontaneously hypertensive rats. *Journal of Pharmacology and Experimental Therapeutics*, **231**, 23–34.

Kawasaki, H., Takasaki, K., Cline, W.H. and Su, C. (1988). Effect of angiotensin III (des-Asp^1-angiotensin II) on the vascular adrenergic neurotransmission in spontaneously hypertensive rats. *European Journal of Pharmacology*, **147**, 125–130.

Kawasaki, H., Nuki, C., Saito, A. and Takasaki, K. (1990). Role of calcitonin gene-related peptide-containing nerves in the vascular adrenergic neurotransmission. *Journal of Pharmacology and Experimental Therapeutics*, **252**, 403–409.

Koss, M.C., Kawari, M. and Ito, T. (1991). Neural activation of α_2-adrenoceptors in cat cutaneous vasculature. *Journal of Pharmacology and Experimental Therapeutics*, **256**, 1126–1131.

Kosterlitz, H.W. and Waterfield, A. (1975). An analysis of the phenomena of acute tolerance to morphine in the guinea-pig isolated ileum. *British Journal of Pharmacology*, **53**, 131–138.

Kosterlitz, H.W., Lydon, R.J. and Watt, A.J. (1970). The effects of adrenaline, noradrenaline and isoprenaline on inhibitory α- and β-adrenoceptors in the longitudinal muscle of the guinea-pig ileum. *British Journal of Pharmacology*, **39**, 398–413.

Kou, K., Ibengwe, J. and Suzuki, H. (1984). Effects of α-adrenoceptor antagonists on electrical and mechanical responses of the isolated dog mesenteric vein to perivascular nerve stimulation and exogenous noradrenaline. *Naunyn Schmiedeberg's Archives of Pharmacology*, **326**, 7–13.

Kubes, P., Melinyshyn, M., Nesbitt, K., Cain, S.M. and Chapler, C.K. (1992). Participation of α_2-adrenergic receptors in neural vascular tone of canine skeletal muscle. *American Journal of Physiology*, **262**, H1705–H1710.

Kyncl, J.J. (1986). Pharmacology of Terazosin. *American Journal of Medicine*, **80**, (Suppl. 5B), 12–19.

Laher, I., Khayal, M.A. and Bevan, J.A. (1986). Norepinephrine-sensitive, phenoxybenzamine-resistant receptor sites associated with contraction in rabbit arterial but not venous smooth muscle: possible role in adrenergic transmission. *Journal of Pharmacology and Experimental Therapeutics*, **237**, 364–368.

Lands, A.M., Arnold, A., McAuliff, J.P., Luduenda, F.P. and Brown, T.G. (1967). Differentiation of receptor systems activated by sympathomimetic amines. *Nature*, **215**, 597–598.

Langer, S.Z. (1974). Commentary; Presynaptic regulation of catecholamine release. *Biochemical Pharmacology*, **23**, 1793–1800.

Langer, S.Z. (1981). Presynaptic regulation of the release of catecholamines. *Pharmacological Reviews*, **81**, 337–362.

Langer, S.Z., Massingham, R. and Shepperson, N.B. (1980). Presence of postsynaptic α_2-adrenoceptors of predominantly extrasynaptic location in the vascular smooth muscle of the dog hindlimb. *Clinical Sciences*, **59**, 225s–228s.

Langer, S.Z., Alder, E., Enero, M.A. and Stefano, F.J.E. (1971). The role of the α receptor in regulating noradrenaline overflow. *Proceedings Of the XXVth International Congress of Physiological Sciences*, 335P.

Le Clerc, G., Rouot, B., Schwartz, J., Velly, J. and Wermuth, C.G. (1980). Studies on some para-substituted clonidine derivatives that exhibit an α-adrenoceptor stimulant activity. *British Journal of Pharmacology*, **71**, 5–9.

Lee, T. J-F., Su, C. and Bevan, J.A. (1976). Neurogenic sympathetic vasoconstriction of the rabbit basilar artery. *Circulation Research*, **39**, 120–126.

Li, G., Regunathan, S., Barrow, C.J., Eshraghi, J., Cooper, R. and Reis, D.J. (1994). Agmatine: an endogenous clonidine-displacing substance in the brain. *Science*, **263**, 966–969.

Li, T. and Zimmerman, B.G. (1991). β-Adrenergic-induced local angiotensin generation in the rabbit hindlimb is dependent on the kidney. *Hypertension*, **17**, 1010–1017.

Limberger, N. and Starke, K. (1983). Partial agonist effect of 2-[2-(1,4-benzodioxanyl)]-2-imidazoline (RX781094) at presynaptic α_2-adrenoceptors in rabbit ear artery. *Naunyn Schmiedeberg's Archives of Pharmacology*, **324**, 75–78.

Limberger, N., Spath, L. and Starke, K. (1991). Subclassification of the presynaptic α_2-autoreceptors in rabbit brain cortex. *British Journal of Pharmacology*, **103**, 1251–1255.

Limberger, N., Trendelenburg, A-U. and Starke, K. (1992). Pharmacological characterization of presynaptic α_2-adrenoceptors in rat submaxillary gland and heart atrium. *British Journal of Pharmacology*, **107**, 246–255.

Limberger, N., Fischer, M.R.G., Wichmann, T. and Starke, K. (1989). Phentolamine blocks presynaptic serotonin autoreceptors in rabbit and rat brain cortex. *Naunyn Schmiedeberg's Archives of Pharmacology*, **340**, 52–61.

Lomasney, J.W., Cotecchia, S., Lefkowitz, R.J. and Caron, M.G. (1991). Molecular biology of α-adrenergic receptors: implications for receptor classification and for the structure-function relationships. *Biochimica Biophysica Acta*, **1095**, 127–139.

MacDonald, A., Daly, C.J., Bulloch, J.M. and McGrath, J.C. (1992). Contribution of α_1-adrenoceptors, α_2-adrenoceptors and purinoceptors to neurotransmission in several rabbit isolated blood vessels: role of neuronal uptake and autofeedback. *British Journal of Pharmacology*, **105**, 347–354.

MacKinnon, A.C., Kilpatrick, A.T., Kenny, B.A., Spedding, M. and Brown, C.M. (1992). [^{3}H]-RS-15385-197, selective and high affinity radioligand for α_2-adrenoceptors: implications for receptor classification. *British Journal of Pharmacology*, **106**, 1011–1018.

MacLean, M.R. and Hiley, C.R. (1988). Effects of enalapril on changes in cardiac output and organ vascular resistances induced by α_1- and α_2-adrenoceptor agonists in pithed normotensive rats. *British Journal of Pharmacology*, **94**, 449–462.

MacLean, M.R. and McGrath, J.C. (1990). Effects of pre-contraction with endothelin-1 on α_2-adrenoceptor and (endothelium-dependent) neuropeptide Y-mediated contractions in the isolated vascular bed of the rat tail. *British Journal of Pharmacology*, **101**, 205–211.

MacLean, M.R., McCulloch, K.M., MacMillan, J.B. and McGrath, J.C. (1993). Influences of the endothelium and hypoxia on neurogenic transmission in the isolated pulmonary artery of the rabbit. *British Journal of Pharmacology*, **108**, 150–154.

Majewski, H., Hedler, L., Schurr, C. and Starke, K. (1984). Modulation of noradrenaline release in the pithed rabbit: a role for angiotensin II. *Journal of Cardiovascular Pharmacology*, **6**, 888–896.

Makita, Y. (1983). Effects of adrenoceptor agonists and antagonists on smooth muscle cells and neuromuscular transmission in the guinea-pig renal artery and vein. *British Journal of Pharmacology*, **80**, 671–679.

Malik, K.U. and Nasjletti, A. (1976). Facilitation of adrenergic transmission by locally generated angiotensin II in rat mesenteric arteries. *Circulation Research*, **38**, 26–29.

Massingham, R., Dubocovich, M.L. and Shepperson, N.B. and Langer, S.Z. (1981). *In vivo* selectivity of prazosin but not WB-4101 for postsynaptic α_1-adrenoceptors. *Journal of Pharmacology and Experimental Therapeutics*, **217**, 467–474.

McCubbin, J.W. and Page, I.H. (1963). Renal pressor system and neurogenic control of arterial pressure. *Circulation Research*, **12**, 553–559.

McGrath, J.C. (1982). Commentary: Evidence for more than one type of postjunctional α-adrenoceptor. *Biochemical Pharmacology*, **31**, 467–484.

McGrath, J.C. and Wilson, V.G. (1987). A comparative study of the α-adrenoceptor antagonism of corynanthine, prazosin and YM-12617 in the rat isolated thoracic aorta. *British Journal of Pharmacology*, **91**, 327P.

McGrath, J.C., Brown, C.M. and Wilson, V.G. (1989). α-adrenoceptors: a critical review. *Medicinal Research Reviews*, **9**, 407–532.

McGrath, J.C., Wilson, V.G., Dunn, W.R. and Templeton, A.G.B. (1991). The interaction between α_1- and α_2-adrenoceptors — the search for vascular α_2-adrenoceptors *in vitro*. In *Adrenoceptors: Structure, Mechanisms, Function — Advances in Pharmacological Sciences*, edited by E. Szabadi and P.M. Bradshaw. pp. 211–220. Basel: Birkhauser Verlag.

McLaughlin, D.P. and MacDonald, A. (1990). Evidence for the existence of 'atypical' β-adrenoceptor (β_3-adrenoceptors) mediating relaxation in the rat distal colon *in vitro*. *British Journal of Pharmacology*, **101**, 569–574.

McPherson, G.A. and Angus, J.A. (1989). Phentolamine and structurally related compounds selectively antagonize the vascular actions of the K^+ channel opener, cromakalin. *British Journal of Pharmacology*, **97**, 941–949.

Medgett, I.C. and Langer, S.Z. (1984). Heterogeneity of smooth muscle α-adrenoceptors in rat tail artery *in vitro*. *Journal of Pharmacology and Experimental Therapeutics*, **229**, 823–830.

Mellander, S., Andersson, P-O., Afzelius, L-E. and Hellstrand, P. (1982). Neural β-adrenergic dilatation of the facial vein in man. *Acta Physiologica Scandanavica*, **114**, 393–399.

Mermet, C., Gonon, F.G. and Stjärne, L. (1990). Online electrochemical monitoring of the local noradrenaline release evoked by electrical stimulation of the sympathetic nerves in isolated rat tail artery. *Naunyn Schmiedeberg's Archives of Pharmacology*, **140**, 323–329.

Michel, A.D., Loury, D.N. and Whiting, R.L. (1989). Differences between the α_2-adrenoceptor in rat submaxillary gland and the α_{2A}- and α_{2B}-adrenoceptor subtypes. *British Journal of Pharmacology*, **98**, 890–897.

Michel, A.D., Loury, D.N. and Whiting, R.L. (1990). Assessment of imiloxan as a selective α_{2B}-adrenoceptor antagonist. *British Journal of Pharmacology*, **99**, 560–564.

Michel, C.M., Philipp, T. and Brodde, O.E. (1992). α- and β-adrenoceptors in hypertension: Molecular biology and pharmacological studies. *Pharmacology and Toxicology*, **70**, (Suppl. II), s1–s10.

Minneman, K.P. (1988). α_1-Adrenergic receptor subtypes, inositol phosphates, and sources of cell Ca^{2+}. *Pharmacological Reviews*, **40**, 87–119.

Molderings, G.J., Likungi, J., Hentrich, F. and Göthert, M. (1988). Facilitatory presynaptic angiotensin receptors on the sympathetic nerves of human saphenous vein and pulmonary artery. Potential involvement in β-adrenoceptor-mediated facilitation of noradrenaline release. *Naunyn Schmiedeberg's Archives of Pharmacology*, **338**, 228–233.

Molderings, G.J., Hentrich, F. and Göthert, M. (1991). Pharmacological characterization of the imidazoline receptor which mediates inhibition of noradrenaline release in the rabbit pulmonary artery. *Naunyn Schmiedeberg's Archives of Pharmacology*, **344**, 630–638.

Morris, J.L. and Gibbins, I.L. (1991). Co-transmission and neuromodulation. In: *Autonomic Neuroeffector Mechanisms*. Eds. Burnstock, G. and Hoyle, C.H.V., pp. 33–120. Chur, Switzerland, Harwood Academic Publishers.

Morrow, A.L. and Creese, I. (1986). Characterisation of α_1-adrenergic receptor subtypes in rat brain: A re-evaluation of [^{3}H]WB4101 and [^{3}H]prazosin binding. *Molecular Pharmacology*, **29**, 321–330.

Moulds, R.F.W. and Worland, P.J. (1980). Potentiation of human vascular smooth muscle contraction by angiotensin. *Journal of Cardiovascular Pharmacology*, **2**, 377–386.

Msghina, M., Mermet, C., Gonon, F. and Stjärne, L. (1992). Electrophysiological and electrochemical analysis of the secretion of ATP and noradrenaline from sympathetic nerves in the rat tail artery: effects of α_2-adrenoceptor agonists and antagonists and noradrenaline uptake blockers. *Naunyn Schmiedeberg's Archives of Pharmacology*, **346**, 173–186.

Mulvany, M.J. and Aalkjaer, C. (1990). Structure and function of small arteries. *Physiological Reviews*, **70**, 921–961.

Murumatsu, I. (1991). Relation between adrenergic neurogenic contraction and α_1-adrenoceptor subtypes in dog mesenteric and carotid and rabbit carotid arteries. *British Journal of Pharmacology*, **102**, 210–214.

Murumatsu, I., Kigoshi, S. and Oshita, M. (1990a). Two distinct α_1-adrenoceptor subtypes involved in noradrenaline contraction of the rabbit thoracic aorta. *British Journal of Pharmacology*, **101**, 662–666.

Murumatsu, I., Ohmura, T. and Oshita, M. (1989). Comparison between sympathetic adrenergic and purinergic transmission in the dog mesenteric artery. *Journal of Physiology*, **411**, 227–243.

Murumatsu, I., Ohmura, T., Kigoshi, S., Hashimoto, S. and Oshita, M. (1990b). Pharmacological subclassification of α_1-adrenoceptors in vascular smooth muscle. *British Journal of Pharmacology*, **99**, 197–201.

Nagao, T. and Szuki, H. (1988). Effects of α-β-methylene ATP on electrical responses produced by ATP and nerve stimulation in smooth muscle cells of the guinea-pig mesenteric artery. *General Pharmacology*, **19**, 799–805.

Nahorski, S.R., Barnett, D.B. and Cheung, Y.D. (1985). α-adrenoceptor-effector coupling affinity states or heterogeneity of the α_2-adrenoceptor. *Clinical Sciences*, **68**, (Suppl. 10), 39s–42s.

Najafipour, H. and Ferrell, W.R. (1993). Sympathetic innervation and α-adrenoceptor profile of blood vessels in the posterior region of the rabbit knee joint. *British Journal of Pharmacology*, **108**, 79–84.

Nakamura, M., Jackson, E.K. and Inagami, T. (1986). β-Adrenoceptor-mediated release of angiotensin II from mesenteric arteries. *American Journal of Physiology*, **250**, H144–H148.

Neild, T.O. and Keef, K. (1985). Measurement of the membrane potential of arterial smooth muscle in anaesthetized animals and its relation to changes in artery diameter. *Microvascular Research*, **30**, 19–28.

Neild, T.O. and Kotecha, N. (1986). Effects of α-β-methylene ATP on membrane potential neuromuscular transmission and smooth muscle contraction in the rat tail artery. *General Pharmacology*, **17**, 461–464.

Nicholas, T.E. (1970). Potentiation of the effects of noradrenaline and of sympathetic stimulation of the perfused rat caudal artery by angiotensin. *Journal of Pharmacy and Pharmacology*, **22**, 37–41.

Nielsen, H., Mortensen, F.V. and Mulvany, M.J. (1990). Differential distribution of postjunctional α_2-adrenoceptors in human omental small arteries. *Journal of Cardiovascular Pharmacology*, **16**, 34–40.

Nielsen, H., Hasenkam, J.M., Pilegaard, H.K., Mortensen, F.V. and Mulvany, M.J. (1991a). α-Adrenoceptors in human resistance arteries from colon, pericardial fat, and skeletal muscle. *American Journal of Physiology*, **261**, H762–H767.

Nielsen, H., Pilegaard, H.K., Hasenkam, J.M., Mortensen, F.V. and Mulvany, M.J. (1991b). Heterogeneity of postjunctional α-adrenoceptors in isolated mesenteric resistance arteries from rats, rabbits, pigs, and humans. *Journal of Cardiovascular Pharmacology*, **18**, 4–10.

Nielsen, H., Thom, S., Hughes, A.D., Martin, G.N., Mulvany, M.J. and Sever, P. (1989). Postjunctional α_2-adrenoceptors mediate vasoconstriction in human subcutaneous resistance arteries. *British Journal of Pharmacology*, **97**, 829–834.

Nielsen, P.J. and Nyborg, N.C.B. (1988). Adrenergic response in retinal resistance vessels. *Ophthalmology*, **13**, 103–107.

Noble, D. and Boyd, C.A.R. (1993). The challenge of integrative physiology. In *The Logic of Life*. Eds., C.A.R. Boyd and D. Noble. pp. 1–15. Oxford University Press. Oxford.

Nunes, J.P. and Guimaraes, S. (1993). Chlorethylclonidine irreversibly activates postjunctional α_2-adrenoceptors in the dog saphenous vein. *Naunyn Schmiedeberg's Archives of Pharmacology*, **348**, 264–268.

Ohyanagi, M., Faber, J.E. and Nishigaki, K. (1991). Differential activation of α_1- and α_2-adrenoceptors on microvascular smooth muscle during sympathetic nerve stimulation. *Circulation Research*, **68**, 232–244.

Oriowo, M.A. and Bevan, J.A. (1990). Chlorethylclonidine unmasks a non-α-adrenoceptor noradrenaline binding site in the rat aorta. *European Journal of Pharmacology*, **178**, 243–246.

Panisset, J.C. and Bourdois, P. (1968). Effect of angiotensin on the response to noradrenaline and sympathetic nerve stimulation, and on the [^{3}H]-noradrenaline uptake in cat mesenteric blood vessels. *Canadian Journal of Physiology and Pharmacology*, **46**, 125–131.

Parkinson, N.A., Thom, S.M., Hughes, A.D., Sever, P.S., Mulvany, M.J. and Nielsen, H. (1992). Neurally evoked responses of human isolated resistance arteries are mediated by both α_1- and α_2-adrenoceptors. *British Journal of Pharmacology*, **106**, 568–573.

Pegram, B.L., Bevan, R. and Bevan, J.A. (1976). Facial vein of the rabbit: neurogenic vasodilation mediated by β-adrenergic receptors. *Circulation Research*, **39**, 854–860.

Perez, D.M., Paiscik, M.T. and Graham, R.M. (1991). Solution-phase library screening for the identification of rare clones: isolation of an α_{1D}-adrenergic receptor cDNA. *Molecular Pharmacology*, **40**, 873–883.

Pernow, J., Saria, A. and Lundberg, J.M. (1986). Mechanisms underlying pre- and postjunctional effects of neuropeptide Y in sympathetic vascular control. *Acta Physiologica Scandanavica*, **126**, 239–249.

Piascik, M.T., Kusiak, J.W., Pitha, J., Butler, B.T., Le, H.T. and Babich, M. (1988). Alkylation of α_1 receptors with a chemically reactive analog of prazosin reveals low affinity sites for norepinephrine in rabbit aorta. *Journal of Pharmacology and Experimental Therapeutics*, **246**, 1001–1011.

Piascik, M.T., Butler, B.T., Kusiak, J.W., Pitha, J. and Holtman, J.R.Jr. (1989). Effect of an alkylating analog of prazosin on α_1 adrenoceptor subtypes and arterial blood pressure. *Journal of Pharmacology and Experimental Therapeutics*, **251**, 878–883.

Piascik, M.T., Butler, B.T., Pruitt, T.A. and Kusiak, J.W. (1990a). Agonist interaction with alkylation-sensitive and -resistant α_1 adrenoceptor subtypes. *Journal of Pharmacology and Experimental Therapeutics*, **254**, 982–991.

Piascik, M.T., Kusiak, J.W. and Barron, K.W. (1990b). α_1-adrenoceptor subtypes and the regulation of peripheral haemodynamics in the conscious rat. *European Journal of Pharmacology*, **186**, 273–278.

Piascik, M.T., Sparks, M.S., Pruitt, T.A. and Soltis, E.E. (1991). Evidence for a complex interaction between the subtypes of the α_1-adrenoceptor. *European Journal of Pharmacology*, **199**, 279–289.

Pickel, V.M., Joh, T.H. and Reis, D.J. (1976). Ultrastructural localization by immunocytochemistry of dopamine-β-hydroxylase within noradrenergic neurons of the rat brain. *Anatomical Record*, **184**, 503.

Ping, P. and Faber, J.E. (1993). Characterization of α-adrenoceptor gene expression and venous smooth muscle. *American Journal of Physiology*, **265**, H1501–H1509.

Powell, C.E. and Slater, I.H. (1958). Blocking of inhibitory adrenergic receptors by a dichloro analogue of isoproterenol. *Journal of Pharmacology and Experimental Therapeutics*, **122**, 480–488.

Purdy, R.E. and Weber, M.A. (1988). Angiotensin II amplification of α-adrenergic vasoconstriction: role of receptor reserve. *Circulation Research*, **63**, 748–757.

Raiteri, M., Bonanno, G., Maura, G., Pende, M., Andriolo, G.C. and Ruelle, A. (1992). Subclassification of release-regulating α_2-autoreceptors in human brain cortex. *British Journal of Pharmacology*, **107**, 1146–1151.

Rajanayagam, M.A.S. and Medgett, I.C. (1987). Greater activation of smooth muscle α_2-adrenoceptors by epinephrine in distal than in proximal segments of rat tail artery. *Journal of Pharmacology and Experimental Therapeutics*, **240**, 679–684.

Rajanayagam, M.A.S., Medgett, I.C. and Rand, M.J. (1990). Vasoconstrictor responses of rat tail artery to sympathetic nerve stimulation contains a component due to activation of postjunctional β- or α_2-adrenoceptors. *European Journal of Pharmacology*, **177**, 35–41.

Ramage, A.G. (1984). The effect of prazosin, indoramin and phentolamine on sympathetic nerve activity. *European Journal of Pharmacology*, **106**, 507–513.

Ramage, A.G. (1986). Evidence of sympathoinhibitory action of prazosin and indoramin. *European Journal of Pharmacology*, **121**, 83–89.

Redfern, W.S. and Clague, R.U. (1991). Effects of RS-15385-197 and other α_2-adrenoceptor antagonists on tail skin temperature in unanesthetized rats. *British Journal of Pharmacology*, **104**, 50P.

Remie, R. and Zaagma, J. (1986). A new technique for the study of vascular presynaptic receptors in freely moving rats. *American Journal of Physiology*, **251**, H463–H467.

Remie, R., Knot, H.J., Kolker, H.J. and Zaagma, J. (1988). Pronounced facilitation of endogenous noradrenaline release by presynaptic β_2-adrenoceptors in the vasculature of freely moving rats. *Naunyn Schmiedeberg's Archives of Pharmacology*, **338**, 215–220.

Roberts, S.P., Kelly, J., Cawthorne, M.A. and Sennitt, M.V. (1992). SKF104078, a postjunctionally selective α_2-adrenoceptor antagonist in the human saphenous vein *in vitro*. *Naunyn Schmiedeberg's Archives of Pharmacology*, **345**, 327–332.

Roesler, J.M., McCafferty, J.P., DeMarinis, R.M., Matthews, W.D. and Hieble, J.P. (1986). Characterization of the antihypertensive activity of SKF86446, a selective α_2-adrenoceptor antagonist in the rat. *Journal of Pharmacology and Experimental Therapeutics*, **236**, 1–7.

Ruffolo, R.R., Sulpizio, A.C., Nichols, A.J., DeMarinis, R.M. and Hieble, J.P. (1987). Pharmacological differentiation between pre- and postjunctional α_2-adrenoceptors by SKF104078. *Naunyn Schmiedeberg' Archives of Pharmacology*, **336**, 415–418.

Saito, A. and Lee, T-J. (1987). Serotonin as an alternative transmitter in sympathetic nerves in large cerebral arteries of the rabbit. *Circulation Research*, **60**, 220–228.

Saito, M., Kojima, C. and Takayanagi, I. (1992). Characterization of α_1-adrenoceptor subtypes labelled by [^{3}H]prazosin in single cells prepared from rabbit thoracic aorta. *European Journal of Pharmacology*, **221**, 35–41.

Saville, V.L., Maynard, K. and Burnstock, G. (1990). Neuropeptide Y potentiates purinergic as well as adrenergic responses of the rabbit ear artery. *European Journal of Pharmacology*, **176**, 117–125.

Saye, J.A., Cassis, L.A., Sturgill, T.W., Lynch, K.R. and Peach, M.J. (1989). Angiotensinogen gene expression in 3T3-L1 cells. *American Journal of Physiology*, **256**, C448–C451.

Schafers, R.F., Elliott, H.L., Howie, C.A. and Reid, J.L. (1991). Studies with abanoquil (UK-52,046) a novel quinoline α_1-adrenoceptor antagonist: I Effects on blood pressure, heart rate and pressor responsiveness in normotensive subjects. *British Journal of Clinical Pharmacology*, **32**, 599–604.

Scheurink, A.J.W., Steffens, A.B., Bouritius, H., Dreteler, G.H., Bruntink, R., Remie, R. and Zaagsma, J. (1989). Adrenal and sympathetic catecholamines in exercising rats. *American Journal of Physiology*, **256**, R155–R160.

Schumman, H-J. and Lues, I. (1983). Postjunctional α-adrenoceptors in the isolated saphenous vein of the rabbit. *Naunyn Schmiedeberg's Archives of Pharmacology*, **323**, 328–334.

Schwartz, D.D. and Malik, K.K. (1992). Characterization of prejunctional α_2 adrenergic receptors involved in modulation of adrenergic transmitter release in the isolated perfused rat kidney. *Journal of Pharmacology and Experimental Therapeutics*, **261**, 1050–1055.

Senaratne, M.P.J., Jakakody, R.L. and Kappagoda, C.T. (1987). Potentiation of the responses to transmural nerve stimulation by α-agonist: a possible role *in vivo*. *Canadian Journal of Physiology and Pharmacology*, **65**, 427–432.

Shen, K-Z., Barajas-Lopez, C. and Surprenant, A. (1990). Functional characterization of neuronal pre- and postsynaptic α_2-adrenoceptor subtypes in guinea-pig submucosal plexus. *British Journal of Pharmacology*, **101**, 925–931.

Shen, Y.-T., Zhang, H. and Vatner, S.T. (1994). Peripheral effects of β_3 adrenergic receptor stimulation in conscious dogs. *Journal of Pharmacology and Experimental Therapeutics*, **268**, 466–473.

Shi, A.G., Kwan, C.Y. and Daniel, E.E. (1989). Relationship between density (maximum binding) of α-adrenoceptor binding sites and contractile response in four canine vascular tissues. *Journal of Pharmacology and Experimental Therapeutics*, **250**, 1119–1124.

Shimamoto, Y., Shimamoto, H., Kwan, C-Y. and Daniel, E.E. (1993). Rauwolscine-induces contraction in the dog mesenteric artery pre-contracted with KCl and endothelin-1: mediation via 5-Hydroxytryptamine$_1$-like receptors. *Journal of Pharmacology and Experimental Therapeutics*, **264**, 201–209.

Simonneaux, V., Ebadi, M. and Bylund, D.B. (1991). Identification and characterization of α_{2D}-adrenergic receptors in bovine pineal gland. *Molecular Pharmacology*, **40**, 235–241.

Sjöblom-Widfeldt, N. and Nilsson, H. (1990). Sympathetic transmission in small mesenteric arteries from the rat: influence of impulse pattern. *Acta Physiologica Scandanavica*, **138**, 525–528.

Skarby, T.V.C., Andersson, K.E. and Edvinsson, L. (1983). Pharmacological characterization of postjunctional α-adrenoceptors in isolated feline cerebral and peripheral arteries. *Acta Physiologica Scandanavica*, **117**, 63–73.

Smith, K., Connaughton, S. and Docherty, J.R. (1992). Investigations of the subtype of α_2-adrenoceptors mediating contractions of the human saphenous vein. *British Journal of Pharmacology*, **106**, 447–451.

Sneddon, P. and Burnstock, G. (1984). ATP as a co-transmitter in rat tail artery. *European Journal of Pharmacology*, **106**, 149–152.

Soltis, E.S. and Cassis, L.A. (1991). Influence of perivascular adipose tissue on rat aortic smooth muscle responsiveness. *Clinical Experiments in Hypertension*, **A13**, 277–296.

Spiers, J.P., Harron, D.W.G. and Wilson, R. (1991). Duration of action and effect on baroreflex function of the antiarrhythmic α_1-adrenoceptor antagonist UK-52,046. *Journal of Pharmacy and Pharmacology*, **43**, 70–72.

Squire, I.B. and Reid, J.L. (1993). Interaction between the renin-angiotensin system and the autonomic nervous system. In: *The Renin-Angiotensin-System* Volume 1. Eds. Robertson, J.I.S. and Nicholls, M.G. pp. 37.1–37.16. Gower London.

Starke, K. (1972). α sympathomimetic inhibition of adrenergic and cholinergic transmission in rabbit heart. *Naunyn Schmiedeberg's Archives of Pharmacology*, **274**, 18–45.

Starke, K. (1977). Regulation of noradrenaline release by presynaptic receptor systems. *Review of Physiology, Biochemistry and Pharmacology*, **77**, 1–124.

Starke, K. (1981). α-Adrenoceptor subclassification. *Review of Physiology, Biochemistry and Pharmacology*, **88**, 199–236.

Starke, K. (1987). Presynaptic α-autoreceptors. *Review of Physiology, Biochemistry and Pharmacology*, **107**, 73–146.

Starke, K., Montel, H., Gayk, W. and Merker, R. (1974). Comparison of the effects of clonidine on pre- and postsynaptic adrenoceptors in the rabbit pulmonary artery. *Naunyn Schmiedeberg's Archives of Pharmacology*, **285**, 133–150.

Starke, K., Borowski, E. and Endo, T. (1975a). Preferential blockade of presynaptic α-adrenoceptors by yohimbine. *European Journal of Pharmacology*, **34**, 385–388.

Starke, K., Endo, T. and Taube, H.D. (1975b). Relative pre- and postsynaptic potencies of α-adrenoceptor agonists in the rabbit pulmonary artery. *Naunyn Schmiedeberg's Archives of Pharmacology*, **291**, 55–78.

Stevens, M.J. and Moulds, R.F.W. (1985). Neuronally released norepinephrine does not preferentially activate postjunctional α_1-adrenoceptors in human blood vessels *in vitro*. *Circulation Research*, **57**, 399–405.

Stephens, N., Bund, S.J., Faragher, E.B. and Heagerty, A.M. (1992). Neurotransmission in human resistance arteries: contribution of α_1- and α_2-adrenoceptors but not P_2-purinoceptors. *Journal of Vascular Research*, **29**, 347–352.

Stjärne, L., Bao, J-X., Gonon, F.G., Msghina, M. and Stjärne, E. (1993). A nonstochastic string model of sympathetic neuromuscular transmission. *News in Physiological Sciences*, **8**, 253–260.

Su, C. (1980). Potentiative effects of α agonistic sympathomimetic amines on vasoconstriction by adrenergic nerve stimulation. *Journal of Pharmacology and Experimental Therapeutics*, **215**, 377–381.

Sulpizio, A. and Hieble, J.P. (1987). Demonstration of α_2-adrenoceptor-mediated contraction in the isolated canine saphenous artery treated with Bay K 8644. *European Journal of Pharmacology*, **135**, 107–110.

Sulpizio, A. and Hieble, J.P. (1991). Lack of a pharmacological distinction between α_1-adrenoceptor mediating intracellular calcium-dependent and independent contractions to sympathetic nerve stimulation in the perfused caudal artery. *Journal of Pharmacology and Experimental Therapeutics*, **257**, 1045–1052.

Suzuki, E., Tsujimoto, G., Tamura, K. and Hashimoto, K. (1990). Two pharmacologically distinct α_1-adrenoceptor subtypes in the contraction of rabbit aorta: Each subtype couples with a different Ca^{2+} signalling mechanism and plays a different physiological role. *Molecular Pharmacology*, **38**, 725–736.

Szabo, B., Hedler, L., Ensinger, H. and Starke, K. (1986). Opioid peptides decrease noradrenaline release and blood pressure in the rabbit at peripheral receptors. *Naunyn Schmiedeberg's Archives of Pharmacology*, **332**, 50–56.

Szemeredi, K., Stull, R., Kopin, I.J. and Goldstein, D.S. (1989). Effects of a peripherally acting α_2-adrenoceptor antagonist (L-659,066) on haemodynamics and plasma levels of catechols in conscious rats. *European Journal of Pharmacology*, **170**, 53–59.

Takaki, M. and Nakayama, S. (1991). Prejunctional modulatory action of neuropeptide Y on responses due to antidromic activation of peripheral terminals of capsaicin-sensitive nerves in the isolated guinea-pig ileum. *British Journal of Pharmacology*, **103**, 1449–1452.

Tham, T.C.K, Guy, S., Shanks, R.G. and Harron, D.W.G. (1992). Dose-dependent α_1-adrenoceptor antagonist activity of anti-arryhthmic drug, abanoquil (UK-52,046), without reduction in blood pressure. *British Journal of Clinical Pharmacology*, **33**, 405–409.

Tan, S. and Curtis-Prior, P.B. (1983). Characterization of the β-adrenoceptor of the adipose cell of the rat. *International Journal of Obesity*, **7**, 409–414.

Templeton, A.G.B., MacMillan, J., McGrath, J.C., Storey, N.D. and Wilson, V.G. (1989). Evidence for prazosin-resistant, rauwolscine-sensitive α-adrenoceptors mediating contractions in the isolated vascular bed of the rat tail. *British Journal of Pharmacology*, **97**, 563–571.

Tian, W-N., Gupta, S. and Deth, R.C. (1990). Species differences in chlorethylclonidine antagonism at vascular α_1 adrenergic receptors. *Journal of Pharmacology and Experimental Therapeutics*, **253**, 877–883.

Tsujimoto, G., Tsujimoto, A., Suzuki, E. and Hashimoto, K. (1989). Glycogen phosphorylase activation by two different α_1-adrenergic receptor subtypes. Methoxamine selectively stimulates a putative α_1-adrenergic receptor subtype (α_{1A}) that couples with Ca^{2+} influx. *Molecular Pharmacology*, **36**, 166–176.

van der Graaf, P.H., Welsh, N.J., Shankley, N.P. and Black, J.W. (1992). Efficacy of idazoxan at α_1-adrenoceptors in rat aorta and small mesenteric artery. *British Journal of Pharmacology*, **107**, 180P.

van Riper, D.A. and Bevan, J.A. (1991). Evidence that neuropeptide Y and norepinephrine mediate electrical filed stimulated vasoconstriction of rabbit middle cerebral artery. *Circulation Research*, **68**, 568–577.

Vincent, J., Elliott, H.L., Meredith, P.A. and Reid, J.L. (1983). Doxazosin, an α_1-adrenoceptor antagonist: pharmacokinetics and concentration-effect relationships in man. *British Journal of Clinical Pharmacology*, **15**, 719–725.

Vizi, E.S. (1977). Presynaptic modulation of neurochemical transmission. *Progress in Neurobiology*, **12**, 181–290.

Vizi, E.S., Harsing, L.G., Gaal, J., Kaposci, J., Bernath, S. and Somogyi, G.T. (1986). CH-38083, a selective, potent antagonist of α_2-adrenoceptors. *Journal of Pharmacology and Experimental Therapeutics*, **238**, 701–706.

von Euler, U.S. (1946). A specific sympathomimetic ergone in adrenergic nerve fibres (sympathin) and its relation to adrenaline and noradrenaline. *Acta Physiologica Scandanavica*, **12**, 73–97.

von Kügelgen, I. and Starke, K. (1985). Noradrenaline and adenosine triphosphate as cotransmitters of neurogenic vasoconstriction in rabbit mesenteric artery. *Journal of Physiology*, **335**, 609–627.

Vu, H.Q., Budai, D. and Duckles, S.P. (1989). Neuropeptide Y preferentially potentiates response to adrenergic nerve stimulation by increasing rate of contraction. *Journal of Pharmacology and Experimental Therapeutics*, **251**, 852–857.

Waeber, B., Nussberger, J. and Brunner, H.R. (1983). Blood pressure dependency on vasopressin and angiotensin II in prazosin-treated conscious normotensive rats. *Journal of Pharmacology and Experimental Therapeutics*, **225**, 442–446.

Webb, D.J., Seidelin, P.H., Benjamin, N., Collier, J.G. and Struthers, A.D. (1988). Sympathetically mediated vasoconstriction is augmented by angiotensin II in man. *Journal of Hypertension*, **6**, (Suppl. 4), S542–S543.

Weiss, R.J., Webb, R.C. and Smith, C.B. (1983). α_2-adrenoceptors on arterial smooth muscle: selective labelling by [^{3}H]-clonidine. *Journal of Pharmacology and Experimental Therapeutics*, **225**, 599–605.

Weitzell, R., Tanaka, T. and Starke, K. (1979). Pre- and postsynaptic effects of yohimbine stereoisomers on noradrenergic transmission in the pulmonary artery of the rabbit. *Naunyn Schmiedeberg's Archives of Pharmacology*, **308**, 127–136.

Wenham, D. and Marshall, I. (1992). α_1-adrenoceptor subtypes in rat thoracic aorta defined using abanoquil and other selective antagonists. *British Journal of Pharmacology*, **107**, 375P.

Westfall, T.C. (1977). Local regulation of adrenergic neurotransmission. *Physiological Reviews*, **57**, 659–728.

Wilffert, B., Timmermans, P.B.M.W.M. and Van Zwieten, P.A. (1982). Extrasynaptic location of α_2- and non-innervated β_2-adrenoceptors in the vascular system of the pithed normotensive rat. *Journal of Pharmacology and Experimental Therapeutics*, **221**, 762–768.

Willette, R.N., Hieble, J.P. and Sauermilch, C.F. (1991). The role of α adrenoceptor subtypes in sympathetic control of the acral-cutaneous microcirculation. *Journal of Pharmacology and Experimental Therapeutics*, **256**, 599–605.

Wilson, V.G., Brown, C.M. and McGrath, J.C. (1991). Are there more than two types of α-adrenoceptors involved in physiological responses? *Experimental Physiology*, **76**, 317–346.

Wong, P.C., Reilly, T.M. and Timmermans, P.B.M.W.M. (1989). Effects of a monoclonal antibody to angiotensin II on haemodynamic response to noradrenergic stimulation in pithed rats. *Hypertension*, **14**, 488–497.

Wong, P.C., Reilly, T.M. and Timmermans, P.B.M.W.M. (1990). Angiotensin II monoclonal antibody: blood pressure effects in normotensive and spontaneously hypertensive rats. *European Journal of Pharmacology*, **186**, 353–358.

Wong-Dusting, H.K. and Rand, M.J. (1988). Pre- and postjunctional effects of neuropeptide Y on rabbit isolated ear artery. *Clinical Experimental Pharmacology and Physiology*, **15**, 411–418.

Woodman, O.L. (1987). The role of α_1- and α_2-adrenoceptor in the coronary vasoconstrictor responses to neuronally released and exogenous noradrenaline in the dog. *Naunyn Schmiedeberg's Archives of Pharmacology*, **336**, 1161–1168.

Wright, I.K., Blaylock, N.A., Kendall, D.A. and Wilson, V.G. (1994). The relationship between density of α-adrenoceptor binding sites and contractile responses in several porcine isolated blood vessels. *British Journal of Pharmacology*, **114**, 678–688.

Yamaguchi, I. and Kopin, I.J. (1980). Differential inhibition of α_1- and α_2-adrenoceptor-mediated pressor responses in pithed rats. *Journal of Pharmacology and Experimental Therapeutics*, **214**, 275–281.

Yamomoto, R., Cline, W.H. and Takasaki, K. (1988). Reassessment of the blocking activity of prazosin at low and high concentrations on sympathetic neurotransmission in the isolated mesenteric vasculature of rats. *Journal of Autonomic Pharmacology*, **8**, 303–309.

Yoshioka, M., Togashi, H., Abe, M., Ikeda, T., Matsumoto, M. and Saito, H. (1990). Central sympathoinhibitory action of a new type of α_1-adrenoceptor antagonist YM-167, in rats. *Journal of Pharmacology and Experimental Therapeutics*, **253**, 427–431.

Zimmerman, B.G. (1962). Effect of acute sympathectomy on responses to angiotensin and norepinephrine. *Circulations Research*, **6**, 27–38.

Zimmerman, B.G. (1979). Adrenergic facilitation by angiotensin II: does it serve a physiological function? *Clinical Sciences*, **60**, 343–348.

2 Cholinergic Vasodilator Mechanisms

Christopher Bell

Department of Physiology, University of Dublin, Trinity College, Dublin 2, Ireland

Despite the fact that acetylcholine is the most well-established neurotransmitter in the mammalian nervous system, there is still doubt about the functional distribution of cholinergic vasodilator nerves. Assessment of the current evidence indicates strongly that there are cholinergic vasodilator supplies, in man and some other species, to resistance vessels of skeletal muscle and the erectile tissue of the penis. Less extensive evidence supports innervation of the vasculature to the uterus, the cerebral circulation and the coronary arterioles. An innervation to exocrine glandular vessels may also exist. In no case, however, is the physiological importance of these nerves established.

KEY WORDS: acetylcholine; vasodilatation; acetylcholinesterase; choline acetyltransferase; erection; exercise; cerebral arteries; coronary arteries; pregnancy.

INTRODUCTION

When I first began studying the autonomic nervous system, the conceptual extent of vasomotor nerves was admirably simple. We knew that vasoconstriction was caused by the release of noradrenaline from vasoconstrictor nerves that supplied all vascular beds, and that some beds also received inputs from cholinergic vasodilator nerves. Most of these were parasympathetic, and their activation was related to local functional hyperaemia of the tissue concerned: this type of cholinergic control was physiologically of most importance in the external genitalia and in exocrine glands. A second set of cholinergic vasodilator neurons originated from the sympathetic nervous system and selectively supplied precapillary vessels in skeletal muscle: these fibres were activated by emotionally orientated cerebral arousal and were probably important in guaranteeing adequate muscle perfusion during the first few seconds of violent exercise. Although certain experimental and clinical findings could not readily be reconciled with this framework, such observations were accepted as denoting exceptions to a generality.

Thirty years later, none of the above certainties remain. The presiding views are that a large number of neuroeffector messengers in addition to noradrenaline and acetylcholine

[ACh] are involved in the regulation of regional vascular resistance, and that at least many of the responses originally attributed to cholinergic nerves are due to other mechanisms. In this critical climate, it might be argued that a survey of cholinergic vasomotor mechanisms has no place. However, it has to be remembered that the progress of ACh from preeminent social status to social outcast as a vasomotor transmitter may, in the future, apply just as much to any of the novel substances for which there is so much current enthusiasm, generally with rather less concrete evidence. Thus, continued monitoring of the status of vasomotor ACh serves as a paradigm for attribution of physiological roles to other substances. It also provides a salutary reminder of the continued need to satisfy the classical criteria of neurotransmitter status (see, for example, Paton, 1958; Curtis, 1961; Bell, 1983a).

The present discussion will be restricted to examination of direct vasomotor innervation by vasodilator cholinergic nerves. The phenomenon of cholinergically mediated vasoconstriction, which has been confirmed only for certain intraabdominal vessels, and which appears to be due to outgrowth of intestinal smooth muscle elements into the vasculature (see Bell, 1969a; Nakazato et al., 1982), will not be considered. Nor will details of the postjunctional mechanism of action of neurogenic ACh, which is addressed authoritatively in other recent reviews (Duckles, 1988; Murray, 1990). This review was completed in 1991.

CRITERIA FOR IDENTIFICATION OF CHOLINERGIC NERVES

MORPHOLOGICAL CRITERIA

Morphological recognition of cholinergic neurons is more contentious than that of most other neuron types, because there is no method capable of directly visualizing endogenous ACh. The nearest available alternatives are staining of acetylcholinesterase (AChE), a hydrolytic enzyme that is involved in normal ACh metabolism and is bound to the membranes of cholinergic neurons and, more recently, immunolocalization of choline acetyltransferase (ChAT), the cytoplasmic enzyme responsible for the synthesis of ACh.

Localization of AChE was regarded for many years as a specific marker for cholinergic neurons, on the basis that the enzyme was found in appreciable concentrations only within these cells (see Gerebtzoff, 1959; Koelle, 1963). However, there is no doubt that, under some circumstances, neurons are stained for AChE that are not functionally cholinergic. In certain species, distinction between AChE in the major neuron classes may be less dramatic than in others: with respect to the rat, in particular, numerous reports exist of AChE staining in known noradrenergic cells. There is some doubt as to whether this does in fact reflect the widespread presence of AChE in rat nerves or whether it is due to non-specificity of staining in some studies (see Bell, 1974). As well as this extreme example, low levels of AChE are certainly present in many neuron classes, and a large number of published reports involve AChE staining obtained with reaction times far in excess of those that are likely to be selective. Where this consideration has made interpretation of the data especially ambiguous, the results have not been considered in this chapter.

Despite these reservations, histochemical visualization of AChE is still a valuable screening technique. For at least most species, including man, staining for the minimum period necessary to visualize known cholinergic elements (such as the somatic motor endplate) identifies nerve populations that are not noradrenergic or sensory in character. However, there remains the uncertainty of whether these cells represent a functionally homogeneous group, limiting the analytical precision of the technique.

While AChE appears to be distributed in a variety of cells in addition to cholinergic neurons, albeit in different concentrations, ChAT is generally thought to be restricted to cells that actively synthesize ACh. At least in theory, therefore, use of antibodies against ChAT should be a technique for selective morphological recognition of cholinergic neurons. In practice, the ChAT antibodies that are available at present have proved to be more generally useful in the brain than in the periphery, due to a lack of peripheral binding. While this may, of course, be a confirmation of the absence of peripheral cholinergic neurons, the lack of binding in Auerbach's plexus of the gut, where there is good functional evidence for cholinergic innervation, suggests that other problems, such as epitopic variation, are involved. Nevertheless, ChAT localization remains in theory the ideal morphological cholinergic marker, once these uncertainties are resolved.

Early studies of peptide localization in various peripheral neurons suggested that the presence of vasoactive intestinal peptide (VIP) might constitute another specific morphological marker for cholinergic neurons. Thus, for instance, VIP is found in the sudomotor neurons, but not in the noradrenergic vasomotor neurons of sympathetic ganglia (Lundberg *et al.*, 1980), and electrical activation of secretomotor parasympathetic axons supplying salivary glands causes overflow of VIP into the venous effluent (Lundberg *et al.*, 1980; Andersson *et al.*, 1982). More recent data, on the other hand, suggest that there is not an absolute correlation of ChAT and VIP. Leblanc, Trimmer and Landis (1987) found in rat ciliary ganglion that every neuron contained ChAT, but most were VIP negative. By contrast, in the sphenopalatine ganglion, a large proportion of ChAT-containing cells also contained VIP. Correlation of the distribution of VIP with that of ChAT in cerebral vasomotor nerves (Saito, Wu and Lee, 1985) showed that ChAT immunoreactivity was predominantly in large axon bundles, while VIP was predominantly in fine varicose fibres. Both groups of axons contained AChE. It is not clear whether this difference in distribution reflects the presence of two fibre populations, or is due to the relative restriction of ChAT to preterminal axons and that of VIP to terminal axons.

At present, there are no techniques for ultrastructural identification of cholinergic axons analogous to the combination of the chromaffin reaction and 5- or 6-hydroxydopamine loading that provides easy discrimination of catecholaminergic axon profiles (see, for instance, Ferguson, Ryan and Bell, 1988). While cholinergic axon vesicles can be predicted to not take up 5- or 6-hydroxydopamine and therefore to be electron lucent after this treatment, an axon profile lacking dense-cored vesicles could represent one of a number of different neuron types, sensory as well as autonomic (Ferguson and Bell, 1988). Ultrastructural localization of AChE has proved a useful confirmatory test (Robinson and Bell, 1967; Esterhuizen *et al.*, 1968; Graham, Lever and Spriggs, 1968; Bell, 1969b), although it has the same notional limitations as have been discussed above for light microscopic studies. Ultrastructural demonstration of ChAT should prove more definitive, but the difficulties in the preservation of enzyme immunoreactivity have so far limited its application.

BIOCHEMICAL CRITERIA

Traditionally, tissue activity of ChAT, active tissue uptake of radiolabelled choline via a hemicholinium-sensitive pathway and the subsequent release of radiolabelled ACh by electrical nerve stimulation have all been taken as good evidence of the presence of cholinergic axons (see, for instance, Fonnum, 1973; Wikberg, 1977; Jope, 1979). All these phenomena are probably of considerable more use than is the tissue level of ACh itself as indices of a cholinergic innervation. Nevertheless, it must be remembered that synthesis of ACh occurs in some non-neural cell and therefore that biochemical data, in isolation, may be misleading (Welsch, 1977). This area has been discussed in detail by Duckles (1988) and the interested reader is referred to her review.

PHARMACOLOGICAL CRITERIA

In catecholaminergic neurons, a wide spectrum of pharmacological agents can be used to manipulate neurotransmitter synthesis, storage and release. In addition, selective neurotoxins such as guanethidine and 6-hydroxydopamine can be used to produce functional and structural destruction of terminal axons or of complete neurons. By contrast, pharmacological manipulation of cholinergic neuronal function is fairly restricted at present, with the most generally useful tools being those that interfere with postsynaptic receptor binding (the atropine-like or antimuscarinic blockers) or with enzymic breakdown by AChE (the antiAChE agents).

To some extent, the relative lack of pharmacological tools for analysis of cholinergic function is balanced by the fact that the postsynaptic antagonists available for application to muscarinic receptors are considerably more selective than are the receptor blockers for any other neurotransmitter. Substances such as hyoscine and atropine, although they have non-specific actions at concentrations in the order of micrograms/ml, can be demonstrated to completely prevent effector responses to postganglionic cholinergic nerve stimulation at concentrations several orders of magnitude below this. It is, therefore, paradoxical that one point of greatest contention concerning the existence of cholinergic vasomotor nerves has centred on the fact that some neurogenic responses of putatively cholinergic origin are partially or entirely resistant to antagonism by antimuscarinic agents.

Atropine resistance of autonomically mediated responses thought to involve parasympathetic (and therefore, by inference, cholinergic) nerves was first reported for the bladder, where in most species the excitatory response to pelvic nerve activation is virtually unaffected by atropine and similar drugs, although it is potentiated by antiAChE agents (Langley and Anderson, 1895; Chesher and Thorp, 1965; Hukovic, Rand and Vanov, 1965; Carpenter, 1981). Subsequent findings have shown similar characteristics of the penile corpora cavernosa, where neither the direct relaxatory effect of pelvic nerve stimulation nor reflex erection are substantially or reproducibly reduced by antimuscarinic agents (Dorr and Brody, 1967; Brindley, 1986; Carati, Creed and Keogh, 1987; and others).

The first theory put forward to explain this apparent paradox was the proximity theory of Dale and Gaddum (1930), which envisaged a situation in which the close apposition of axon terminals and postsynaptic membrane led to extremely high concentrations of transmitter in the region of the receptors, and in which antagonist drugs were inactive because of the constraints of competitive kinetics, and possibly also because of diffusional barriers. This proposal is compatible with later observations that, in contradistinction to the atropine resistance of normal nerve-mediated responses, the enhancement of response produced by antiAChE treatment is reversed entirely by atropine (Chesher and Thorp, 1965; Hukovic, Rand and Vanov, 1965). Furthermore, recent denervation studies in rat bladder have shown that, during early Wallerian degeneration, when nerve terminals are known to start retracting, the motor response of the bladder becomes highly sensitive to atropine (Hammarström and Sjöstrand, 1984). Nevertheless, the basic refractoriness of a response to atropine-like agents must still raise a serious doubt as to whether the neuroeffector junction involved does in fact utilize ACh as a neurotransmitter.

A further complication to interpretation of pharmacological data involving cholinoceptive agents is the possibility that atropine-sensitive vasodilator responses may be due to inhibition of tonic noradrenergic constriction, rather than to direct dilatation of smooth muscle. Evidence for the presence of inhibitory muscarinic receptors on noradrenergic axon terminals was first put forward over 20 years ago (Haeusler et al., 1968; Lindmar, Löffelholz and Muscholl, 1968; Rand and Varma, 1970) and has recently been confirmed electrophysiologically by Kuriyama and his colleagues (Kuriyama and Suzuki, 1981). While the participation of these presynaptic receptors must be considered a possible source of interference in studies of putative cholinergic vasomotor mechanism *in vivo*, they are less likely to interfere with *in vitro* experimentation, because tissue treatment with sympatholytic drugs is commonly used to prevent vasoconstrictor responses to field stimulation.

ASSESSMENT OF CURRENT STATUS

SKELETAL MUSCLE

Pharmacologically, extremely convincing evidence exists for a powerful cholinergic innervation to the precapillary resistance vessels of limb skeletal muscle in cat and dog. Electrical activation of specific pathways in forebrain and midbrain, or of the peripheral sympathetic trunk, leads, in animals pretreated with sympatholytics, to substantial muscle vasodilatation which is completely abolished by low doses of atropine methonitrate or similar, peripherally active, antimuscarinic agents (Bülbring and Burn, 1935; Eliasson, Lindgren and Uvnäs, 1952; Abrahams, Hilton and Zbrozyna, 1964; Lang et al., 1976). Nevertheless, the mediation of this vasodilator action via postganglionic sympathetic axons has never been definitively confirmed by morphological techniques. Although there are several reports of AChE-positive nerve fibres associated with skeletal muscle of the tongue (El-Rakhawy and Bourne, 1961; Bell and Burnstock, 1971), only one report exists of AChE-positive fibres in limb muscle (Bolme and Fuxe, 1970).

The pathway through the forebrain and midbrain that mediates the vasodilator response is known to be close to that which is associated with the 'fright, flight or fight' reaction in cats (Abrahams et al., 1964). Later studies have, however, shown that functional activation of vasodilator responses is more complex than this geographical correlation might suggest. In an elegant series of experiments using chronically instrumented cats, Zanchetti's group showed that the cholinergic outflow to the hindlimb could be activated in two ways. During generalized alerting prior to exercise there was a bilateral vasodilatation and, coincident with the initial movements of motor patterns associated with aggression or avoidance, there was selective dilatation in the working limb (Mancia, Baccelli and Zanchetti, 1972; Ellison and Zanchetti, 1973). Somewhat similar experiments in conscious dogs have demonstrated cholinergic vasodilatation at the onset of exercise in response to conditioned stimuli (Bolme and Novotny, 1969). In this study, however, it could not be determined whether the response was bilateral or unilateral. In all these studies the doses of atropine used were low, and not likely to have been acting non-specifically, but in no case were the animals pretreated with sympatholytics, so it must be considered possible that the cholinergically mediated vasodilatation involved prejunctional rather than postjunctional actions (see Pharmacological Criteria).

Bülbring and Burn (1936) found that sympathetic trunk stimulation in hare and monkey did not elicit the somatic limb vasodilatation seen in cats and dogs, and Uvnäs and colleagues (Uvnäs, 1966; Bolme et al., 1970) were unable to find central pathways in non-human primates that corresponded to the ones that evoked similar responses in cats and dogs. Similar negative results for monkey were reported by Schramm, Honig and Bignall (1971), who could demonstrate vasodilator effects of adrenal medullary activation due to central stimulation, but could not obtain evidence for vasodilator nerves. However, studies of normal human volunteers have demonstrated clearly that emotionally oriented arousal produces a forearm vasodilatation that is at least partially reversed by peripheral administration of atropine (Blair et al., 1959; Fencl et al., 1959). The characteristics of the systemic circulatory responses elicited in these studies, together with later findings, indicate that the atropine-insensitive portion of the vasodilator response can be attributed to β-adrenoceptor activation due to adrenal medullary secretion (Greenfield, 1966). A more recent study has extended these findings and provided a more complete parallel with the data from cat and dog. During isometric forearm exercise, the onset of contraction is associated with a contralateral, atropine-sensitive vasodilatation (Sanders, Mark and Ferguson, 1989). While all these observations in humans are consistent with vasodilator inputs to muscle resistance vessels, the possibility must be borne in mind, as in the animal studies, that the atropine-sensitive effects observed could be due to inhibition of sympathetic tone rather than to an action on the vascular smooth muscle.

Although the pharmacological data outlined above comprise moderately unequivocal evidence for the existence of sympathetic cholinergic innervation to muscle vasculature, there is still absolutely no evidence for any physiological role for these nerves. The association of their activation with central pathways mediating arousal led to suggestions that they may exist in order to provide optimal nutritive perfusion of somatic muscles during the first few seconds of emotionally orientated exercise, before interstitial metabolites have accumulated sufficiently to induce metabolic hyperaemia (Abrahams et al., 1964; Folkow and Neil, 1971). Zanchetti's observation that vasodilatation was restricted to exercising muscle during a variety of alerting responses (Ellison and Zanchetti, 1973) suggests that they could also help to ensure perfusion of small muscles during intermittent activation that never leads to appreciable metabolite build-up, such as may occur in the hand of a musician (Bell, 1983b). However, there are no data whatsoever to demonstrate that either of these phenomena, if they do normally occur in man, confer any functional advantage. Although it would be possible to assess whether or not efficiency of some types of muscle activation was altered by the administration of antimuscarinic agents, the complexity of neuroendocrine responses to emotion and to associated exercise makes it likely that no useful conclusions could be reached.

UTERUS

The extrinsic (parametrial) uterine arterial supply in guinea-pig is densely innervated by pelvic axons that contain high levels of AChE (Bell, 1968) and release ACh on electrical stimulation (Bell, 1970). Preconstricted arteries from virgin guinea-pigs show no vasodilator response to ACh, although they dilate in the presence of other relaxatory agents and, after treatment with sympatholytics, respond to electrical field stimulation with a weak vasodilatation that is entirely resistant to antimuscarinic drugs. By contrast, arteries from guinea-pigs during the latter half of pregnancy, or after chronic treatment with oestradiol, respond to ACh with marked vasodilatation (Bell, 1968, 1973a; Bell and Coffey, 1982). Sympatholytic-treated vessels from pregnant animals also exhibit a marked vasodilator response to field stimulation that is potentiated by antiAChE agents and attenuated, but not abolished, by hyoscine (Bell, 1968). These data suggest strongly the existence of a cholinergic nerve supply to the parametrial vasculature, although there appears to be an additional non-cholinergic input. Perivascular nerves staining for AChE have also been seen around the parametrial vessels of dog and pig (Bell, 1971) and, in dog, these vessels exhibit hyoscine-sensitive vasodilator responses to ACh and to field stimulation in both pregnant and non-pregnant animals (Ryan, Clark and Brody, 1974). The parametrial arteries of rat, rabbit, pig, cow and sheep contain no AChE-positive nerves (Bell, 1971) and little is known about vasomotor response to nerve stimulation in these species, although it has been reported for sheep that parasympathetic stimulation *in vivo* has no effect in either pregnant or non-pregnant animals (Greiss *et al.*, 1967). The situation in primates is confused. In the macaque, arteries from non-pregnant individuals dilate to ACh but exhibit a hysocine-resistant vasodilator response to field stimulation (Bell, 1976). Arteries from non-pregnant women, by contrast, show no vasodilator response to either ACh or field stimulation (Bell, 1969c). However, AChE-containing nerves are associated with the vessels in both species.

The observations in guinea-pig that parametrial vessels dilate to ACh only during pregnancy, or after oestrogen priming, suggest that, if cholinergic vasodilator neurons have a functional role in control of uterine vascular resistance, this is associated with the maintenance of foetoplacental blood flow (Bell, 1974). In agreement with this, administration of atropine to guinea-pigs in late pregnancy was observed to result in constriction of the parametrial vasculature (Bell and Brown, 1971). Furthermore, animals in which pelvic nerve section had been performed prior to cenception or that had been given atropine methonitrate during the last half of the pregnancy, showed foetal retardation and an increased incidence of stillbirths (Bell, 1973b). In dogs also, pelvic parasympathectomy during pregnancy has been reported to cause foetal death (Toth, McEwan and Shabanah, 1964). All these observations could, however, have explanations quite independent of any effects on uterine blood flow. No direct documentation of a tonic vasodilator influence on parametrial resistance exists; nor are any data available on the effects of antimuscarinic agents on uterine flow or foetal outcome in man (but see Bell, 1973b).

PENIS

The traditional view of penile erection being mediated by cholinergic vasodilator inputs was primarily due to the known importance of pelvic parasympathetic pathways in erectile function. On the other hand, evidence concerning the involvement of ACh in the vascular processes of erection is much more confused. In both animals and man, atropine and similar drugs have usually been reported not to prevent erections (Langley and Anderson, 1895; Dorr and Brody, 1967; Brindley and Craggs, 1975; Brindley, 1986). However, several analyses of the progression of erection have confirmed both for dog (Andersson, Bloom and Mellander, 1984; Carati, Creed and Keogh, 1987; Vardi, Belur and Siroky, 1987) and man (Bancroft and Bell, 1985) that establishment of full tumescence involves two separate processes; arterial vasodilatation and engorgement of the corporal spaces. For dog, while the arterial response is at least predominantly resistant to atropine, the corporal response is abolished or considerably attenuated by atropine. AChE-positive nerve fibres have been described within penile tissue of man and several other species (Shirai, Sazaki and Rikimaru, 1972; McConnell, Benson and Wood, 1979) and Blanco et al. (1988) have demonstrated the existence of ACh synthesis and release from isolated strips of human corpus cavernosum. Moreover, Saenz de Tejada and colleagues (1988) reported that these strips responded to field stimulation with relaxations that were enhanced by antiAChE treatment and attenuated, although not abolished, by atropine.

On balance, the available data indicate that cholinergic inputs probably do contribute to erection in man and in dog. The controversy concerning atropine sensitivity may be due in part to different criteria for assessing erection — for example, arterial blood flow versus intracavernosal pressure, tissue tumescence versus penile diameter, and cavernosal as opposed to spongiosal engorgement. We have noted, in an extensive series of normal human volunteers, that the absolute and temporal relationship of arterial vasodilatation (as assessed by transcutaneous photometry) and corporal engorgement (as assessed by penile diameter changes) varied considerably between subjects (Bancroft and Bell, 1985). It is possible that this also has contributed to the uncertainties evident in the literature: if active relaxation in corporal tissue constitutes a prominent component of erection only in some individuals, then only these individuals will respond dramatically to atropine blockade.

CEPHALIC VASCULATURE

Numerous reports have documented the innervation of cerebral and pial arterial vessels by AChE-positive nerve fibres in a variety of species (see, for example, Kobayashi et al., 1983; Hara, Hamill and Jacobowitz, 1985; Saito, Wu and Lee, 1985; Estrada et al., 1988). As well, biochemical evidence for the existence of perivascular cholinergic mechanisms has been strengthened by findings of VIP-containing axons (Hara, Hamill and Jacobowitz, 1985; Saito, Wu and Lee, 1985), of ChAT activity (Duckles, 1981; Bevan et al., 1982a;

Estrada, Hamel and Krause, 1983; Saito, Wu and Lee, 1985; Estrada *et al.*, 1988), choline uptake and ACh release (Florence and Bevan, 1979; Duckles, 1981; Hamel *et al.*, 1986).

Some studies have reported, for several species, the presence of active vasodilator responses to field stimulation of isolated segments of various cephalic arteries, which are abolished by atropine (see Bevan *et al.*, 1982b; Brayden and Bevan, 1985). Conversely, other studies, using closely similar preparations and techniques, have reported complete resistance to atropine-induced attenuation of these vasodilator responses (Lee *et al.*, 1978; Duckles, 1979; Lee, 1982). In addition, Duckles (1980) noted that, while β-bungarotoxin abolished the neurogenic release of ACh from cerebral arterial preparations, it did not affect the relaxatory response similarly. It is difficult to draw any useful conclusions from these contradictory data.

The putatively cholinergic pathways that have been described histochemically have their origins in the cranial parasympathetic ganglia. There are also additional data that suggest the possibility of intracerebral cholinergic projections to the cerebral vasculature. In several animal species, electrical stimulation of the cerebellar fastigial nucleus has been shown to cause a short-latency, widespread vasodilatation in the cerebral cortex, which is not secondary to local metabolic activation (McKee, Denn and Stone, 1976; Nakai *et al.*, 1983). A similar response has been demonstrated to stimulation of the basal nucleus of Meynert (Sato and Sato, 1990). Both types of response have been shown to be attenuated by atropine (Arneric *et al.*, 1986; Sato and Sato, 1990). There is, however, some doubt as to whether or not these effects are due to direct vasomotor innervation of the cerebral vessel by cholinergic nerves. The vasodilator response to stimulation of the basal nucleus is abolished only when atropine is administered in combination with a nicotinic antagonist (Sato and Sato, 1990), while that to cerebellar stimulation is reduced considerably more by systemically administered atropine than by atropine applied to the cortical surface (Arneric *et al.*, 1986). These observations suggest that the cholinergic synapse involved may be an interneuronal one within the ascending pathways being activated, rather than a final vasomotor one. It is of some interest that a similar, atropine-sensitive cortical vasodilator response has been reported to be elicited by intravenous administration of thyrotropin-releasing hormone (Inanami *et al.*, 1988).

CORONARY VASCULATURE

Localization of substantial amounts of AChE to non-sympathetic perivascular fibres around the coronary arteries has been documented for a variety of species, including man (Navaratnam and Palkama, 1965; Schenk and El-Badawi, 1968; Malor, Griffin and Taylor, 1973; Denn and Stone, 1976; Pillay and Reid, 1982). A number of physiological studies in anaesthetized dogs have reported coronary vasodilatation following vagal nerve stimulation (Berne, DeGuest and Levy, 1965; Daggett *et al.*, 1967; Feigl, 1969; Tiedt and Religa, 1979), which is attenuated by atropine (Daggett *et al.*, 1967; Feigl, 1969). In addition, activation of intracardiac chemoreceptors in both anaesthetized and conscious dogs has been reported to induce reflex, atropine-sensitive vasodilatation (Feigl, 1975; Zucker *et al.*, 1987). The same fibres appear to be activated by an elevation of the carotid sinus pressure (Ito and Feigl, 1985). Any physiological role of these fibres remains obscure. It is also important to note that a number of other studies have been unable to demonstrate vasodilator responses to the same stimuli (see Kalsner, 1989 for references). In view of the experimental and physiological complexity of separating specific vasomotor neural influences from metabolic and mechanical constraints on coronary perfusion, the cynic could equally well argue for either the positive or the negative findings being artefactual (see Van Winckle and Feigl, 1989 for one presentation of this scenario).

EXOCRINE GLANDS

The difficulty of divorcing metabolic influences from directly mediated neural inputs, mentioned above for the coronary vasculature, presents an even greater interpretative problem with respect to cholinergically innervated exocrine glands. Activation of the neural inputs will necessarily result in recruitment of glandular metabolic processes that themselves cause local vasodilatation, and any distinction between these effects and the action of specific vasodilator fibres relies on the possibility that the two modalities of input have different frequency dependencies or different susceptibilities to pharmacological agents.

In the case of the salivary gland, which is the exocrine tissue that has been most fully analysed, there is good ultrastructural evidence for a direct parasympathetic innervation to the vasculature (Garrett, 1966), but the identity of these nerves is uncertain. As long ago as 1872, Heidenhain noted that atropine abolished secretory responses of the cat salivary gland to parasympathetic nerve stimulation without abolishing the concomitant increase in glandular blood flow, and his finding has been confirmed many times since for this species (e.g. Fox and Hilton, 1958; Schachter and Beilenson, 1968). However, vascular responses in some other species are sensitive to atropine (Morley, Schachter and Smaje, 1966). In the cat, it has been suggested, because of the atropine resistance of the vasodilator response to parasympathetic activation, that this is mediated by neurally released VIP rather than by ACh (Lundberg et al., 1980; Andersson et al., 1982). On the other hand, examination of the relevant data casts some doubt on the physiological relevance of these atropine-resistant responses. Fox and Hilton (1958) and Skinner and Webster (1968) noted that the vasodilatation following stimulation of the chorda tympani at submaximal voltages was highly sensitive to atropine, while that initiated by stimulation at supramaximal voltages was predominantly atropine resistant. Similarly, the experiments of Lundberg et al. (1980) and Andersson et al. (1982) showed that vascular responses to low frequencies of nerve stimulation, such as are likely to occur under natural conditions, were reduced considerably by atropine, and that the atropine-resistant response was elicited primarily at supraphysiological frequencies (see Bell, 1983a). The evidence is therefore consistent with some involvement of ACh in functional vasodilatation, although its importance, relative to that of other factors, is not known. To my knowledge, no studies have assessed the atropine sensitivity of vasodilator responses to reflexly induced activation of exocrine glands.

Shen et al. (1989) recently reported that stimulation of ChAT-positive neurons in isolated preparations of guinea-pig submucous plexus induced vasodilatation of submucosal arterioles: this response was enhanced by topical antiAChE treatment and abolished by topical atropine. Such a response could be related to an absorptive or to a secretory mucosal function of the gut.

LUNG

Sparse AChE-containing nerve fibres, distinct from bronchomotor nerves, have been seen around intrapulmonary arterial and arteriolar vessels in cat, dog and rabbit (Daly and Hebb, 1966; Fillenz, 1970; El-Bermani, Bloomquist and Montvilo, 1982), although they have been reported to be absent from the equivalent vessels of man (Partanen *et al.*, 1982). Ultrastructurally, non-catecholaminergic axon profiles containing small, electron-lucent vesicles have been described around pulmonary arteries in cat, but no AChE localization was carried out (Knight *et al.*, 1981).

Early functional studies, in particular by Daly and Hebb, suggested the existence of vagal inhibitory effects on pulmonary vascular resistance in the dog, but the difficulties of excluding the effects of concomitant bronchomotor activation prevented any definite conclusions being drawn (Daly and Hebb, 1966). More recently, a study in anaesthetized cats has been reported that strongly suggests the existence of cholinergically mediated vagal inputs to the pulmonary resistance vessels in this species (Nandiwada, Hyman and Kadowitz, 1983). There is, however, no indication of whether this response can be elicited reflexly, nor is there any indication as to what useful purpose it might serve.

CONCLUSIONS

On balance, there is good evidence that vasodilator cholinergic nerve fibres directly supply the resistance beds of some skeletal muscles, and supply some components of the erectile system of the penis in man and certain other species. Sparser evidence supports similar inputs to the uterine circulation, to resistance vessels in the cerebral and coronary circulations, and to the nutritive precapillary beds of exocrine glands. In no case, however, is it possible at present to estimate the physiological advantage, if any, conferred by these nerves. The state of the evidence is summarized in Table 2.1.

TABLE 2.1

Ratings of the extent to which different criteria support the existence of cholinergic vasodilator nerves in specific areas. See text for further details

Organ	Species	Morphology	Pharmacology	Reflex activation	Functional importance
Skeletal muscle	Cat, dog	Poor	Excellent	Good	?
	Man	?	Moderate	Moderate	?
Uterus	Guinea-pig, dog	Good	Excellent	?	?
	Man	Moderate	?	?	?
Penis	Dog	Good	Moderate	Poor	Poor
	Man	Good	Good	Poor	Poor
Cerebral vessels	Rat, cat	Excellent	Moderate	?	?
Coronary vessels	Dog, primates	Moderate	Moderate	Moderate	?
Exocrine glands	Various	Good	Moderate	?	?

Excellent: convincing evidence by classical criteria;
Good: convincing evidence with less extensive documentation;
Moderate: evidence sparse, or contradictory in different studies;
Poor: predominantly negative evidence;
?: no known data available.

ACKNOWLEDGEMENTS

Original research cited in the text was supported by the National Health and Medical Research Council of Australia, the National Heart Foundation of Australia and the Helen M. Schutt Trust. I thank Rachel Dowling for assistance in preparation of the manuscript.

REFERENCES

Abrahams, V.C., Hilton, S.M. and Zbrozyna, A. (1964). Role of active muscle vasodilatation in the alerting stage of the defence reaction. *Journal of Physiology, London*, **171**, 189–202.

Andersson, P.O., Bloom, S.R., Edwards, A.V. and Järhult, J. (1982). Effects of stimulation of the chorda tympani in bursts on submaxillary responses in the cat. *Journal of Physiology, London*, **322**, 469–481.

Andersson, P.O., Bloom, S.R. and Mellander, S. (1984). Haemodynamics of pelvic nerve induced penile erection in the dog: possible mediation by vasoactive intestinal peptide. *Journal of Physiology, London*, **350**, 209–224.

Arneric, S.P., Iadecola, C., Honig, M.A., Underwood, M.D. and Reis, D.J. (1986). Local cholinergic mechanisms mediate the cortical vasodilatation elicited by electrical stimulation of the fastigial nucleus. *Acta Physiologica Scandinavica*, Supplement **552**, 70–73.

Bancroft, J. and Bell, C. (1985). Simultaneous recording of penile diameter and penile arterial pulse during laboratory-based erotic stimulation in normal subjects. *Journal of Psychosomatic Research*, **29**, 303–313.

Bell, C. (1968). Dual vasoconstrictor and vasodilator innervation of the uterine arterial supply in the guinea pig. *Circulation Research*, **23**, 279–289.

Bell, C. (1969a). Indirect cholinergic vasomotor control of intestinal blood flow in the domestic chicken. *Journal of Physiology, London*, **205**, 317–327.

Bell, C. (1969b). Fine structural localization of acetylcholinesterase at a cholinergic vasodilator nerve–arterial smooth muscle synapse. *Circulation Research*, **24**, 61–70.

Bell, C. (1969c). Evidence for dual innervation of the human extrinsic uterine arteries. *Journal of Obstetrics and Gynaecology of the British Commonwealth*, **76**, 1123–1128.

Bell, C. (1970). Effects of circulating oestrogen on function of the cholinergic dilator nerves supplying the guinea-pig uterine artery. *British Journal of Pharmacology*, **39**, 190P.

Bell, C. (1971). Distribution of cholinergic vasomotor nerves to the parametrial arteries of some laboratory and domestic animals. *Journal of Reproduction and Fertility*, **27**, 53–58.

Bell, C. (1973a). Oestrogen-induced sensitization of the uterine artery of the guinea-pig to acetylcholine. *British Journal of Pharmacology*, **49**, 595–601.

Bell, C. (1973b). Obstetric prevention of mental retardation. *British Medical Journal*, **II**, 246.

Bell, C. (1974). Control of uterine blood flow in pregnancy. *Medical Biology*, **52**, 219–228.

Bell, C. (1976). Innervation and responses to vasoactive drugs of the extrinsic uterine artery of the macaque. *Cardiovascular Research*, **10**, 482–486.

Bell, C. (1983a). Problems and ambiguities in the identification of autonomic neurotransmitters. *Journal of the Autonomic Nervous System*, **8**, 79–87.

Bell, C. (1983b). Vasodilator neurones supplying skin and skeletal muscle of the limbs. *Journal of the Autonomic Nervous System*, **7**, 257–262.

Bell, C. and Brown, M.J. (1971). Arteriographic evidence for a cholinergic dilator mechanism in uterine hyperaemia of pregnancy in the guinea-pig. *Journal of Reproduction and Fertility*, **27**, 59–65.

Bell, C. and Burnstock, G. (1971). Cholinergic vasomotor neuroeffector junctions. In *Physiology and Pharmacology of Vascular Neuroeffector Systems*, edited by J.A. Bevan, R.J. Furchgott, R.A. Maxwell and A.P. Somlyo, pp. 37–46. Basel: S. Karger.

Bell, C. and Coffey, C. (1982). Factors influencing oestrogen-induced sensitization to acetylcholine of guinea-pig uterine artery. *Journal of Reproduction and Fertility*, **66**, 166–172.

Berne, R.M., DeGuest, H. and Levy, M.N. (1965). Influence of the cardiac nerves on coronary resistance. *American Journal of Physiology*, **208**, 763–769.

Bevan, J.A., Buga, G.M., Florence, V.M., Gonslaves, A. and Snowden, A. (1982a). Distribution of choline acetyltransferase in cerebral and extracranial arteries of the cat. *Circulation Research*, **50**, 470–476.

Bevan, J.A., Buga, G.M., Jope, C.A., Jope, R.S. and Moritoki, H. (1982b). Further evidence for a muscarinic component to the neural vasodilator innervation of cerebral and cranial extracerebral arteries of the cat. *Circulation Research*, **51**, 421–429.

Blair, D.A., Glover, W.E., Greenfield, A.D.M. and Roddie, I.C. (1959). Excitation of cholinergic vasodilator nerves to human skeletal muscle during emotional stress. *Journal of Physiology, London*, **148**, 633–647.

Blanco, R., Saenz de Tejada, I., Goldstein, I., Krane, R.J., Wotiz, H.H. and Cohen, R.A. (1988). Cholinergic neurotransmission in human corpus cavernosum. II. Acetylcholine synthesis. *American Journal of Physiology*, **254**, H468–H472.

Bolme, P. and Fuxe, R. (1970). Adrenergic and cholinergic nerve terminals in skeletal muscle vessels. *Acta Physiologica Scandinavica*, **78**, 52–59.

Bolme, P. and Novotny, J. (1969). Conditioned reflex activation of the sympathetic cholinergic vasodilator nerves in the dog. *Acta Physiologica Scandinavica*, **77**, 58–67.

Bolme, P., Novotny, J., Uvnäs, B. and Wright, P.J. (1970). Species distribution of sympathetic cholinergic vasodilator nerves in skeletal muscle. *Acta Physiologica Scandinavica*, **78**, 60–64.

Brayden, J.E. and Bevan, J.A. (1985). Neurogenic muscarinic vasodilatation in the cat. *Circulation Research*, **56**, 205–221.

Brindley, G.S. (1986). Pilot experiments on the actions of drugs injected into the human corpus cavernosum penis. *British Journal of Pharmacology*, **87**, 495–500.

Brindley, G.S. and Craggs, M.D. (1975). The effect of atropine on the urinary bladder of the baboon and of man. *Journal of Physiology, London*, **256**, 55P.

Bülbring, E. and Burn, J.H. (1935). The sympathetic dilator fibres in the muscles of the cat and dog. *Journal of Physiology, London*, **83**, 483–501.

Bülbring, E. and Burn, J.H. (1936). Sympathetic vasodilator fibres in the hare and the monkey compared with other species. *Journal of Physiology, London*, **88**, 341–360.

Carati, C.J., Creed, K.E. and Keogh, E.J. (1987). Autonomic control of penile erection in the dog. *Journal of Physiology, London*, **384**, 525–538.

Carpenter, F.G. (1981). Atropine and micturition responses by rats with intact and partially innervated bladders. *British Journal of Pharmacology*, **73**, 837–842.

Chesher, G.B. and Thorp, R.H. (1965). The atropine resistance of the response to intrinsic nerve stimulation of the guinea-pig bladder. *British Journal of Pharmacology and Chemotherapy*, **25**, 288–294.

Curtis, D.R. (1961). The pharmacology of central and peripheral inhibition. *Pharmacological Reviews*, **15**, 333–363.

Daggett, W.M., Nugent, G.C., Carr, P.W., Powers, P.C. and Harada, Y. (1967). Influence of vagal stimulation on ventricular contractility, O_2 consumption and coronary flow. *American Journal of Physiology*, **212**, 8–18.

Dale, H.H. and Gaddum, J.H. (1930). Reactions of denervated voluntary muscle, and their bearing on the mode of action of parasympathetic and related nerves. *Journal of Physiology, London*, **70**, 109–144.

Daly, I. de B. and Hebb, C. (1966). *Pulmonary and Bronchial Vascular Systems*. London: Edward Arnold.

Denn, M.J. and Stone, H.L. (1976). Autonomic innervation of dog coronary arteries. *Journal of Applied Physiology*, **41**, 30–34.

Dorr, L.D. and Brody, M.J. (1967). Haemodynamic mechanisms of erection in the canine penis. *American Journal of Physiology*, **213**, 1526–1531.

Duckles, S.P. (1979). Neurogenic dilator and constrictor responses of pial arteries *in vitro*. Differences between dogs and sheep. *Circulation Research*, **44**, 482–490.

Duckles, S.P. (1980). Vasodilator innervation of cerebral blood vessels. In *Mechanisms of Vasodilatation*, edited by P.M. Vanhoutte and I. Leusen, pp. 27–38. New York: Raven Press.

Duckles, S.P. (1981). Evidence for a functional cholinergic innervation of cerebral arteries. *Journal of Pharmacology and Experimental Therapeutics*, **217**, 544–548.

Duckles, S.P. (1988). Acetylcholine. In *Nonadrenergic Innervation of Blood Vessels*, Vol. I, edited by G. Burnstock and S.G. Griffith, pp. 15–26. Boca Raton: CRC Press.

El-Bermani, A.W., Bloomquist, E. and Montvilo, J. (1982). Distribution of pulmonary cholinergic nerves in the rabbit. *Thorax*, **37**, 703–710.

Eliasson, S., Lindgren, P. and Uvnäs, B. (1952). Representation in the hypothalamus and the motor cortex in the dog of the sympathetic vasodilator outflow to the skeletal muscle. *Acta Physiologica Scandinavica*, **27**, 18–37.

Ellison, G.D. and Zanchetti, A. (1973). Diffuse and specific activation of sympathetic cholinergic fibres of the cat. *American Journal of Physiology*, **225**, 142–149.

El-Rakhawy, M.T. and Bourne, G.H. (1961). Cholinesterases in the human tongue. *Bibliotheca Anatomica*, **2**, 243–255.

Esterhuizen, A.C., Graham, J.D.P., Lever, J.D. and Spriggs, T.L.B. (1968). Catecholamine and acetylcholinesterase distribution in relation to noradrenaline release. An enzyme histochemical and autoradiographic study on the innervation of the cat nictitating membrane. *British Journal of Pharmacology*, **32**, 46–56.

Estrada, C., Hamel, E. and Krause, D.N. (1983). Biochemical evidence for cholinergic innervation of intracerebral vessels. *Brain Research*, **266**, 261–270.

Estrada, C., Triguero, D., Muñoz, J. and Sureda, A. (1988). Acetylcholinesterase-containing fibres and choline acetyltransferase activity in isolated cerebral microvessels from goats. *Brain Research*, **453**, 275–280.

Feigl, E.O. (1969). Parasympathetic control of coronary blood flow in dogs. *Circulation Research*, **25**, 509–519.

Feigl, E.O. (1975). Reflex parasympathetic vasodilatation elicited from cardiac receptors in the dog. *Circulation Research*, **37**, 175–182.

Fencl, V., Heijl, J., Madlafousek, J. and Brod, J. (1959). Changes of blood flow in forearm muscle and skin during an acute emotional stress (mental arithmetic). *Clinical Science*, **18**, 491–498.

Ferguson, M. and Bell, C. (1988). The ultrastructural localization and characterization of sensory nerves in the rat kidney. *Journal of Comparative Neurology*, **294**, 9–16.

Ferguson, M., Ryan, G.B. and Bell, C. (1988). The innervation of the dog renal cortex: an ultrastructural study. *Cell and Tissue Research*, **253**, 539–546.

Fillenz, M. (1970). Innervation of pulmonary and bronchial blood vessels of the dog. *Journal of Anatomy*, **106**, 449–461.

Florence, V.M. and Bevan, J.A. (1979). Biochemical determination of cholinergic innervation in cerebral arteries. *Circulation Research*, **45**, 212–218.

Folkow, B. and Neil, E. (1971). *Circulation*. Oxford: Oxford University Press.

Fonnum, F. (1973). A rapid radiochemical method for the determination of choline acetyltransferase. *Journal of Neurochemistry*, **24**, 407–409.

Fox, R.H. and Hilton, S.M. (1958). Bradykinin formation in human skin as a factor in heat vasodilatation. *Journal of Physiology, London*, **142**, 219–232.

Garrett, J.R. (1966). The innervation of salivary glands IV. The effects of certain procedures on the ultrastructure of nerves in glands of the cat. *Journal of the Royal Microscopical Society*, **86**, 15–31.

Gerebtzoff, M.A. (1959). *Cholinesterases: A Histochemical Contribution to the Solution of Some Functional Problems*. London: Pergamon Press.

Graham, J.D.P., Lever, J.D. and Spriggs, T.L.B. (1968). An examination of adrenergic axons around pancreatic arterioles of the cat for the presence of acetylcholinesterase by high resolution autoradiographic and histochemical methods. *British Journal of Pharmacology*, **33**, 15–20.

Greenfield, A.D.M. (1966). Survey of the evidence for active neurogenic vasodilatation in man. *Federation Proceedings*, **25**, 1607–1610.

Greiss, F.C., Gobble, F.L., Anderson, S.G. and McGuirt, W.F. (1967). Effect of parasympathetic nerve stimulation on the uterine vascular bed. *American Journal of Obstetric and Gynecology*, **99**, 1067–1072.

Haeusler, G., Thoenen, H., Haefely, W. and Huerlimann, A. (1968). Electrical events in cardiac adrenergic nerves and noradrenaline release from the heart induced by acetylcholine and KCl. *Archiv für Experimentalle Pathologie und Pharmakologie*, **261**, 389–411.

Hamel, E., Assumel-Lundin, C., Edvinsson, L. and MacKenzie, E.C. (1986). Cholinergic innervation of small pial vessels: specific uptake and release processes. *Acta Physiologica Scandinavica*, Supplement **552**, 13–16.

Hammarström, M. and Sjöstrand, N.O. (1984). Comments on the atropine resistance of the neurogenic contractile response of the rat detrusor muscle. *Acta Physiologica Scandinavica*, **122**, 475–481.

Hara, H., Hamill, G.S. and Jacobowitz, D.M. (1985). Origin of cholinergic nerves to the rat major cerebral arteries: coexistence with vasoactive intestinal polypeptide. *Brain Research Bulletin*, **14**, 179–188.

Heidenhaim, R. (1872). Über die Wirkung einiger Gifte auf die Nerven der Glandula submaxillaris. *Pflüger's Archiv für Physiologie*, **5**, 309–318.

Hukovic, S., Rand, M.J. and Vanov, S. (1965). Observations on an isolated, innervated preparation of rat urinary bladder. *British Journal of Pharmacology*, **24**, 178–188.

Inanami, O., Meguro, K., Ohno, K. and Sato, A. (1988). Contribution of cholinergic vasodilation on the increase in cerebral cortical blood flow responses to the intravenous administration of thyrotropin releasing hormone in anaesthetized rats. *Neuroscience Letters*, **88**, 184–188.

Ito, B.R. and Feigl, E.O. (1985). Carotid baroreceptor reflex coronary vasodilation in the dog. *Circulation Research*, **56**, 486–495.

Jope, R.S. (1979). High-affinity choline transport and acetylCoA production in brain and their roles in the regulation of acetylcholine synthesis. *Brain Research Reviews*, **1**, 313–344.

Kalsner, S. (1989). Cholinergic constriction in the general circulation and its role in coronary artery spasm. *Circulation Research*, **65**, 237–257.

Knight, D.S., Ellison, P.J., Hibbs, G.R., Hyman, A.L. and Kadowitz, P.J. (1981). A light and electron microscopic study of the innervation of pulmonary arteries in the cat. *Anatomical Record*, **201**, 513–521.

Kobayashi, S., Kyoshima, K., Olschowka, J.A. and Jacobowitz, D.M. (1983). Vasoactive inhibitory peptide immunoreactive and cholinergic nerves in the whole mount preparation of the major cerebral arteries of the rat. *Histochemistry*, **79**, 377–381.

Koelle, G.B. (1963). Cytological distribution and physiological functions of cholinesterase. In *Cholinesterases and Anticholinesterase Agents*, edited by G.B. Koelle, pp. 187–298. Heidelberg: Springer.

Kuriyama, H. and Suzuki, H. (1981). Adrenergic transmissions in the guinea-pig mesenteric artery and their cholinergic modulations. *Journal of Physiology, London*, **317**, 383–396.

Lang, W.J., Bell, C., Conway, E.L. and Padanyi, R. (1976). Cutaneous and muscular vasodilatation in the canine hindlimb evoked by central stimulation. *Circulation Research*, **38**, 560–566.

Langley, J.L. and Anderson, H.K. (1895). The innervation of the pelvic and adjoining viscera. III. The external generative organs. *Journal of Physiology, London*, **19**, 85–121.

Leblanc, C.G., Trimmer, B.A. and Landis, S.C. (1987). Neuropeptide Y-like immunoreactivity in rat cranial parasympathetic neurons: coexistence with vasoactive intestinal peptide and choline acetyltransferase. *Proceedings of the National Academy of Sciences of the USA*, **84**, 3511–3515.

Lee, T.J.-F. (1982). Cholinergic mechanisms in the large cat cerebral artery. *Circulation Research*, **50**, 870–879.

Lee, T.J.-F, Hume, W.R., Su, C. and Bevan, J.A. (1978). Neurogenic vasodilatation of cat cerebral arteries. *Circulation Research*, **42**, 535–542.

Lindmar, R., Löffelholz, K. and Muscholl, E. (1968). A muscarinic mechanism inhibiting the release of noradrenaline from peripheral adrenergic nerve fibres by nicotinic agents. *British Journal of Pharmacology and Chemotherapy*, **32**, 280–294.

Lundberg, J.M., Änggård, A., Fahrenkrug, J., Hökfelt, T. and Mutt, V. (1980). Vasoactive intestinal polypeptide in cholinergic neurons of exocrine glands: functional significance of coexisting transmitters for vasodilatation and secretion. *Proceedings of the National Academy of Sciences of the USA*, **77**, 1651–1655.

McConnell, J.A., Benson, G.S. and Wood, J. (1979). Autonomic innervation of the mammalian penis: a histochemical and physiological study. *Journal of Neural Transmission*, **45**, 227–238.

McKee, J.C., Denn, M.J. and Stone, H.L. (1976). Neurogenic cerebral vasodilatation from electrical stimulation of the cerebellum in the monkey. *Stroke*, **17**, 179–186.

Malor, R., Griffin, J. and Taylor, S. (1973). Innervation of the blood vessels in guinea-pig atria. *Circulation Research*, **7**, 95–104.

Mancia, G., Baccelli, G. and Zanchetti, A. (1972). Haemodynamic responses to different emotional stimuli in the cat: patterns and mechanisms. *American Journal of Physiology*, **223**, 925–933.

Morley, J., Schachter, M. and Smaje, L.H. (1966). Vasodilatation in the submaxillary gland of the rabbit. *Journal of Physiology, London*, **187**, 595–602.

Murray, K.J. (1990). Cyclic AMP and mechanisms of vasodilatation. *Pharmacology and Therapeutics*, **47**, 329–346.

Nakai, M., Iadecola, C., Ruggiero, D.A., Tucker, L.W. and Reis, D.J. (1983). Electrical stimulation of cerebellar fastigial nucleus increases cerebral cortical blood flow without change in local metabolism: evidence for an intrinsic system in brain for primary vasodilation. *Brain Research*, **260**, 35–49.

Nakazato, Y., Ohga, A., Shigei, T. and Uematsu, T. (1982). Extrinsic innervation of the canine abdominal vena cava and the origin of cholinergic vasoconstrictor nerves. *Journal of Physiology, London*, **328**, 191–203.

Nandiwada, P.A., Hyman, A.L. and Kadowitz, P.J. (1983). Pulmonary vasodilator responses to vagal stimulation and acetylcholine in the cat. *Circulation Research*, **53**, 86–95.

Navaratnam, V. and Palkama, A. (1965). Cholinesterases in the walls of the great arterial trunks and coronary arteries. *Acta Anatomica*, **60**, 445–448.

Partanen, M., Laitinen, A., Hervonen, A., Toivanen, M. and Laitinen, L.A. (1982). Catecholamine and acetylcholinesterase-containing nerves in human lower respiratory tract. *Histochemistry*, **76**, 175–186.

Paton, W.D.M. (1958). Central and synaptic transmission in the nervous system (pharmacological aspects). *Annual Review of Physiology*, **20**, 431–470.

Pillay, C.V. and Reid, J.V.O. (1982). Histochemical localization of acetylcholinesterase in the wall of cardiac blood vessels in the baboon, dog and vervet monkey. *Basic Research in Cardiology*, **77**, 213–219.

Rand, M.J. and Varma, B. (1970). The effects of cholinomimetic drugs on responses to sympathetic nerve stimulation and noradrenaline in the rabbit ear artery. *British Journal of Pharmacology*, **38**, 758–770.

Robinson, P.M. and Bell, C. (1967). The localization of acetylcholinesterase at the autonomic neuromuscular junction. *Journal of Cell Biology*, **33**, 93–102.

Ryan, M.J., Clark, K.E. and Brody, M.J. (1974). Neurogenic and mechanical control of canine uterine vascular resistance. *American Journal of Physiology*, **227**, 547–555.

Saenz de Tejada, I., Blanco, R., Goldstein, I., Azadzoi, K., Morenas, A. de las, Krane, R.J. and Cohen, R.A. (1988). Cholinergic neurotransmission in human corpus cavernosum. I. Responses of isolated tissue. *American Journal of Physiology*, **254**, H459–H467.

Saito, A., Wu, J.-Y. and Lee, T.J.-F. (1985). Evidence for the presence of cholinergic nerves in cerebral arteries: an immunohistochemical demonstration of choline acetyltransferase. *Journal of Cerebral Blood Flow and Metabolism*, **5**, 527–534.

Sanders, J.S., Mark, A.L. and Ferguson, D.W. (1989). Evidence for cholinergically mediated vasodilatation at the beginning of isometric exercise in humans. *Circulation*, **79**, 815–824.

Sato, A. and Sato, Y. (1990). Cerebral cortical vasodilatation in response to stimulation of cholinergic fibres originating in the nucleus basalis of Meynert. *Journal of the Autonomic Nervous System*, **30**, S137–S140.

Schachter, M. and Beilenson, S. (1968). Mediator of vasodilatation in the submaxillary gland. *Federation Proceedings*, **27**, 73–75.

Schenk, E.A. and El-Badawi, A. (1968). Dual innervation of arteries and arterioles: a histochemical study. *Zeitschrift für Zellforschung und Mikroskopische Anatomie*, **91**, 170–177.

Schramm, L.P., Honig, C.R. and Bignall, K.E. (1971). Active muscle vasodilatation in primates homologous with sympathetic cholinergic vasodilatation in carnivores. *American Journal of Physiology*, **221**, 768–777.

Shen, K.-Z., Neild, T.O., Surprenant, A. and Galligan, J.J. (1989). Neurogenic cholinergic vasodilatation of arterioles in guinea-pig submucosa. *British Journal of Pharmacology*, **96**, 113P.

Shirai, M., Sasaki, K. and Rikimaru, A. (1972). Histochemical investigation on the distribution of adrenergic and cholinergic nerves in human penis. *Tohoku Journal of Experimental Medicine*, **107**, 403–404.

Skinner, N.S. Jr. and Webster, M.E. (1968). Kinins, β-adrenergic receptors and functional vasodilatation in the submaxillary gland of the cat. *Journal of Physiology, London*, **195**, 505–519.

Tiedt, N. and Religa, A. (1979). Vagal control of coronary blood flow in dogs. *Basic Research in Cardiology*, **74**, 267–276.

Toth, A., McEwan, R. and Shabanah, E.H. (1964). Role of the autonomic nervous system in the nutrition of the products of conception. Effects of pelvic parasympathectomy on uterine and subplacental decidual blood flow. *Fertility and Sterility*, **15**, 263–271.

Uvnäs, B. (1966). Cholinergic vasodilator nerves. *Federation Proceedings*, **25**, 1618–1622.

Van Winckle, D.M. and Feigl, E.O (1989). Acetylcholine causes coronary vasodilatation in dogs and baboons. *Circulation Research*, **65**, 1580–1593.

Vardi, Y., Belur, R. and Siroky, M.B. (1987). Pelvic nerve induced relaxation of canine corporal smooth muscle is blocked by atropine. *Federation Proceedings*, **46**, 338.

Welsch, F. (1977). The cholinergic system in tissues without innervation. *Biochemical Pharmacology*, **26**, 1281–1286.

Wikberg, J. (1977). Release of [³H] acetylcholine from isolated guinea-pig ileum. A radiochemical method for studying the release of cholinergic neurotransmitter in the intestine. *Acta Physiologica Scandinavica*, **101**, 302–317.

Zucker, I.H., Cornish, K.G., Hackley, J. and Bliss, K. (1987). Effects of left ventricular receptor stimulation on coronary blood flow in conscious dogs. *Circulation Research*, **61**, II.54–II.60.

3 Efferent Function — Non-Adrenergic, Non-Cholinergic Mechanisms

Anders Franco-Cereceda

Department of Thoracic Surgery, Karolinska Hospital, S-171 76 Stockholm, Sweden

The contribution of neurogenic mediator candidates apart from noradrenaline (NA) and acetylcholine (ACh) to the control of vascular tone has attracted enormous — and sometimes disputed — attention during the past decades. Today there is an abundance of evidence suggesting that adenosine 5'-triphosphate (ATP) and neuropeptide Y (NPY) are co-localized with NA in sympathetic perivascular nerves while in parasympathetic nerve terminals vasoactive intestinal polypeptide (VIP) is present in certain vascular beds. Direct application of NPY as well as ATP to various vascular bed preparations confirms their vasoconstrictor action. Stimulation of sympathetic nerves *in vitro* and *in vivo* causes nonadrenergic vasoconstriction which can be blocked by experimental manipulations that inhibit ATP or NPY mechanisms. Thus, the vasopressor response to stimulation of sympathetic nerves can be attenuated by the sequential use of chemical or surgical sympathectomy, reserpine treatment or α-adrenoceptor blockade and tachyphylaxis to α, βmethyleneATP ($\alpha\beta$metATP), irrespective of the order of administration. VIP, with potent vasodepressor effects, seems to be a candidate for the observed atropine-resistant vasodilatation that occurs upon stimulation of parasympathetic nerves. It should be emphasized, though, that the discovery of nitric oxide synthase (NOS) in postganglionic parasympathetic nerves suggests an important role for nitric oxide (NO) in the neuronal control of vascular homeostasis.

Here, some ideas from the literature on the relative contributions of these agents to vascular control are reviewed, bearing in mind that NA and ACh are the principal transmitters regulating the neuronal control of vascular tone.

KEY WORDS: ATP; co-transmission; NO; NPY; non-adrenergic; non-cholinergic; VIP.

INTRODUCTION

At the end of the 19th century Langley developed the concept of an involuntary, autonomic nervous system consisting of sympathetic and parasympathetic divisions in which stimulation evoked respectively pressor and depressor effects on the cardiovascular system (see Langley, 1921). The idea of nerves acting on effector organs through the release of chemically active agents gained support at the beginning of this century when Elliott was able to demonstrate that the effects of nerve stimulation were mimicked by injections of adrenaline (Elliott, 1905). At about the same time, Dixon presented evidence that vagus nerve stimulation released a muscarine-like substance (Dixon, 1906). The actual release of a transmitter substance from nerves was later demonstrated by Loewi in 1921, in an experiment in which perfusate from a frog heart, in which the vagal nerves were stimulated, evoked a similar inhibitory effect in a recipient heart (Loewi, 1921), an effect caused by acetylcholine (ACh; Witanowski, 1925; Dale and Dudley, 1929). Early experiments had also revealed that sympathetic nerve stimulation lead to the release of a chemical substance, originally thought to be adrenaline, into the blood stream (Cannon and Bacq, 1931). Noradrenaline (NA) was later shown to be the principal cathecolamine released from sympathetic nerves (von Euler, 1946).

Today there is an abundance of experimental evidence suggesting that "Dale's principle" of "one neuron — one transmitter"-hypothesis (Dale, 1935) is inaccurate (although it also seems clear that the possibility of co-transmitters was never excluded by Dale; see Burnstock, 1982). The concept of co-transmission was originally presented by Burnstock who, through comparative studies on the evolution of the autonomic nervous system and in a series of experiments has provided evidence of adenosine $5'$-triphosphate (ATP) being a co-transmitter in sympathetic nerves (Burnstock, 1976; see Burnstock, 1988). However, recent findings also suggest that neuropeptides occur in both sympathetic and parasympathetic nerves (see Lundberg and Hökfelt, 1986). Immunohistochemical techniques have revealed that somatostatin-like immunoreactivity (-LI; Hökfelt et al., 1977), enkephalin-LI (Schultzberg et al., 1979) and neuropeptide Y-LI (NPY; Lundberg et al., 1982) co-exist with NA in a subpopulation of sympathetic nerves. Furthermore, vasoactive intestinal polypeptide (VIP) and peptide histidine isoleucine (PHI) are presumably co-stored with ACh in parasympathetic nerves (Lundberg et al., 1979, 1981a,b, 1984c). Somatostatin has also been suggested to be present in a population of peripheral cholinergic nerves of the cardiovascular system (Campbell et al., 1982; Day, Polak and Bloom, 1985; Franco-Cereceda, Lundberg and Hökfelt, 1986). Other peptides postulated to be present in perivascular nerves include neurotensin (Reinecke et al., 1982), galanin (Ekblad et al., 1985), cholecystokinin (Hendry, Jones and Beinfeld, 1983) gastrin-releasing peptide (Uddman et al., 1983), vasopressin-like peptide (Hanley et al., 1984), dynorphin (Morris et al., 1985), gastrin (Schultzberg et al., 1980) and endothelin (Giaid et al., 1989), as well as calcitonin gene-related peptide and tachykinins (Holzer, 1988). There are, in addition to polypeptides and ATP, other substances present together with the classical transmitters NA and ACh in perivascular nerves. Thus, γ-aminobutyric acid (Jessen et al., 1979) and 5-hydroxytryptamine (5-HT; Scheibel, Tomiyasu and Scheibel, 1975; Wood and Mayer, 1979) are other transmitter candidates in the autonomic nervous system. Interestingly, neuronal nitric oxide synthase (NOS) is present in both postganglionic parasympathetic nerves (Kummer et al., 1992) and preganglionic sympathetic nerves (Blottner and Baumgarten 1992).

The present paper will discuss the possible relative contributions of some of these compounds in the nervous control of blood vessels. The emphasis will be on ATP and NPY in sympathetic nerves and VIP, PHI and NO in parasympathetic nerves in relation to non-adrenergic, non-cholinergic mechanisms. This overview will be restricted to the peripheral innervation of blood vessels and will focus on efferent functions and not deal with the integration of cardiovascular reflexes or the central regulation of cardiovascular functions. Moreover, the "efferent function" of capsaicin-sensitive C-fibre afferents involving calcitonin gene-related peptide and substance P and related tachykinins

(Franco-Cereceda, 1988; Holzer, 1988; Maggi and Meli, 1988) will not be discussed in this context.

NON-ADRENERGIC MECHANISMS

NA is generally considered to be the classical transmitter in the sympathetic nervous system. The effects of NA are mediated through interaction with α-adrenoceptors (α_{1A}, α_{1B}, α_{2A}, α_{2B}, α_{2C}) and β-adrenoceptors (β_1, β_2, β_3). Of the vascular effects evoked by NA, vasoconstriction is accomplished by stimulation of α_1- as well as α_2-adrenoceptors, while β-adrenoceptor stimulation results in vasodilatation in some vascular beds.

There have been many reports of both *in vivo* and *in vitro* experiments suggesting the occurrence of α-adrenoceptor-resistant vasoconstriction upon sympathetic nerve stimulation. As early as 1948 Folkow and Uvnäs reported that sympathetic nerve stimulation caused an adrenoceptor-resistant vasoconstriction in the cat hindlimb (Folkow and Uvnäs, 1948). Reserpine pretreatment, which depletes the tissue content of NA (Carlsson, 1965), attenuated the vasoconstrictor response and this diminished vasopressor effect could be reversed to a large extent by simultaneous preganglionic denervation (Rosell and Sedvall, 1962), although the NA content was almost totally depleted after denervation (Sedvall and Thorson, 1965). However, reserpine pretreatment depletes not only NA but also the co-stored vasoconstrictor NPY from sympathetic nerve terminals, an effect dependent on intact nerve activity (Lundberg *et al.*, 1985c,d), thus suggesting that the remaining response may not be caused by incomplete blockade of adrenoceptors as initially proposed (Folkow and Uvnäs, 1948) or different fractions of NA stores with different sensitivities to reserpine (Sedvall and Thorson, 1965). Interestingly, the vasoconstrictor response to nerve stimulation after sympathetic decentralization combined with reserpine administration disappeared after continuous nerve stimulation (Rosen and Sedvall, 1962). Furthermore, the vasoconstrictor response to sympathetic nerve stimulation in the rabbit basilar artery and cat submandibular gland consists of an initial NA component and a slowly developing second component attributed to another transmitter (Lee, Su and Bevan, 1976; Lee, Chiuch and Adam, 1980; Lundberg and Tatemoto, 1982). The release of this transmitter is inhibited by presynaptic α_2-adrenoceptor stimulation and the vasoconstriction is enhanced by exogenous NA. In addition, the vasoconstriction to sympathetic nerve stimulation in the human forearm is partly resistant to α-adrenoceptor blockade (Taddei, Salvetti and Pedrinelli, 1989). Several recent reports have demonstrated the existence of non-adrenergic vasoconstriction upon sympathetic nerve stimulation in a variety of species, as shown in Table 3.1.

A general characteristic feature of these results is the total inhibition, by α-adrenoceptor antagonism, of the vasoconstrictor effects exerted by applied NA, although a substantial guanethidine- or 6-hydroxydopamine (6-OHDA)- sensitive portion of the vasoconstrictor response remained upon nerve stimulation. However, the involvement of ATP or NPY in these effects varies considerably.

Apart from vasoconstriction, sympathetic nerve stimulation evokes a rapid excitatory junction potential (EJP) in the systemic arteries of most mammals (Bell, 1969; Hirst, 1977).

TABLE 3.1

Some recent demonstrations of non-adrenergic vasoconstriction upon sympathetic nerve stimulation in different organs and blood vessels from various species under *in vivo* and *in vitro* conditions in which ATP or NPY have been suggested to be involved

Tissue	Postulated transmitter	Publication
In vitro		
Rabbit		
basilar artery	ATP	Lee, Su and Bevan, 1976
central ear artery	ATP	Suzuki and Kou, 1983
tail artery	ATP	Sneddon and Burnstock, 1984
mesenteric artery	ATP	Kügelgen and Starke, 1985
saphenous artery	ATP	Burnstock and Warland, 1987
skeletal muscle	NPY	Öhlen *et al.*, 1990
Rat		
kidney	ATP	Malik, 1980
tail artery	ATP	Sneddon and Burnstock, 1984
mesenteric artery	ATP	Sjöblom-Widfelt, 1990
Dog		
basilar artery	ATP	Muramatsu *et al.*, 1981
mesenteric artery	ATP	Muramatsu, Kigoshi and Oshita, 1984
Guinea-pig		
saphenous artery	ATP	Cheung and Fujioka, 1986
mesenteric artery	ATP	Hottenstein and Kreulen 1986
uterine artery	NPY	Morris and Murphy, 1988
vena cava	NPY	Morris, 1991
In vivo		
Cat		
submandibular gland	NPY	Lundberg and Tatemoto, 1982
spleen	NPY	Lundberg *et al.*, 1984a
intestine	NPY	Hellström, Olerup and Tatemoto, 1985
oral mucosa	NPY	Edwall *et al.*, 1987
nasal mucosa	NPY	Lundblad *et al.*, 1987
intestine	ATP	Taylor and Parsons, 1989
Pig		
spleen	NPY	Lundberg *et al.*, 1989
nasal mucosa	NPY	Lacroix *et al.*, 1988b
kidney	NPY	Pernow and Lundberg, 1989a
bronchi and lungs	NPY	Franco-Cereceda *et al.*, 1995
Rabbit		
hindquarter	ATP	Hirst and Lew, 1987
Dog		
skeletal muscle	NPY	Pernow, 1988
Pithed rat	ATP	Bulloch and McGrath, 1986
Pithed bullfrog	NPY	Stofer, Fatherazi and Horn, 1990

The EJP can evoke an action potential which is usually, but not always, necessary to achieve a contraction (see Speden, 1975). The EJP is not influenced by α-adrenoceptor blocking agents but it can be abolished by drugs like guanethidine and tetrodotoxin that interfere with transmitter release (Hirst and Neild, 1980; Cheung, 1982; Sneddon, Westfall and Fedan, 1982). This has been interpreted by some to be due to the release of a substance co-stored with NA, presumably ATP (see Burnstock, 1988), while others have suggested that NA is indeed the sole transmitter released and the EJPs are due to stimulation of a specific, pharmacologically distinct, receptor called the γ-receptor, which is activated at high NA concentrations (Hirst and Neild, 1980). It is of interest in this context that in many of these blood vessels, exogenously applied ATP, but not NA, mimics the nerve stimulation-induced EJP (Karashima and Kuriyama, 1981; Fujiwara, Itoh and Suzuki, 1982; Suzuki, 1985). The EJP can also be evoked in tissues depleted of NA (Suzuki, Mishima and Miyahara, 1984).

When evaluating the results obtained by sympathetic nerve stimulation, complex situations often exist which make the interpretation of the results difficult. For instance, both in the control situation and after chemical or surgical sympathectomy, one must consider the possible involvement of other neurogenic vasoactive components, including cholinergic sympathetic vasodilator fibres (Bülbring and Burn, 1935; Folkow, 1955), antidromic activation of C-fibre afferents running parallel with sympathetic fibres (Holzer, 1988) as well as tetrodotoxin-resistant vasodilatation, suggested to be mediated by intramural nerves (Senaratne and Kappagoda, 1986). In addition, transmural nerve stimulation can cause non-neuronal vasodilatation through the production of free radicals (Lamb and Webb, 1984).

ATP

The co-transmitter hypothesis (Burnstock, 1976) is now widely accepted, although the functional significance of the putative messengers co-existing in neurons remains essentially unknown. An abundance of evidence suggests that ATP is a transmitter candidate and may act as a co-transmitter with NA in perivascular nerves, at least in some species.

SYNTHESIS/STORAGE

ATP is present in both small and large dense-cored vesicles together with NA (Lagercrantz, 1971). The molar ratio of NA:ATP varies in different tissues and species and may also vary within different portions of nerves but has been estimated to be 50:1 in the terminal region (see Stjärne, 1989). ATP is synthesized in mitochondria and incorporated into the vesicles by carrier-mediated transport. Therefore, sympathetic nerve terminals contain ATP distributed in a transmitter pool and ATP in a cytosolic, non-transmitter pool used for energy metabolism (Stjärne, 1989). ATP is probably only secreted from the storage vesicles and not from the cytosol, together with NA, upon nerve stimulation (Stjärne and Åstrand, 1984).

RELEASE

By using tritium-labelled adenosine and NA, Su has demonstrated that ATP is released together with NA from sympathetic nerves supplying the rabbit aorta and portal vein

(Su, 1975, 1978). Similar results were obtained with other blood vessel preparations (Levitt and Westfall, 1982; Westfall, Sedaa and Bjur, 1987; Sedaa et al., 1990). The molar ratio of released ATP and NA correspond to that observed in the sympathetic nerve terminal (Kirkpatrick and Burnstock, 1987; Kasakov et al., 1988). Moreover the release is tetrodotoxin- and guanethidine-sensitive and can be abolished by Ca^{2+} removal or 6-OHDA pretreatment (Katsuragi and Su, 1980, 1982), as expected, for release from vesicularly stored transmitters. After release and activation of purinergic receptors (see below), ATP is rapidly broken down to adenosine. Adenosine is then taken up into the nerve terminals by a high-affinity system, converted to ATP and reincorporated into physiological stores. Under normal conditions, the basal levels of purines in the blood are therefore low and the influence of circulating purines is negligible. Increased intraluminal concentrations have been detected during hypoxia and vessel wall damage but because of the rapid degradation and uptake, the actual concentrations at the site of release are probably considerably higher (see Burnstock and Kennedy, 1985b).

ATP release is favored by high, irregular stimulation frequencies (Kennedy, Saville and Burnstock, 1986), but ATP is also released during low-frequency stimulation (Schwartz and Malik, 1989) and even a single nerve stimulation can release ATP (Kennedy, Saville and Burnstock, 1986; Angus, Broughton and Mulvany, 1988; Sjöblom-Widfeldt, 1990). In the rat kidney low frequencies release ATP preferentially, compared to NA, while at higher frequencies mainly NA is released (Sjöblom-Widfeldt, 1990). These findings suggest that the mechanism of release of the transmitters from nerve fibres may be different (Schwartz and Malik, 1989).

Nerve-stimulation-evoked NA release from a number of blood vessels is inhibited by stimulation of the A_1-receptor (De Mey, Burnstock and Vanhoutte 1979; see Fredholm et al., 1983; Burnstock, 1989). ATP release is also autoinhibited through negative feedback on prejunctional receptors (Katsuragi and Su, 1982; Sneddon, Meldrum and Burnstock, 1984; Bao, Eriksson and Stjärne, 1990) and the release of ATP is attenuated by NA (Stjärne, 1989).

In addition to inhibiting NA and ATP release, ATP may also attenuate the release of other substances from perivascular sympathetic nerves (Bao, Eriksson and Stjärne, 1990) and it modulates ACh release in skeletal muscle, intestines and the brain (see Burnstock, 1989).

RECEPTORS

Burnstock has presented evidence for subgroups of purinoceptors (Burnstock, 1978). Originally, the existence of two receptors, named P_1 and P_2, was suggested based on an agonist potency order of adenosine > AMP > ADP > ATP for the P_1 receptor and ATP > ADP > AMP > adenosine for the P_2 receptor. Since this classification, several subtypes have been proposed and the receptors have now been further subdivided into A_1 and A_2 for the P_1-receptor and P_{2x} and P_{2y} for the P_2-receptor (Londos, Cooper and Wolff, 1980; Burnstock and Kennedy, 1985a). There is much support for this classification from findings on the characteristics of P_1 and P_2-receptors with regard to different modes of action and agonist and antagonist potency as well as specific second messenger system activation (see Burnstock, 1989; Olsson and Pearson, 1990), although the existance of additional purinoreceptors with modulatory effects on transmitter release has recently been proposed (Shinozuka, Bjur and Westfall, 1990). The most important effects of P_{2x}-receptor stimulation is contraction of vascular smooth muscle while P_{2y} and A_2-receptors cause vasodilatation and A_1 attenuates transmitter release. In blood vessels, P_{2y}-purinoceptors are present on endothelial cells and act by releasing endothelium-derived relaxing factor (EDRF) and prostacyclin while P_{2x}-purinoceptors are located on vascular smooth muscle and are particularly concentrated at sympathetic nerve endings (Burnstock, 1989). Naturally, the distribution of different receptor subtypes will determine the functional effects observed by released or applied ATP in a given preparation.

VASCULAR EFFECTS

In a number of different vascular beds, the response to sympathetic nerve stimulation consists of two components; a fast constriction followed by a slow, sustained constriction. The major effect of neuronally released ATP on blood vessels tone is constriction, although the rapid degradation of ATP to adenosine complicates the interpretation of ATP effects.

Generally, the effects of both exogenous and released ATP are short-lived (Figure 3.1) and ATP appears to be most important in the initiation of the contraction since this phase is usually reduced after desensitization with the stable ATP analogue $\alpha\beta$methylene ATP ($\alpha\beta$metATP; see below). The contribution of ATP to the response to sympathetic nerve stimulation varies considerably in different vessels as determined by the presence of a remaining $\alpha\beta$metATP-sensitive vasoconstrictor component after adrenoceptor blockade. This is especially apparent in the rabbit saphenous artery (Figure 3.1; Burnstock and Warland, 1987), rabbit (Ramme et al., 1987) and dog (Muramatsu et al., 1981; Machaly, Dalziel and Sneddon, 1988) mesenteric artery, the rat tail artery (Sneddon and Burnstock, 1984) and mesenteric arteries from the rat (Angus, Broughton and Mulvany, 1988; Sjöblom-Widfeldt, 1990) where a portion of the vasoconstrictor response has been attributed to ATP. The pattern of nerve stimulation is of importance for the relative contribution of ATP in vasoconstrictor responses (Kennedy, Saville and Burnstock, 1986; Schwartz and Malik, 1989; Sjöblom-Widfeldt 1990). Thus, there is an inverse relationship between the frequency and the ATP component since at low frequencies ATP is the principal vasoconstrictor while at higher frequencies the purinergic component diminishes, whereas that of NA is enhanced (Burnstock and Warland, 1987; Schwartz and Malik, 1989).

Pretreatment with reserpine depletes the peripheral tissue content of NA and NPY from sympathetic nerve terminals (Lundberg et al., 1985c,d) while it does not influence adenine nucleotides in storage vesicles (see below) or nerve-stimulated (Kirkpatrick and Burnstock, 1987) or potassium-evoked purine release (Katsuragi and Su, 1980). After reserpine pretreatment, a nerve-stimulation-evoked, $\alpha\beta$metATP-sensitive vasoconstrictor response remains, which is similar in magnitude to that in prazosin-incubated controls (Muramatsu, 1987; Warland and Burnstock, 1987; Saville and Burnstock, 1988). Reserpine treatment may therefore be used to reveal a remaining purinergic component in sympathetic vascular control.

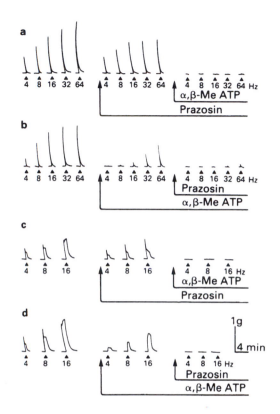

Figure 3.1   In the isolated rabbit saphenous artery, transmural nerve stimulation for 1 sec (a,b) or 1 min (c,d) causes a rapidly developing contraction which is totally abolished after α-adrenoceptor blockade (prazosin) combined with desensitization of P_2-purinoceptors (αβmetATP). Note the additive effects of αβmetATP and prazosin regardless of order of administration. (From Burnstock and Warland, 1987. With permission.)

Upon repeated exposure to or in the presence of αβmetATP there is a desensitization of P_2-receptors with subsequent loss of the vasoconstrictor effects of ATP (Figures 3.1, 3.2). The effects of αβmetATP are not inhibited by guanethidine, prazosin or 8-phenyltheophyl-line, suggesting that ATP and αβmetATP produce contractions through activation of postsynaptic P_{2x}-purinoceptors (Muramatsu, 1987). Desensitization of P_{2x}-purinoreceptors following αβmetATP *in vitro* seems to be specific for the vasoconstrictor effects of ATP without any influence on responses to exogenous NA (Kügelgen and Starke, 1985; Kennedy, Saville and Burnstock, 1986), tyramine (Muramatsu, 1987), angiotensin II (Schwartz and Malik, 1989), potassium ions (Bao, Eriksson and Stjärne, 1990) or NPY (Sjöblom-Widfeldt, 1990). Furthermore, in arteries from the rabbit (Ishikawa, 1985; Kügelgen and Starke, 1985; Miyahara and Suzuki, 1987, Ramme *et al.*, 1987), dog (Muramatsu and Kigoshi, 1987), guinea-pig (Ishikawa, 1985) and rat (Vidal, Hicks and Langer, 1986; Kotecha and Neild, 1987; Yamamoto and Cline, 1987; Shinozuka, Bjur and Westfall, 1990), αβmetATP has been shown not to influence NA release. An abundance of evidence thus

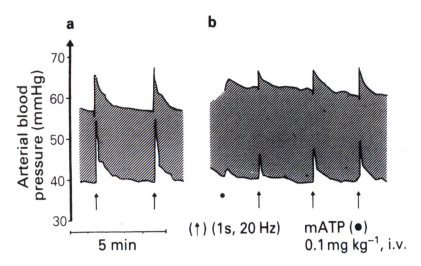

Figure 3.2 Stimulation of the spinal sympathetic outflow in the pithed rat evokes a short-lived pressor response (a) which after desensitization of P_2-purinoceptors (dot in b) is attenuated with maximum blockade at 1 min after tachyphylaxis to $\alpha\beta$metATP (first arrow in b). (From Bulloch and McGrath, 1988. With permission.)

suggests that $\alpha\beta$metATP does not affect the nerve-stimulation-evoked release of NA. However, the possibility that $\alpha\beta$metATP inhibits the release of NA (Bao, Eriksson and Stjärne, 1990) and NPY (Lacroix, 1989) as well as other unknown substances from perivascular nerves should not be dismissed (Stjärne and Åstrand, 1985). It has also been demonstrated that $\alpha\beta$metATP can increase NA release in the rat tail artery upon high-frequency stimulation (Shinozuka, Bjur and Westfall, 1990). The actual site at which $\alpha\beta$metATP activates the cell has also been questioned (Byrne and Large, 1986; Nagao and Suzuki, 1988). Another disadvantage with $\alpha\beta$metATP is the relatively rapid recovery of the desensitization *in vivo*.

Intra-arterially or intravenously administered ATP usually evokes only vasodilatation (Torregrosa *et al.*, 1988; Taylor *et al.*, 1989), mediated by activation of purinergic receptors, by release of EDRF and prostacyclin, or through its breakdown to adenosine. The ATP released upon nerve stimulation is likely to reach other receptors than those activated when given systemically (see Burnstock, 1989). By using $\alpha\beta$metATP, Taylor and co-workers were able to evoke a pressor effect in resistance vessels in the rabbit ear and cat intestinal vasculature (Taylor *et al.*, 1989), thus demonstrating P_{2x}-mediated vasoconstriction under *in vivo* conditions. However, the attenuation of the sympathetic nerve-mediated pressor response *in vivo* seems to be non-selective since a general unresponsiveness to other vasoconstrictor agents occurs after $\alpha\beta$metATP desensitization, (Taylor and Parsons, 1989; Dalziel *et al.*, 1990). In the pithed rat, the vasopressor response to sympathetic nerve stimulation was not altered by $\alpha\beta$metATP-desensitization while after α-adrenoceptor blockade or reserpine pretreatment the remaining response was reduced by $\alpha\beta$metATP (Flavahan *et al.*, 1985). Whether this is due to inhibition of ATP mechanisms or an attenuation of a residual NPY-release (Lundberg *et al.*, 1989) is not clear. Somewhat contradictorily, other reports demonstrate that a major portion of the sympathetic vasopressor effect in the pithed rat is indeed sensitive to $\alpha\beta$metATP (Figure 3.2) regardless of α-adrenoceptor blocking agents (Bulloch and McGrath, 1988). A striking difference between *in vitro* and *in vivo* conditions is also apparent in the pithed rabbit model (Bulloch and McGrath, 1988) in which $\alpha\beta$metATP had no effect on the pressor response to sympathetic nerve stimulation, whereas in many isolated rabbit blood vessels there is clearly an important purinergic vasoconstriction (see Burnstock, 1988). However, it was recently demonstrated that the P_{2x}-antagonist suramine did not influence the sympathetic vasoconstriction in the human saphenous vein (Rump and von Kügelgen, 1994).

The other principal effect of ATP in vessels is the generation of the EJP, which has been demonstrated in a large number of arteries (see Kennedy, 1988). A single EJP may if sufficiently large, or in combination with successive EJPs, activate voltage-dependent calcium channels and contraction follows (Hirst and Jobling, 1989). The EJP is not influenced by α-adrenoceptor blockade (Holman and Surprenant, 1980; Suzuki and Kou, 1983), or reserpine pretreatment (Warland and Burnstock, 1987) but can be abolished by $\alpha\beta$metATP (Sneddon and Burnstock, 1984; Angus, Broughton and Mulvany, 1988). EJPs can be evoked in tissues depleted of NA (Suzuki, Mishima and Miyahara, 1984) and application of ATP produces electrical responses similar to the EJP (Suzuki, 1985; Miyahara and Suzuki, 1987). The postulated γ-adrenoceptor therefore does not seem to be involved in the generation of arterial EJPs, but may have a function in modulating Ca^{2+}-influx into arterial smooth muscle cells (Hirst and Jobling, 1989). The importance of the ATP-evoked EJP could be, like KCl, to elicit a membrane depolarization which would act synergistically with NA with increased ion permeability adding to the vasoconstrictor response (Ralevic and Burnstock, 1990).

In addition to sympathetic vasoconstrictor effects, there is evidence that ATP acts as a non-sympathetic vasodilator in the rabbit portal vein (Reilly, Saville and Burnstock, 1987) and skeletal muscle vasculature (Shimada and Stitt, 1984) and contributes to non-sympathetic pulmonary vasoconstriction (Inoue and Kannan, 1988). ATP may also exert powerful vasoactive effects after release from endothelial cells (and release of EDRF), C-fibre afferents or intrinsic cardiac neurons (see Burnstock, 1989). The activation of P_{2y} purinoceptors located on the endothelium mediates vasodilatation and the activation of P_{2x}-purinoceptors located on vascular smooth muscle cells mediates vasoconstriction, which implies that ATP elicits different responses in vessels depending on the concentration used, the vascular tone of the vessel and also the degree of endothelial integrity.

INTERACTION WITH NA AND NPY

Apart from their own vasoconstrictor effects, NA and ATP can modulate vascular tone synergistically through prejunctional interaction with the release (see above), or postjunctionally with the potentiation of vasoconstriction (Lukacsko and Blumberg, 1982; Krishnamurty and Kadowitz, 1983). This potentiation can occur at subthreshold concentrations of ATP and is likely to involve mobilization of intracellular or extracellular calcium (Ralevic and Burnstock, 1990). In some preparations where NPY exerts no effect *per se*, the response to both nerve stimulation and $\alpha\beta$metATP was enhanced by NPY, suggesting that the ATP response can be postjunctionally modulated by NPY (Saville, Maynard and Burnstock, 1990).

PHYSIOLOGICAL AND PATHOPHYSIOLOGICAL IMPLICATIONS OF ATP IN SYMPATHETIC TRANSMISSION

The exact importance of the involvement of ATP in sympathetic transmission is still unclear, but there are findings which indicate that ATP could be an important contributor to vascular control. Thus, in normotensive rats, the major neurogenic contraction in the tail artery is mediated by NA while in the spontaneously hypertensive rat, ATP effects are more pronounced, which suggests an involvement of ATP in hypertensive disease (Vidal, Hicks and Langer, 1986). Interestingly, the purinergic modulation of adrenergic transmitter release is attenuated in these rats (Kamikawa, Cline and Su, 1980). Subsensitivity of presynaptic A_1-receptors suggests that enhanced transmitter release could contribute to increases in vascular resistance in hypertensive rats (Illes *et al.*, 1989) However, this hypothesis has been challenged in a recent paper by Dalziel and co-workers who found that in tail arteries from hypertensive rats *in vitro* there is a hyperreactivity to exogenously applied NA and $\alpha\beta$metATP as well as to sympathetic nerve stimulation (Dalziel, Machaly and Sneddon, 1989), but they found no differences in the responses to nerve stimulation after α-adrenoceptor blockade in normotensive or hypertensive pithed rats. In addition, the pressor response to intravenously administered NA and $\alpha\beta$metATP did not differ in these rats.

The contractile effects of ATP, $\alpha\beta$metATP and the purinergic component of contractions evoked by sympathetic nerve stimulation are dependent on an influx of extracellular Ca^{2+} since it can be blocked by Ca^{2+}-entry-blocking agents like nifedipine (Bulloch and McGrath, 1988), verapamil, diltiazem (Omote, Kigoshi and Muramatsu, 1989) and nicardipine (Torregrosa *et al.*, 1990). It is noteworthy in this context that in both the pithed rat (Bulloch and McGrath, 1988) and dog mesenteric artery (Omote, Kigoshi and Muramatsu, 1989) the purinergic, rather than adrenergic, nerve-mediated vasoconstriction was attenuated by nifedipine. In view of the beneficial clinical effects of Ca^{2+}-channel blocking agents, an involvement of ATP in hypertension and vasospasm has been postulated (Burnstock, 1989).

Reactive hyperaemia is the well known physiological event following reperfusion after arterial occlusion (Gaskell, 1877; Bayliss, 1902). This phenomenon is considered to be due to both physical and metabolic factors (see Olsson, 1975). ATP release and activation of endothelial P_{2y}-purinoceptors may be involved in post-occlusive hyperaemia (Burnstock, 1977). The actual involvement of ATP is, however, difficult to evaluate, owing to the complex mixture of released/formed agents co-operating with basic myogenic wall tension in this reaction. The vasodilator effects of ATP may also be beneficial in the treatment of hypoxic pulmonary hypertension (Benumof, Fukunaga and Trousdale, 1982) and chronic obstructive pulmonary disease (Gaba *et al.*, 1986; Gaba and Préfant, 1990).

Unfortunately, most of the studies on ATP have been conducted under *in vitro* conditions and the confirmation that these findings also take place *in vivo* is a key to defining the significance of ATP in sympathetic neurotransmission. If ATP contributes to the physiological regulation of vascular tone, the effects observed should also occur in a wide variety of vascular beds and include small arteries, arterioles and precapillary sphincters in many species. At the present time a purinergic component appears to play an important part in some vessels while in others no purine component can be observed. The possible contribution of ATP, originating from non-neuronal sources, in cardiovascular homeostasis should also be clarified. These questions are likely to be answered in more detail in the near future. Moreover, before assigning an important role to ATP in cardiovascular control, ATP mechanisms must be confirmed in man (see also Holmquist, Hedlund and Andersson, 1990).

NPY

The 36-amino acid residue peptide NPY was originally isolated from the porcine brain (Tatemoto, Carlquist and Mutt, 1982) and belongs to the pancreatic polypeptide family. NPY shares considerable sequence homology with pancreatic polypeptide, produced by cells of the endocrine pancreas, and it was subsequently discovered that the avian pancreatic polypeptide immunoreactivity observed in neuronal tissue was actually NPY (Lundberg et al., 1982).

SYNTHESIS/STORAGE

NPY is generated from a precursor form, 97 amino acids in length (Minth et al., 1984), and is one of the most widely distributed peptides yet discovered. NPY is found in a variety of species with marked homology. The nerve cell body synthesizes NPY, whereupon it is stored in large dense-cored vesicles and transported to the peripheral nerve terminal by axonal transport (Fried, Lundberg and Theodorsson-Norheim, 1985; see Lundberg et al., 1989). The molar ratio of NA:NPY has been estimated to be approximately 1:150 in sympathetic nerve terminals while in the cell body region the ratio is around 1:10 (Fried, Lundberg and Theodorsson-Norheim, 1985). In situ hybridization techniques have been used to localize high levels of NPY mRNA in the stellate ganglia which contain a population of NPY immunoreactive cell bodies (Schalling et al., 1988). The relative amount of NPY in sympathetic ganglia varies considerably, suggesting that NPY occurs in a subpopulation of noradrenergic neurons (Lundberg et al., 1983). NPY is generally co-stored with NA, but there have been reports of co-existence of NPY and ACh and adrenaline as well as various peptides such as dynorphin, somatostatin, vasoactive intestinal polypeptide and calcitonin gene-related peptide (see McDonald, 1988; Lacroix, 1989).

NPY occurs in high concentrations in the cardiovascular system and NPY-immuno-reactive, noradrenergic nerve fibres densely innervate the blood vessels, being more numerous around arteries than around the corresponding veins. NPY fibres are not only present within perivascular nerves but are also associated with myocardial cells and adrenaline-containing chromaffin cells of the adrenal medulla (Lundberg et al., 1982, 1983, 1986b). The tissue content of NPY can be depleted by surgical sympathectomy as well as by treatment with 6-OHDA or reserpine, the latter effect in perivascular nerves being dependent on intact nerve activity since it can be blocked by preganglionic nerve transection or by ganglionic blocking agents like chlorisondamine (Lundberg et al., 1984a, 1985d). The degree of neuronal activity also determines the extent of depletion (Nagata et al., 1987). Reserpine pretreatment simultaneously results in a compensatory increase in synthesis of NPY, as indicated by increased NPY mRNA followed by elevated NPY in the supply region, i.e. sympathetic ganglia (Schalling et al., 1988).

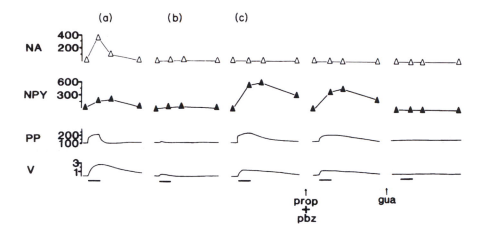

Figure 3.3 The effects of postganglionic nerve stimulation (bar is 10 Hz, 10V, 5ms for 2 min) on volume reduction (V; ml) and perfusion pressure (PP; mm Hg) as well as release of NPY (fmol/min) and NA (pmol/min) from the cat spleen. The effects of nerve stimulation in controls (a) are abolished after reserpine pretreatment (b) while after preganlionic denervation, in combination with reserpine pretreatment (c) there is a substantial, adrenoceptor antagonist-resistant (prop = propranolol; pbz = phenoxy-benzamine) but guanethidine-sensitive (gua), residual functional effect, and release of NPY but not NA. (From Lundberg *et al.*, 1986b. With permission.)

RELEASE

NPY is released in a guanethidine-sensitive manner from a variety of organs upon sympathetic nerve stimulation (Lundberg *et al.*, 1986b; Figure 3.3; see also Table 3.1). NPY release is favoured by high stimulation frequencies, i.e. strong sympathetic activation, and the NPY-overflow under *in vivo* conditions is strongly correlated with the vasoconstriction observed (see Lundberg *et al.*, 1986a; Pernow, 1988; Lacroix, 1989; Lundberg *et al.*, 1989). Circulating NPY is probably primarily cleared over the splanchnic region (Ahlborg, Lundberg and Sollevi, 1991). Pharmacological studies suggest a common Ca^{2+}-dependent exocytotic co-release of NA and NPY from sympathetic nerve terminals (Richardt *et al.*, 1988; Haass *et al.*, 1989). The release is enhanced after α-adrenoceptor blockade, or β-adrenoceptor stimulation, and is reduced by α-adrenoceptor stimulation, indicating that NPY release is regulated prejunctionally by NA (Figure 3.3; Lundberg *et al.*, 1984a; Dahlöf, Dahlöf and Lundberg, 1986; Lundberg *et al.*, 1986b; Rudehill *et al.*, 1987; Linton-Dahlöf, 1989). Conversely, NPY inhibits NA release from perivascular sympathetic nerves (Dahlöf *et al.*, 1985b; Lundberg *et al.*, 1985b; Pernow, 1988). NPY also inhibits cholinergic transmission (Franco-Cereceda, Lundberg and Dalhöf, 1985; Potter, 1985). The co-stored substances NPY and NA thus interact reciprocally in modulating their release from sympathetic nerve terminals. This also implies that agents and conditions that influence NA release and receptor binding will have effects on NPY. There is, in addition, pharmacological evidence that prejunctional NPY mechanisms attenuate NPY release from sympathetic nerve terminals (see Modin, 1994).

RECEPTORS

After investigating the direct vasoconstrictor effects, potentiation of NA-evoked vaso-constriction and inhibition of NA release by NPY and related peptides, Håkansson and co-workers postulated the existence of separate pre- and postjunctional NPY-receptors named Y_1 and Y_2 (Wahlestedt, Yanaihara and Håkansson, 1986, Wahlestedt et al., 1987). The Y_1-receptor is mainly located postjunctionally, causes vasoconstriction and is coupled to phospholipase C with subsequent rises in intracellular Ca^{2+} after activation, while the Y_2 receptor is presynaptically located, inhibits NA release and is associated with the inhibition of the adenylate cyclase system. Both receptors are activated by the whole NPY molecule and the homologous peptide YY, but the Y_1-receptor is not stimulated by C-terminal fragments of less than 24 amino acids in length, whereas the Y_2 receptor is activated by smaller C-terminal fragments. This classification was challenged by Lundberg et al. (1988), who demonstrated receptors with Y_2 characteristics postjunctionally. Furthermore, Michel and co-workers raised several important questions regarding the second messenger systems involved in the respective Y_1- and Y_2-receptor response (Michel et al., 1990). Interestingly, in heart myocytes NPY(18–36) competitively inhibits ^{125}I-NPY binding and also attenuates NPY-evoked inhibition of adenylate cyclase activity and is devoid of any agonist activity per se (Balasubramaniam and Sheriff, 1990) suggesting the existence of an Y_3-receptor (Balasubramaniam et al., 1990).

VASCULAR EFFECTS

A possible physiological role of NPY was originally suggested in a study on the cat submandibular gland where a peptide-like, i.e. slowly developing and long-lasting, α-adrenoceptor antagonist-resistant vasoconstriction was observed after sympathetic stim-ulation (Lundberg and Tatemoto, 1982). A similar effect could be reproduced by injections of NPY. Later this phenomenon was described in several preparations (see Table 3.1). The existence of a large non-adrenergic component is especially apparent following sympathetic nerve stimulation with high frequencies and irregular bursts, which also favour NPY release (Lacroix et al., 1988a; Pernow et al., 1989).

NPY causes profound pressor effects when administered in vivo. The increase in blood pressure by NPY is due to increased vascular resistance as well as increased cardiac stroke volume secondarily to an increased venous return (MacLean and Hiley, 1990). The sensitivity of different organs to i.v. administered NPY largely depends on the species investigated. In the rabbit (Minson, McRitchie and Chalmers, 1989) and rat (Gardiner, Bennett and Compton, 1988), the renal vascular bed is most sensitive while the splenic circulation is most sensitive in the pig (Rudehill et al., 1987). Supersensitivity to the pressor effects of NPY following chemical or surgical sympathectomy has been demonstrated both in the rat (Mabe et al., 1987; Nield, 1987; Benarroch et al., 1990) and pig (Lacroix, 1989). Since in the pig nasal mucosa $\alpha\beta$metATP- and α_2-agonist-evoked vasoconstriction were also enhanced, the observed supersensitivity could reflect changes in intracellular pathways rather than specific up-regulation of receptors.

Reserpine is a useful tool in evaluating the effects of NPY under in vivo conditions (Lundberg et al., 1985c,d). Thus, reserpine pretreatment depletes the peripheral tissue stores of NA while leaving those of NPY largely unaffected if the neuronal activity has been impaired pharmacologically (by clonidine, guanethidine or chlorisondamine) or surgically (by denervation). High-frequency stimulation of sympathetic nerves in a variety of organs under *in vivo* conditions while there is still NPY (and ATP, see above) in the peripheral nerve terminals reveals only a long-lasting vasoconstriction strongly correlated with NPY outflow and subject to fatigue upon repeated stimulation, probably owing to restricted terminal resupply of NPY by axonal transport (Lundberg *et al.*, 1986b; see Pernow, 1988; Lacroix, 1989). However, taking into account that NA inhibits NPY release, the nerve stimulation-evoked NPY release after NA depletion by reserpine is likely to be overestimated.

ATP mechanisms have been evaluated in some of these *in vivo* models. In the pig nasal mucosa (Lacroix *et al.*, 1988b), $\alpha\beta$metATP mimicked the vascular responses to sympathetic nerve stimulation after α-adrenoceptor blockade combined with reserpine pretreatment, while ATP given intra-arterially caused a short-lasting vasoconstriction followed by vasodilatation. It should be emphasized, however, that endogenously released ATP is likely to reach receptors other than those activated by exogenous ATP. Furthermore, since $\alpha\beta$metATP inhibited NPY release in reserpine-pretreated pigs but not in controls, it is difficult to draw conclusions about the contribution of ATP to reserpine-resistant sympathetic porcine nasal vasoconstriction. It seems clear that after depletion of NA and NPY by reserpine pretreatment, no ATP component can be demonstrated in many vascular preparations (Lundberg *et al.*, 1987). Although exogenous NPY causes vasoconstriction in the rat mesenteric artery, a possible NPY component in the vascular response to sympathetic nerve stimulation could only be demonstrated after increasing basal vascular tone with vasopressin suggesting that in this preparation NPY release mainly modulated the response to other transmitters (Sjöblom-Widfeldt, 1990).

It has been difficult to consistently show vasoconstrictor effects of NPY *in vitro* while, *in vivo*, NPY is almost always a potent vasocontrictor regardless of the vascular bed studied (Rudehill *et al.*, 1986). This may be related to the fact that experiments using *in vitro* techniques study relatively large blood vessels while NPY exerts its main effects on small resistance vessels (Hughes *et al.*, 1988; Franco-Cereceda, 1989). The vascular reactivity to NPY is also rapidly lost in isolated organ models (Allen *et al.*, 1983; Franco-Cereceda, Lundberg and Dahlöf, 1985). There have been, however, reports on potent vasoconstrictor effects of NPY in several different isolated blood vesssel preparations, including cat cerebral arteries (Edvinsson *et al.*, 1983), rabbit blood vessels (Edvinsson *et al.*, 1984), human coronary arteries (Franco-Cereceda and Lundberg, 1987), human mesenteric veins, renal and skeletal muscle arteries (Pernow, Svenberg and Lundberg, 1987), guinea-pig uterine artery (Figure 3.4) and vena cava (Morris and Murphy, 1988; Morris, 1991) and the rat femoral artery (Lundberg *et al.*, 1985b). The vasoconstrictor effect of NPY is slow in onset, long lasting, endothelium-independent and repeated administration of NPY induces tachyphylaxis.

Strong evidence for direct participation of NPY in sympathetic vasoconstriction *in vitro* has been presented by Morris and Murphy in experiments on guinea-pig uterine arteries (Figure 3.4) and vena cava where vasodilator axons had been surgically removed prior to the experiments (Morris and Murphy, 1988; Morris, 1991). Thus, the neurogenic contraction and the contraction evoked by exogenous NPY, but not NA, were reduced by trypsin (which cleaves peptides containing the amino acids lysine or arginine) and

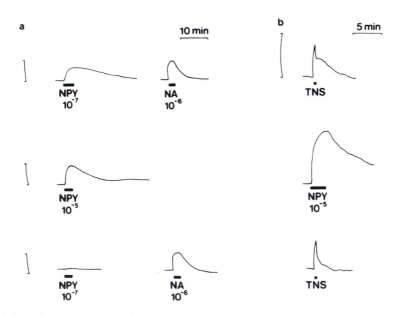

Figure 3.4   In isolated guinea-pig uterine arteries, NPY (a) evokes a contraction subject to tachyphylaxis upon repeated administration. Desensitization to NPY does not influence the NA-evoked contractions (a) while the vasoconstrictor response to transmural nerve stimulation (TNS) is markedly reduced (b). (From Morris and Murphy 1988. With permission.)

following NPY desensitization the slow phase of the neurogenic vasoconstriction, but not the prazosin-sensitive portion, was reduced. Interestingly, the recently developed Y_1-receptor antagonist BIBP 3226 attenuated the sympathetic vasoconstriction in the guinea-pig vena cava (Malmström and Lundberg, 1995).

The vasoconstrictor effect of NPY is not influenced by α- or β-adrenoceptor blocking agents (Lundberg and Tatemoto, 1982; Lundberg et al., 1984a; Figure 3.4) but can be attenuated by Ca^{2+}-channel blockers like nifedipine, verapamil, diltiazem and nimodipine (Edvinsson et al., 1983; Edvinsson, 1985; Pernow, 1988). Subsequently, the sustained contractions of NPY have been suggested to be mediated through a prolonged smooth muscle depolarization with continuous refilling of calcium stores (Fallgren et al., 1990).

NPY also inhibits vasodilatation evoked by ACh, substance P, adenosine and β-adrenoceptor stimulation and may thus have a function of opposing vasodilatation (Han and Abel, 1987; Fallgren, Ekblad and Edvinsson, 1989). The possibility that NPY may produce some of its effects through the release of other endogenous substances such as prostaglandins (Martin and Patterson, 1989) requires further investigation (Rioux et al., 1986).

INTERACTION WITH NA

Although direct contractile in vitro effects of NPY are usually not as apparent as in vivo, NPY often enhances the vasoconstrictor effect of NA in vitro (Edvinsson et al., 1984;

Ekblad *et al.*, 1984; Glower, 1985; Wahlestedt *et al.*, 1985) as well as *in vivo* (Dahlöf, Dahlöf and Lundberg, 1985a; Revington and McCloskey, 1988). NPY also potentiates the vasoconstriction of phenylephrine, sympathetic nerve stimulation (Dahlöf *et al.*, 1985b), histamine (Ekblad *et al.*, 1984; Han and Abel, 1987), tyramine and angiotensin II but not vasopressin (Waeber *et al.*, 1988), and $\alpha\beta$metATP (Saville, Maynard and Burnstock, 1990). In other vessels, NPY does not influence the effects of prostaglandin $F_{2\alpha}$, serotonin or high potassium concentrations (Edvinsson *et al.*, 1984), indicating that the potentiation is dependent on the vascular preparation studied. Therefore, this effect may not be caused by a general change in smooth muscle reactivity with increased Ca^{2+}-influx (Glower, 1986; Andriantsitohaina and Stoclet, 1988) but, rather, suggests that NPY induces specific changes in receptor characteristics and/or second messenger systems. NPY-evoked contractions are not influenced by removal of the endothelium (Pernow and Lundberg, 1988; Fallgren *et al.*, 1990) and a possible involvement of the endothelium in the NPY-induced enhancement of NA-evoked contractions (Daly and Hieble, 1987) seems unlikely (Budai, Vu and Duckles, 1989). NPY inhibits forskolin-induced adenylate cyclase stimulation (Fredholm, Jansen and Edvinsson 1985) and this pertussis-toxin-sensitive inhibitory pathway has been suggested to be involved in the potentiating effect of NPY on NA-evoked vasoconstriction (Kassis *et al.*, 1987). Although the vasoconstrictor effect of NPY is highly dependent on calcium influx, the potentiating effect is not influenced by nifedipine but seems to require sodium influx followed by mobilization of intracellular Ca^{2+} and increased phospholipase C activity, which would be an alternative explanation for the synergism between NPY and NA (Wahlestedt *et al.*, 1985, 1990). Nifedipine does not influence NPY-evoked inhibition of NA release, which excludes any presynaptic action of this drug (Pernow, 1988).

PHYSIOLOGICAL AND PATHOPHYSIOLOGICAL IMPLICATIONS OF NPY IN SYMPATHETIC TRANSMISSION

Plasma levels of NPY are correlated with those of NA and an increase in plasma NA by reflex sympathetic discharge is accompanied by a parallel increase in NPY levels with an increasing NPY ratio the higher the frequencies (Lundberg *et al.*, 1985a; Pernow, 1988). The actual contribution of various possible sources, such as the brain, peripheral nervous system, enteric nervous system and the adrenals, to plasma NPY may differ under various conditions, however. Resting NPY plasma levels are low in most species, including man (around 20 pM; Pernow, 1988), with a biphasic disappearance curve and half-lives of 4 and 20 min for the two respective slopes (Pernow, Lundberg and Kaiser, 1987). Sympathetic activation by exercise releases NPY (Lundberg *et al.*, 1985a; Morris *et al.*, 1986), but the actual contribution of NPY in sympathetic transmission under physiological conditions remains to be established. With regard to pathophysiological situations, there are many reports on possible NPY involvement in a variety of cardiovascular disorders. Thus, experimental ligation of the coronary arteries reduces cardiac levels of NPY (Han *et al.*, 1989) and an increased NPY outflow from the heart is observed in response to ischaemia (Franco-Cereceda *et al.*, 1990) . Since the peripheral plasma NPY- and NA-levels were also increased, it is likely that an enhanced sympathetic discharge, rather than an energy deficiency, caused the alterations in NPY levels and the release from the heart. This is supported by the finding that total stop-flow ischaemia of isolated hearts does not release

NPY (Franco-Cereceda, 1988). Furthermore, elevated plasma levels of NPY are found in patients with left heart failure, angina pectoris and myocardial infarction, indicating that NPY may contribute to the clinical signs of haemodynamic disturbance observed in these conditions (Maisel *et al.*, 1989; Hulting *et al.*, 1990). Intracoronarily administered NPY in humans with angina pectoris causes cardiac ischaemia (Clarke *et al.*, 1987). The potent direct coronary vasoconstrictor effect of NPY can be prevented by Ca^{2+}-channel blocking agents (Franco-Cereceda, Lundberg and Dahlöf, 1985; Franco-Cereceda, 1989) while α-adrenoceptor blockade is ineffective (Allen *et al.*, 1983; Aizawa *et al.*, 1985), implying that NPY may be involved in coronary vasospasm, which is known to respond to inhibition of Ca^{2+} influx but poorly to α-adrenoceptor blockade (see Corr *et al.*, 1990). Subarachnoid haemorrhage is associated with increased NPY levels in the cerebrospinal fluid (Abel *et al.*, 1988) and decreased neuronal levels of NPY, suggesting that NPY may also contribute to cerebral vasospasm (Jackowski *et al.*, 1989).

In spontaneously hypertensive rats, the inhibitory effect of NPY on NA release is weaker and the vasoconstrictor effect of NPY is stronger than in normotensive rats, which is supporting evidence of a role for NPY in the development and maintenance of hypertension (Westfall *et al.*, 1988). Recently elevated plasma levels of NPY have been detected in patients with hypertension (Edvinsson, Ekman and Thulin, 1991). Hypertension in phaeochromocytoma is also associated with highly elevated plasma levels of NPY (up to nM; see Adrian *et al.*, 1983; Lundberg *et al.*, 1986c).

NPY is preferentially released by high-frequency stimulation and the vasoconstrictor activity of NPY is most important during stimulation of high sympathetic nerve activity. Adrenergic desensitization by increased neuronal discharge is reversed by NPY and this may represent an additional modulation of sympathetic transmitter effects, which could be of use in restoring therapeutically induced desensitization to adrenergic drugs (Wahlestedt *et al.*, 1990). The vasoconstrictor effect of NPY may also be beneficial in the treatment of hypotension induced by, for instance, endotoxaemia (Evéquoz *et al.*, 1988), a condition in which plasma NPY levels are elevated (Watson *et al.*, 1988).

NON-CHOLINERGIC MECHANISMS

As long ago as 1872, Heidenhahn proposed the existence of a separate set of vasodilator nerves supplying the salivary glands, based on the ability of atropine to block parasympathetic nerve stimulation-induced salivary secretion, but not vasodilatation (see Lundberg, 1981). The atropine-resistant component was especially apparent at higher-frequency stimulations (Darke and Smaje, 1972). A variety of interpretations has been put forward to explain this residual atropine-insensitive vasodilator response, but it seems likely that it is mediated by VIP (Lundberg, 1981).

Evidence for the occurrence of non-cholinergic non-adrenergic vasodilator nerves in the blood vessels of the nasal mucosa has also been presented some years ago (Änggård, 1974). More recent experiments have established that stimulation of parasympathetic nerves to the nasal mucosa and laryngo-tracheal circulation of the cat, dog and pig evokes an increase in blood flow that is partly resistant to atropine but is attenuated by ganglionic blocking agents (Lundblad *et al.*, 1983; Lung *et al.*, 1984; Martling, Änggård and Lundberg, 1985; Laitinen, Laitinen and Widdicombe, 1987; Stjärne *et al.*, 1991), and thus increasing evidence, particularly from the respiratory tract, suggests the involvement of a non-cholineric vasodilator component in the regulation of blood flow (see Widdicombe, 1990).

Another area of great interest in this context is the cerebral circulation, in which Lee and co-workers have demonstrated a neurogenic vasodilatation that was not influenced by agents inhibiting ACh mechanisms (Lee, Su and Bevan, 1975; Lee, Saito and Berezin, 1984).

VIP/PHI

VIP is a 28 amino acid residue peptide first isolated from the porcine intestine and given its name because of its potent and long-lasting vasodilator activity (Said and Mutt, 1970a,b). It was later shown that the human and porcine forms of VIP are identical (Carlqvist *et al.*, 1982).

STORAGE/SYNTHESIS

Originally, VIP was considered to be a gut hormone but immunohistochemical studies revealed that it may also be a transmitter (Bryant *et al.*, 1976; Fahrenkrug, 1979, 1981; Edvinsson and Uddman, 1988). Later the presence of VIP in a population of cholinergic nerves (Lundberg *et al.*, 1979; Uddman *et al.*, 1981) was established (Lundberg *et al.*, 1984c). These nerves probably also contain a 27 amino acid residue peptide, peptide histidine-isoleucine (PHI) (Yanaihara *et al.*, 1983), derived from the VIP-precursor (Christofides *et al.*, 1982) or peptide histidine-methionine (PHM) in man, which differs in 2 amino acids from porcine PHI (Itoh *et al.*, 1983). VIP-immunoreactive perivascular nerve terminals are widespread and particularly abundant in the upper respiratory, gastrointestinal and urogenital tract, as well as in cerebral vessels (see Owman, 1990).

Like most polypeptides, VIP is synthesized in the neuronal cell body as a larger precursor molecule, cleaved to a final form and transported along the axon to the terminal where it is stored in large dense-cored vesicles (Johansson and Lundberg, 1981; Lundberg *et al.*, 1981).

RELEASE

VIP release by activation of peripheral parasympathetic nerves has been demonstrated in the venous effluent from various parts of the gastrointestinal tract (Fahrenkrug *et al.*, 1978). submandibular gland (Figure 3.5; Lundberg *et al.*, 1980; Uddman *et al.*, 1980), nasal mucosa (Uddman *et al.*, 1981) and cerebrovascular circulation (Bevan *et al.*, 1984). The release of VIP is abolished by ganglionic blocking agents like chlorisondamine, indicating a neuronal origin. Moreover, the basal outflow of VIP is diminished upon muscarinic receptor blockade (Fahrenkrug *et al.*, 1978) while upon stimulation, atropine can enhance VIP release (Figure 3.5; Lundberg *et al.*, 1984b), suggesting a regulatory action of ACh on VIP release. The release is favoured by high-frequency stimulation which enhances the atropine-resistant vasodilatation in the salivary gland (Lundberg *et al.*, 1984b). Resting

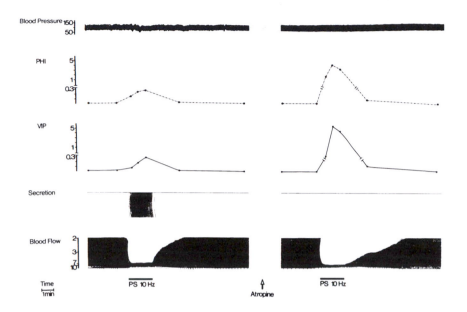

Figure 3.5 Parasympathetic nerve stimulation (chorda-lingual nerve; 10 Hz, 1 ms, 10V, for 2 min) evokes an increase in blood flow (ml/min) in the cat submandibular gland and salivary secretion (drops) concurrently with increased venous plasma levels of VIP and PHI (pmol/min/g). Atropine prolongs the vasodilator response in combination with enhanced release of VIP and PHI. (From Lundberg *et al.*, 1984b. With permission.)

plasma levels of VIP are low (Fahrenkrug and Schaffalitsky de Muckadell, 1977) owing to a half-life of approximately 1–2 min (Domschke *et al.*, 1978).

RECEPTORS

Specific VIP-binding sites have been identified in human, bovine, rat and guinea-pig pulmonary vessels (Robberecht *et al.*, 1982; Barnes *et al.*, 1986; Carstairs and Barnes, 1986) as well as in bovine cerebral arteries (Suzuki *et al.*, 1985) located in the media. VIP receptors have been subdivided into VIP1 (Ishihara *et al.*, 1992) and VIP2 (Lutz *et al.*, 1993) receptors. Activation of VIP receptors in cardiac and vascular membrane preparations is associated with stimulation of the adenylate cyclase system (Cohen and Schwab-Landry, 1980; Chatelain *et al.*, 1983; Christophe *et al.*, 1984) which mediates the relaxation of precontracted arteries by VIP (Huang and Rorstad, 1983; Edvinsson *et al.*, 1985).

VASCULAR EFFECTS

VIP is a potent, endothelium-independent vasodilator acting directly on the vascular smooth muscle (see Wharton and Gulbenkian, 1989; Owman, 1990). The potency of VIP varies in

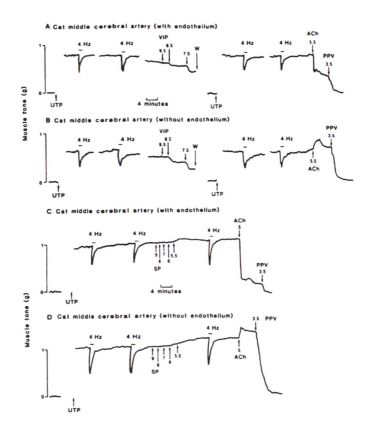

Figure 3.6   Transmural nerve stimulation of cat cerebral arteries evokes an endothelium-independent vaso-dilatation (a,b) similar in appearance to the effect of VIP but not substance P(c,d). (From Lee, Saito and Berezin, 1984. With permission.)

different vascular beds studied and, interestingly, the cerebral and salivary gland circulation are among the most sensitive to VIP (Said and Mutt, 1970b; Lundberg *et al.*, 1981; Lee, 1986). On a molar basis, VIP is about 50–100 times more potent than ACh as a vasodilator. The relaxant effect of VIP is not restricted to arteries, but also capacitance vessels dilate in response to VIP (Järhult, Hellstrand and Sundler, 1980).

Electrical field stimulation of various isolated arteries from many species, including the rabbit (Duckles and Said, 1982), cat (Figure 5.6; Lee *et al.*, 1978; Lee, 1986; Bevan *et al.*, 1986; Kubota *et al.*, 1988), guinea-pig (Kubota *et al.*, 1986, 1988), dog, monkey (Toda, 1982) and man (Toda, 1981) evokes an atropine-resistant vasodilatation which does not occur after blockade of neurogenic transmission by either tetrodotoxin or ganglionic blocking agents. The relaxation of the arteries is frequency-dependent, is mimicked by exogenous VIP and remains unchanged after α- and β-adrenoceptor blockade. Furthermore, the vasodilator response induced by ACh, but not by nerve stimulation, depends on the presence of the endothelium (Figure 5.6) and the neurogenic vasodilatation also remains after sympathetic denervation (Lee, 1986). Taken together with the presence of VIP nerve terminals in the adventitia-media layer, but not in the intima, it is likely that the nerve stimulation induced relaxation is due to VIP.

Further convincing evidence of VIP mediating a neurogenic vasodilatation is the finding that a specific VIP antiserum markedly reduced the nerve stimulation-induced vasodilatation in the cat submandibular gland *in vivo* (Lundberg *et al.*, 1980) and cat cerebral arteries *in vitro* (Bevan *et al.*, 1984; Brayden and Bevan, 1986).

The magnitude of VIP-induced vasodilatation and increased blood flow *in vivo* varies at different sites. The potency and efficacy of VIP as a vasodilator are greater in the coronary and extracranial circulation than in the pulmonary or renal circulation (Brum *et al.*, 1986). This widespread vasodilatation by VIP results in decreased blood pressure and increased cardiac output (Domschke and Domschke, 1982; Smitherman *et al.*, 1982). VIP administered i.v. to man evokes a marked vasodilatation concomitantly with an increase in heart rate (Domschke and Domschke, 1982), the latter effect possibly being related to both reflex sympathetic activation and a direct effect of VIP on cardiac contractility (Said and Mutt 1970a; Franco-Cereceda, Bengtsson and Lundberg, 1987). Thus, the abundance of VIP-immunoreactive nerve fibres in the cardiac (Weihe, Reinecke and Forssmann, 1984), cerebral (Uddman *et al.*, 1981) and laryngo-tracheal circulation (Martling *et al.*, 1990) parallels VIP receptor mechanisms *in vivo*, i.e. potent tissue-selective vasodilatation of exogenous VIP. Following parasympathetic nerve stimulation *in vivo* there is a markedly increased venous effluent of VIP in parallel with a vasodilator response (Figures 3.5). Interestingly, the duration of this response is prolonged after atropine when a further increase in VIP outflow is observed (Lundberg *et al.*, 1984b).

PHI is released in a 1:1 ratio with VIP upon parasympathetic nerve stimulation and the release is enhanced by atropine (Figure 3.5; Lundberg *et al.*, 1984c). PHI also exerts atropine-resistant vasodilatation, although usually with a significantly lower potency than VIP. Furthermore, there are considerable regional variations in the relative amounts of VIP and PHI, with the heart and lung containing more VIP (Fahrenkrug *et al.*, 1985). To what extent PHI also contributes to the non-cholinergic vasodilatation remains unclear.

PHYSIOLOGICAL AND PATHOPHYSIOLOGICAL IMPLICATIONS OF VIP IN CHOLINERGIC TRANSMISSION

Based on the potent effects of VIP in the pulmonary circulation a role for VIP in maintaining low vascular resistance in the pulmonary circulation has been suggested (Kubota *et al.*, 1983). Disturbances of this relaxatory system would promote pulmonary hypertension as observed in various pathophysiological conditions.

Since VIP enhances cardiac output (Said and Mutt, 1970a), potently dilates human coronary arteries (Franco-Cereceda and Rudehill, 1989) and plasma levels of VIP are increased in patients with acute heart failure (Clark *et al.*, 1983), the possibility remains that VIP may have a pathophysiological role in cardiac disorders. Furthermore, the inotropic effects of VIP are attenuated in left ventricular hypertrophy due to hypertension (Fouad *et al.*, 1986). Perivascular cerebral VIP nerve fibre decrease following experimental subarachnoidal haemorrhage and VIP could therefore counteract the pathophysiological processes inducing cerebral vasospasm (Uemura *et al.*, 1986). In the dog, the venous plasma levels of VIP are not increased in response to hypoxia or hypercapnia, while the local blood flow increases up to 300% (Wilson *et al.*, 1981), and thus the proper stimulus for VIP release remains unclear.

NO

Nitric oxide (NO) has been demonstrated to mediate the endothelium-dependent relaxation evoked by certain stimuli, e.g. ACh, substance P (Furchgott and Zawadski, 1980; Palmer, Ferrige and Moncada, 1987). However, recent findings of NOS in neuronal tissue and the co-existance of NO and VIP in parasympathetic postganglionic nerve terminals suggest that NO may be synthesised and released from cholinergic vascular nerve terminals (Kummer *et al.*, 1992; Blottner and Baumgarten, 1994). Thus, inhibition of NO-production attenuates parasympathetic, non-cholinergic vasodilatation (Garthwaite, 1991).

SYNTHESIS/RELEASE

NO is produced from L-arginine by NOS which is present in an inducible form (in macrophages) and a constitutive form (in endothelial and neuronal cells; Mayer *et al.*, 1989; Busse and Mülch, 1990; Bredt and Snyder, 1990). In contrast to ACh and VIP/PHI, NO is not vesicularly stored but locally produced on demand (shear stress; Moncada, Palmer and Higgs, 1991) and thereafter "released" by diffusion. After release NO is bound to the heme region in soluble gyanylyl cyclase which activates the enzyme, thereby increasing cGMP levels (Wolin, Wood and Ignarro, 1982). This may cause vascular relaxation through activation of a protein kinase (Rapaport, Draznin and Murad, 1983), or through reduction in intracellular calcium (Rashatwar, Cornwell and Lincoln, 1987). Interestingly, neuronal depolarization induces NO-synthesis (Bredt and Snyder, 1990). NOS can be inhibited by several L-arginine analogues which act as false substrates. Unfortunately, however, these compounds are non-selective with regards to endothelial and neuronal NOS which make interpretation of data difficult. Furthermore, it was recently demonstrated that several of the L-arginine analogues used to inhibit NO-synthesis and NO-effects also influenced the responses to e.g. VIP (Gaw *et al.*, 1991; Edwards and Garrett, 1991; see Modin, 1994). Moreover, these analogues may attenuate peptide release upon parasympathetic nerve stimulation (Modin, 1994).

PHYSIOLOGICAL AND PATHOPHYSIOLOGICAL IMPLICATIONS

Apart from indirect evidence using L-arginine analogues to inhibit NO-mediated vaso-dilatation *in vivo* and *in vitro*, the administration of inhaled NO has revealed potent vasodilator actions of NO in the pulmonary circulation (Frostell *et al.*, 1993). This effect is restricted to the pulmonary circulation in a low concentration range while increasing the concentration causes systemic vasodilatation. Endothelial NOS is stimulated by shear stress which indicates that NO may represent a major regulator of vascular tone (Moncada, Palmer and Higgs, 1991). Naturally, the use of nitrovasodilators (as NO donors) in cardiovascular disorders further support the importance of NO in vascular homeostasis.

SUMMARY AND CONCLUDING REMARKS

Transmitter criteria should include: synthesis and storage in presynaptic neurons; Ca^{2+}-dependent release upon nerve terminal depolarization; interaction with specific receptors at post- and prejunctional sites; inactivation mechanisms, i.e. uptake or enzymatic degradation after release; nerve-stimulation responses should mimic those of the exogenous substance; there should be similar modulation of the response to nerve stimulation and to the exogenous substance by drugs. Some of these criteria have been fulfilled by several of the substances co-stored with NA and ACh in the autonomic nervous system. However, the mere existence and co-release of a substance in perivascular nerve fibres does not necessarily imply a role as a co-transmitter since the agent could be involved in a variety of other mechanisms, including regulation of transmitter release. Co-transmission therefore should include effects on target cells in which co-released transmitters interact.

When studying vascular responses, the conclusions drawn depend on the type of organs and blood vessels investigated and on the experimental conditions imposed. Unfortunately, marked species differences exist, which make it difficult to extrapolate findings from one investigation to another. The relevance of an observed effect may also be affected when comparing *in vitro* findings with *in vivo* observations upon which reflex systems impinge. The functional significance of co-existence could also depend on the activity of the nerve terminal, high-frequency stimulation often being needed to evoke peptide release. It is also clear that general conclusions regarding co-existence are difficult to draw since there are different pools of nerves, some peptide-containing nerve terminals being predominant in visceral organs but not in blood vessels and *vice versa*. The lack of specific receptor antagonists for many of these agents and the fact that their metabolism, release and functional effects are influenccd by agents considered to specifically influence the classical transmitters NA and ACh further obscure the findings.

It may be concluded that ATP and NPY seem to fulfil all of the above-mentioned requirements for transmitters: synthesis and storage of ATP and NPY in sympathetic nerves is obvious; Ca^{2+}-dependent release occurs upon nerve stimulation; exogenous ATP or NPY mimic some of the non-adrenergic effects of nerve stimulation in several experimental models; after release, ATP is rapidly degraded enzymatically while NPY diffuses away; distinct receptors exist both pre- and postjunctionally; and pharmacological interventions influence ATP as well as NPY mechanisms. As for VIP and NO, the situation is more uncertain but it is tempting to claim that VIP as well as NO are peripheral neurotransmitters in the non-cholinergic vasodilatation observed upon stimulation of parasympathetic nerves to vascular smooth muscle.

It is indeed true that enormous advances in technology and methodology in the last few decades have opened up new possibilities for studying biologically active agents previously unknown (Carlsson, 1988). To what extent these agents actually have important effects and possibly contribute to neurotransmission under physiological and pathophysiological conditions is largely unclear but deserves further investigation. A functional change in haemodynamics following selective removal or blockade of the actions exerted by the compounds discussed in this article must be demonstrated but this will require the development of selective antagonists.

ACKNOWLEDGEMENTS

The support of the Swedish Heart-Lung Foundation, the Wallenberg Foundation and the Swedish Medical Research Council (9896) is gratefully acknowledged.

REFERENCES

Abel, P.W., Han, C., Noe, B.D. and McDonald, J.K. (1988). Neuropeptide Y: vasoconstrictor effects and possible role in cerebral vasospasm after experimental subarachnoid haemorrhage. *Brain Research*, **463**, 250–258.

Adrian, T.E., Terenghi, G., Brown, M.J., Allen, J.M., Bacarese-Hamilton, A.J., Polak, J.M., *et al.* (1983). Neuropeptide Y in phaeocromocytomas and ganglioneuroblastomas. *Lancet*, **ii**, 540–542.

Ahlborg, G., Lundberg, J.M. and Sollevi, A. (1991). Vasoconstriction and metabolic effects of neuropeptide Y in man with special reference to splanchnic and renal clearance at rest and during exercise. *Acta Physiologica Scandinavica*, in press.

Aizawa, Y., Murata, M., Hayashi, M., Funazaki, T., Ito, S. and Shibata, A. (1985). Vasoconstrictor effects of neuropeptide Y (NPY) on canine coronary circulation. *Japanese Circulation Journal*, **49**, 584–588.

Allen, J.M., Bircham, P.M.M., Edwards, A.V., Tatemoto, K. and Bloom, S.R. (1983). Neuropeptide Y (NPY) reduces mycardial perfusion and inhibits the force of contraction of the isolated rabbit heart. *Regulatory Peptides*, **6**, 247–252.

Andriantsitohaina, R. and Stoclet, J.C. (1988). Potentiation by neuropeptide Y of vasoconstriction in rat resistance arteries. *British Journal of Pharmacology*, **95**, 419–428.

Änggård, A. (1974). The effects of parasympathetic nerve stimulation on the microcirculation and secretion in the nasal mucosa of the cat. *Acta Oto-Laryngologica*, **78**, 98–105.

Angus, J.A., Broughton, A. and Mulvany, M.J. (1988). Role of α-adrenoceptors in constrictor responses of rat, guinea-pig and rabbit small arteries to neural activation. *Journal of Physiology*, **403**, 495–510.

Balasubramaniam, A. and Sheriff, S. (1990). Neuropeptide Y (18–36) is a competitive antagonist of neuropeptide Y in rat cardiac ventricular membranes. *Journal of Biological Chemistry*, **265**, 14724–14727.

Balasubramaniam, A., Sheriff, S., Rigel, D.F. and Fisher, J.E. (1990). Characterization of neuropeptide Y binding sites in rat cardiac ventricular membranes. *Peptides*, **11**, 545–550.

Bao, J.X., Eriksson, I.E. and Stjärne, L. (1990). Neurotransmitters and pre- and post-junctional receptors involved in the vasoconstrictor response to sympathetic nerve stimulation in rat tail artery. *Acta Physiologica Scandinavica*, **140**, 467–479.

Barnes, P.J., Cadieux, A., Carstairs, J.R., Greenberg, B. Polak, J.M. and Rhoden, K. (1986). Vasoactive intestinal peptide bovine in pulmonary artery: localisation, function and receptor autoradiography. *British Journal of Pharmacology*, **89**, 157–162.

Bayliss, W.M. (1902). On the local reaction of the arterial wall to changes in internal pressure. *Journal of Physiology*, **28**, 220–231.

Bell, C. (1969). Transmission from vasoconstrictor and vasodilatator nerves to single smooth muscle cells of the guinea-pig uterine artery. *Journal of Physiology*, **205**, 695–708.

Benumof, J.L., Fukunaga, A.F. and Trousdale, F.R. (1982). ATP inhibits hypoxic pulmonary vasoconstriction. *Anesthesiology*, **57**, A474.

Benarroch, E.E., Schmelzer, J.D., Ward, K.K.,. Nelson, D.K. and Low, P.A. (1990). Noradrenergic and neuropeptide Y mechanisms in guanethidine-sympathectomized rats. *American Journal of Physiology*, **205**, R371–R375.

Bevan, J.A., Buga, G.M., Moskowitz, M.A. and Said, S.I. (1986). *In vitro* evidence that vasoactive intestinal peptide is a transmitter of neuro-vasodilatation in the head of the cat. *Neuroscience*, **19**, 597–604.

Bevan, J.A., Moscowitz, M.A., Said, S.I. and Buga, G. (1984). Evidence that vasoactive intestinal polypeptide is a dilator transmitter to some cerebral and extracerebral cranial arteries. *Peptides*, **5**, 385–388.

Blottner, D. and Baumgarten, H.G. (1992). Nitric oxide synthase (NOS)-containing sympathoadrenal cholinergic neurons in the rat IML-cell column: evidence from histochemistry, immuno-histochemistry and reterograde labelling. *Journal of Comparative Neurolgy*, **316**, 45–55.

Brayden, J.E. and Bevan, J.A. (1986). Evidence that vasoactive intestinal polypeptide (VIP) mediates neurogenic vasodilatation of feline cerebral arteries. *Stroke*, **17**, 1189–1192.

Bredt, D.S. and Snyder, S.H. (1992). Nitric oxide, a novel neuronal messenger. *Neuron*, **8**, 3–11.

Brum, J.M., Bove, A.A. Sufan, Q., Reilly, W. and Go, V.L.W. (1986). Action and localization of vasoactive intestinal peptide in the coronary circulation: Evidence for nonadrenergic, noncholinergic coronary regulation. *Journal of the American College of Cardiology*, **7**, 406–413.

Bryant, M.G., Bloom, S.R., Polak, J.M., Albuquerque, R.H., Modlin, I. and Pearse, A.G.E. (1976). Possible dual role for vasoactive intestinal peptide as gastrointestinal hormone and neurotransmitter substance. *Lancet*, **i**, 991–993.

Budai, D., Vu, H.Q. and Duckles, S.P. (1989). Endothelium removal does not affect potentiation by neuropeptide Y in rabbit ear artery. *European Journal of Pharmacology*, **168**, 97–100.

Bülbring, E. and Burn, J.H. (1935). The sympathetic dilator fibre in the muscle of the cat and dog. *Journal of Physiology*, **83**, 483–501.

Bulloch, J.M. and McGrath, J.C. (1988). Selective blockade by nifedipine of "purineric" rather than adrenergic nerve-mediated vasopressor responses in the pithed rat. *British Journal of Pharmacology*, **95**, 695–700.

Bulloch, J.M. and McGrath, J.C. (1986). Blockade of vasopressor and vas deferens responses by α,β-methylene ATP in the pithed rat. *British Journal of Pharmacology*, **89**, 577P.

Burnstock, G. (1976). Do some nerve cells release more than one transmitter? *Neuroscience*, **1**, 239–248.

Burnstock, G. (1977). Autonomic neuroeffector junctions — Reflex vasodilatation of the skin. *Journal of Investigative Dermatology*, **69**, 47–57.

Burnstock, G. (1978). A basis for distinguishing two types of purinergic receptors. In *Cell Membrane Receptors for Drugs and Hormones: A Multidisciplinary Approach*, edited by R.W. Straub and L. Bolis, pp. 107–163. New York: Raven Press.

Burnstock, G. (1982). The co-transmitter hypothesis, with special reference to the storage and release of ATP with noradrenaline and acetylcholine. In *Co-transmission*, edited by A.C. Cuello, pp. 151–163. London: McMillan Press Ltd.

Burnstock, G. (1988). Some historical perspectives and future directions. In *Nonadrenergic Innervation of Blood Vessels*, edited by G. Burnstock and S.G. Griffith, pp. 1–14. Boca Raton: CRC Press, Inc.

Burnstock, G. (1989). Vascular control by purines with emphasis on the coronary system. *European Heart Journal*, **10** (Suppl. F), 15–21.

Burnstock, G. and Kennedy, C. (1985a). Is there a basis for distinguishing two types of P_2-purinoceptor? *General Pharmacology*, **16**, 433–440.

Burnstock, G. and Kennedy, C. (1985b). A dual function for adenosine 5'-triphosphate in the regulation of vascular tone. *Circulation Research*, **58**, 319–330.

Burnstock, G. and Warland, J.J.I. (1987). A pharmacological study of the rabbit saphenous artery *in vitro*: a vessel with a large purinergic contractile response to sympathetic nerve stimulation. *British Journal of Pharmacology*, **90**, 111–120.

Busse, R. and Mülch, A. (1990). Calcium-dependent nitric oxide synthesis in endothelial cytosol is mediated by calmodulin. *FEBS Letters*, **265**, 133–136.

Byrne, N.G. and Large, W.A. (1986). The effect of $\alpha\beta$-methylene ATP on the depolarization evoked by noradrenaline (γ-adrenoceptor response) and ATP in the immature rat basilar artery. *British Journal of Pharmacology*, **88**, 6–8.

Campbell, G.C., Gibbins, I.L., Morris, J.L., Furness, J.B., Costa, M., Oliver, J., *et al.* (1982). Somatostatin in contained in and released from cholinergic nerves in the heart of the toad *Bufo marinus*. *Neuroscience*, **7**, 2012–2023.

Cannon, W.B. and Bacq, Z.M. (1931). Studies on the conditions of activity in endocrine organs. *American Journal of Physiology*, **96**, 392–412.

Carlsson. A. (1965). Drugs which block the storage of 5-hydroxytryptamine and related amines. In *Handbook of Experimental Pharmacology*, edited by V.R. Erspamer, pp. 529–592. Berlin: Springer.

Carlsson, A. (1988). Peptide neurotransmitters — redundant vestiges? *Pharmacology and Toxicology*, **62**, 241–242.

Carlqvist, M., Jörnvall, H., Tatemoto, K. and Mutt, V. (1982). A porcine brain polypeptide identical to the vasoactive intestinal polypeptide. *Gastroenterology*, **83**, 245–249.

Carstairs, J.R. and Barnes P.J. (1986). Visualization of vasoactive intestinal peptide receptors in human and guinea pig lung. *The Journal of Pharmacology and Experimental Therapeutics*, **239**, 249–255.

Chatelain, P., Robberecht, P., Waelbroeck, M., De Neef, P., Camus, J-C., Huu, A.N., *et al.* (1983). Topographical distribution of the secretin- and VIP-stimulated adenylate cyclase system in the heart of five animal species. *Pflügers Archives*, **397**, 100–105.

Cheung, D.W. (1982). Two components in the cellular response of rat tail arteries to nerve stimulation. *Journal of Physiology*, **328**, 461–468.

Cheung, D.W. and Fujioka, M. (1986). Inhibition of the excitatory junction potential in the guinea-pig saphenous artery by ANAPP$_3$. *British Journal of Pharmacology*, **89**, 3–5.

Christofides, N.D., Yiangou, Y., Blank, M.A., Tatemoto, K., Polak, J.M. and Bloom, S.R. (1982). Are peptide histidine isoleucine and vasoactive intestinal peptide co-synthesised in the same prohormone? *The Lancet*, **ii**, 1398.

Christophe, J., Waelbroeck, M., Chatelain, P. and Robberecht, P. (1984). Heart receptors for VIP, PHI and secretin are able to activate adenylate cyclase and to mediate inotropic and chronotropic effects. Species variations and physiopathology. *Peptides*, **5**, 341–353.

Clark, A.J.L., Adrian, T.E., McMichael, H.B. and Bloom, S.R. (1983). Vasoactive intestinal peptide in shock and heart failure. *The Lancet*, **i**, 539.

Clarke, J.G., Davies, G.I., Kerwin, R., Hackett, D., Larkin, S., Dawbarn, D., *et al.* (1987). Coronary artery infusion of neuropeptide Y in patients with angina pectoris, *The Lancet*, **i**, 1057–1059.

Cohen, M.L. and Schwab-Landry, A. (1980). Vasoactive intestinal polypeptide: increased tone, enhancement of acetylcholine release and stimulation of adenylate cyclase in intestinal smooth muscle. *Life Science*, **26**, 811–822.

Corr, L.A., Aberdeen, J.A., Milner, P., Lincoln, J. and Burnstock, G. (1990). Sympathetic and nonsympathetic neuropeptide Y-containing nerves in the rat myocardium and coronary arteries. *Circulation Research*, **66**, 1602–1609.

Dahlöf, C., Dahlöf, P. and Lundberg, J. (1985a). Neuropeptide Y (NPY): enhancement of blood pressure increase upon α-adrenoceptor activation and direct pressor effects in pithed rat. *European Journal of Pharmacology*, **109**, 289–292.

Dahlöf, C., Dahlöf, P. and Lundberg, J.M. (1986). α_2-adrenoceptor-mediated inhibition of nerve stimulation-evoked release of neuropeptide Y (NPY)-like immunoreactivity in the pithed guinea-pig. *European Journal of Pharmacology*, **131**, 279–283.

Dahlöf, C., Dahlöf, P., Tatemoto, K. and Lundberg, J.M. (1985b). Neuropeptide Y (NPY) reduces field stimulation-evoked release of noradrenaline and enhances the force of contraction in the rat portal vein. *Naunyn-Schmiedeberg's Archives of Pharmacology*, **328**, 327–330.

Dale, H.H. (1935). Pharmacology and nerve-endings. *Proceedings of the Royal Society of Medicine*, **28**, 319–332.

Dale, H.H. and Dudley, H.W. (1929). The presence of histamine and acetylcholine in the spleen of the ox and horse. *Journal of Physiology*, **68**, 97–113.

Daly, R.N. and Hieble, J.P. (1987). Neuropeptide Y modulates adrenergic neurotransmission by an endothelium dependent mechanism. *European Journal of Pharmacology*, **138**, 445–446.

Dalziel, H.H., Gray, G.A., Drummond, R.M., Furman, B.L. and Sneddon, P. (1990). Investigation of the selectivity of α,β-methylene ATP in inhibiting vascular responses of the rat *in vivo* and *in vitro*. *British Journal of Pharmacology*, **99**, 820–824.

Dalziel, H.H., Machaly, M. and Sneddon, P. (1989). Comparison of the purinergic contribution to sympathetic vascular responses in SHR and WKY rats *in vitro* and *in vivo*. *European Journal of Pharmacology*, **173**, 19–26.

Darke, A.C. and Smaje, L.H. (1972). Dependence of functional vasodilatation in the cat submaxillary gland upon stimulation frequency. *Journal of Physiology*, **226**, 191–203.

Day, S.M., Polak, J.M. and Bloom, S.R. (1985). Somatostatin in the human heart and comparison with guinea-pig and rat heart. *British Heart Journal*, **53**, 153–157.

De Mey, J., Burnstock, G. and Vanhoutte, P.M. (1979). Modulation of the evoked release of noradrenaline in canine saphenous vein via presynaptic receptors for adenosine but not ATP. *European Journal of Pharmacology*, **55**, 401–405.

Dixon, W.E. (1906). Vagus inhibition. *British Medical Journal*, **2**, 1806.

Domschke, S. and Domschke, W. (1982). Biological actions of vasoactive intestinal peptide in man. In: *Vasoactive Intestinal Peptide*, edited by S.I. Said, pp. 201–209. New York: Raven Press.

Domschke, S., Domschke, W., Bloom, S.R., Mitznegg, P., Mitchell, S.J., Lux, G., *et al.* (1978). Vasoactive intestinal peptide in man: pharmacokinetics, metabolic and circulatory effects. *Gut*, **19**, 1049–1053.

Duckles, S.P. and Said, S.I. (1982). Vasoactive intestinal peptide as a neurotransmitter in the cerebral circulation. *European Journal of Pharmacology*, **78**, 371–374.

Edwall, B., Gazelius, B., Fazekas, A., Theodorsson-Norheim, E. and Lundberg, J.M. (1987). Neuropeptide Y (NPY) and sympathetic control of blood flow in oral mucosa and dental pulp in the cat. *Acta Physiologica Scandinavica*, **25**, 253–264.

Edwards, A.V. and Garrett, J.R. (1993). Nitric oxide-related vasodilator responses to parasympathetic stimulation of the submandibular gland in the cat. *Journal of Physiology (London)*, **464**, 379–392.

Edvinsson, L. (1985). Characterization of the contractile effect of neuropeptide Y in feline cerebral arteries. *Acta Phyiologica Scandinavica*, **125**, 33–41.

Edvinsson, L., Ekblad, R., Håkansson, R. and Wahlestedt, C. (1984). Neuropeptide Y potentiates the effect of various vasoconstrictor agents on rabbit blood vessels. *British Journal of Pharmacology*, **83**, 519–525.

Edvinsson, L., Ekman, R. and Thulin, T. (1991). Increased plasma levels of neuropeptide Y-like immunoreactivity and catecholamines in severe hypertension remain after treatment to normotension in man. *Regulatory Peptides*, **32**, 287–297.

Edvinsson, L., Emson, P., McCulloch, J., Tatemoto, K. and Uddman, R. (1983). Neuropeptide Y: cerebrovascular innervation and vasomotor effects in the cat. *Neuroscience Letters*, **43**, 79–84.

Edvinsson, L., Fredholm, B.B., Hamel, E., Jansem, I. and Verrechia (1985). Perivascular peptides relax cerebral arteries concomitant with stimulation of cAMP accumulation or release of an endothelium-derived relaxing factor. *Neuroscience Letters*, **58**, 213–217.

Edvinsson, L. and Uddman, R. (1988). Vasoactive intestinal polypeptide (VIP): Putative neurotransmitter in the cardiovascular system. In: *Nonadrenergic Innervation of Blood Vessels*, edited by G. Burnstock and S.G. Griffith, pp. 101–127. Boca Raton: CRC Press, Inc.

Ekblad, E., Edvinsson L., Wahlestedt, C., Uddman, R., Håkansson, R. and Sundler, F. (1984). Neuropeptide Y co-exists and co-operates with noradrenaline in perivascular nerve fibers. *Regulatory Peptides*, **8**, 225–235.

Ekblad, E., Rökaeus, A., Håkansson, R. and Sundler, F. (1985). Galanin nerve fibres in the rat gut: distribution, origin and projections. *Neuroscience*, **16**, 355–363.

Elliott, T.R. (1905). The action of adrenalin. *Journal of Physiology*, **32**, 401–467.

Euler, U.S.von (1946). A specific sympathomimetic ergone in adrenergic nerve fibers (sympathin) and its relations to adrenaline and nor-adrenaline. *Acta Physiologica Scandinavica*, **12**, 73–97.

Evéquoz, D., Waeber, B., Aubert, J-F., Flückiger, J.P., Nussberger, J. and Brunner, H.R. (1988). Neuropeptide Y prevents the blood pressure fall induced by endotoxin in conscious rats with adrenal medullectomy. *Circulation Research*, **62**, 25–30.

Fahrenkrug, J. (1979). Vasoactive intestinal polypeptide: measurement, distribution and putative neurotransmitter function. *General Review*, **19**, 149–169.

Fahrenkrug, J. (1981). VIP as a neurotransmitter in the peripheral nervous system. In: *Vasoactive Intestinal Polypeptide*, edited by S.I. Said, pp. 361–372. Raven Press, New York.

Fahrenkrug, J., Bek, T., Lundberg, J.M. and Hökfelt, T. (1985). VIP and PHI in cat neurons: Co-localization but variable tissue content possible due to different processing. *Regulatory Peptides*, **12**, 21–34.

Fahrenkrug, J., Galbo, H., Holst, J.J. and Schaffalitsky de Muckadell, O.B. (1978). Influence of the autonomic nervous system on the release of vasoactive intestinal polypeptide from the porcine gastrointestinal tract. *Journal of Physiology (Lond)*, **280**, 405–422.

Fahrenkrug, J. and Schaffalitsky de Muckadell, O.B. (1977). Radioimmunoassay of vasoactive intestinal polypeptide (VIP) in plasma. *Journal of Laboratory and Clinical Medicine*, **89**, 1379–1388.

Fallgren, B., Ekblad, E. and Edvinsson, L. (1989). Co-existence of neuropeptides and differential inhibition of vasodilator responses by neuropeptide Y in guinea pig uterine arteries. *Neuroscience Letters*, **100**, 71–76.

Fallgren, B., Arlock, P., Jansen, I. and Edvinsson, L. (1990). Neuropeptide Y in cerebrovascular function: comparison of membrane potential changes and vasomotor responses evoked by NPY and other vasoconstrictors in the guinea pig basilar artery. *Neuroscience Letters*, **114**, 117–122.

Flavahan, N.A., Grant, T.L., Gried, J. and McGrath, J.C. (1985). Analysis of the α-adrenoceptor-mediated and other components in the sympathetic vasopressor responses of the pithed rat. *British Journal of Pharmacology*, **86**, 265–274.

Folkow, B. (1955). Nervous control of the blood vessels. *Physiological Reviews*, **35**, 629–663.

Folkow, B. and Uvnäs, B. (1948). The chemical transmission of vasoconstrictor impulses to the hind limbs and the splanchnic region of the cat. *Acta Physiologica Scandinavica*, **15**, 365–388.

Fouad, F.M., Shimamatsu, K., Said, S.I. and Tarazi, R.C. (1986). Inotropic responsiveness in hypertensive left ventricular hypertrophy: Impaired inotropic response to glucagon and vasoactive intestinal peptide in renal hypertensive rats. *Journal of Cardiovascular Pharmacology*, **8**, 398–405.

Franco-Cereceda, A. (1988). Calcitonin gene-related peptide and tachykinins in relation to local sensory control of cardiac contractility and coronary vascular tone. *Acta Physiologica Scandinavica*, **133**, (Suppl. 569), 1–63.

Franco-Cereceda, A. (1989). Endothelin- and neuropeptide Y-induced vasoconstriction of human epicardial coronary arteries *in vitro*. *British Journal of Pharmacology*, **97**, 968–972.

Franco-Cereceda, A. and Lundberg, J.M. (1987). Potent effects of neuropeptide Y and calcitonin gene-related peptide on human coronary vascular tone *in vitro*. *Acta Physiologica Scandinavica*, **131**, 159–160.

Franco-Cereceda, A. and Rudehill, A. (1989). Capsaicin-induced vasodilatation of human coronary arteries *in vitro* is mediated by calcitonin gene-related peptide rather than substance P or neurokinin A. *Acta Physiologica Scandinavica*, **136**, 575–580.

Franco-Cereceda, A., Bengtsson, L. and Lundberg, J.M. (1987). Inotropic effects of calcitonin gene-related peptide, vasoactive intestinal polypeptide and somatostatin on human right atrium *in vitro*. *European Journal of Pharmacology*, **134**, 69–76.

Franco-Cereceda, A., Lundberg, J.M. and Dahlöf, C. (1995). Neuropeptide Y and sympathetic control of heart contractility and coronary vascular tone. *Acta Physiologica Scandinavica*, **124**, 361–369.

Franco-Cereceda, A., Lundberg, J.M. and Hökfelt, T. (1986). Somatostatin: an inhibitory parasympathetic transmitter in the human heart. *European Journal of Pharmacology*, **132**, 101–102.

Franco-Cereceda, A., Öwall, A., Settergren, G., Sollevi, A. and Lundberg, J.H.M. (1990). Release of neuro-peptide Y and noradrenaline from the human heart by aortic occlusion during coronary artery surgery. *Cardiovascular Research*, **24**, 242–246.

Franco-Cereceda, A., Martran, R., Alving, K. and Lundberg, J.M. (1995). Sympathetic vascular control of the laryngeo-tracheal, bronchial and pulmonary circulation in the pig: Evidence for non-adrenergic mechanisms involving neuropeptide Y. *Acta Physiologica Scandinavica*, **155**, 193–204.

Fredholm, B.B., Gustafsson, L.E., Hedqvist, P. and Sollevi, A. (1983). Adenosine in the regulation of neurotrans-mitter release in the peripheral nervous system. In: *Regulatory function of adenosine*, edited by R.M. Berne, T.W. Rall and R. Rubio, pp. 479–495. The Hague; Martinus Nijhoff.

Fredholm, B.B., Jansen, I. and Edvinsson, L. (1985). Neuropeptide Y is a potent inhibitor of cyclic AMP accumulation in feline cerebral blood vessels. *Acta Physiologica Scandinavica*, **124**, 467–469.

Fried, G., Lundberg, J.M. and Theodorsson-Norheim, E. (1985a). Subcellular storage and axonal transport of neuropeptide Y (NPY) in relation to catecholamines in the cat. *Acta Physiologica Scandinavica*,**125**, 145–154.

Frostell, C.G., Blomqvist, H., Hedenstierna, G., Zapol, W.M. (1993). Inhaled nitric oxide selectively reverses human hypoxic pulmonary vasoconstriction without causing systemic vasodilatation. *Anesthesiology*, **78**, 427–435.

Furchgott R.F. and Zawadski, J.V. (1980). The obligatory role of endothelial cells in the relaxation of arterial smooth muscle by acetylcholine. *Nature*, **288**, 373–376.

Fujiwara, S., Itoh, T. and Suzuki, H. (1982). Membrane properties and exitatory neuromuscular transmission in the smooth muscle of the dog cerebral arteries. *British Journal of Pharmacology*, **77**, 197–208.

Gaba, S.J.M., Bourgouin-Karaouni, D., Dujols, P., Michel, F.B. and Prefaut, C. (1986). Effects of adenosine triphosphate on pulmonary circulation in chronic obstructive pulmonary disease. *American Review of Respiratory Disease*, **134**, 1140–1144.

Gaba, S.J.M. and Préfaut, C. (1990). Comparison of pulmonary and systemic effects of adenosine triphosphate in chronic ohstructive pulmonary disease — ATP: a pulmonary controlled vasoregulator? *European Respiratory Journal*, **3**, 450–455.

Gardiner, S.M., Bennett, T. and Compton, A.M. (1988). Regional haemodynamic effects of neuropeptide Y, vasopressin and angiotensin II in conscious, unrestrained, Long Evans and Brattleboro rats. *Journal of the Autonomic Nervous System*, **24**, 15–27.

Garthwaite, J. (1991). Glutamate, nitric oxide and cell-cell signalling in the nervous system. *Trends in Neuroscience*, **14**, 60–67.

Gaskell, W.H. (1877). The changes in the blood stream in muscles through stimulation of their nerves. *Journal of Anatomy*, **11**, 360–402.

Gaw, A.J., Aberdeen, J., Humphrey, P.P.A., Wadsworth, R.M. and Burnstock, G. (1991). Relaxation of sheep cerebral arteries by vasoactive intestinal polypeptide and neurogenic stimulation: inhibition by L-N^G-monomethylarginine in endothelium-denuded vessels. *British Journal of Pharmacology*, **102**, 567–572.

Giaid, A., Gibson, S.J., Ibrahim, N.B.N., Legon, S., Bloom, S.R. Yanagisawa, M., *et al.* (1989). Endothelin 1, an endothelium-derived peptide, is expressed in neurons of the human spinal cord and dorsal root ganglia. *Proceedings of the National Academy of Science of the United States of America*, **86**, 7634–7638.

Glower, W.E. (1985). Increased sensitivity of the rabbit ear artery to noradrenaline following perivascular nerve stimulation may be a response to neuropeptide Y released as cotransmitter. *Clinical and Experimental Pharmacology and Physiology*, **12**, 227–230.

Glower, W.E. (1986). Effect of neuropeptide Y (NPY) on calcium permeability in vascular smooth muscle. *Proceedings of International Congress of Physiology Sciences*, P318.06.

Haass, M., Hock, M., Richardt, G. and Schömig, A. (1989). Neuropeptide Y differentiates between exocytotic and nonexocytotic noradrenaline release in guinea-pig heart. *Naunyn-Schmiedeberg's Archives of Pharmacology*, **340**, 509–515.

Han, S. and Abel, P.W. (1987). Neuropeptide Y potentiates contraction and inhibits relaxation of rabbit coronary arteries. *Journal of Cardiovascular Pharmacology*, **9**, 675–681.

Han, C., Wang, X., Fiscus, R.R., Gu, J. and McDonald, J.K. (1989). Changes in cardiac neuropeptide Y after experimental myocardial infarction in rat. *Neuroscience Letters*, **104**, 141–146.

Hanley, M.R., Benton, H.P., Lightman S.L., Todd, K., Bone, E.A., Fretten, P., *et al.* (1984). A vasopressin-like peptide in the mammalian sympathetic nervous system. *Nature*, **309**, 258–261.

Heidenhahn, R. (1872). Uber die Wirkung eineger Gifte auf die nerven der glandula submaxillaris. *Pflügers Archives*, **5**, 309–318.

Hellström, P.M., Olerup, O. and Tatemoto, K. (1985). Neuropeptide Y may mediate effects of sympathetic nerve stimulations on colonic motility and blood flow in the cat. *Acta Physiologica Scandinavica*, **124**, 613–624.

Hendry, S.H.C., Jones, E.G. and Beinfeld, M.C. (1983). Cholecystokinin-immunoreactive neurons in rat and monkey cerebral cortex make symmetric synapses and have intimate associations with blood vessels. *Proceedings of the National Academy of Sciences of the United States of America*, **80**, 2400–2404.

Hirst, G.D.S. (1977). Neuromuscular transmission in arterioles of guinea-pig submucosa. *Journal of Physiology*, **273**, 263–275.

Hirst, G.D.S. and Jobling, P. (1989). The distribution of γ-adrenoceptors and P_2 purinoceptors in mesenteric arteries and veins of the guinea-pig. *British Journal of Pharmacology*, **96**, 993–999.

Hirst, G.D.S. and Lew, M.J. (1987). Lack of involvement of α-adrenoceptors in sympathetic neural vasoconstriction in the hindquarters of the rabbit. *British Journal of Pharmacology*, **90**, 51–60.

Hirst, G.D.S. and Neild, T.O. (1980). Evidence for two populations of excitatory receptors for noradrenaline on arteriolar smooth muscle. *Nature*, **283**, 767–768.

Hökfelt, T., Elvin, L.G., Elde, R., Schultzberg, M., Goldstein, N. and Luft, R. (1977). Occurrence of somatostatin-like immuno-reactivity in some peripheral sympathetic noradrenergic neurons. *Proceedings of the National Academy of Sciences of the United States of America*, **74**, 3587–3591.

Holman, M.E. and Surprenant, A.M. (1980). An electrophysiological analysis of the effects of noradrenaline and α-receptor antagonists on neuromuscular transmission in mammalian muscular arteries. *British Journal of Pharmacology*, **71**, 651–661.

Holmquist, F., Hedlund, H and Andersson, K.E. (1990). Effects of the α-adrenoceptor agonist R-(–)-YM 12617 on isolated human penile erective tissue and vas deferens. *European Journal of Pharmacology*, **186**, 87–93.

Holzer, P. (1988). Local effector function of capsaicin-sensitive sensory nerve endings: involvement of tachykinins, calcitonin gene-related peptide and other neuropeptides. *Neuroscience*, **24**, 739–768.

Hottenstein, O.D. and Kreulen, D.C. (1986). Evidence for cotransmission using adrenergic, purinergic and non-adrenergic (peptide-like) responses in mesenteric arteries of the guinea-pig. *Abstract. Neuroscience Society*, **12**, 628.

Huang, M. and Rorstad, O.P. (1983). Effects of vasoactive intestinal polypeptide, monoamines, prostaglandins, and 2-chloroadenosine on adenylate cyclase in rat cerebral microvessels. *Journal of Neurochemistry*, **40**, 719–726.

Hughes, A.D., Thom, S.A.M., Martin, G.N., Nielsen, H., Hair, W.M., Schachter, M., *et al.* (1988). Size and site-dependent heterogeneity of human vascular responses *in vitro*. *Journal of Hypertension*, **6**, (Suppl. 4) S173–S175.

Hulting, J., Sollevi, A., Ullman, B., Franco-Cereceda, A., and Lundberg, J.M. (1990). Plasma neuropeptide Y on admission to a coronary care unit. Raised levels in patients with left heart failure. *Cardiovascular Research*, **24**, 102–108.

Illes, P., Rickman, H., Brod, I., Bucher, B. and Stoclet, J-C. (1989). Subsensitivity of presynaptic adenosine A_1-receptors in caudal arteries of spontaneously hypertensive rats. *European Journal of Pharmacology*, **174**, 237–251.

Inoue, T. and Kannan, M.S. (1988). Noradrenergic and non-cholinergic excitatory neurotransmission in rat intrapulmonary artery. *American Journal of Physiology*, **254**, H1142–H1148.

Ishihara, T., Shigemoto, R., Mori, K., Takahashi, K. and Nagata, S. (1992). Functional expression and tissue distribution of a novel receptor for vasoactive intestinal polypeptide. *Neuron*, **8**, 811–819.

Ishikawa, S. (1985). Actions of ATP and α,β-methylene ATP on neuromuscular transmission and smooth muscle membrane of the rabbit and guinea-pig mesenteric arteries. *British Journal of Pharmacology*, **86**, 777–787.

Itoh, N., Obata, K., Yanaihara, N. and Okamoto, H. (1983). Human preprovasoactive intestinal polypeptide contains a novel PHI-27-like peptide, PHM-27. *Nature*, **304**, 547–549.

Jackowski, A., Crockard, A., Burnstock, G. and Lincoln, J. (1989). Alterations in serotonin and neuropeptide Y content of cerebrovascular sympathetic nerves following experimental subarachnoid haemorrhage. *Journal of Cerebral Blood Flow and Metabolism*, **9**, 271–279.

Järhult, J., Hellstrand, P. and Sundler, F. (1980). Immunohistochemical localization of VIP-like immunoreactivity in large dense-core vesicles of 'cholinergic type' nerve terminals in cat exocrine glands. *Neuroscience*, **5**, 847–862.

Jessen, K.R., Mirsky, R., Dennison, M.E. and Burnstock, G. (1979). GABA may be neurotransmitter in the vertebrate peripheral nervous system. *Nature*, **81**, 71–74.

Johansson, O. and Lundberg J.M. (1981). Ultrastructural localization of VIP-like immunoreactivity in large dense-core vesicles of 'cholinergic-type' nerve terminals in cat exocrine glands. *Neuroscience*, **6**, 847–862.

Kamikawa, Y., Cline, W.H. and Su, S. (1980). Diminished purinergic modulation of the vascular adreneric neurotransmission in spontaneously hypertensive rats. *European Journal of Pharmacology*, **66**, 347–353.

Karashima, T. and Kuriyama, H. (1981). Electrical properties of smooth muscle cell membrane and neuromuscular transmission in the guinea-pig basilar artery. *British Journal of Pharmacology*, **74**, 495–504.

Kasakov, L., Ellis, J., Kirkpatrick, I.C., Milner, P. and Burnstock, G. (1988). Direct evidence for concomitant release of noradrenaline, adenosine 5'-triphosphate and neuropeptide Y from sympathetic nerve supplying the guinea-pig vas deferens. *Journal of Autonomic Nervous System*, **22**, 75–82.

Kassis, S., Olasmaa, M., Terenius, L. and Fishman, P.H. (1987). Neuropeptide Y inhibits cardiac adenylate cyclase through a pertussis toxin-sensitive G protein. *Journal of Biological Chemistry*, **262**, 3429–3431.

Katsuragi, T. and Su, C. (1982). Purine release from vascular adrenergic nerves by high potassium and a calcium ionophore A-23187. *Journal of Pharmacology and Experimental Therapeutics*, **215**, 685–690.

Katsuragi, T. and Su, C. (1982). Augmentation by theophylline of (^{3}H)-purine release from vascular adrenergic nerves: evidence for presynaptic autoinhibition. *Journal of Pharmacology and Experimental Therapeutics*, **220**, 152–156.

Kennedy, C. (1988). Possible roles for purine nucleotides in perivascular neurotransmission. In *Nonadrenergic Innervation of Blood Vessels*, edited by G. Burnstock and S.G. Griffith, pp. 65–76. Boca Raton: CRC Press, Inc.

Kennedy, C., Saville V.L. and Burnstock, G. (1986). The contributions of noradrenaline and ATP to the responses of the rabbit central ear artery to sympathetic nerve stimulation depend on the parameters of stimulation. *European Journal of Pharmacology*, **122**, 291–300.

Kirkpatrick, K. and Burnstock, G. (1987). Sympathetic nerve-mediated release of ATP from the guinea-pig vas deferens is unaffected by reserpine. *European Journal of Pharmacology*, **138**, 207–214.

Kotecha, N. and Neild, T.O. (1987). Effects of denervation on the responses of the rat tail artery to α,β-methylene ATP. *General Pharmacology*, **18**, 535–537.

Krishnamurty, V.S.R. and Kadowitz, P.J. (1983). Influence of adenosine triphosphate on the isolated perfused mesenteric artery of the rabbit. *Canadian Journal of Physiology and Pharmacology*, 61, 409–1417.

Kubota, E., Hamasaki, Y., Sata, T., Saga, T. and Said, S.I. (1988). Autonomic innervation of pulmonary artery: Evidence for a nonadrenergic noncholinergic inhibitory system. *Experimental Lung Research*, **14**, 349–358.

Kubota, E., Sata, T., Soas, A.H., Paul, S. and Said, S.I. (1986). Vasoactive intestinal peptide as a possible transmitter of nonadrenergic, noncholinergic relaxation of pulmonary artery. *Transactions of the Association of American Physicians*, **98**, 233–242.

Kügelgen, I.V. and Starke, K. (1985). Noradrenaline and adenosine triphosphate as co-transmitters of neurogenic vasoconstriction in rabbit mesenteric artery. *Journal of Physiology*, **367**, 435–455.

Kummer, W., Fischer, A., Mundel, P. Mayer, B. Hoba, B., Philippin, B. and Preissler, U. (1992). Nitric oxide synthase in VIP-containing vasodilator nerve fibres in the guinea-pig. *Neuroreport*, **3**, 653–655.

Lacroix, J.-S. (1989). Adrenergic and non-adrenergic mechanisms in sympathetic vascular control of the nasal mucosa. *Acta Physiologica Scandinavica*, **136**, (Suppl. 581), 1–63.

Lacroix, J.S., Stjärne, P., Änggård, A. and Lundberg, J.M. (1988a). Sympathetic vascular control of the pig nasal mucosa: (I) increased resistance and capacitance vessel responses upon stimulation with irregular bursts compared to continuous impulses. *Acta Physiologica Scandinavica*, **132**, 83–90.

Lacroix, J.S., Stjärne, P., Änggård, A. and Lundberg, J.M.. (1988b). Sympathetic vascular control of the pig nasal mucosa (2): resderpine-resistant, non-adrenergic nervous responses in relation to neuropeptide Y and ATP. *Acta Physiologica Scandinavica*, **133**, 183–197.

Lagercrantz, H. (1971). Isolation and characterization of sympathetic nerve trunc vesicles. *Acta Physiologica Scandinavica*, **82** (Suppl 366), 1–40.

Laitinen, L., Laitinen M.A. and Widdicombe, J.G. (1987). Dose-related effects of pharmacological mediators on tracheal vascular resistance in dogs. *British Journal of Pharmacology*, **92**, 703–709.

Lamb, F.S. and Webb, R.C. (1984). Vascular effects of free radicals generated by electrical stimulation. *American Journal of Physiology*, **247**, H709–H714.

Langley, J.N. (1921). The Autonomic Nervous System. Part I. Cambridge: Heffer.

Lee, T.J.-F. (1986). Sympathetic and nonsympathetic transmitter mechanisms in cerebral vasodilatation and constriction. In: *Neural Regulation of Brain Circulation*, edited by C. Owman and J.E. Hardebo, pp. 285–296. Elseviere Science Publishers B.V. (Biomedical Division).

Lee, T.J.-F., Chiuch, C.C. and Adam, T. (1980). Synaptic transmission of vasoconstrictor nerves in rabbit basilar artery. *European Journal of Pharmacology*, **61**, 55–70.

Lee, T.J.-F., Hume, W.R., Su, C. and Bevan, J.A. (1978). Neurogenic vasodilatation of cat cerebral arteries. *Circulation Research*, **42**, 535–542.

Lee, T.J.-F., Saito, A. and Berezin, A. (1984). Vasoactive intestinal polypeptide-like substance: The potential transmitter for cerebral vasodilatation. *Science*, **224**, 898–890.

Lee, T.J.F., Su, C. and Bevan, J.A. (1975). Nonsympathetic dilator innervation of cat cerebral arteries. *Experientia*, **31**, 1424–1426.

Lee, T.J.F., Su, C. and Bevan, J.A. (1976). Neurogenic sympathetic vasoconstriction of the rabbit basilar artery. *Circulation Research*, **39**, 120–126.

Levitt, B. and Westfall, D.P. (1982). Factors influencing the release of purines and norepinephrine in the rabbit portal vein. *Blood Vessels*, **19**, 30–40.

Linton-Dahlöf, P. (1989). Modulatory interactions of neuropeptide Y (NPY) on sympathetic. *Acta Physiologica Scandinavica*, **137** (Suppl 586), 1–85.

Londos, C., Cooper, D.M.F. and Wolff, J. (1980). Subclasses of external adenosine receptors. *Proceedings of the National Academy of Sciences of the United States of America*, **77**, 2551–2554.

Loewi, O. (1921). Über humorale Übertragbarkeit der Herznervenwirkung. *Pflügers Archives*, **189**, 239–242.

Lukacsko, R. and Blumberg, A. (1982). Modulation of the vasoconstrictor response to adrenergic stimulation by nucleosides and nucleotides. *Journal of Pharmacology and Experimental Therapeutics*, **222**, 344–349.

Lundberg, J.M. (1981). Evidence for coexistence of vasoactive intestinal polypeptide (VIP) and acetylcholine in neurons of cat exocrine glands. *Acta Physiologica Scandinavica*, (Suppl. 496), 1–57.

Lundberg, J.M., Änggård, A., Emson, P., Fahrenkrug, J. and Hökfelt, T. (1981a). Vasoactive intestinal polypeptide and cholinergic mechanisms in cat nasal mucosa: Studies on choline acetyltransferase and release of vasoactive intestinal polypeptide. *Proceedings of the National Academy of Sciences of the United States of America*, **78**, 5255–5259.

Lundberg, J.M., Änggård, A., Fahrenkrug, J. Hökfelt, T. and Mutt, V. (1980). Vasoactive intestinal polypeptide in cholinergic neurons of exocrine glands: Functional significance of co-existing transmitters for vasodilatation and secretion. *Proceedings of the National Academy of Sciences of the United States of America*, **77**, 1651–1655.

Lundberg, J.M., Änggård, A., Theodorsson-Norheim, E. and Pernow, J. (1984a). Guanethidine-sensitive release of neuropeptide Y-like immunoreactivity in the cat spleen by sympathetic nerve stimulation. *Neuroscience Letters*, **52**, 175–180.

Lundberg, J.M., Fahrenkrug, J., Larsson O. and Änggård, A. (1984b). Corelease of vasoactive intestinal polypeptide and peptide histidine isoleucine in relation to atropine-resistant vasodilatation in cat submandibular salivary gland. *Neuroscience Letters*, **52**, 37–42.

Lundberg, J.M., Fahrenkrug, J., Hökfelt, T., Martling, C-R., Larsson O., Tatemoto, K., *et al.* (1984c). Co-existence of peptide HI (PHI) and VIP in nerves regulating blood flow and bronchial smooth muscle tone in various mammals including man. *Peptides*, **5**, 593–606.

Lundberg, J.M., Fried, G., Fahrenkrug, J., Holmstedt, B., Hökfelt, T., Lagercrantz, H., *et al.* (1981b). Subcellular fractionation of cat submandibular gland: comparative studies on the distribution of acetylcholine and vasoactive intestinal polypeptide (VIP). *Neuroscience*, **6**, 1001–1010.

Lundberg, J.M., Fried, G., Pernow, J. and Theodorsson-Norheim, E. (1986a). Corelease of neuropeptide Y and catecholamines upon adrenal activation in the cat. *Acta Physiologica Scandinavica*, **126**, 231–238.

Lundberg, J.M., Fried, G., Pernow, J., Theodorsson-Norheim, E. and Änggård, A. (1986b). NPY- a mediator of reserpine-resistant non-adrenergic vasoconstriction in cat spleen after preganglionic denervation? *Acta Physiologica Scandinavica*, **126**, 151–152.

Lundberg, J.M., Hemsén, A., Rudehill, A., Härfstrand, A., Larsson, O., Sollevi, A., *et al.* (1988). Neuropeptide Y and α-adrenergic receptors in pig spleen: localization, binding characteristics, cyclic AMP effects and functional responses in control and denervated animals. *Neuroscience*, **24**, 659–672.

Lundberg, J.M. and Hökfelt, T. (1986). Multiple co-existence of peptides and classical transmitters in peripheral autonomic and sensory neurons — Functional and pharmacological implications. In: *Progress in Brain Research*, edited by T. Hökfelt, K. Fuxe and B. Pernow, pp. 241–262. Elsevier Science Publishers B.V. (Biomedical Division).

Lundberg, J.M., Hökfelt, T., Hemsén, A., Theodorsson-Norheim, E., Pernow, J., Hamberger, B., *et al.* (1986c). Neuropeptide Y-like immunoreactivity in adrenaline cells of adrenal medulla and in tumors and plasma of pheochromocytoma patients. *Regulatory Peptides*, **13**, 169–182.

Lundberg, J.M., Hökfelt, T., Schultzberg, M., Uvnäs-Wallensten, K., Kohler, C. and Said, S.I. (1979). Occurrence of vasoactive intestinal polypeptide (VIP)-like immunoreactivity in certain cholinergic neurons of the cat: Evidence from combined immunohistochemistry and acetylcholinesterase staining. *Neuroscience*, **4**, 1539–1559.

Lundberg, J.M., Martinsson, A., Hemsén, A., Theodorsson-Norheim, E., Svedenhag, J., Ekblom, B., *et al.* (1985a). Co-release of neuropeptide Y and catecholamines during physical exercise in man. *Biochemical and Biophysical Research Communications*, **133**, 30–36.

Lundberg, J.M., Pernov, J., Franco-Cereceda, A. and Rudehill, A. (1987). Effects of antihypertensive drugs on sympathetic vascular control in relation to neuropeptide Y. *Journal of Cardiovascular Pharmacology*, **10**, S51–S58.

Lundberg, J.M., Pernow, J., Tatemoto, K. and Dahlöf, C. (1985b). Pre- and postjunctional effects of NPY on sympathetic control of rat femoral artery. *Acta Physiologica Scandinavica*, **123**, 511–513.

Lundberg, J.M., Rudehill, A., Sollevi, A. and Hamberger, B. (1989). Evidence for co-transmitter role of neuropeptide Y in the pig spleen. *British Journal of Pharmacology*, **96**, 675–687.

Lundberg, J.M., Saria, A., Franco-Cereceda, A., Hökfelt, T., Terenius, L. and Goldstein, M. (1985c). Differential effects of reserpine and 6-hydroxydopamine on neuropeptide Y (NPY) and noradrenaline in peripheral neurones. *Naunyn-Schmiedeberg's Archives of Pharmacology*, **328**, 331–340.

Lundberg, J.M., Saria, A., Franco-Cereceda, A. and Theodorsson-Norheim, E. (1985d). Mechanisms underlying changes in the contents of neuropeptide Y in cardiovascular nerves and adrenal gland induced by sympatholytic drugs. *Acta Physiologica Scandinavica*, **124**, 603–611.

Lundberg, J.M. and Tatemoto, K. (1992). Pancreatic polypeptide family (APP, BPP, NPY and PYY) in relation to sympathetic vasoconstriction resistant to α-adrenoceptor blockade. *Acta Physiologica Scandinavica*, **116**, 393–402.

Lundberg, J.M., Terenius, L., Hökfelt, T. and Goldstein, M. (1983). High levels of neuropeptide Y in peripheral noradrenergic neurons in various mammals including man. *Neuroscience Letters*, **42**, 167–172.

Lundberg, J.M., Terenius, L., Hökfelt, T., Martling, C.R., Tatemoto, K, Mutt, V., et al. (1982). Neuropeptide Y (NPY)-like immunoreactivity in peripheral noradrenergic nerves and effects of NPY on sympathetic function. *Acta Physiologica Scandinavica*, **116**, 477–480.

Lundblad, L. Saria, A., Lundberg, J.M. and Änggård, A. (1983). Increased vascular permeability in rat nasal mucosa induced by substance P and stimulation of capsaicin-sensitive trigeminal neurons. *Acta Oto-Laryngologica*, **96**, 479–494.

Lundblad, L., Änggård, A., Saria, A. and Lundberg, J.M. (1987). Neuropeptide Y and non-adrenergic sympathetic vascular control of the cat nasal mucosa. *Journal of the Autonomic Nervous System*, **20**, 189–197.

Lung, M.A., Phipps, R.J., Wang, J.C. and Widdicombe, J.G. (1984). Control of nasal vasculature and airflow resistance in the dog. *Journal of Physiology*, **349**, 535–551.

Lutz, E.M., Sheward, W.J., West, K.M., Morrow, J.A., Fink, G. and Harmar, A.J. (1993). The VIP_2 receptor: molecular characterization of a cDNA encoding a novel receptor for vasoactive intestinal peptide. *FEBS Letters*, **334**, 3–8.

Mabe, Y., Pérez, R., Tatemoto, K. and Huidobro-Toro, J.P. (1987). Chemical sympathectomy reveals pre- and postsynaptic effects of neuropeptide Y (NPY) in the cardiovascular system. *Experientia*, **43**, 1018–1020.

Machaly, M., Dalziel, H.H. and Sneddon, P. (1988). Evidence for ATP as a cotransmitter in dog mesenteric artery. *European Journal of Pharmacology*, **147**, 83–92.

MacLean, M.R. and Hiley, C.R. (1990). Effect of neuropeptide Y on cardiac output, its distribution, regional blood flow and organ vascular resistances in the pithed rat. *British Journal of Pharmacology*, **99**, 340–342.

Maggi, C.A. and Meli, A. (1988). The sensory efferent function of capsaicin-sensitive sensory neurons. *General Pharmacology*, **19**, 1–43.

Maisel, A.S., Scott, N.A., Motulsky, H.J, Michel, M.C., Boublik, J.H., Rivier, J.E., et al. (1989) Elevation of plasma neuropeptide Y levels in congestive heart failure. *American Journal of Medicine*, **86**, 43–48.

Malik, K.U. (1980). Differential effect of α-adrenergic blocking agents on the vasoconstrictor responses to periarterial nerve stimulation and to injected norepinephrine in the isolated rat kidney. *Federation Proceedings*, **39**, 1004.

Malmström, R. and Lundberg, J.M. (1995). Endongenous NPY acting on the Y_1 receptor account for major part of the sympathetic vasoconstriction on guinea-pig vena cava: evidence using BIBP 3226 and 3435. *European Journal of Pharmacology*, **294**, 661–668.

Martin, E.S. and Patterson, R.E. (1989). Coronary constriction due to neuropeptide Y: alleviation with cyclooxygenase blockers. *American Journal of Physiology*, **257**, H927–H934.

Martling, C.-R., Alving, K., Hökfelt, T. and Lundberg, J.M. (1990). Innervation of the lower airways and neuropeptide effects on bronchial and vascular tone in the pig. *Cell and Tissue Research*, **260**, 223–233.

Martling, C.-R., Änggård, A. and Lundberg, J.M. (1985). Non-cholinergic vasodilatation in the tracheobronchial tree of the cat induced by vagal nerve stimulation. *Acta Physiologica Scandinavica*, **125**, 343–346.

Mayer, B., Schmidt, K., Humbert, P. and Böhme, E. (1989). Biosynthesis of endothelium-derived relaxing factor. *Biochemical and Biophysical Research Communications*, **164**, 678–685.

McDonald, J.K. (1988). NPY and related substances. *Critical Reviews in Neurobiology*, **4**, 97–135.

Michel, M.C., Schlickcr, E., Fink, K., Boublik, J.H., Göthert, M., Willette, R.N., et al. (1990). Distinction of NPY receptors *in vivo* and *in vitro*. NPY (18–36) discriminates NPY-receptor subtypes *in vitro*. *American Journal of Physiology*, **259**, E131–E139.

Minson, R, McRitchie, R. and Chalmers, J. (1989). Effects of neuropeptide Y on renal, mesenteric and hindlimb vascular beds of the conscious rabbit. *Journal of the Autonomic Nervous System*, **27**, 139–146.

Minth, C., Bloom, S., Polak, J.M. and Dixon, J. (1984). Cloning, characterization and DNA sequence of a human cDNA encoding neuropeptide tyrosine. *Proceedings of the National Academy of the Sciences of the United States of America*, **81**, 4577–4581.

Miyahara, H. and Suzuki, H. (1987). Pre- and post-junctional effects of adenosine triphosphate on noradrenergic transmission in the rabbit ear artery. *Journal of Physiology*, **389**, 423–440.

Modin, A. (1994). Non-adrenergic, non-cholinergic vascular control with reference to neuropeptide Y, vasoactive intestinal polypeptie and nitric oxide. *Acta Physiologica Scandinavica*, **151**, (Suppl. 622) 1–74.

Moncada, S., Palmer, R.M.J. and Higgs, E.A. (1991). Nitric oxide: physiology, pathophysiology and pharmacology. *Pharmacological Reviews*, **43**, 109–142.

Morris, J.L. (1991). Roles of neuropepide Y and noradrenaline in sympathetic neurotransmission to the thoracic vena cava and aorta of guinea-pig. *Regulatory Peptides*, **32**, 297–310.

Morris, J.L., Gibbins, I.L., Furness, J.B., Costa, M. and Murphy, R. (1985). Co-localization of neuropeptide Y, vasoactive intestinal polypeptide and dynorphin in non-noradrenergic axons of the guinea-pig uterine artery. *Neuroscience Letters*, **62**, 31–37.

Morris, J.L. and Murphy, R. (1988). Evidence that neuropeptide Y released from noradrenergic axons causes prolonged contraction of the guinea-pig uterine artery. *Journal of the Autonomic Nervous System*, **24**, 241–249.

Morris, J.L., Russel, A.E., Kapoor, V., Cain, M.D., Elliott J.M., *et al.* (1986). Increases in plasma neuropeptide Y concentrations during sympathetic activation in man. *Journal of the Autonomic Nervous System*, **17**, 143–149.

Muramatsu, I. (1987). The effect of reserpine on sympathetic, purinergic neurotransmission in the isolated mesenteric artery of the dog: a pharmacological study. *British Journal of Pharmacology*, **91**, 467–474.

Muramatsu, I., Fujiwara, M., Miura, A. and Sakakibara, Y. (1981). Possible involvement of adenine nucleotides in sympathetic neuroeffector mechanisms of dog basilar artery. *Journal of Pharmacology Experimental Therapeutics*, **216**, 401–409.

Muramatsu, I. and Kigoshi, S. (1987). Purinergic and non-purinergic innervation in the cerebral arteries of the dog. *British Journal of Pharmacology*, **92**, 901–908.

Muramatsu, I., Kigoshi, S. and Oshita, M. (1984). Nonadrenergic nature of prazonin-resistant, sympathetic contraction in the dog mesenteric artery. *Journal of Pharmacology and Experimental Therapeutics*, **229**, 532–538.

Nagao, T. and Suzuki, H. (1988). Effects of α,β-methylene ATP on electrical responses produced by ATP and nerve stimulation in smooth muscle cells of the guinea-pig mesenteric artery. *General Pharmacology*, **19**, 799–805.

Nagata, M., Franco-Cereceda, A., Saria, A., Amann, R. and Lundberg, J.M. (1987). Reserpine-induced depletion of neuropeptide Y in the guinea-pig: tissue-specific effects and mechanisms of action. *Journal of the Autonomic Nervous System*, **20**, 257–263.

Nield, T.O. (1987). Actions of neuropeptide Y on innervated and denervated rat tail arteries. *Journal of Physiology*, **386**, 19–30.

Öhlén, A., Persson, M.G., Lindbom, L., Gustafsson, L.E. and Hedqvist, P. (1990). Nerve-induced nonadrenergic vasoconstriction and vasodilatation in skeletal muscle. *American Journal of Physiology*, **258**, H1334–H1338.

Olsson, R.A. (1975). Myocardial reactive hyperaemia. *Circulation Research*, **37**, 263–269.

Olsson, R.A. and Pearson (1990). Cardiovascular purinoceptors. *Physiological Reviews*, **70**, 761–845.

Omote, S., Kigoshi, S. and Muramatsu, I. (1989). Selective inhibition by nifedipine of the purinergic component of neurogenic vasoconstriction in the dog mesenteric artery. *European Journal of Pharmacology*, **160**, 239–245.

Owman, C. (1990). Peptidergic vasodilator nerves in the peripheral circulation and in the vascular beds of the heart and brain. *Blood Vessels*, **27**, 73–93.

Palmer, R.M.J., Ferrige, A.G. and Moncada, S. (1987). Nitric oxide release accounts for the biological activity of endothelium-derived relaxing factor. *Nature*, **327**, 524.

Pernow, J. (1988). Co-release and functional interactions of neuropeptide Y and noradrenaline in peripheral sympathetic vascular control. *Acta Physiologica Scandinavica*, **133**, (Suppl 568), 1–56.

Pernow, J. and Lundberg, J.M. (1988). Neuropeptide Y induces potent contraction of arterial vascular smooth muscle via an endothelium-independent mechanism. *Acta Physiologica Scandinavica*, **134**, 157–158.

Pernow, J. and Lundberg, J.M. (1989). Release and vasoconstrictor effects of neuropeptide Y in relation to non-adrenergic sympathetic control of renal blood flow in the pig. *Acta Physiologica Scandinavica*, **136**, 507–517.

Pernow, J., Lundberg, J.M. and Kjaiser, L. (1987a). Vasoconstrictor effects *in vivo* and plasma disappearance rate of neuropeptide Y in man. *Life Sciences*, **40**, 47–54.

Pernow, J., Schwieler, J., Kahan, T., Hjemdahl, P., Oberle, J., Wallin, B.G., *et al.* (1989). Influence of sympathetic discharge pattern on norepinephrine and neuropeptide Y release. *American Journal of Physiology*, **257**, H866–H872.

Pernow, J., Svenberg, T. and Lundberg, J.M. (1987b). Action of calcium antagonists in pre- and post-junctional effects of neuropeptide Y on human peripheral blood vessels *in vitro*. *European Journal of Pharmacology*, **136**, 207–218.

Potter, E. (1985). Prolonged non-adrenergic inhibition of cardiac vagal action following sympathetic stimulation: neuromodulation by neuropeptide Y? *Neuroscience Letters*, **54**, 117–121.

Ralevic, V. and Burnstock, G. (1990). Postjunctional synergism of noradrenaline and adenosine 5'-triphosphate in the mesenteric arterial bed of the rat. *European Journal of Pharmacology*, **175**, 291–299.

Ramme, D., Regenold, J.T., Starke, K., Busse, R. and Illes, P. (1987). Identification of the neuroeffector transmitter in jejunal branches of the rabbit mesenteric artery. *Naunyn-Schmiedeberg's Archives of Pharmacology*, **336**, 267–273.

Rapaport, R.M., Draznin, M.B. and Murad, F. (1983) Endothelium-dependent relaxation in the rat aorta may be mediated through cGMP-dependent phosphorylation. *Nature*, **306**, 174-176.

Rashatwar, S., Cornwell, T.L. and Lincoln. T.M. (1987) Effects of 8- bromo-cGMP on calcium-levels in vascular smooth muscle cells: possible regulation of calcium-ATPase by cGMP-dependent protein kinase. *Proceedings of the National Academy of Sciences of the United States of America*, **84**, 5685–5689.

Reilly, W.M., Saville, V.L., Burnstock, G. (1987). An assessment of the antagonist activity of reactive blue 2 at P_1- and P_2-purinoceptors: supporting evidence for purinergic innervation of the rabbit portal vein. *European Journal of Pharmacology*, **40**, 47–53.

Reinecke, M., Weihe, E., Carraway, R.E., Leeman, S.E. and Forssmann, W.G. (1982). Localization of neurotensin immunoreactive nerve fibres in the guinea-pig heart: evidence derived by immunohistochemistry radio immunoassay and chromatography. *Neuroscience*, **7**, 1785–1795.

Revington, M. and McCloskey, D.I. (1988). Neuropeptide Y and control of vascular resistance in skeletal muscle. *Regulatory Peptides*, **23**, 331–342.

Richardt, G., Haass, M., Neeb, S., Hock, M., Lang, R.E. and Schömig, A. (1988). Nicotine-induced release of noradrenaline and neuropeptide Y in guinea pig heart. *Klinische Wochenschrift*, **66**, (Suppl XI), 21–27.

Rioux, F., Bachelard, H., Martel, J.C. and Pierre, S.St. (1986). The vasoconstrictor effect of neuropeptide Y and related peptides in the guinea pig isolated heart. *Peptides*, **7**, 27–31.

Robberecht, P., Tatemoto, K., Chatelain, P., Waelbroeck, M, Delhaye, M., Taton, G., *et al.* (1982). Effects of PHI on vasoactive intestinal peptide receptors and adenylate cyclase activity in lung membranes. A comparison in man, rat, mouse and guinea pig. *Regulatory Peptides*, **4**, 241–250.

Rosell, S. and Sedvall, G. (1962). The rate of disappearance of vasoconstrictor responses to sympathetic chain stimulation after reserpine treatment. *Acta Physiologica Scandinavica*, **56**, 306–314.

Rudehill, A., Olcén, M., Sollevi, A., Hamberger, B., and Lundberg, J.M. (1987). Release of neuropeptide Y upon haemorrhagic hypovolaemia in relation to vasoconstrictor effects in the pig. *Acta Physiologica Scandinavica*, **131**, 517–523.

Rudehill, A., Sollevi, A., Franco-Cereceda, A. and Lundberg, J.M. (1986). Neuropeptide Y (NPY) and the pig heart: release and coronary vasoconstrictor effects. *Peptides*, **7**, 821–826.

Rump, L.C. and von Kügelgen, I. (1994). A study of ATP as a sympathetic cotransmitter in human saphenous vein. *Br J Pharmacology*, **111**, 65–72.

Said, S.I. and Mutt, V. (1970a). Polypeptide with broad biological activity: Isolation from small intestine. *Science*, **169**, 1217–1218.

Said, S.I. and Mutt, V. (1970b). Potent peripheral and splanchnic vasodilator peptide from normal gut. *Nature*, **225**, 863–864.

Said, S.I. and Mutt, V. (1972). Isolation from porcine-intestinal wall of a vasoactive octacosapeptide related to secretin and to glucagon. *European Journal of Biochemistry*, **28**, 199–215.

Saville, V.L. and Burnstock, G. (1988). Use of reserpine and 6-hydroxydopamine supports evidence for purinergic cotransmission in the rabbit ear artery. *European Journal of Pharmacology*, **155**, 271–277.

Saville, V.L., Maynard, K.I. and Burnstock, G. (1990). Neuropeptide Y potentiates purinergic as well as adrenergic responses of the rabbit ear artery. *European Journal of Pharmacology*, **176**, 117–125.

Schalling, M., Franco-Cereceda, A., Hökfelt, T., Persson, H. and Lundberg, J.M. (1988). Increased neuropeptide Y messenger RNA and peptide content in sympathetic ganglia after reserpine pretreatment. *European Journal of Pharmacology*, **156**, 419–420.

Scheibel, E.M., Tomiyasu, U. and Scheibel, A.B. (1975). Do raphe nuclei of the reticular formation have a neurosecretory or vascular sensor function? *Experimental Neurology*, **47**, 316–329.

Schultzberg, M., Hökfelt, T., Nilsson, G., Terenius, L., Rehfeld, J.F., Brown, M., *et al.* (1980). Distribution of peptide- and catecholamine-containing neurons in the gastrointestinal tract of rat and guinea-pig: immunohistochemical studies with antisera to substance P, vasoactive intestinal poly-peptide, enkephalins, somatostatin, gastrin/cholecystokinin, neurotensin and dopamine β-hydroxylase. *Neuroscience*, **5**, 689–744.

Schultzherg, M., Hökfelt, T., Terenius, L. Elfvin, L-G., Lundberg, J.M., Brandt, J., *et al.* (1979). Enkephalin immunoreactive nerve fibres and cell bodies in sympathetic ganglia of the guinea-pig and rat. *Neuroscience*, **4**, 249–270.

Schwartz, D.D. and Malik, K.U. (1989). Renal periarterial nerve stimulation-induced vasoconstriction at low frequencies is primarily due to release of a purinergic transmitter in the rat. *Journal of Pharmacology and Experimental Therapeutics*, **250**, 764–771.

Sedaa, K.O., Bjur, R.A., Shinozuka, K. and Westfall, D.P. (1990) Nerve and drug-induced release of adenosine nucleotides and nucleotides from rabbit aorta. *Journal of Pharmacology and Experimental Therapeutics*, **252**, 1060–1067.

Sedvall, G. and Thorson, J. (1965). Adrenergic transmission at vasoconstrictor nerve terminals partially depleted of noradrenaline. *Acta Physiologica Scandinavica*, **64**, 251–258.

Senaratne, M.P.J. and Kappaoda, T. (1986). Tetrodotoxin-resistant relaxation to transmural nerve stimulation in canine saphenous veins: a possible neural origin. *Canadian Journal of Physiology and Pharmacology*, **64**, 1328–1334.

Shimada, S.G. and Stitt, J.T. (1984). An analysis of the purinergic component of active muscle vasodilatation obtained by electrical stimulation of the hypothalamus in rabbits. *British Journal of Pharmacology*, **83**, 577–589.

Shinozuka, K., Bjur, R.A. and Westfall, D.P. (1990). Effects of α,β-methylene ATP on the prejunctional purinoceptors of the sympathetic nerves of the rat caudal artery. *Journal of Pharmacology and Experimental Therapeutics*, **254**, 900–904.

Sjöblom-Widfeldt, N. (1990). Neuro-muscular transmission in blood vessels: phasic and tonic components. *Acta Physiologica Scandinavica*, **138**, (Suppl 587), 1–52.

Smitherman, T.C., Sakio, H., Geumei, A.M., Yoshida, T., Oyamada, M. and Said, S.I. (1982). Coronary vasodilator action of VIP. In: *Vasoactive Intestinal Peptide*, edited by. S.I. Said, pp. 169–176, Raven Press, New York.

Sneddon, P. and Burnstock, G. (1984). ATP as a co-transmitter in rat tail artery. *European Journal of Pharmacology*, **106**, 149–152.

Sneddon, P., Meldrum, L.A. and Burnstock, G. (1984). Control of transmitter release in guinea-pig vas deferens by prejunctional P_1-purinoceptors. *European Journal of Pharmacology*, **105**, 293–299.

Sneddon, P., Westfall, D.P. and Fedan, J.S. (1982). Cotransmitters in the motor nerves of the guinea pig vas deferens: electrophysiological evidence. *Science*, **218**, 693–695.

Speden, R.N. (1975). Excitation of vascular smooth muscle. In *Smooth Muscle*, edited by E. Bülbring, A.F. Brading, A.W. Jones and T. Tomita, pp. 558–612. London: Edward Arnold Ltd.

Stjärne, L. (1989). Basic mechanisms and local modulation of nerve impuse-induced secretion of neurotransmitters from individual sympathetic nerve varicosities. *Review of Physiology Biochemistry and Pharmacology*, **112**, 1–137.

Stjärne, L. and Åstrand, P. (1984). Discrete events measure single quanta of ATP secreted from sympathetic nerves of guinea-pig and mouse vas deferens. *Neuroscience*, **13**, 21–28.

Stjärne, L. and Åstrand, P. (1985). Relative pre- and postjunctional roles of noradrenaline and adenosine 5′-triphosphate as neurotransmitters of the sympathetic nerves of guinea-pig and mouse vas deferens. *Neuroscience*, **14**, 929–946.

Stjärne, P., Lacroix, J.-S., Änggård, A. and Lundberg, J.M. (1991). Release of CGRP by trigeminal nerve stimulation and capsaicin in relation to changes in nasal vascular resistance and capacitance function. *Regulatory Peptides*, in press.

Stofer, W.D., Fatherazi, S. and Horn, J.P. (1990). Neuropeptide Y mimics a non-adrenergic component of sympathetic vasoconstriction in the bullfrog. *Journal of the Autonomic Nervous System*, **31**, 141–152.

Su, C. (1975). Neurogenic release of purine compounds in blood vessels. *Journal of Pharmacology and Experimental Therapeutics*, **195**, 159–166.

Su, C. (1978). Purinergic inhibition of adrenergic transmission in rabbit blood vessels. *Journal of Pharmacology and Experimental Therapeutics*, **204**, 351–361.

Suzuki, H. (1985). Electrical responses of smooth muscle cells of the rabbit ear artery to adenosine and adenosine triphosphate. *Journal of Physiology*, **359**, 401–415.

Suzuki, H. and Kou, K. (1983). Electrical components contributing to the nerve-mediated contractions in the smooth muscles of the rabbit ear artery. *Japanese Journal of Physiology*, **33**, 743–756.

Suzuki, Y., McMaster, D., Huang, M., Lederis, K. and Rorstad, O.P. (1985). Characterization of functional receptors for vasoactive intestinal peptide in bovine cerebral arteries. *Journal of Neurochemistry*, **45**, 890–899.

Suzuki, H., Mishima, S. and Miyahara, H. (1984). Effects of reserpine on electrical responses evoked by perivascular nerve stimulation in the rabbit ear artery. *Biomedical Research*, **5**, 259–266.

Taddei, S., Salvetti, A. and Pedrinelli, R. (1989). Persistence of sympathetic-mediated forearm vasoconstriction after α-blockade in hypertensive patients. *Circulation*, **80**, 485–490.

Tatemoto, K., Carlquist, M. and Mutt, V. (1982). Neuropeptide Y — a novel brain peptide with structural similarities to peptide YY and pancreatic polypeptide. *Nature*, **296**, 659–660.

Taylor, E.M. and Parsons, M.E. (1989). Adrenergic and purinergic neurotransmission in arterial resistance vessels of the cat intestinal circulation. *European Journal of Pharmacology*, **164**, 23–33.

Taylor, E.M., Parsons, M.E., Wright, P.W., Pepkin, M.A. and Howson, W. (1989). The effects of adenosine triphosphate and related purines on arterial resistance vessels *in vitro* and *in vivo*. *European Journal of Pharmacology*, **161**, 121–133.

Toda, N. (1981). Non-adrenergic, non-cholinergic innervation in monkey and human cerebral arteries. *British Journal of Pharmacology*, **72**, 281–283.

Toda, N. (1982). Relaxant responses to transmural stimulation and nicotine of dog and monkey cerebral arteries. *American Journal of Physiology*, **243**, H145–H153.

Torregrosa, G., Miranda, F.J., Salom, J.B., Alabadi, J.A., Alvarez, C. and Alborch, E.H. (1990). Heterogeneity of P_2-purinoceptors in brain circulation. *Journal of Cerebral Blood Flow and Metabolism*, **10**, 572–579.

Torregrosa, G., Terassa, J.C., Salom, J.B., Miranda, F.J., Campos, V. and Alborch, E. (1988). P_1-purinoceptors in the cerebrovascular bed of the goat *in vivo*. *European Journal of Pharmacology*, **149**, 17–24.

Uddman, R., Alumets, J., Edvinsson, L., Håkansson, R. and Sundler, F. (1981). VIP nerve fibres around peripheral blood vessels. *Acta Physiologica Scandinavica*, **112**, 65–70.

Uddman, R., Edvinsson, L., Owman, C. and Sundler, F. (1983). Nerve fibres containing gastrin-releasing peptide around pial vessels. *Journal of Cerebral Blood Flow and Metabolism*, **3**, 386–390.

Uddman, R., Fahrenkrug, J., Malm, L., Alumets, J., Håkansson, R. and Sundler, F. (1980). Neuronal VIP in salivary glands: distribution and release. *Acta Physiologica Scandinavica*, **110**, 31–42.

Uddman, R., Malm, L. Fahrenkrug, J. and Sundler, F. (1981). VIP increases in nasal blood flow during stimulation of the Vidian nerve. *Acta Oto-Laryngologica*, **91**, 135–142.

Uemura, Y., Sugimoto, T., Okamoto, S., Handa, H. and Mizuno, N. (1986). Changes of vasoactive intestinal polypeptide-like immunoreactivity in cerebrovascular nerve fibers after subarachnoid haemorrhage: an experimental study in the dog. *Neuroscience Letters*, **71**, 137–141.

Vidal, M., Hicks, P.E. and Langer, S.Z. (1986). Differential effects of α,β-methylene ATP on responses to nerve stimulation in SHR and WKY tail arteries. *Naunyn-Schmiedeberg's Archives of Pharmacology*, **332**, 384–390.

Waeber, B., Aubert, J.-F., Corder, R., Evéquoz, D., Nussberger, J., Gaillard, R., *et al.* (1988). Cardiovascular effects of neuropeptide Y. *American Journal of Hypertension*, **1**, 193–199.

Wahlestedt, C., Edvinsson, L., Ekblad, E. and Håkansson, R. (1985). Neuropeptide Y potentiates noradrenaline-evoked vasoconstriction: mode of action. *Journal of Pharmacology and Experimental Therapeutics*, **234**, 735–741.

Wahlestedt, C., Edvinsson, L., Ekblad, E. and Håkansson, R. (1987). Effects of neuropeptide Y at sympathetic neuroeffector junctions: existence of Y_1- and Y_2-receptors. In: *Neuronal Messengers in Vascular Function*, edited by A. Nobin, C. Owman and B. Arneklo-Nobin, pp. 231–242. Amsterdam: Elsevier Science.

Wahlestedt, C., Håkansson, R., Vaz, C.A. and Zukowska-Grojec Z. (1990). Norepinephrine and neuropeptide Y: vasoconstrictor cooperation *in vivo* and *in vitro*. *American Journal of Physiology*, **258**, R736–R742.

Wahlestedt, C., Yanaihara, N. and Håkansson, R. (1986). Evidence for different pre- and post-junctional receptors for neuropeptide Y and related peptides. *Regulatory Peptides*, **13**, 307–318.

Warland, J.J.I. and Burnstock, G. (1987). Effects of reserpine and 6-hydroxydopamine on the adrenergic and purinergic components of sympathetic nerve responses of the rabbit saphenous artery. *British Journal of Pharmacology*, **92**, 871–880.

Watson, J.D., Sury, M.R., Corder, R., Carson, R., Bouloux, P.M., Lowry, P.J., *et al.* (1988). Plasma levels of neuropeptide Y are increased in human sepsis but are unchanged during canine endotoxin shock despite raised catecholamine concentrations. *Journal of Endocrinology*, **116**, 421–426.

Weihe, E., Reinecke, M. and Forssmann, W.G. (1984). Distribution of vasoactive intestinal polypeptide-like immunoreactivity in the mammalian heart. *Cell and Tissue Research*, **236**, 527–540.

Westfall, D.P., Sedaa, K. and Bjur, R.A. (1987). Release of endogenous ATP from rat caudal artery. *Blood Vessels*, **24**, 125–127.

Westfall, T.C., Martin, J., Chen, X., Ciarleglio A., Carpentier, S., Henderson, K., *et al.* (1988). Cardiovascular effects and modulation of noradrenergic neurotransmission following central and peripheral administration of neuropeptide Y. *Synapse*, **2**, 299–307.

Wharton, J. and Gulbenkian, S. (1989). Peptides in the mammalian cardiovascular system. *Experientia*, **56**, 292–316.

Widdicombe, J.G. (1990). The NANC system and airway vasculature. *Archives Internationales de Pharmacodynamie*, **303**, 83–99.

Wilson, D.A., O'Neill, J.T., Said, S.I. and Traystman, R.J. (1981). Vasoactive intestinal polypeptide and the canine cerebral circulation. *Circulation Research*, **48**, 138–148.

Witanowski, W.R. (1925). Über humorale Übertragbarkeit der Herznervenwirkung. *Pflügers Archives*, **208**, 694–704.

Wolin, M.S., Wood, K.S. and Ignarro, L.J. (1982). Guanylate cyclase from bovine lung. A kinetic analysis of the regulation of unpurified soluble enzyme by protoporphyrin IX, heme and nitrosyl-heme. *Journal of Biological Chemistry*, **267**, 11312–11320.

Wood, J.D. and Mayer, C.J. (1979). Serotonergic activation of tonic-type enteric neurons in guinea-pig small bowel. *Journal of Neurophysiology*, **42**, 582–593.

Yamamoto, R. and Cline, W.H. JR. (1987). Release of endogenous NE from mesenteric vasculature of WKY and SHR in response to PNS. *Journal of Pharmacology and Experimental Therapeutics*, **241**, 826–832.

Yanaihara, N., Nokihara, K., Yanaihara, C., Iwanaga, T. and Fujita, T. (1983). Immunocytochemical demonstration of PHI and its co-existence with VIP in intestinal nerves of the rat and pig. *Archivum Histologicum Japonicum*, **46**, 575–581.

4 Vascular Afferent Nerves: Involved in Local Blood Flow Regulation?

Lars Edvinsson,[1] Inger Jansen-Olesen,[2] Sergio Gulbenkian[3] and Rolf Uddman[4]

[1] *Department of Internal Medicine, University Hospital of Lund,*
  S-221 85 Lund, Sweden
[2] *Department of Experimental Research, and*
[3] *Department of Cell Biology, Gulbenkian Institute of Science,*
  2781 Oeiras, Portugal
[4] *Department Otorhinolaryngology, University of Lund,*
  Malmö General Hospital, S-214 01 Malmö, Sweden

Blood vessels are invested by sensory afferent nerves containing calcitonin gene-related peptide (CGRP), substance P (SP) and neurokinin A (NKA). The three peptides co-exist both in the perivascular nerve fibres and in the sensory ganglia. Studies of isolated vessels have revealed that all three peptides are potent vasodilators. CGRP appears to be the more important vasodilator, and is released upon activation of the sensory fibres, as judged from blockade experiments with a CGRP antagonist, CGRP (8-37), and with a tachykinin antagonist, spantide. Stimulation of the trigeminal ganglion, the major cranial sensory ganglion, elicits dilatation of cranial blood vessels and increases cerebral blood flow. Lesion experiments have revealed that the trigemino-vascular fibres have no tonic influence on cerebral blood flow, but may modify vasoconstrictor responses as elicited *in situ*. The sensory-vascular system may thus be involved in local blood flow regulation by sensing and buffering sudden and marked alterations in vessel tone.

KEY WORDS: sensory nerves; blood vessels; substance P; calcitonin gene-related peptide; blood flow regulation.

INTRODUCTION

Cell bodies of primary afferent (sensory) neurons are located in the spinal (dorsal root) and cranial sensory ganglia (trigeminal, nodose — jugular) and send fibres in both the central and the peripheral directions. These neurons not only transmit information to the central nervous system but also act as "effector" neurons which control blood flow and other vascular functions (for reviews see Holzer, 1988; Lembeck and Holzbauer, 1988; Maggi and Meli, 1988). This latter function is exerted by release of peptide transmitters from the peripheral nerve terminals (Szolcsányi, 1984; Holzer, 1988; Maggi and Meli, 1988). This was first demonstrated by the finding that stimulation of the peripheral ends of cut dorsal roots induced vasodilatation in the skin area supplied by the respective neurons, "antidromic vasodilatation" (Stricker, 1876; Bayliss, 1901). The present review points to the possible role of sensory neurons in local control of blood flow.

INNERVATION OF BLOOD VESSELS

Immunocytochemical studies have shown that the peripheral autonomic nervous system contains numerous regulatory peptides in addition to the "classical" neurotransmitters, nor-adrenaline (NA) and acetylcholine (ACh). In sympathetic perivascular fibres neuropeptide tyrosine (NPY) coexists with a subpopulation of the NA-containing neurons (Uddman et al., 1985). NPY may induce constriction, potentiate the post-synaptic action of NA, and inhibit the release of endogenous NA (Ekblad et al., 1984; Lundberg and Stjärne, 1984; Wahlestedt et al., 1985, 1987). In the parasympathetic system, the main neuropeptide is vasoactive intestinal peptide (VIP). VIP has been shown to coexist with ACh (Lundberg et al., 1981; Lundberg, Änggård and Fahrenkrug, 1981) as well as NPY and in some species dynorphin (Morris et al., 1985). In perivascular nerve fibres belonging to the sensory nervous system, substance P (SP), neurokinin A (NKA) and calcitonin gene-related peptide (CGRP) have been demonstrated (Furness et al., 1982; Uddman et al., 1986; Wharton et al., 1986; Gibbins, Furness and Costa, 1987; O'Brien et al., 1989). The peptides are synthesized in the somata of sensory neurons (Keen et al., 1982; Rosenfeld et al., 1983; Nakanishi, 1987) and brought to the nerve endings by way of axonal transport. Stimulus-induced exocytotic release of the peptides from synaptic vesicles in the peripheral terminals depends on the presence of extracellular Ca^{2+} (Maggi et al., 1989; Amann et al., 1990). Due to their ability to dilate blood vessels, it is thought that one of the primary objectives of CGRP, SP and NKA is to mediate the vascular effects of sensory nerve stimulation (see Holzer, 1988). This has been confirmed by the fact that the vascular actions of exogenous and endogenous CGRP, SP and NKA can be blocked by the use of specific antibodies or antagonists. The simultaneous release of several co-existing sensory neuropeptides (Saria et al., 1986) is likely to exert an intricate control of vascular functions (see Brain and Williams, 1989).

Although SP, NKA and CGRP induce vasodilatation there is considerable variation in the responsiveness of different vascular regions to these neuropeptides. Furthermore, there is only scattered information about the reactions of the venous system to perivascular peptides. In the following sections a comparison of the perivascular innervation pattern will be given for two regions.

MORPHOLOGY

The general neuronal marker protein gene product (PGP 9.5), has revealed that blood vessels (arteries and veins) possess a rich supply of nerve fibres and fascicles forming a loose network in the adventitia and at the adventitial-medial border (for references see Edvinsson et al., 1989a). In general, arteries have a slightly richer nerve supply as compared to the veins, but the nerve plexus in the latter often appears to display a more regular arrangement with a predominant circular orientation around the vessel.

The distribution of peptide-containing nerve fibres to blood vessels has been studied on large arteries of the conduit and large muscular types. The proximal part of such vessels contains a dense supply of nerve fibres forming a network whereas the distal part only harbours few or single fibres. In the superior mesenteric artery (SMA), the proximal or central portion is of the conduit type, and the distal or peripheral portion, in the vicinity of the intestine, where the vessel has a diameter around 200–300 μm, can be considered a resistance vessel (Edvinsson et al., 1989b). Thus, the proximal part of the SMA possesses a rich supply of NPY- and tyrosine hydroxylase (TH)-immunoreactive nerve fascicles and fibres forming a loose network in the wall of the artery. The fibres containing CGRP, SP and NKA appear to form a somewhat less dense plexus, while the supply of VIP-containing fibres is moderate. The perivascular nerve fibres in the distal part of the SMA display a different distribution pattern and density compared to that of the proximal part. NPY- and TH-immunoreactive nerves are numerous, forming a dense perivascular network, with a predominant circular or spiral orientation along the long axis of the vessel (Figures 4.1a, b). SP-, NKA- and CGRP-immunoreactive nerves are less numerous and distributed mainly parallel to the long axis of the distal SMA (Figures 4.1c–e). Only a few fibres containing VIP can be seen in the distal SMA (Figure 4.1f).

ELECTRON MICROSCOPY

Electron microscopical immunocytochemistry of the guinea pig SMA has revealed a moderate amount of NPY- and a few VIP-containing nerve terminals close to the adventitial-medial border in both proximal and distal regions of the artery (Edvinsson et al., 1989b) (Figure 4.2d). CGRP-, SP- and NKA-immunoreactive nerve terminals also occur in the adventitia, but are less closely associated with smooth muscle cells of the medial layer (Figures 4.2a–c). The NPY-, CGRP-, SP- and NKA-immunoreactivities consistently occur in the large vesicle population of nerve terminals (70–100 nm in diameter) (Edvinsson et al., 1989b).

When comparing an artery of the conduit type with a resistance vessel it appears that the sympathetic component (NPY and TH) is richer in the resistance part, as compared to the conduit vessel. The number of parasympathetic fibres (VIP) is moderate in proximal arteries and few in the small resistance vessels. For the sensory fibres the pattern is again different, although the density of CGRP-, SP- and NKA-containing nerve fibres appears to be similar in both proximal and distal regions of the SMA, there is a different spatial arrangement. In the proximal SMA the fibres show a predominantly circular orientation around the vessel circumference, whereas in the distal SMA they run parallel to the long axis of the vessel. Another important observation is that the CGRP-/tachykinin-immunoreactive nerve terminals, are fairly widely separated from the smooth muscle cells in the adventitia. It is possible that the peptides released in response to sensory nerve stimulation act on adjacent nerve terminals. This indicates a slightly different role as compared with the NPY/TH-immunoreactive nerve terminals, which are preferentially located at the adventitial-medial border, close to smooth muscle cells of the media. At the ultrastructural level, SP-, NKA- and CGRP-immunoreactivity have been shown to occur in the same

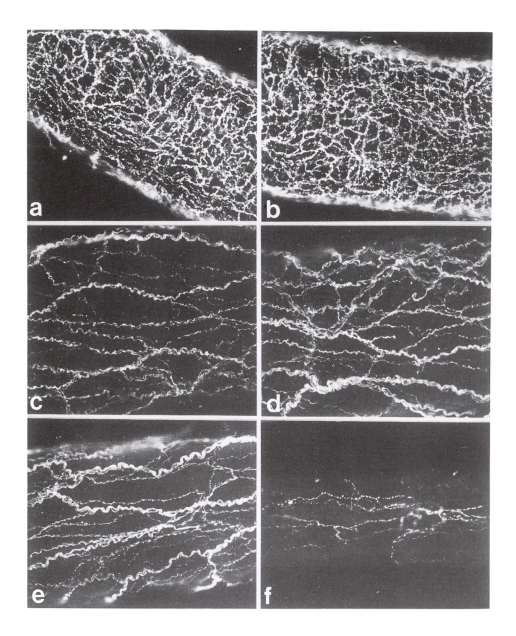

Figure 4.1 Whole mount preparations of distal branches of the superior mesenteric artery (SMA) (close to the small intestine) immunostained for (a) NPY, (b) TH, (c) CGRP, (d) SP (e) NKA, and (f) VIP. The density and distribution pattern of the immunostained innervation differ from that seen in the proximal SMA. The density of the NPY- and TH-immunoreactive plexus is very similar and increases dramatically with declining vessel size. The distribution pattern of CGRP, SP and NKA immunoreactivities is also very similar, however, the density of nerves displaying these immunoreactivities falls as the vessels are followed distally towards the intestine. VIP-immunoreactive fibres are few and run mainly along the vessel wall. Magnification ×175.

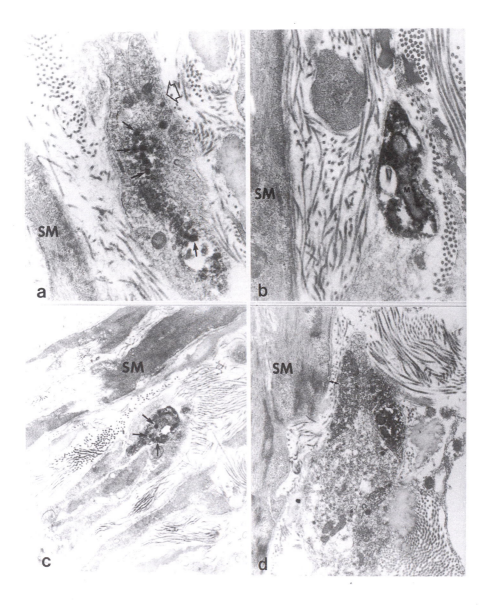

Figure 4.2   Photomicrographs of transverse sections of the superior mesenteric artery (SMA), at the adventitial-medial junction, immunostained for (a) CGRP, (b) NKA, (c) SP, and (d) NPY using the pre-embedding PAP technique. Labelled and unlabelled axon profiles (open arrows) occur together in the adventitia and contain secretory vesicles (arrows); similar observations were made in proximal and distal segments. CGRP, NKA A- and SP-immunoreactive axons have a similar distribution and were rarely seen in close proximity to the vascular smooth muscle (SM). NPY-immunoreactive axons occurred more frequently and in closer proximity to the media with the junctional cleft being as little as 50–100 nm wide (double arrow). Magnification ×16.195.

vesicles (Gulbenkian *et al.*, 1986); this has possible implications for co-release and interaction between these peptides in evoking the smooth muscle response to sensory nerve stimulation.

ORIGIN OF PERIVASCULAR SENSORY NERVES

Most, if not all, CGRP-containing nerve fibres in, e.g. the rat stomach represent extrinsic sensory neurons which originate in dorsal root ganglia (Sternini, Reeve and Brecha, 1987; Su *et al.*, 1987; Green and Dockray, 1988; Varro *et al.*, 1988) whilst vagal sensory fibres contribute little to the CGRP content of the rat stomach (Green and Dockray, 1988; Varro *et al.*, 1988). Vagal, CGRP-containing, sensory neurons innervate the oesophagus (Rodrigo *et al.*, 1985). SP, NKA and CGRP co-exist in the perivascular sensory axons, but the overlap is not complete in as much as more fibres contain CGRP than SP and NKA (Gibbins *et al.*, 1985; Lee *et al.*, 1985; Rodrigo *et al.*, 1985; Uddman *et al.*, 1986; Su *et al.*, 1987; Green and Dockray, 1988).

In the cranial circulation of the cat there is a moderate supply of SP- and NKA-immunoreactive nerves (Edvinsson, McCulloch and Uddman, 1981; Uddman *et al.*, 1981), and a rich supply of CGRP-containing nerve fibres (Edvinsson, 1985; Hanko *et al.*, 1985; Uddman *et al.*, 1986). Retrograde axonal tracing and denervation studies have shown that the SP, NKA and CGRP fibres to cranial blood vessels originate in the trigeminal ganglion, but with contributions also from dorsal root ganglion and internal carotid mini-ganglia (Mayberg *et al.*, 1981; Liu-Chen, Han and Moskowitz, 1983; Liu-Chen, Mayberg and Moskowitz, 1983; Mayberg, Zervas and Moskowitz, 1984; Saito, Liu-Chen and Moskowitz, 1987; Edvinsson, Hara and Uddman, 1989; Suzuki, Hardebo and Owman, 1989). The amount of sensory nerve fibres diminishes in distal vessels (smaller size). In addition, there are fewer fibres in the more caudally located pial vessels than in the vessels located in the rostral part of the circle of Willis. The caudal third of the basilar artery and the vertebral artery have been shown to be innervated from the upper cervical dorsal root ganglia (Edvinsson, Hara and Uddman, 1989; Saito and Moskowitz, 1989; Suzuki, Hardebo and Owman, 1989). The general distribution of NKA-containing nerve fibres resembles that of SP. The coexistence of SP and NKA in sensory ganglia and in perivascular nerve fibres has been demonstrated by immunocytochemical staining methods (Dalsgaard *et al.*, 1985; Sundler *et al.*, 1985). CGRP-immunoreactivity is present in the perikarya of neurons in the trigeminal ganglion of all species examined, including man. It is frequently co-localized with SP and NKA in trigeminal cell bodies and perivascular nerve fibres, although the number of CGRP-containing cells exceeds the number of SP-containing cells (Rosenfeld *et al.*, 1983; Lee *et al.*, 1985; Uddman *et al.*, 1985; McCulloch *et al.*, 1986; Edvinsson, Hara and Uddman, 1989; Jansen-Olesen *et al.*, 1995).

RELEASE OF SENSORY NEUROPEPTIDES

The release of SP from peripheral sensory nerve endings was first demonstrated in dental pulp. In these experiments, the inferior alveolar nerve was stimulated electrically using stimulation parameters known to activate C-fibres and to increase pulp blood flow (Olgart *et al.*, 1977; Gazelius and Olgart, 1980). An enhanced release of SP was noted in the superfusate of an exposed dental pulp (Brodin *et al.*, 1981). Similarily, electrical or mechanical stimulation of the trigeminal nerve resulted in an increase in the SP concentration in the aqueous humour of the eye (Bill *et al.*, 1979) and skin (White and Helme, 1985). In cerebral vessels and pial membranes, electrical field stimulation, capsaicin or potassium-induced depolarization caused an enhanced release of SP (Edvinsson, Rosendahl-Helgesen and Uddman, 1983; Moskowitz, Brody and Liu-Chen, 1983). CGRP has been shown to be released by stimulation of the perivascular nerves of rat mesenteric resistance blood vessels (Kawasaki *et al.*, 1988). Electrical stimulation of the trigeminal ganglion results in an increase of SP- and CGRP-immunoreactivity in blood samples taken from the external jugular vein (Goadsby, Edvinsson and Ekman, 1988).

A property of the sensory neurons associated with the circulatory system is their sensitivity to capsaicin. Capsaicin, the pungent ingredient of red peppers, is chemically related to vanillyl amide (8-methyl-N-vanillyl-6-nonenamide). In cerebral and coronary vessels capsaicin causes local release of CGRP from primary sensory afferents (Franco-Cereceda *et al.*, 1987; Jansen *et al.*, 1990). Capsaicin has a specific action on a subpopulation of neuropeptide-containing primary afferent neurones involving the activation of a specific receptor — the vanilloid receptor (Szállási and Blumberg, 1990). Activation of this receptor leads to an influx of sodium (Na) and calcium ions (Ca) which at low doses (in the μg/kg range) excites afferent neurons, which have small cell bodies, and unmyelinated (C-fibre) or thinly myelinated (A-fibre) axons, an action which is soon followed by desensitisation or defunctionalization of the primary afferent neurons (see Kaufman *et al.*, 1982; Longhurst *et al.*, 1984; Szolcsányi, 1984, 1990; Holzer, 1991). Systemic administration of high doses of capsaicin (in the mg/kg range) damages these neurons, and the extent of damage (ultrastructural changes or degeneration of C-fibre and A-fibre afferent neurons) depends on the dosage, route of administration, animal species, and the age of the animals (see Szolcsányi, 1990; Holzer, 1991). This population of neurons is connected to chemonociceptors, polymodal nociceptors and warmth receptors (Szolcsányi, 1990; Holzer, 1991). Capsaicin's specificity for sensory neurons is not absolute, and particularly the acute actions of capsaicin are not restricted to afferent neurons (see Holzer, 1991); some of the acute effects on blood vessels appear to be the result of a direct action at the vanilloid receptor on the vascular smooth muscle (Duckles, 1986; Bény, Brunet and Huggel, 1989; Edvinsson *et al.*, 1990a; Jansen *et al.*, 1990) and endothelium (Kenins, Hurley and Bell, 1984). The label "capsaicin-sensitive" is applied to those afferent neurons which, acutely, are excited and in the long term, damaged, by the drug.

In cats subjected to cronic unilateral trigeminal ganglionectomy and equipped with a cranial window it has been shown that the vasodilator responses to nitroprusside and nitroglycerin (NTG) were markedly depressed on the denervated side (Wei *et al.*, 1992). Application of the CGRP antagonist α-CGRP 8-37 on the innervated side reduced the response to nitrovasodilators to the same extent as denervation. It was suggested that nitrovasodilators exerted their action via activation of sensory fibres which released CGRP (Wei *et al.*, 1992). However, experiments performed on isolated arteries *in vitro*, which provides a model situation where the effect of NTG on vascular receptors and perivascular nerves can be studied in isolation. NTG induced relaxation of cerebral vessels without involving the sensory neuropeptides substance P and CGRP (Jansen-Olesen *et al.*, 1994). These results are supported by *in vivo* studies of experimental headache in man, in which NTG was administered by intravenous infusion, but no change was observed in levels of CGRP in blood from the external jugular vein drawn before, during and after NTG infusion (Iversen *et al.*, 1993).

PHARMACOLOGY OF SENSORY NEUROPEPTIDES

CHARACTERIZATION OF NEUROKININ RECEPTORS

The tachykinins, SP, NKA, neuropeptide K (NPK) and neurokinin B (NKB) induce strong relaxation of precontracted cerebral arteries from guinea pig and man (Jansen *et al.*, 1991). In the guinea pig basilar artery, the tachykinin receptors appear to be of the NK-1 type (Edvinsson and Jansen, 1987; Jansen *et al.*, 1991). In human pial arteries, and pig and cat middle cerebral arteries, the receptors seem to be a non NK-1 subtype or a mixture of NK-1 and NK-2 subtypes (Jansen *et al.*, 1991). In the rat and rabbit basilar arteries, SP is more potent than NKA. In rat cerebral arteries, the tachykinins act as weak dilators, while the responses are stronger in the rabbit (Edvinsson *et al.*, 1988). In guinea pig basilar arteries, devoid of endothelium, none of the tachykinins cause relaxation. Perivascular microinjection of SP, NKA and NKB to cat cerebral arterioles *in situ* results in increases in the arteriolar calibre. The change in calibre to NKB is 9% while that to SP and NKA is 15–20%; relaxations occur at the same peptide concentrations *in vitro* and *in situ* (Jansen *et al.*, 1991).

In guinea pig basilar arteries, the SP antagonist, spantide (10^{-7}–10^{-5} M), induces a parallel shift to the right of the relaxant responses induced by SP, NKA and NPK without alteration of the maximum response (Edvinsson and Jansen, 1987; Jansen *et al.*, 1991). Schild plot analysis shows regression lines with slopes that do not differ from unity, resulting in pA_2 values of 6.9 for SP and NKA, and 6.7 for NPK. In contrast, spantide (10^{-5} M) has no competitive antagonistic effect on the relaxation induced by NKB, although a reduction in maximum effect is seen. Spantide does not block dilatations induced by CGRP in the same preparations.

SP, NKA, NPK and NKB induce endothelium-dependent relaxations of precontracted cerebral vessel segments (Edvinsson and Jansen, 1987; Edvinsson *et al.*, 1988; Jansen *et al.*, 1991). The order of potency does not fit perfectly the suggested order of potency for different tachykinin receptor subtypes (Regoli *et al.*, 1987). Spantide shifts the concentration-response curves of the SP- and NKA-induced relaxations (NK-1 and NK-2) competitively. However, the maximum response induced by NKB (NK-3) is markedly depressed by spantide with no alteration in the sensitivity to the tachykinins, this suggests a non-competitive manner of action. Thus, spantide may be of value in characterisation of some neurokinin receptor subtypes.

During the last few years new nonpeptide neurokinin 1 (NK-1) and NK-2 receptor antagonists appeared. CP 96, 345 is selective for the NK-1 receptor and has been shown to attenuate SP and capsaicin-induced plasma extravasation in the hamster cheek pouch

(Gao *et al.*, 1993). SR 140 333 is another NK-1 receptor antagonist which blocks the [Sar9, Met(02) 11] SP induced relaxation of rabbit pulmonary artery while it has no antagonistic effect on relaxations induced by NK-2 or NK-3 selective agonists (Emonds *et al.*, 1993). In the cerebral circulation of guinea pig the NK-1 receptor antagonist RP 675 40 blocks substance P induced relaxations while the NK-2 antagonist SR 48968 has no such effect even in concentrations up to 10^{-5} M (Jansen-Olesen, I. and Edvinsson, L., unpublished observations). Thus, these findings further support that the tachykinin receptors in the guinea pig basilar artery is of the NK-1 type.

CHARACTERISATION OF CGRP RECEPTORS

CGRP dilates peripheral (Brain *et al.*, 1985) and cerebral blood vessels (Edvinsson, 1985) through the activation of adenylyl cyclase (Edvinsson *et al.*, 1985; Jansen, Mortensen and Edvinsson, 1992). CGRP seems to act on receptors located on the cerebrovascular smooth muscle, since removal of the endothelium does not attenuate its response (Edvinsson *et al.*, 1985). There is limited information on the receptor pharmacology of different CGRP analogs in a given system. Investigations on vascular and non-vascular smooth muscle have suggested that human (h)-βCGRP is most potent followed by rat (r)-αCGRP which is more potent than h-αCGRP (Holman, Craig and Marshall, 1986; Marshall *et al.*, 1986a, b; Chakder and Rattan, 1990). Furthermore, in the internal anal sphincter smooth muscle [Tyr^0]CGRP 28-37 is a stronger antagonist on the effects of the α- and β-forms of hCGRP as compared to that of r-αCGRP (Chakder and Rattan, 1990). Recently, a C-terminal fragment of h-αCGRP, hCGRP(8-37), has been shown to act as a competitive h-αCGRP receptor antagonist in the cardiovascular system of the rat, in the guinea pig atrium and guinea pig ileum. The antagonistic activity of hCGRP(8-37) is weak in the rat vas deferens and ineffective against h-αCGRP-induced hyperthermia. Consequently, the existence of at least two classes of CGRP receptors has been suggested (Dennis *et al.*, 1990; Donoso *et al.*, 1990), one being sensitive to hCGRP(8-37) and the other being insensitive to hCGRP(8-37). The antagonist was found in conscious Long Evans rats to block the hypertensive, tachycardic and common and internal carotid artery vasodilator effects of h-αCGRP but had no effect on resting blood pressure, heart rate or common or internal carotid haemodynamics (Gardiner *et al.*, 1991). In this system h-αCGRP 28-37 was ineffective.

The effects of five CGRP related peptides and two calcitonin analogs have been studied in the cerebral circulation. r-αCGRP, r-βCGRP, h-αCGRP, h-βCGRP and [Tyr^0]CGRP all induce strong (I_{max}: 80–87%) and potent (pD$_2$: 8.1–8.9) relaxations of guinea pig basilar arteries (Jansen, 1992). Human and salmon calcitonin relax in the same concentration interval as the CGRP analogs (pD$_2$; 8.6 and 8.1, respectively), but with much weaker maximum responses (I_{max} 12%). The order of potency is: r-αCGRP > r-βCGRP > human calcitonin > h-αCGRP > h-βCGRP > [Tyr^0]CGRP > salmon calcitonin.

In guinea pig basilar arteries; hCGRP(8-37) (10^{-6} M) has significant antagonistic effects on the relaxation induced by the α-forms but not the β-forms of CGRP. The calculated pA$_2$ values are 6.93 (r-αCGRP) and 7.11 (h-αCGRP). [Tyr^0]CGRP 28-37 does not block any of the agonists tested (Jansen, 1992). If anything, there is a slight potentiation of the relaxation induced by the two β-forms of CGRP. The responses to SP and NKA are not blocked by these putative CGRP antagonists. A concentration of NKA (3×10^{-9} M), SP (10^{-10} M) or CGRP (10^{-9} M), which elicits a dilator response of approximately 5–20% of maximum relaxation, does not potentiate or block the relaxant effect of any of the other peptides. In the guinea pig basilar artery, the maximum relaxations induced by the CGRP analogs are superior to those of calcitonin. There is no excessive difference in potency of relaxation induced by calcitonin as compared to CGRP. This suggests that calcitonin may act as a partial agonist at CGRP receptors.

In the guinea pig basilar artery, hCGRP(8-37) blocks the relaxant responses induced by h- and r-αCGRP but not relaxations induced by their β-forms. Thus, the guinea pig basilar artery appears to be equipped with the CGRP-1 subtype of CGRP receptors. The strong relaxant responses induced by β-CGRP (rat and human forms) are not blocked by this antagonist. This suggests that the α- and β-forms of CGRP act via different subtypes of CGRP receptors. Furthermore, the other antagonist studied, [Tyr^0]CGRP 28-37, is devoid of antagonistic effect on the α- and β-forms of CGRP. It is in this context interesting to note that [Tyr^0]CGRP 28-37 blocks responses induced by h-αCGRP, r-αCGRP and h-βCGRP in the internal anal sphincter muscle (Chakder and Rattan, 1990). These findings further support the existence of more than one subtype of receptors for CGRP. However, in the rat kidney (Castellucci, Maggi and Evangelista, 1993), and mesenteric small arteries (Lei, Mulvany and Nyborg, 1994) the responses to αCGRP and βCGRP was shifted to the right in the presence of 10^{-6} M human αCGRP(8-37). In the mesenteric small arteries the pA_2 values were calculated to be 7.2 and 7.0 respectively, which is close to that found in the guinea pig basilar arteries mentioned above. Furthermore, still recent unpublished studies (Jansen-Olesen, Nilsson and Edvinsson, unpublished observations) have shown that in the guinea pig cerebral blood vessels the cyclic AMP formation induced by αCGRP and βCGRP is blocked by 10^{-6} M CGRP 8-37. These results indicates that βCGRP might act on two different receptors in the guinea pig cerebral circulation — the well known CGRP-1 receptor which mediates the relaxant response via activation of adenylyl cyclase and perhaps another receptor not associated to adenylyl cyclase which can mask the inhibitory effect by CGRP 8-37 on CGRP-1 receptors. However, further studies need to be performed to unravel this possibility.

EFFECTS OF CAPSAICIN ON CEREBRAL ARTERIES *IN VITRO*

Capsaicin in high concentrations (10^{-5}–3×10^{-4} M) elicits weak contractions of guinea pig basilar artery segments at the resting level of tension (Jansen *et al.*, 1991). The contraction amounts to 17% of the potassium-induced contraction with a pD_2 of 5.6×10^{-5} M. In precontracted artery segments, capsaicin induces concentration-dependent biphasic relaxations. The first phase is seen in low capsaicin concentrations (10^{-10}–10^{-6} M) and has an I_{max} of 70% of the histamine precontraction. The second phase of response (I_{max} 100%) is seen in high capsaicin concentrations (10^{-5}–10^{-4} M). Repeated capsaicin administrations to vessel segments decrease the I_{max} of the first phase to $24\pm5\%$ while the second phase is unaltered with an I_{max} of $96\pm3\%$. Experiments performed in the presence of spantide (3×10^{-6} M) do not reveal any significant variation as compared to control experiments. Removal of the endothelium abolishes the relaxant response to ACh, SP and NKA but does not alter the responses to capsaicin or CGRP (Jansen *et al.*, 1990).

The administration of capsaicin (10^{-8}–10^{-5} M) to vessel segments in cat middle cerebral arteries at their resting level of tension causes a concentration-dependent contraction (Edvinsson et al., 1990a). The contractile response is reproducible upon a second exposure. The contraction is unaffected by the presence of the α-adrenoceptor blocker phentolamine (10^{-6} M) or the 5-hydroxytryptamine antagonist ketanserin (10^{-6} M), but significantly reduced in calcium-free medium. A dihydropyridine calcium entry blocker, nimodipine, (10^{-11}–10^{-6} M) causes a complete concentration-dependent reversal of capsaicin-induced precontraction of arterial segments. In precontracted cerebral arteries, capsaicin elicits a concentration-dependent relaxation. The concentration of capsaicin causing half-maximal relaxation is $3.7 \pm 1.3 \times 10^{-14}$ M, and the maximal relaxation is $25 \pm 7\%$ relative to precontraction. The relaxation induced by low concentrations of capsaicin is unaffected by propranolol, cimetidine atropine or spantide. The presence of 10^{-6} M CGRP 8-37 or repeated exposure of cerebral arteries to capsaicin successively reduces the relaxant response to capsaicin (Jansen et al., 1990; Edvinsson et al., 1995).

The dilator response to periarterial nerve stimulation is reduced by the addition of CGRP 8-37 (Kawasaki et al., 1991), desensitization to CGRP (Han, Naes and Westfall, 1990a) and CGRP immunoblockade (Han, Naes and Westfall, 1990b). These findings indicate a mediator role of CGRP in sensory nerve-mediated dilatation of mesenteric arteries in rat (Holzer, 1993).

The effects of capsaicin have also been tested in guinea pigs after subcutaneous injections of capsaicin to deplete the sensory nerve fibres of stored neurotransmitters (Duckles and Buck, 1982; Duckles and Levitt, 1984; Saito and Goto, 1986). In vessel segments from these animals biphasic responses are not seen (Jansen et al., 1991); only relaxation is observed at capsaicin concentrations 10^{-5}–10^{-4} M. As compared to vessel segments from control animals there is no change in maximum dilatory response to capsaicin after chronic capsaicin treatment. The relaxant responses to SP, NKA, NPK and CGRP are unaltered in histamine-precontracted basilar arteries showing no postjunctional alterations in response to the sensory nerve associated peptides.

EFFECT OF CAPSAICIN ON CEREBRAL ARTERIES IN SITU

The perivascular microapplication of capsaicin results in a biphasic response when tested in situ (Edvinsson et al., 1990a). This reaction consists of an initial reduction in arteriolar calibre lasting for less than 1 min, and is followed by a sustained increase in arteriolar calibre lasting for more than 15 min. The constriction is seen at capsaicin concentrations of 10^{-6} to 10^{-5} M, while the dilatation occurs at capsaicin concentrations of 10^{-7} to 10^{-5} M. Repeated microapplications of capsaicin (10^{-6} M) give an unaltered vasoconstrictor response while the delayed vasodilator response is markedly reduced already after a single prior microapplication of capsaicin at the same site. Thus, the vasodilator response is probably due to released peptides from sensory nerve fibres, while the vasoconstrictor effect is non-specific.

Experiments performed in cats, in which the ipsilateral trigeminal ganglion has been surgically removed, reveal that perivascular microapplication of capsaicin (10^{-6} M) elicits an initial vasoconstriction of a magnitude similar to that observed in sham-operated cats.

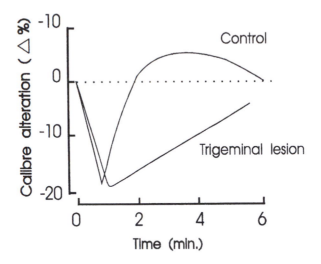

Figure 4.3 Schematic illustration of responses of pial arterioles to the perivascular microinjection of a vasoconstrictor agent in sham-operated and in trigeminal-lesioned animals. The constrictor response has returned to baseline within 2 min in controls while the process is markedly prolonged in lesioned animals. Sometimes a slight overshoot in the response (i.e. dilatation above baseline) can be seen in sham-operated animals.

However, the duration of the initial vasoconstriction in the sham-operated animals is significantly less than in cats with trigeminal lesions (Figure 4.3). Moreover, delayed vasodilatation is not observed in cats in which the trigeminal nerve has been surgically ablated before capsaicin microapplication.

The findings indicate that vasodilator substances are released from sensory fibres which originate in the trigeminal ganglion. These substances act via a non-endothelium-dependent mechanism. Furthermore, the dilatation is not related to an action via cholinergic, adrenergic, histaminergic or tachykinin receptors. At present, the results suggest that CGRP or a similarly active substance is responsible for the first phase of the capsaicin-evoked relaxation in guinea pig and for the dilatory response induced by capsaicin in cat. The findings are in concert with previous studies on coronary arteries, where the capsaicin-induced coronary vasodilatation was dependent neither on endothelium removal nor on SP-tachyphylaxis (Franco-Cereceda et al., 1987; Franco-Cereceda and Rudehill, 1989).

RELEASE OF SP AND CGRP IN MAN

MIGRAINE

A decade ago it was suggested that the fifth cranial nerve is involved in the headache phase of migraine (Moskowitz et al., 1979). Evidence in favour of this view came from several sources. The first and second divisions of the trigeminal nerve have unilateral projections in man (Cushing, 1904). Headache evoked by internal carotid injection of histamine is strictly localized to the ipsilateral forehead or behind the eye of that side (Wolff, 1963), which requires an intact trigeminal pathway (Pickering and Hess, 1933). Pain can be evoked by distending large cerebral blood vessels mechanically or by electrical stimulation of their immediate surroundings (Ray and Wolff, 1940). Furthermore, interruption of the trigeminal ganglia appear to be the single most effective surgical procedure for relieving migraine headaches (White and Sweet, 1955).

It seems that the trigemino-cerebrovascular system provides the brain with a neurogenic mechanism capable of an immediate, local, sustained response under emergency conditions, where excessive constriction of the larger arteries threatens the function of the central nervous system. Direct stimulation of the trigeminal ganglion affects both the cerebral and the extracerebral circulation. In the cat, stimulation of the trigeminal ganglion increases extracerebral blood flow and facial temperature (Lambert et al., 1984). In man, the facial temperature is increased upon trigeminal ganglion thermocoagulation (Drummond, Gonski and Lance, 1983). Furthermore, trigeminal activation in both man and cat causes an increase in the plasma levels of CGRP and SP in cranial vasculature effluent (Goadsby, Edvinsson and Ekman, 1988). Electrical stimulation of the superior sagittal sinus, a trigeminally innervated vascular structure, increases cerebral blood flow (Lambert et al., 1988) and causes release of SP and CGRP into the cranial circulation (Zagami, Goadsby and Edvinsson, 1990). It was recently shown in man that there is a marked increase in craniovascular levels of CGRP, but not of NPY, VIP and SP, during the headache phase of migraine with and without aura (Goadsby, Edvinsson and Ekman, 1990).

SUBARACHNOID HAEMORRHAGE

Subarachnoid haemorrhage (SAH) is often accompanied by vasospasm which reaches a maximum several days after the start of the bleed (Kågström et al., 1966; Bergvall and Galera, 1969; Bergvall, Steiner and Forster, 1973; Weir et al., 1978). About one half of the patients with spasm following aneurysmal SAH develop signs of cerebral ischaemia, a major cause of morbidity and mortality (Fletcher, Taveras and Pool, 1959; Allock and Drake, 1965; Griffith, Cummins and Thomson, 1972; Weir et al., 1975; Saito, Ueda and Sano, 1977; Sano and Saito, 1978; Sundt, Kobayashi and Fobe, 1982). The headache in the course of SAH has often been interpreted as due to increased intracranial pressure, or meningeal irritation by blood or cerebral ischemia. However, it could well be caused by an activation of the trigemino-cerebrovascular system (McCulloch et al., 1986). The concomitant release of stored CGRP and tachykinins would then dilate cerebral vessels (or reduce the degree of vasoconstriction) to alleviate the vasoconstriction induced by SAH. This hypothesis is supported by observations that blood in the subarachnoid space causes a depletion of SP from perivascular nerve fibres (Hara, Nosko and Weir, 1986; Uemura et al., 1987), and by an increase in ganglionic content of the preprotachykinin mRNA that codes for SP (Linnik et al., 1989).

Experimentally induced vasospasm is biphasic, with a short-lived acute phase and a late phase reaching a maximum two to seven days after SAH, depending on the species examined (Brawley, Strandness and Kelly, 1968; Kågström, Nilsson and Svendgaard, 1969; Kuwayama et al., 1972; Nagai et al., 1974; Barry, Gogjian and Stein, 1979; Peerless et al.,

1982). In recent studies (Edvinsson *et al.*, 1990b, 1991), we observed decreased levels of CGRP in cerebral vessels after SAH; this was seen both in cerebral blood vessels of rats exposed to experimental SAH and in cerebral blood vessels from humans that had suffered a fatal SAH. These data are in concert with previous experiments on dogs where a significant reduction of the CGRP fibre network was reported after a cisternal injection of blood (Nozaki, Kikuchi and Mizuno, 1989). CGRP induced stronger dilatations in cerebral arteries from rats exposed to SAH than in controls (Edvinsson *et al.*, 1990b). In man, human αCGRP and human βCGRP are strong vasodilators whether the vessels are precontracted with $PGF_{2\alpha}$ or by human blood (Edvinsson *et al.*, 1991).

Many patients suffering from SAH develop a delayed ischaemic neurologic deficit which sometimes is manifested as a vasoconstriction on the angiogram (cerebral vasospasm). The time of onset is debated; the symptoms are not clinically significant until at least on the third day (Jennet and Teasdale, 1981), and not all patients recovering from SAH develop this complication. A few years ago, a reflex protecting the brain against excessive vasoconstriction was suggested by McCulloch and co-workers (McCulloch *et al.*, 1986; Edvinsson *et al.*, 1987b). The suggestion was based on the observation that a number of vasoconstrictor agents showed a prolonged effect after trigeminal lesions. During SAH, spasmogens such as 5-HT, haemoglobin, catecholamines, blood, fibrin, fibrinogen degradation products or prostaglandins could be responsible for the development of the vasoconstriction. This may lead to activation of the protective trigemino-cerebrovascular reflex to compensate for cerebral vasospasm. This reflex is normally able to cope with the increase in tone by an enhanced release and/or synthesis of CGRP during the first days no matter what the stimulus, but with time the system becomes ineffective in some patients (Juul *et al.*, 1990). The reason for this inability may reside in the peptidergic nature of the system. CGRP cannot be synthetised rapidly enough, the stores are inadequate to maintain the supply, or the contractile stimuli in combination with the factors listed above simply overpower the protective response. The failure of the system is manifested by intense vasoconstriction, cerebral symptoms and finally in ischaemia and cell death in a number of patients. In one study of patients it was seen that cerebral vessels were depleted of CGRP after a fatal SAH (Edvinsson *et al.*, 1990b). This indicates failure in the system. Recent studies have shown that i.v. administration of CGRP dilates cerebral vessels in humans (Martin, Perry and Pickard, 1991; Juul *et al.*, 1991). Furthermore, in one patient who developed an ischaemic deficit postoperatively (after clipping of an aneurysm and nimodipine treatment) the infusion of CGRP resulted in marked improvement of the clinical condition (Juul *et al.*, 1991).

GENERAL PRINCIPLES

Sensory peptides display two different modes of action: SP and NKA having a focus on the endothelium and CGRP on the smooth muscle cells. Furthermore, there are significant differences in potency of SP, NKA and CGRP; this varies among the cranial arteries in man and indicates that the trigeminal system modulates the responses in the intra- and extracranial circulations differently. It is possible that SP causes an inflammatory response in the dura mater while such a reaction is not seen in the cerebral circulation (Markowitz,

Saito and Moskowitz, 1987). CGRP is involved in a dynamic reflex aimed to protect the brain against vasoconstriction. The magnitude of the arteriolar responses to the perivascular microapplication of a number of vasoactive substances does not change following surgical lesions of the trigeminal nerve (McCulloch *et al.*, 1986; Edvinsson *et al.*, 1987b). However, the duration of the vasoconstriction induced by such substances is markedly prolonged. Furthermore, trigeminal lesions do not modify resting local blood flow nor metabolism, or change the coupling between flow or metabolism (Lou, Edvinsson and MacKenzie, 1987). This speaks in favour of the view that the trigemino-cerebrovascular system may be involved in a reflex response to vasoconstriction which is designed to restore the normal vascular diameter. Such a system would have important pathophysiological implications (McCulloch *et al.*, 1986) (Figure 4.3) both in SAH and in migraine (Barkley *et al.*, 1990; Edvinsson *et al.*, 1990b, 1991).

Support for this view is given by Moskowitz *et al.* (1988) who demonstrated that during increases or decreases in arterial PCO_2, and in hypoxia, vasoconstrictor and vasodilator responses were symmetrical following chronic unilateral sectioning of the trigeminal ganglia. However, superfusion of vessels with NA constricts large and small pial arterioles to a greater extent on the denervated side. After severe hypertension, small and large arterioles dilate on both sides although to greater extent on the innervated side. Furthermore, it has been noted that in acutely hypertensive animals, extravasation is greater in the intact, than in the deafferented, hemisphere. In a parallel study, Sakas *et al.* (1989) provided further support for a trigeminovascular reflex-like mechanism operating during acute severe hypertension and seizures. This reflex seems to be present also in postocclusive cerebral hyperaemia (Moskowitz *et al.*, 1989; Macfarlane *et al.*, 1991).

Involvement of sensory neuropeptides has been also noted in patients with severe hypertension (Edvinsson, Ekman and Thulin, 1989; Edvinsson, *et al.*, 1992) and with congestive heart failure (Edvinsson *et al.*, 1990c). However, the pattern of changes in CGRP and SP levels are different in these two circulatory disorders. Hence there is a dynamic role of the sensory afferent nervous system in regulating local vascular changes in many circulatory disorders in man. Details of the reflex changes as outlined for the trigeminovascular system, will undoubtedly be analysed also in great detail for the peripheral circulation.

ACKNOWLEDGEMENTS

This work was supported by the Swedish Medical Research Council (grant no 05958 and grant no 06859), the Söderberg Foundation and the Faculty of Medicine, University of Lund, Sweden.

REFERENCES

Allock, J.M. and Drake, C.G. (1965). Ruptured intracranial aneurysms: the role of arterial spasm. *Journal of Neurosurgery*, **22**, 21–29.

Amann, R., Maggi, C.A., Giuliani, S., Donnerer, J. and Lembeck, F. (1990). Effects of carbonyl cyanide p-trichloro-methoxy-phenylhydrazone (CCP) and of ruthenium red (RR) on capsaicin-evoked neuropeptide release from peripheral terminals of primary afferent neurones. *Archiv der Pharmazie*, **341**, 534–537.

Barkley, G.L., Tepley, N., Nagel-Leiby, S., Moran, J.E., Simkins, R.T. and Welch, K.M. (1990). Magneto-encephalographic studies of migraine. *Headache*, **7**, 428–434.

Barry, K.J., Gogjian, M.A. and Stein, B.M. (1979). Small animal model for investigation of subarachnoid haemorrhage and cerebral vasospasm. *Stroke*, **10**, 538–541.

Bayliss, W.M. (1901). On the origin from the spinal cord of the vasodilator fibres of the hindlimb and the nature of these fibres. *Journal of Physiology*, **26**, 173–209.

Bény, J.-L., Brunet, P.C. and Huggel, H. (1989). Effects of substance P, calcitonin gene-related peptide and capsaicin on tension and membrane potential of pig coronary artery *in vitro*. *Regulator Peptides*, **25**, 25–36.

Bergvall, U. and Galera, R. (1969). Time relationship between subarachnoid haemorrhage, arterial spasm, changes in cerebral circulation and posthaemorrhagic hydrocephalus. *Acta Radiologica*, **9**, 229–237.

Bergvall, U., Steiner, L. and Forster, D.M.C. (1973). Early pattern of cerebral circulatory disturbances following subarachnoid haemorrhage. *Neuroradiology*, **5**, 24–32.

Bill, A., Stjernschantz, J., Mandahl, A., Brodin, E. and Nilsson, G. (1979). Substance P. Release on trigeminal nerve stimulation, effects in the eye. *Acta Physiologica Scandinavica*, **106**, 371–373.

Brain, S.D. and Williams, T.J. (1989). Interactions between the tachykinins and calcitonin gene-related peptide lead to the modulation of oedema formation and blood flow in rat skin. *British Journal of Pharmacology*, **97**, 77–82.

Brain, S.D., Williams, T.J., Tippins, J.R., Morris, H.R. and MacIntyre, I. (1985). Calcitonin gene-related peptide is a potent vasodilator. *Nature (Lond)*, **313**, 54–56.

Brawley, B.W., Strandness, D.E. Jr. and Kelly W.A. (1968). The biphasic response of cerebral vasospasm in experimental subarachnoid haemorrhage. *Journal of Neurosurgery*, **28**, 1–8.

Brodin, E., Gazelius, B., Olgart, L. and Nilsson, G. (1981). Tissue concentration and release of substance P-like immunoreactivity in the dental pulp. *Acta Physiologica Scandinavica*, **111**, 141–149.

Castellucci, A., Maggi, C.A. and Evangelista, S. (1993). Calcitonin gene-related peptide (CGRP-1) receptor mediates vasodilatation in the rat isolated and perfused kidney. *Life Science*, **53**, 153–158.

Chakder, S. and Rattan, S. (1990). [Tyr^0]-calcitonin gene-related peptide 28-37 (rat) as a putative antagonist of calcitonin gene-related peptide response on opossum internal anal sphincter smooth muscle. *Journal of Pharmacology and Experimental Therapeutics*, **253**, 200–206.

Cushing, H. (1904). The sensory distribution of the fifth cranial nerve. *Bulletin of John Hopkins Hospital*, **15**, 213–232.

Dalsgaard, C.-J., Hägerstrand, A., Theodorsson, E., Brodin, E. and Hökfelt, T. (1985). Neurokinin A-like immunoreactivity in rat primary sensory neurons: Coexistence with SP. *Histochemistry*, **83**, 37–39.

Dennis, T., Fournier, A., Cadieux, A., Pomerleau, F.B., Jolicoeur, F.B., St. Pierre, S. *et al.* (1990). hCGRP 8-37, a calcitonin gene-related peptide antagonist revealing calcitonin gene-related pepide receptor heterogeneity in brain and periphery. *Journal of Pharmacology and Experimental Therapeutics*, **254**, 123–128.

Donoso, V.M., Fournier, A., St. Pierre, S. and Huidobro-Toro, J.P. (1990). Pharmacological characterization of CGRP$_1$ receptor subtype in the vascular system in the rat: studies with hCGRP fragments and analogs. *Peptides*, **11**, 885–889.

Drummond, P.D., Gonski, A. and Lance, J.W. (1983). Facial flushing after thermocoagulation of the Gasserian ganglion. *Journal of Neurology Neurosurgery Psychiatry*, **46**, 611–616.

Duckles, S.P. and Buck, S.H. (1982). Substance P in the cerebral vasculature: depletion by capsaicin suggests a sensory role. *Brain Research*, **245**, 171–174.

Duckles, S.P. and Levitt, B. (1984). Specificity of capsaicin treatment in the cerebral vasculature. *Brain Research*, **308**, 141–144.

Duckles, S.P. (1986). Effects of capsaicin on vascular smooth muscle. *Naunyn Schmiedeberg's Archives of Pharmacology*, **333**, 59–64.

Edvinsson, L. (1985). Functional role of perivascular peptides in the control of cerebral circulation. *Trends in Neuroscience*, **8**, 126–131.

Edvinsson, L. and Jansen, I. (1987). Characterization of tachykinin receptors in isolated cerebral arteries of guinea pig. *British Journal of Pharmacology*, **90**, 553–559.

Edvinsson, L., Brodin, E., Jansen, I. and Uddman, R. (1988). Neurokinin A in cerebral vessels: characterization, localization and effects *in vitro*. *Regulatory Peptides*, **20**, 181–197.

Edvinsson, L., Delgado-Zygmunt, T., Ekman, R., Jansen, I., Svendgaard, N.-Aa. and Uddman, R. (1990b). Involvement of perivascular sensory fibers in the pathophysiology of cerebral vasospasm following subarachnoid haemorrhage. *Journal of Cerebral Blood Flow and Metabolism*, **10**, 602–607.

Edvinsson, L., Ekman, R., Hedner, P. and Valdemarsson, S. (1990c). Congestive heart failure: Involvement of perivascular peptides reflecting activity in sympathetic, parasympathetic and afferent fibres. *European Journal of Clinical Investigation*, **20**, 85–89.

Edvinsson, L., Ekman, R., Jansen, I., McCulloch, J., Mortensen, A. and Uddman, R. (1991). Reduced levels of calcitonin gene-related peptide-like immunoreactivity in human brain vessels after subarachnoid haemorrhage. *Neuroscience Letters*, **121**, 151–154.

Edvinsson, L., Ekman, R. and Thulin, T. (1989). Reduced levels of calcitonin gene-related peptide (CGRP) but not substance P during and after treatment of severe hypertension in man. *Journal of Human Hypertension*, **3**, 267–270.

Edvinsson, L., Ekman, R., Jansen, I., McCulloch, J. and Uddman, R. (1987a). Calcitonin gene-related peptide and cerebral blood vessels: Distribution and vasomotor effects. *Journal of Cerebral Blood Flow and Metabolism*, **7**, 720–728.

Edvinsson, L., Fredholm, B.B., Hamel, E., Jansen, I. and Verrecchia, C. (1985). Perivascular peptides relax cerebral arteries concomitant with stimulation of cyclic adenosine monophosphate accumulation or release of an endothelium-derived relaxing factor in the cat. *Neuroscience Letters*, **58**, 213–217.

Edvinsson, L., Gulbenkian, S., Wharton, J., Jansen, I. and Polak, J.M. (1989a). Peptide-containing nerves in the rat femoral artery and vein. *Blood Vessels*, **26**, 254–271.

Edvinsson, L., Gulbenkian, S., Jansen, I., Wharton, J., Cervantes, C. and Polak, J.M. (1989b). Comparison of peptidergic mechanisms in different parts of the guinea pig superior mesenteric artery: immunocytochemistry at the light and ultrastructure levels and responses *in vitro* of large and small arteries. *Journal of the Autonomic Nervous System*, **28**, 141–154.

Edvinsson, L., Hara, H. and Uddman, R. (1989). Retrograde tracing of nerve fibers to the rat middle cerebral artery with True Blue: colocalization with different peptides. *Journal of Cerebral Blood Flow and Metabolism*, **9**, 212–218.

Edvinsson, L., Erlinge, D., Ekman, R. and Thulin, T. (1992). Sensory nerve terminal activity in severe hypertension as reflected by circulating calcitonin gene-related peptide (CGRP) and substance P. *Blood Pressure*, **1**, 223–229.

Edvinsson, L., Jansen, I., Kingman, T.A. and McCulloch, J. (1990a). Cerebrovascular responses to capsaicin *in vitro* and *in situ*. *British Journal of Pharmacology*, **100**, 312–318.

Edvinsson, L., Jansen-Olesen, I., Kingman, T.A., McCulloch, J. and Uddman, R. (1995). Modification of vasoconstrictor responses in cerebral blood vessels by lesioning of the trigeminal nerve: possible involvement of CGRP. *Cephalagia*, **15**, 373–383.

Edvinsson, L., McCulloch, J., Kingman, T.A. and Uddman, R. (1987b). Functional significance of the trigeminal innervation: involvement in cerebrovascular disorders. In *Advances in Headache Research* edited by F. Clifford Rose, pp. 87–93. London, England: Libbey & Co Ltd.

Edvinsson, L., McCulloch, J. and Uddman, R. (1981). Substance P: immunohistochemical localization and effect upon cat pial arteries *in vitro* and *in situ*. *Journal of Physiology*, **318**, 251–258.

Edvinsson, L., Rosendahl-Helgesen, S. and Uddman, R. (1983). Substance P: localization, concentration and release in cerebral arteries, choroid plexus and dura mater. *Cell and Tissue Research*, **234**, 1–7.

Ekblad, E., Edvinsson, L., Wahlestedt, C., Uddman, R., Håkanson, R., and Sundler, F. (1984). Neuropeptide Y co-exists and co-operates with noradrenaline in perivascular nerve fibres. *Regulatory Peptides*, **8**, 225–235.

Emonds Alt, X., Doutremepuich, J.D., Heaulme, M., Neliat, G., Santucci, V., Steinberg, R., *et al.* (1993). *In vitro* and *in vivo* biological activities of SP 140 333, a novel potent non-peptide tachykinin NK-1 receptor antagonist. *European Journal of Pharmacology*, **250**, 403–413.

Fletcher, T.M., Taveras, J.M. and Pool, J.L.C. (1959). Cerebral vasospasm in angiography for intracranial aneurysms: incidence and significance in one hundred consecutive angiograms. *Archives of Neurology*, **1**, 38–47.

Franco-Cereceda, A. and Rudehill, A. (1989). Capsaicin-induced vasodilatation of human coronary arteries *in vitro* is mediated by calcitonin gene-related peptide rather than substance P or neurokinin A. *Acta Physiologica Scandinavica*, **136**, 575–580.

Franco-Cereceda, A., Henke, H., Lundberg, J.M., Petermann, J.B., Hökfelt, T. and Fischer, J.A. (1987). Calcitonin gene-related peptide (CGRP) in capsaicin-sensitive substance P-immunoreactive sensory neurons in animals and man: distribution and release by capsaicin. *Peptides*, **8**, 399–410.

Furness, J.B., Papka, R.E., Della, N.G., Costa, M. and Eskay, R.L. (1982). Substance P-like immunoreactivity in nerves associated with the vascular system of guinea-pigs. *Neuroscience*, **7**, 447–459.

Gao, X.P., Robbins, R.A., Snider, R.M., Lowe, J., Rennard, S.I., Anding, P., *et al.* (1993). NK-1 receptors mediate tachykinin-induced increase in microvascular clearance in hamster cheek and pouch. *American Journal of Physiology*, **265**, H593–H598.

Gardiner, S.M., Compton, A.M., Kemp, P.A., Bennett, T., Bose, C., Foulkes, R., *et al.* (1991). Human α-calcitonin gene-related peptide (CGRP)-(8-37), but not -(28-37), inhibits carotid vasodilator effects of human α-CGRP *in vivo*. *European Journal of Pharmacology*, **199**, 375–378.

Gazelius, B. and Olgart, L. (1980). Vasodilatation in the dental pulp produced by electrical stimulation of the inferior alveolar nerve in the cats. *Acta Physiologica Scandinavica*, **108**, 181–186.

Gibbins, I.L., Furness, J.B. and Costa, M. (1987). Pathway-specific patterns of the co-existence of substance P, calcitonin gene-related peptide, cholecystokinin and dynorphin in neurons of the dorsal root ganglia of the guinea-pig. *Cell and Tissue Research*, **248**, 417–437.

Gibbins, I.L., Furness, J.B., Costa, M., MacIntyre, I., Hillyard, C.J., and Girgis, S. (1985). Co-localization of calcitonin gene-related peptide-like immunoreactivity with substance P in cutaneous, vascular and visceral sensory neurons of guinea pigs. *Neuroscience Letters*, **57**, 125–130.

Goadsby, P.J., Edvinsson, L. and Ekman, R. (1988). Release of vasoactive peptides in the extracerebral circulation of man and cat during activation of the trigeminovascular system. *Annals of Neurology*, **23**, 193–196.

Goadsby, P.J., Edvinsson, L. and Ekman, R. (1990). Vasoactive peptide release in the extracerebral circulation of human during migraine headache. *Annals of Neurology*, **28**, 183–187.

Green, T. and Dockray, G.J. (1988). Characterization of the peptidergic afferent innervation of the stomach in the rat, mouse and guinea-pig. *Neuroscience*, **25**, 181–193.

Griffith, H.B., Cummins, B.H. and Thomson, J.L.G. (1972). Cerebral arterial spasm and hydrocephalus in leaking arterial aneurysms. *Neuroradiology*, **4**, 212–214.

Gulbenkian, S., Merighi, A., Wharton, J., Varndell, I.M. and Polak, J.M. (1986). Ultrastructural evidence for the coexistence of calcitonin gene-related peptide and substance P in secretory vesicles of peripheral nerves in the guinea pig. *Journal of Neurocytology*, **15**, 535–542.

Han, S.-P., Naes, L. and Westfall, T.C. (1990a). Inhibition of periarterial nerve stimulation-induced vasodilatation of the mesenteric arterial bed by CGRP 8-37 and CGRP receptor desensitization. *Biochemical Biophysical Research Communications*, **168**, 786–791.

Han, S.-P., Naes, L. and Westfall, T.C. (1990b). Calcitonin gene-related peptide is the endogenous mediator of nonadrenergic-noncholinergic vasodilatation in rat mesentery. *Journal of Pharmacology and Experimental Therapeutics*, **255**, 423–428.

Hanko, J., Hardebo, J.E., Kåhrström, J., Owman, C. and Sundler, F. (1985). Calcitonin gene-related peptide is present in mammalian cerebrovascular nerve fibres and dilates pial and peripheral arteries. *Neuroscience Letters*, **57**, 91–95.

Hara, H., Nosko, M. and Weir, B. (1986). Cerebral perivascular nerves in subarachnoid haemorrhage. A histochemical and immunological study. *Journal of Neurosurgery*, **65**, 531–539.

Holman, J.J., Craig, R.K. and Marshall, I. (1986). Human α- and β-CGRP and rat α-CGRP are coronary vasodilators in rat. *Peptides*, **7**, 231–235.

Holzer, P. (1988). Local effector functions of capsaicin-sensitive sensory nerve endings: involvement of tachykinins, calcitonin gene-related peptide and other neuropeptides. *Neuroscience*, **24**, 739–768.

Holzer, P. (1991). Capsaicin: cellular targets, mechanisms of action, and selectivity for thin sensory neurons. *Pharmacological Reviews*, **43**, 143–201.

Holzer, P. (1993). Capsaicin-sensitive nerves in the control of vascular effector mechanisms. In *Capsaicin in the Study of Pain*, edited by John Wood, pp. 191–218. London: Academic Press.

Iversen, H.K., Jansen, I., Edvinsson, L. and Olesen, J. (1993). Calcitonin gene-related peptide levels during nitroglycerin-induced headache. *Cephalalgia*, **13**, 185.

Jansen, I. (1992). Characterization of calcitonin gene-related peptide (CGRP) receptors in guinea pig basilar artery. *Neuropeptides*, **21**, 73–79.

Jansen, I., Alafaci, C., McCulloch, J., Uddman, R. and Edvinsson, L. (1991). Tachykinins (substance P, neurokinin A, neuropeptide K and neurokinin B) in the cerebral circulation: Vasomotor responses *in vitro* and *in situ*. *Journal of Cerebral Blood Flow and Metabolism*, **11**, 567–575.

Jansen, I., Alafaci, C., Uddman, R. and Edvinsson, L. (1990). Evidence that calcitonin gene-related peptide contributes to capsaicin-induced relaxation of guinea pig cerebral arteries. *Regulatory Peptides*, **31**, 167–178.

Jansen, I., Mortensen, A. and Edvinsson, L. (1992). Characterization of calcitonin gene-related peptide (CGRP) receptors in human cerebral vessels. Vasomotor responses and cAMP accumulation. *Annals of New York Academy of Science*, **657**, 435–441.

Jansen-Olesen, I., Iversen, H.K., Olesen, J. and Edvinsson, L. (1994). The effect of nitroglycerin on sensory neuropeptides in isolated guinea pig basilar arteries. In *The Biology of Nitric Oxide vol. 3 Physiology and Clinical Aspects*, edited by Moncada, Feelisch, Busse and Higgs, pp. 368–373. London: Portland Press Ltd.

Jansen-Olesen, I., Gulbenkian, S., Valenca, A., Antunes, J.L., Wharton, J., Polak, J.M. and Edvinsson, L. (1995). The peptidergic innervation of the human superficial temporal artery: immunohistochemistry, ultrastructure and vasomotility. *Peptides*, **16**, 275–287.

Jennet, B. and Teasdale, G. (1981). *Management of Head Injuries*, pp. 1–361. Philadelphia: F.A. Davies Company.

Juul, R., Edvinsson, L., Gisvold, S.E., Ekman, R., Brubakk, O. and Fredriksen, T.A. (1990). Calcitonin gene-related peptide-LI in subarachnoid haemorrhage in man. Signs of activation of the trigemino-cerebrovascular system? *British Journal of Neurosurgery*, **4**, 171–180.

Juul, R., Edvinsson, L., Ekman, R., Brubakk, A.O., Hara, H., Fredriksen, T.A., *et al.* (1991). Perivascular neuropeptides in human subarachnoid haemorrhage. *Journal of Cerebral Blood Flow and Metabolism*, **11**(suppl. 2), S643.

Kågström, E., Greitz, T., Hansson, J. and Galera, R. (1966). Changes in cerebral arterial blood flow after subarachnoid haemorrhage. *Excerpta Medical International Congress Series*, **110**, 629–633.

Kågström, E., Nilsson, P.E. and Svendgaard, N.-Aa. (1969). Clinical and experimental spasm of the cerebral vessels. *Excerpta Medical International Congress Series*, **193**, 60.

Kaufman, M.P., Iwamoto, G.A., Longhurst, J.C. and Mitchell, J.H. (1982). Effects of capsaicin and bradykinin on afferent fibres with endings in skeletal muscle. *Circulation Research*, **50**, 133–139.

Kawasaki, H., Nuki, C., Saito, A. and Takasaki, K. (1991). NPY modulates neurotransmission of CGRP-containing vasodilator nerves in rat mesenteric arteries. *American Journal of Physiology*, **261**, H683–H690.

Kawasaki, H., Takasaki, K., Saito, A. and Goto, K. (1988). Calcitonin gene-related peptide acts as a novel vasodilator neurotransmitter in mesenteric resistance vessels of the rat. *Nature*, **335**, 164–167.

Keen, P., Harmar, A.J., Spears, F. and Winter, E. (1982). Biosynthesis, axonal transport and turnover of neuronal substance P. In *Substance P in the Nervous System*, edited by R. Porter and M. O'Connor, pp. 145–160. London: Pitman.

Kenins, P., Hurley, J.V. and Bell, C. (1984). The role of substance P in the axon reflex in the rat. *British Journal of Dermatology*, **111**, 551–559.

Kuwayama, A., Zervas, N.T., Belson, R., Shintani, A. and Pickren, K. (1972). A model for experimental cerebral arterial spasm. *Stroke*, **3**, 49–56.

Lambert, G.A., Bogduk, N., Goadsby, P.J., Duckworth, J.W. and Lance, J.W. (1984). Decreased carotid arterial resistance in cats in response to trigeminal stimulation. *Journal of Neurosurgery*, **61**, 307–315.

Lambert, G.A., Goadsby, P.J., Zagami, A.S. and Duckworth, J.W. (1988). Comparative effects of stimulation of the trigeminal ganglion and the superior sagittal sinus on cerebral blood flow and evoked potentials in the cat. *Brain Research*, **453**, 143–149.

Lee, T., Kawai, Y., Shiosaka, S., Takami, K., Kiyama, H., Hillyard, C.J., *et al.* (1985). Coexistence of calcitonin gene related peptide and substance P-like peptide in single cells of the trigeminal ganglion of the rat: Immunohistochemical analysis. *Brain Research*, **330**, 194–196.

Lei, S., Mulvany, M.J. and Nyborg N.C. (1994). Characterization of the CGRP receptor and mechanisms of action in rat mesenteric small arteries. *Pharmacology and Toxicology*, **74**, 130–135.

Lembeck, F. and Holzbauer, M. (1988). Neuronal mechanisms of cutaneous blood flow. In *Nonadrenergic Innervation of Blood Vessels, Volume II: Regional Innervation*, edited by G. Burnstock and S.G. Griffith, pp. 119–132, Boca Raton: CRC Press.

Linnik, M.D., Sakas, D.E., Uhl, G.R. and Moskowitz, M.A. (1989). Subarachnoid blood and headache: altered trigeminal tachykinin gene expression. *Annals of Neurology*, **25**, 179–184.

Liu-Chen, L.-Y., Han, D.H. and Moskowitz, M.A. (1983). Pial arachnoid contains substance P originating from trigeminal neurons. *Neuroscience*, **9**, 803–808.

Liu-Chen, L.-Y., Mayberg, M.R. and Moskowitz, M.A. (1983). Immunohistochemical evidence for a substance P-containing trigeminovascular pathway to pial arteries in cats. *Brain Research*, **268**, 162–166.

Longhurst, J.C., Kaufman, M.P., Ordway, G.A. and Musch, T.I. (1984). Effects of bradykinin and capsaicin on endings of afferent fibres from abdominal visceral organs. *American Journal of Physiology*, **247**, R552–R559.

Lou, H.C., Edvinsson, L. and MacKenzie, E.T. (1987). The concept of coupling blood flow to brain function: Revision required? *Annals of Neurology*, **22**, 289–297.

Lundberg, J.M., Änggård, A., Emson, P., Fahrenkrug, J. and Hökfelt, T. (1981). Vasoactive intestinal polypeptide and cholinergic mechanisms in cat nasal mucosa. Studies on choline acetyl transferase and release of vasoactive intestinal polypeptide. *Proceedings of the National Academy of Sciences of the United States of America*, **78**, 5255–5259.

Lundberg, J.M., Änggård, A. and Fahrenkrug, J. (1981). Complementary role of vasoactive intestinal polypeptide (VIP) and acetylcholine for cat submandibular gland blood flow and secretion. II. Effects of cholinergic antagonists and VIP antiserum. *Acta Physiologica Scandinavica*, **113**, 329–336.

Lundberg, J.M. and Stjärne, L. (1984). Neuropeptide Y (NPY) depresses the secretion of ^{3}H-noradrenaline and the contractile response evoked by field stimulation in rat vas deferens. *Acta Physiologica Scandinavica*, **120**, 477–479.

Macfarlane, R., Tasdemiroglu, E., Moskowitz, M.A., Uemura, Y., Wei, E.P. and Kontos, H.A. (1991). Chronic trigeminal ganglionectomy or topical capsaicin application to pial vessels attenuates postocclusive cortical hyperemia but does not influence postischemic hypoperfusion. *Journal of Cerebral Blood Flow and Metabolism*, **11**, 261–291.

Maggi, C.A. and Meli, A. (1988). The sensory-efferent function of capsaicin-sensitive sensory neurons. *General Pharmacology*, **19**, 1–43.

Maggi, C.A., Santicioli, P., Geppetti, P., Parlani, M, Astolfi, M., Del Bianco, E., *et al.* (1989). The effect of calcium free medium and nifedipine on the release of substance P-like immunoreactivity and contractions induced by capsaicin in the isolated guinea pig and rat bladder. *General Pharmacology*, **20**, 445–456.

Markowitz, S., Saito, S. and Moskowitz, M.A. (1987). Neurogenically mediated leakage of plasma protein occurs from blood vessels in dura but not brain. *Journal of Neuroscience*, **7**, 4129–4136.

Marshall, I., Al-Kazwini, S.J., Roberts, P.M., Shepperson, N.B., Adams, M. and Craig, P.K. (1986a). Cardiovascular effects of human and rat CGRP compared in the rat and other species. *European Journal of Pharmacology*, **123**, 207–216.

Marshall, I., Al-Kazwini, S.J., Holman, J.J. and Craig, P.K. (1986b). Human and rat α-CGRP but not calcitonin cause mesenteric vasodilatation in rats. *European Journal of Pharmacology*, **123**, 217–222.

Martin, J.L., Perry, S and Pickard, J.D. (1991). Cerebral blood flow and doppler flow velocity: Different responses to three vasodilators. *Journal of Cerebral Blood Flow and Metabolism*, **11** (Suppl. 2), S455.

Mayberg, M.R., Langer, R.S., Zervas, N.T. and Moskowitz, M.A. (1981). Perivascular meningeal projections from cat trigeminal ganglia: possible pathway for vascular headaches in man. *Science*, **213**, 228–230.

Mayberg, M.R., Zervas, N.T. and Moskowitz, M.A. (1984). Trigeminal projections to supratentorial pial and dura blood vessels in cats demonstrated by horseradish peroxidase histochemistry. *Journal of Comparative Neurology*, **223**, 46–56.

McCulloch, J., Uddman, R., Kingman, T.A. and Edvinsson, L. (1986). Calcitonin gene-related peptide: Functional role in cerebrovascular regulation. *Proceedings of the National Academy of Sciences of the United States of America*, **83**, 5741–5745.

Morris, J.L., Gibbins, I.L., Furness J.B., Costa, M. and Murphy, R. (1985). Co-localization of neuropeptide Y, vasoactive intestinal polypeptide and dynorphin in non-adrenergic axons of the guinea-pig uterine artery. *Neuroscience Letters*, **62**, 31–37.

Moskowitz, M.A., Brody, M. and Liu-Chen, L.-Y. (1983). *In vitro* release of immunoreactive substance P from putative afferent nerve endings in bovine pial arachnoid. *Neuroscience*, **9**, 809–814.

Moskowitz, M.A., Wei, E.P., Saito, K. and Kontos, H.A. (1988). Trigeminalectomy modifies pial arteriolar response to hypertension or norepinephrine. *American Journal of Physiology*, **255**, H1–H6.

Moskowitz, M.A., Reinhard, J.F. Jr., Romero J., Melamed, E. and Pettibone, D.J. (1979). Neurotransmitters and the fifth cranial nerve: is there a relation to the headache phase of migraine? *Lancet*, **ii**, 883–885.

Moskowitz, M.A., Sakas, D.E., Wei, E.P., Kano, M., Buzzi, M.G., Ogilvy, C., *et al.* (1989). Postocclusive cerebral hyperemia is markedly attenuated by chronic trigeminal ganglionectomy. *American Journal of Physiology*, **257**, H1736–H1739.

Nagai, H., Suzuki, Y., Sugiura, M., Noda, S. and Mabe, H. (1974). Experimental cerebral vasospasm. Part 1: Factors contributing to early spasm. *Journal of Neurosurgery*, **41**, 285–292.

Nakanishi, S. (1987). Substance P precursor and kininogen their structures, gene organizations, and regulation. *Physiological Reviews*, **67**, 1117–1142.

Nozaki, K., Kikuchi, H. and Mizuno, N. (1989). Change of calcitonin gene-related peptide like immunoreactivity in cerebrovascular nerve fibers in the dog after experimentally produced subarachnoid haemorrhage. *Neuroscience Letters*, **102**, 27–32.

O'Brien, C., Woolf, C.J., Fitzgerald, M., Lindsay, R.M. and Molander, C. (1989). Differences in the chemical expression of rat primary afferent neurons which innervate skin, muscle or joint. *Neuroscience*, **32**, 493–502.

Olgart, L., Gazelius, B., Brodin, E. and Nilsson, G. (1977). Release of substance P-like immunoreactivity from the dental pulp. *Acta Physiologica Scandinavica*, **101**, 510–512.

Peerless, S.J., Fox, A.J., Komatsu, K. and Hunter, I.G. (1982). Angiographic study of vasospasm following subarachnoid haemorrhage in monkeys. *Stroke*, **13**, 473–479.

Pickering, G.W. and Hess, W. (1933). Observations on the mechanism of headache produced by histamine. *Clinical Science*, **1**, 77–101.

Ray, B.S. and Wolff, H.G. (1940). Experimental studies on headache. *Archives of Surgery*, **41**, 813–856.

Regoli, D., Drapeau, G., Dion, S. and D'Orleans-Juste, P. (1987). Pharmacological receptors for substance P and neurokinins. *Life Science*, **40**, 109–117.

Rodrigo, J., Polak, J.M., Fernandez, L., Ghatei, M.A., Mulderry, P. and Bloom, S.R. (1985). Calcitonin gene-related peptide immunoreactive sensory and motor nerves of the rat, cat, and monkey esophagus. *Gastroenterology*, **88**, 444–451.

Rosenfeld, M.G., Mermod, J.-J., Amara, S.G., Swanson, L.W., Sawchenko, P.E. and Rivier, J., *et al.* (1983). Production of a novel neuropeptide encoded by the calcitonin gene via tissue-specific RNA processing. *Nature*, **304**, 129–135.

Saito, A. and Goto, K. (1986). Depletion of calcitonin gene-related peptide (CGRP) by capsaicin in cerebral arteries. *Journal of Pharmacobio-Dynamics*, **9**, 613–619.

Saito, I., Ueda, Y. and Sano, K. (1977). Significance of vasospasm in the treatment of ruptured intracranial aneurysms. *Journal of Neurosurgery*, **47**, 412–429.

Saito, K. and Moskowitz, M.A. (1989) Contributions from the upper cervical dorsal roots and the trigeminal ganglia to the feline circle of Willis. *Stroke*, **20**, 524–526.

Saito, K., Liu-Chen, L.-Y. and Moskowitz, M.A. (1987). Substance P-like immunoreactivity in rat forebrain leptomeninges and cerebral vessels originates from the trigeminal but not sympathetic ganglia. *Brain Research*, **403**, 66–71.

Sakas, D.E., Moskowitz, M.A., Wei, E.P., Kontos, H.A., Kano, M. and Ogilvy, C.S. (1989). Trigeminovascular fibres increase blood flow in cortical gray matter by axon reflex-like mechanisms during acute severe hypertension or seizures. *Proceedings of the National Academy of Sciences of the United States of America*, **86**, 1401–1405.

Sano, K. and Saito, I. (1978). Timing and indication of surgery for ruptured intracranial aneurysms with regard to cerebral vasospasm. *Acta Neurochirurgica*, **41**, 49–60.

Saria, A., Gamse, R., Petermann, J., Fischer, J.A., Theodorsson-Norheim, E. and Lundberg, J.M. (1986). Simultaneous release of several tachykinins and calcitonin gene-related peptide from rat spinal cord slices. *Neuroscience Letters*, **63**, 310–314.

Sternini, C., Reeve, J.R. and Brecha, N. (1987). Distribution and characterization of calcitonin gene-related peptide immunoreactivity in the digestive system of normal and capsaicin-treated rats. *Gastroenterology*, **93**, 852–862.

Stricker, S. (1876). Untersuchungen über die gefässwurzeln des ischadicus. Stitz.Ber.Kaiserl.Acad.Wiss. (Wien) 3, 173–185.

Su, H.C., Bishop, A.E., Power, R.F., Hamada, Y. and Polak, J.M. (1987). Dual intrinsic and extrinsic origins of CGRP- and NPY-immunoreactive nerves of rat gut and pancreas. *Journal of Neuroscience*, **7**, 2674–2687.

Sundler, F., Brodin, E., Ekblad, E., Håkanson, R. and Uddman, R. (1985). Sensory nerve fibers: Distribution of substance P, neurokinin A and calcitonin gene-related peptide. In *Tachykinin Antagonists*, Fernström Symp., Vol. 6, edited by Håkanson, R. and Sundler, F., pp. 3–14, Amsterdam: Elsevier Science Publishers.

Sundt, T.M. Jr., Kobayashi, S. and Fobe, N.C. (1982). Results and complications of surgical management of 809 intracranial aneurysms in 722 patients. *Journal of Neurosurgery*, **56**, 753–765.

Suzuki, N., Hardebo, J.E. and Owman, C. (1989). Origins and pathways of cerebrovascular nerves storing substance P and calcitonin gene-related peptide in rat. *Neuroscience*, **31**, 427–438.

Szállási, A. and Blumberg, P.M. (1990). Resiniferatoxin and its analogs provide novel insight into the pharmacology of the vanilloid (capsaicin) receptor. *Life Science*, **47**, 1399–1408.

Szolcsányi, J. (1984). Capsaicin-sensitive chemoceptive neuronal system with dual sensory-efferent function. In *Antidromic Vasodilatation and Neurogenic Inflammation*, edited by L.A. Chachl, J. Szolcsányi and F. Lembeck, pp. 27–52. Budapest: Akadémiai Kiadó.

Szolcsányi, J. (1990). Capsaicin, irritation, and desensitization. Neurophysiological basis and future perspectives. In *Irritation*, edited by B.G. Green, J.R. Mason and M.R. Kare, Chemical Senses, Vol. 2, pp. 141–168. New York and Basel: Marcel Dekker.

Uddman, R., Edvinsson, L., Ekblad, E., Håkanson, R. and Sundler, F. (1986). Calcitonin gene-related peptide (CGRP): perivascular distribution and vasodilatory effects. *Regulatory Peptides*, **15**, 1–23.

Uddman, R., Ekblad, E., Edvinsson, L., Håkanson, R. and Sundler, F. (1985). Neuropeptide Y (NPY)-like immunoreactivity in perivascular nerves of the guinea-pig. *Regulatory Peptides*, **12**, 243–257.

Uddman, R., Edvinsson, L., Owman, C. and Sundler, F. (1981). Perivascular substance P: occurrence and distribution in mammalian pial vessels. *Journal of Cerebral Blood Flow and Metabolism*, **1**, 227–232.

Uemura, Y., Sugimoto, T., Okamoto, S., Handa, H. and Mizuno, N. (1987). Changes of neuropeptide immuno-reactivity in cerebrovascular nerve fibers after experimentally produced SAH. *Journal of Neurosurgery*, **66**, 741–747.

Varro, A., Green, T., Holmes, S. and Dockray, G.J. (1988). Calcitonin gene-related peptide in visceral afferent nerve fibres: quantification by radioimmunoassay and determination of axonal transport rates. *Neuroscience*, **26**, 927–932.

Wahlestedt, C., Edvinsson, L., Ekblad, E. and Håkanson, R. (1985). Neuropeptide Y potentiates noradrenaline-evoked vasoconstriction: mode of action. *Journal of Pharmacology and Experimental Therapeutics*, **234**, 735–741.

Wahlestedt, C., Edvinsson, L., Ekblad, E. and Håkanson, R. (1987). Effects of neuropeptide Y at sympathetic neuroeffector junctions: existence of Y1- and Y2-receptors. In *Neuronal Messengers in Vascular Function*, edited by A. Nobin, C. Owman and B. Arneklo-Nobin, pp. 231–242. Amsterdam: Elsevier.

Wei, E.P., Moskowitz, M.A., Boccalini, P. and Kontos, H.A. (1992). Calcitonin gene-related peptide mediates nitroglycerin and sodium nitroprusside-induced vasodilatation in feline cerebral arterioles. *Circulation Research*, **70**, 1313–1319.

Weir, B., Grace, M., Hansen, J. and Rothberg, C. (1978). Time course of vasospasm in man. *Journal of Neurosurgery*, **48**, 173–178.

Weir, B., Rothberg, C., Grace, M. and Davis, F. (1975). Relative prognostic significance of vasospasm following subarachnoid haemorrhage. *Canadian Journal of Neurological Science*, **2**, 109–114.

Wharton, J., Gulbenkian, S., Mulderry, P.K., Ghatei, M.A., McGregor, G.P., Bloom, S.R., *et al.* (1986). Capsaicin induces depletion of calcitonin gene-related peptide (CGRP) immunoreactive nerves in the cardiovascular system of the guinea pig and rat. *Journal of the Autonomic Nervous System*, **16**, 289–309.

White, D.M. and Helme, R.D. (1985). Release of substance P from peripheral nerve terminals following electrical stimulation of the sciatic nerve. *Brain Research*, **336**, 27–31.

White, J.C. and Sweet, W.H. (1955). *Pain. Its Mechanism and Neurological Control*. Springfield: Charles Thomas.

Wolff, H.G. (1963). *Headache and Other Head Pain*. New York: Oxford University Press.

Zagami, A.S., Goadsby, P.J. and Edvinsson, L. (1990). Stimulation of the superior sagittal sinus in the cat causes release of vasoactive peptides. *Neuropeptides*, **16**, 69–75.

5 Interactions Between Perivascular Nerves and Endothelial Cells in Control of Local Vascular Tone

V. Ralevic and G. Burnstock

Department of Anatomy and Developmental Biology and
Centre for Neuroscience, University College London,
London WC1E 6BT, UK

Perivascular nerves, once considered simply adrenergic or cholinergic, release many types of neurotransmitters, including peptides, purines and nitric oxide. Cotransmission (synthesis, storage and release of more than one transmitter by a single nerve) commonly takes place. Some afferent nerves have an efferent (motor) function and axon reflex control of vascular tone by these "sensory-motor" nerves is more widespread than once thought.

The endothelium mediates both vasodilatation and vasoconstriction via specific membrane-bound receptors and subsequent release of endothelium-derived vasoactive factors. Endothelial cells can store and release vasoactive substances such as adenosine 5'-triphosphate, acetylcholine and substance P (vasodilators) and endothelin (vasoconstrictor). The origins and functions of such vasoactive substances are discussed. Endothelial vasoactive substances may be of greater significance in the response of blood vessels to local changes while perivascular nerves may be more concerned with integration of blood flow in the whole organism.

Under short-term physiological conditions there is a dynamic balance between sympathetic nerve-mediated vasoconstrictor tone and endothelial-mediated vasodilator tone. The balance of dual regulation of vascular tone by perivascular nerves and endothelial cells may be altered by long-term changes such as ageing, hypertension, diabetes and atherosclerosis, as well as by trauma and surgery. Studies of vascular tone in disease, and after denervation or mechanical injury, suggest possible trophic interactions between perivascular nerves and endothelial cells. Such trophic interactions may be important for growth and development of the two control systems, particularly in the microvasculature where neural-endothelial separation is small.

KEY WORDS: endothelium; parasympathetic nerves; perivascular nerves; sensory-motor nerves; sympathetic nerves; vasoconstriction; vasodilatation.

INTRODUCTION

Studies of neurohumoral control of the vasculature were for many years concerned largely with the role of catecholamines released from sympathetic perivascular nerves and from the adrenal medulla into the bloodstream. However, recent discoveries, following the introduction of improved techniques in immunohistochemistry, electron microscopy, electrophysiology and pharmacology, have profoundly reshaped our understanding of the autonomic nervous system (Burnstock, 1986a). Many new putative neurotransmitters have been proposed and neuromodulatory mechanisms have been recognised, including prejunctional inhibition or enhancement of release, postjunctional modulation of transmitter action, and the secondary involvement of locally synthesized hormones and prostaglandins. The existence of more than one transmitter substance in some nerves, or cotransmission, is now also widely recognized (Burnstock, 1976, 1990a). Endothelial regulation of vascular tone is now an integral part of our view of cardiovascular physiology, stemming from the seminal discovery that this innermost layer of all blood vessels plays a crucial role in the vasodilator response of the vessel to acetylcholine (ACh) (Furchgott and Zawadzki, 1980) and to other substances via the release of endothelial nitric oxide (NO) (Vanhoutte and Rimele, 1983; Palmer, Ferrige and Moncada, 1987). It is now known that endothelial cells are able to sense and respond to changes in haemodynamic forces, and circulating or locally produced vasoactive substances, by synthesizing and/or releasing biologically active substances (including a number of established transmitters such as ACh, adenosine 5'-triphosphate (ATP) and substance P) which mediate vasoconstriction or vasodilatation.

The present article focuses in particular on the interactions of the various perivascular nerve types and the more recently recognised roles of endothelial cells in controlling vascular tone. Both short-term interactions between perivascular nerve and endothelial cell mechanisms in relation to physiological events, and long-term interactions that occur in old age and as a consequence of disease and trauma, will be considered.

PERIVASCULAR NERVES

Perivascular nerves at the adventitial-medial border of most blood vessels form an extensive plexus of branching terminal fibres. These terminal axons are devoid of Schwann cell covering and are rich in varicosities (1–2 μm diameter) separated by intervaricose regions (0.1–0.3 μm diameter) (Burnstock, 1986a). The varicosities are the main sites of storage of neurotransmitters, which are released "en passage" by the depolarizing effect of nerve impulses passing along the axons, to act on vascular smooth muscle cells in electrical continuity with each other via gap junctions (Burnstock and Griffith, 1988; Dhital and Burnstock, 1989). The varicosities do not have a fixed relationship with particular smooth muscle cells and the junctional cleft varies between 60–2000 nm, with greater separations being associated with larger blood vessels. There is a lack of postjunctional specialization of the smooth muscle at the vascular neuromuscular junction, unlike "synapses" at the motor end plate in striated muscle or within ganglia. Modification of the process of neurotransmission characteristically takes place by the actions of "neuromodulators" which may be circulating hormones; local agents such as prostanoids, bradykinin or histamine; or neurotransmitter substances released from the same varicosity or from varicosities of adjacent nerve terminals.

For more than 50 years, the only transmitters considered in perivascular nerves were noradrenaline (NA) and ACh. Since the discovery of non-adrenergic, non-cholinergic

TABLE 5.1
Established and putative transmitters in perivascular nerves

Noradrenaline (NA)
Acetylcholine (ACh)
Adenosine 5'-triphosphate (ATP)
5-Hydroxytryptamine (5-HT)
Dopamine (DA)
Enkephalin-Dynorphin (ENK-DYN)
Vasoactive intestinal polypeptide (VIP)
Peptide histidine isoleucine (PHI)
Substance P (SP)
Gastrin-releasing peptide (GRP)
Somatostatin (SOM)
Neurotensin (NT)
Vasopressin (VP)
Cholecystokinin-Gastrin (CCK-GAS)
Neuropeptide Y-Pancreatic polypeptide (NPY-PPP)
Galanin (GAL)
Angiotensin (Ag)
Adrenocorticotrophic hormone (ACH)
Calcitonin gene-related peptide (CGRP)
Nitric oxide (NO)

nerves in the early 1960s, more than 12 new chemical messengers have been identified, including monoamines, purines, amino acids, polypeptides, and NO (Table 5.1).

The concept of cotransmission, i.e., that nerves synthesize, store, and release more than one transmitter, first proposed by Burnstock in 1976, is now generally accepted to be a widespread phenomenon involving virtually all known transmitter systems (Cuello, 1982; Burnstock, 1983; Osborne, 1983; Chan-Palay and Palay, 1984; Hökfelt, Fuxe and Pernow, 1986; Bartfai, Iverfeldt and Fisone, 1988; Burnstock, 1990a; Kupfermann, 1991). Despite the complexity provided by the growing list of established and putative transmitters and the formidable number of possible combinations of cotransmitters, patterns are emerging that indicate a considerable degree of organization within the autonomic nervous system. This has led to the concept that autonomic nerves have a "chemical coding", i.e., individual neurons contain particular combinations of transmitter substances, have processes that project to identifiable target sites, and have defined central connections. This concept has been developed fully for the enteric nervous system (Furness and Costa, 1987), but it also applies to perivascular nerves.

SYMPATHETIC NERVES

There is now a substantial body of evidence showing that NA, ATP and neuropeptide Y (NPY) act as cotransmitters, being released from sympathetic nerves in variable proportions depending on the tissue, the species and on the parameters of stimulation (Burnstock, 1986b) (Figure 5.1). Most of the early studies were made on the vas deferens (Stjärne, 1989),

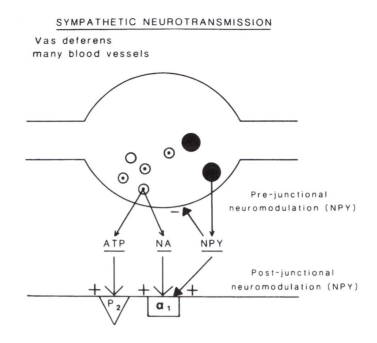

Figure 5.1 Diagram showing that noradrenaline (NA), adenosine 5′-triphosphate (ATP) and neuropeptide Y (NPY) are released as cotransmitters from sympathetic nerves supplying the vas deferens and many blood vessels. NA and ATP, released from small (and large) granular vesicles, act on the smooth muscle to elicit contraction (+) via smooth muscle α_1-adrenoceptors and P_2-purinoceptors respectively. NPY, preferentially released from large vesicles, generally has little direct action on the muscle cell, but exerts potent neuromodulatory actions: both prejunctional inhibition (−) of the release of NA and ATP, and postjunctional enhancement of the action of NA. (Prejunctional α_2-adrenoceptors and P_1-purinoceptors can also reduce transmitter release when activated by NA and adenosine respectively). (Adapted from Burnstock, 1987).

but sympathetic cotransmission involving NA and ATP has now also been described in a number of different large blood vessels (Burnstock, 1986b, 1988a), including the rat tail artery (Sneddon and Burnstock, 1984; Bao, Eriksson and Stjärne, 1989), rabbit ear artery (Kennedy and Burnstock, 1985; Suzuki, 1985; Saville and Burnstock, 1988), dog basilar artery (Muramatsu and Kigoshi, 1987), mesenteric artery of various species (Ishikawa, 1985; Von Kügelgen and Starke, 1985; Ramme et al., 1987; Muir and Wardle, 1988; Machalay, Dalziel and Sneddon, 1988; Muramatsu, 1992), rabbit pulmonary artery (Katsuragi and Su, 1982), guinea-pig and rabbit saphenous artery (Cheung and Fujioka, 1986; Burnstock and Warland, 1987; Warland and Burnstock, 1987), and rabbit hepatic artery (Brizzolara and Burnstock, 1990). Sympathetic cotransmission involving NA and ATP has also been shown in rat mesenteric resistance vessels (Sjöblom-Widfeldt, 1990), in the circulation of skeletal muscle (Shimada and Stitt, 1984), arterial resistance vessels of the cat intestine (Taylor and Parsons, 1989), rat kidney (Schwartz and Malik, 1989), dog skin (Flavahan and Vanhoutte, 1986), and in the pithed rat (Bulloch and McGrath, 1988; Schlicker, Urbanek and Göthert, 1989).

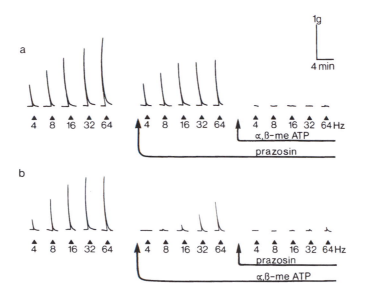

Figure 5.2   Contractions produced in the isolated saphenous artery of the rabbit on neurogenic transmural stimulation (0.08–0.1 ms; supramaximal voltage) for 1 sec (a, b) at the frequencies (Hz) indicated (▲). Nerve stimulations were repeated in the presence of 10 μM prazosin added before (a) or after (b) desensitization of the P_2-purinoceptor with α, β-methylene ATP (α, β-meATP) as indicated on the figure by the arrowed lines.
(From Burnstock and Warland, 1987).

Purinergic cotransmission has been identified from several lines of investigation: sympathetic nerve stimulation elicits a response which is only partially blocked by the α_1-adrenoceptor antagonist prazosin, while the prazosin-resistant component is blocked by the ATP antagonist, arylazido aminoproprionyl-ATP (ANAPP$_3$), or by selective desensitization of the P_{2X}-purinoceptor with α, β-methylene ATP (Figure 5.2); ATP is released during sympathetic nerve stimulation and this release is prevented by tetrodotoxin, by the sympathetic blocker guanethidine, or following destruction of sympathetic nerves with 6-hydroxydopamine (6-OHDA), but is unaffected by selective depletion of NA by reserpine; ATP, but not NA, mimics the excitatory junction potentials (EJPs). It has also emerged from these studies that ATP is characteristically released during short bursts of sympathetic stimulation (1 s or less) whereas during prolonged periods of stimulation the NA component dominates the mechanical responses (Kennedy, Saville and Burnstock, 1986).

Considerable variation exists in the ratio of NA:ATP released in different vessels. For example, ATP is the major component of sympathetic cotransmission in the rabbit saphenous artery and mesenteric arteries (Burnstock and Warland, 1987; Ramme et al., 1987), but appears to be a relatively minor component in the rabbit ear artery and rat tail artery. In guinea-pig submucosal arterioles, vasoconstriction and EJPs recorded in response to sympathetic nerve stimulation are mediated exclusively by ATP, with the role of NA being to act as a prejunctional neuromodulator via α_2-adrenoceptors, causing depression of

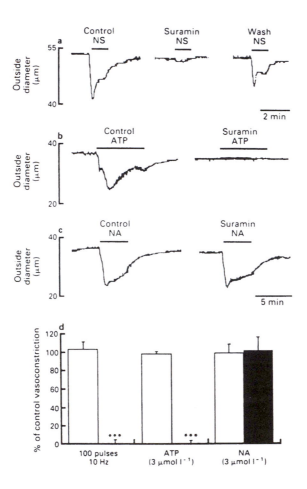

Figure 5.3 Constrictions of guinea-pig submucosal arterioles in response to nerve stimulation are mediated through the activation of P_2-purinoceptors. (a) Nerve-evoked constrictions (100 pulses at 10 Hz) were abolished by the putative P_2-purinoceptor antagonist, suramin (100 μM); the response is partially reversed on washout (20 min). (b) Constrictions to exogenously applied ATP (3 μM) were abolished by suramin (100 μM). (c) Suramin (100 μM) had no effect on the contraction evoked by the exogenous application of noradrenaline (NA, 3 μM). (d) Summary of the effects of suramin, data are expressed as mean ($\pm$ s.e.mean shown by vertical bar) of the % of constriction before suramin application in response to nerve stimulation ($n = 6$), and the response to exogenously applied ATP ($n = 4$) or NA ($n = 4$). Open columns = control responses; solid = suramin. Periods of nerve stimulation (NS) or the superfusion of ATP or NA are indicated by bars. *** $P < 0.001$. (From Evans and Surprenant, 1992).

transmitter release (Evans and Surprenant, 1992) (Figure 5.3). The purinergic component of sympathetic cotransmission is selectively affected by the dihydropyridines, nifedipine and Bay K 8644 (Stone, 1981; MacKenzie, Manzini and Burnstock, 1988). A model depicting sympathetic cotransmission is shown in Figure 5.1.

Cotransmission provides the potential for greater functional complexity and fine tuning via multiple postjunctional actions and pre- and postjunctional neuromodulatory mechanisms. The postjunctional synergism which occurs for instance between NA and ATP (Kennedy, Delbro and Burnstock, 1985; Kennedy and Burnstock, 1986; Ralevic and Burnstock, 1990) provides justification for cotransmission in terms of transmitter economy.

NPY is also stored in, and released from, sympathetic nerves (Lundberg et al., 1983, 1984a). Electron microscopy and fractionation studies carried out in some non-vascular tissues have demonstrated that NPY is preferentially localized, along with NA and ATP, in large dense-cored vesicles (80–90 nm), while no NPY is found in the small dense-cored vesicles which are major storage sites for NA and ATP (Stjärne, Lundberg and Åstrand, 1986). Again the pattern of sympathetic stimulation appears to be an important determinant of release, with preferential release of NPY occurring in response to high frequency intermittent bursts of stimulation (Lundberg et al., 1986). In many vessels, NPY has little direct postjunctional action (Pernow, Saria and Lundberg, 1986; Stjärne, Lundberg and Åstrand, 1986). Its major role appears to be that of a neuromodulator: NPY has potent prejunctional actions reducing the release of NA and ATP; postjunctionally it enhances the actions of NA and ATP (Wahlestedt, Yanaihara and Håkanson, 1986; Stjärne, 1989; Saville, Maynard and Burnstock, 1990). The geometry of particular sympathetic neuromuscular junctions appears to influence the type of neuromodulation, i.e., with wide junctions, postjunctional potentiation by NPY dominates, while narrow clefts favour prejunctional inhibition by NPY (Burnstock, 1990a). Since cleft size in turn may vary with the size of the vessel this has implications for the role of NPY in the microvasculature. NPY has direct constrictor actions in some vessels, including those in the heart, brain, spleen and skeletal muscle, but its origin may be from intrinsic or local neurons rather than sympathetic nerves.

In a study of blood vessels in guinea-pig skin, a different chemical coding for sympathetic nerves has been demonstrated that varies with the size of the vessel: in precapillary arteries, sympathetic nerves contain only dynorphin (DYN), and not NPY, as a cotransmitter with NA; in the smaller arteries DYN, NPY and NA are present, while the distributing arteries contain the classic combination of NPY and NA (Gibbins and Morris, 1990). ATP is likely to be present at all levels.

5-Hydroxytryptamine (5-HT) immunofluorescent nerves have been localized in a number of vessels (Griffith and Burnstock, 1983; Burnstock and Griffith, 1988). However, it seems that, for the most part, 5-HT is not synthesized and stored in separate nerves, but is taken up, stored in, and released as a "false transmitter" from sympathetic nerves (Jackowski, Crockard and Burnstock, 1989). The effect of 5-HT on blood vessels depends on the size of the vessel and the prevailing level of vascular tone. Large vessels are usually constricted by 5-HT, while 5-HT in the microcirculation causes dilatation of arterioles, together with constriction of venules, and may cause plasma extravasation due to the rise in capillary pressure.

NO may act as a non-adrenergic, non-cholinergic transmitter in some sympathetic neurons. Immunoreactivity for NO synthase (NOS; the enzyme responsible for synthesis of NO and used as a marker for NO) has been shown in preganglionic sympathetic neurons in the rat (Anderson et al., 1993) and in post-synaptic elements of rat (Dun et al., 1993) and bovine superior cervical ganglia (Sheng et al., 1993). Positive staining for nicotinamide-adenine dinucleotide hydrogen phosphate-diaphorase (NADPH-d; used as a marker for

NOS) has also been shown in preganglionic sympathetic neurons (Anderson, 1992; Morris *et al.*, 1993).

PARASYMPATHETIC NERVES

Our basic concept of parasympathetic cotransmission in perivascular nerves is largely derived from classic studies of parasympathetic transmission in vessels of the cat salivary gland. In parasympathetic nerves in this gland, vasoactive intestinal polypeptide (VIP) is co-stored and co-released with ACh. During low-frequency stimulation ACh is released to increase salivary secretion from acinar cells and to elicit some dilatation of blood vessels in the gland (Bloom and Edwards, 1980; Lundberg, 1981). VIP is released from the same nerves, especially at high stimulation frequencies, to produce marked dilatation and, although it has no direct effect on acinar cells, it acts as a neuromodulator to substantially enhance the postjunctional effect of ACh on acinar cell secretion and to increase the release of ACh from the nerve varicosities via prejunctional receptors (Figure 5.4). The differential release of ACh and VIP at low- and high-frequency stimulation may be related to the different ratios of these transmitters within storage vesicles in the nerve terminal; ACh is preferentially found in small clear vesicles and VIP in large dense-cored vesicles, with the latter apparently needing stronger frequencies of stimulation to release their transmitter content (Lundberg, 1981).

The picture of parasympathetic cotransmission in vessels of the salivary gland and elsewhere in the cardiovascular system may be more complex given that peptide histidine isoleucine (PHI; derived from the same precursor molecule as VIP, namely prepro-VIP) (Lundberg *et al.*, 1984b), NPY (Leblanc, Trimmer and Landis, 1987; Leblanc and Landis, 1988), calcitonin gene-related peptide (CGRP) (Mione, Ralevic and Burnstock, 1990) and NO (Bredt and Snyder, 1992) have been colocalized with VIP/choline acetyltransferase (ChAT) in parasympathetic perivascular nerves or parasympathetic ganglia with vascular targets. Indeed, NOS-immunoreactivity has recently been colocalized with VIP, PHI and NPY in parasympathetic neurons of the submandibular salivary gland (Modin, 1994). In the urinary bladder, ATP is a cotransmitter with ACh in parasympathetic nerves and it remains to be seen whether this combination is more widely distributed in parasympathetic nerves supplying blood vessels.

Parasympathetic cotransmission involving NO may be particularly important in cerebral vessels. Lesion of postganglionic parasympathetic nerve fibres showed that NOS-containing nerve fibres in the adventitia of rat cerebral arteries originated from parasympathetic cell bodies in the sphenopalatine ganglia, many of which also contain VIP (Nozaki *et al.*, 1993; Minami *et al.*, 1994). Iadecola and coworkers (1993) have suggested that NOS-containing nerve fibres of peripheral origin (sphenopalatine ganglia) innervate large cerebral arteries, while the NOS-containing fibres associated with arterioles and capillaries are from neural processes of central origin (dendrites). An inhibitor of NOS, N^G-nitro-L-arginine, attenuated the increase in cerebral blood flow to stimulation of postganglionic parasympathetic nerves in the rat (Morita-Tsuzuki, Hardebo and Bouskela, 1993). NO-mediated neurogenic relaxation has been shown in endothelium-denuded cat pial arteries and NADPH-d immunopositive nerve fibres were detected in the adventitial layer; however, the staining of scattered ganglion-like neuronal cell bodies raised the possibility of

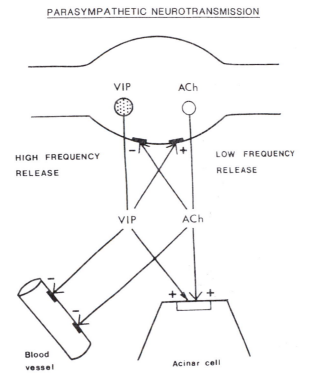

Figure 5.4   A classic transmitter acetylcholine (ACh) coexists with vasoactive intestinal polypeptide (VIP) in parasympathetic nerves supplying the cat salivary gland. ACh and VIP are stored in separate vesicles; they can be released differentially at different stimulation frequencies to act on acinar cells and glandular blood vessels. Cooperation is achieved by selective release of ACh at low-impulse frequencies, and of VIP at high frequencies. Pre- and postjunctional modulation is indicated. (From Burnstock, 1983).

an intrinsic origin for these fibres (Estrada, Mengual and Gonzalez, 1993). Neuronal NO-mediated relaxation has been shown in dog (Toda *et al.*, 1993; Toda, Ayajiki and Okamura, 1993; Yoshida *et al.*, 1993) and cat (Ayajiki, Okamura and Toda, 1994) cerebral arteries, and the fibres suggested to arise from the pterygopalatine ganglion. Neuronal NO-mediated relaxation has also been described in porcine (Lee and Sarwinski, 1991; Chen and Lee, 1993), bovine (Gonzalez and Estrada, 1991; Ayajiki, Okamura and Toda, 1993) and human (Toda, 1993) cerebral arteries. NADPH-d immunopositive fibres have recently been shown in human cerebral vessels (Tomimoto *et al.*, 1994).

NOS-immunoreactivity was demonstrated in VIP/ACh-containing perivascular nerve fibres of intralingual arteries and arterioles, and VIP/NOS-containing cell bodies were located in parasympathetic intralingual ganglia of the guinea-pig (Kummer *et al.*, 1992). The fast and slow components of neurogenic vasodilatation of the guinea-pig uterine artery have been suggested to be mediated by NO and VIP respectively, acting as cotransmitters (Morris, 1993).

Autonomic control of penile erection, involving relaxation of the smooth muscle of the corpus cavernosum as well as dilatation of other penile vascular beds, has traditionally been attributed to the vasodilator effects of ACh and VIP. NO may have a role in this since NOS and NADPH-d immunoreactivity was shown in neuronal plexuses in the adventitial layer of penile arteries, axons of the penile cavernous nerve and in the associated pelvic ganglia (Burnett *et al.*, 1992; Keast, 1992). Further, a functional correlate is shown by the ability of inhibitors of NO formation to block non-adrenergic non-cholinergic relaxation of the bovine penile artery (Liu, Gillespie and Martin, 1991) and isolated strips of rabbit and human corpus cavernosum (Ignarro *et al.*, 1990; Kim *et al.*, 1991; Pickard, Powell and Zar, 1991; Rajfer *et al.*, 1992).

In the vasculature of the rat eye, NOS-containing nerve fibres were chiefly parasympathetic in nature, coexisting with VIP and arising from the pterygopalatine ganglion (Yamamoto *et al.*, 1993). NO-containing nerves in the adventitia and media of the dog retinal artery were also suggested to arise from the pterygopalatine ganglion and relaxations to electrical stimulation were abolished by an inhibitor of NOS (Toda *et al.*, 1993; Toda, Kitamura and Okamura, 1994). Non-adrenergic, non-cholinergic vasodilatation in the bovine ciliary artery has been shown to be mediated by CGRP from sensory nerves and by NO from nitrergic nerves (Wiencke *et al.*, 1994). Numerous NOS-positive ganglion cells accompanied the NADPH-d-positive perivascular nerves in the human eye suggesting a possible intrinsic nitrergic innervation (Flugel *et al.*, 1994).

SENSORY-MOTOR NERVES

The neuropeptides substance P, neurokinin A (NKA) and CGRP, potent vasodilators in many systems, are the principal transmitters in primary afferent nerves and have been shown to coexist in the same perivascular terminals (Gibbins *et al.*, 1985; Lee *et al.*, 1985; Lundberg *et al.*, 1985; Uddman *et al.*, 1985) in the same large granular vesicles (Gulbenkian *et al.*, 1986; Wharton and Gulbenkian, 1987). There is also evidence that ATP may have a role as a transmitter in sensory nerves, possibly acting as a cotransmitter with substance P and/or CGRP (Jahr and Jessel, 1983; Salt and Hill, 1983; Fyffe and Perl, 1984; Krishtal, Marchenko and Obukhov, 1988) (Figure 5.5). Many other peptides and non-peptides including somatostatin and VIP, have been claimed to be transmitters in sensory neurons (Maggi and Meli, 1988). Unmyelinated sensory neurons containing cholecystokinin/CGRP/DYN/substance P have been shown to project to cutaneous arterioles in guinea-pig skin (Gibbins, Furness and Costa, 1987), although the precise roles of each of these substances remains to be determined.

Primary afferent nerves are widely distributed throughout the cardiovascular system having been identified extensively in the heart, around large arteries and veins, and in smaller vessels supplying vascular beds (Duckles and Buck, 1982; Furness *et al.*, 1982; Barja, Mathison and Huggel, 1983; Lundberg *et al.*, 1985; Terenghi *et al.*, 1986; Franco-Cereceda *et al.*, 1987; Mione, Ralevic and Burnstock, 1990). In addition to their afferent (sensory) function, whereby they convey signals from the periphery to the central nervous system, primary afferents have an efferent (motor) function on target tissues which may take place by the axon reflex arrangement (see Figure 5.5), or by the release of transmitter from the same terminal that is excited by the environmental stimulus (Maggi and Meli, 1988;

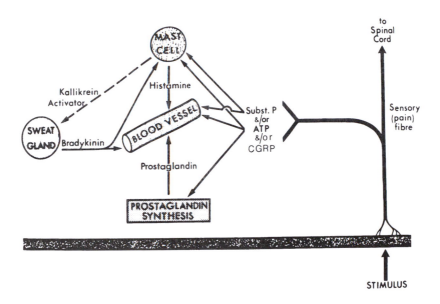

Figure 5.5 Diagram showing the basis of the "axon reflex" in the skin leading to vasodilatation and in-flammation. It is suggested that calcitonin gene-related peptide (CGRP), substance P (Subst. P), and adeno-sine 5'-triphosphate (ATP) are released during antidromic activation of sensory collaterals. (Adapted from Burnstock, 1977).

Szolcsanyi, 1988). In recognition of their dual function, and to distinguish them from that population of afferents with an entirely sensory role, the term "sensory-motor" has been used for these nerves (Burnstock, 1985).

The functional consequences of sensory cotransmission are illustrated by the pre- and postjunctional neuromodulatory interactions that have been described for substance P and CGRP. When substance P is injected with CGRP into human skin, it is able to convert the CGRP-mediated long-lasting vasodilatation into a transient response by a mechanism which is dependent on the action of proteases released from mast cells by substance P (Brain and Williams, 1988). On the other hand, CGRP potentiates tachykinin-induced plasma protein extravasation in rat and rabbit skin (Gamse and Saria, 1985). By analogy with other systems, it seems likely that modulatory interactions between substance P, CGRP, ATP and other putative sensory cotransmitters will increasingly be described.

Sensory-motor nerves appear to contribute importantly in vasodilator control of the rat mesenteric arterial vasculature via release of CGRP (Kawasaki et al., 1988) (Figure 5.6). Pre-junctional modulation of sensory-motor nerve-mediated vasodilatation of the rat mesenteric arterial bed by adenosine (a breakdown product of ATP) (Rubino, Ralevic and Burnstock, 1993), opioid peptides (Li and Duckles, 1991; Ralevic, Rubino and Burnstock, 1994), NPY (Kawasaki et al., 1991; Li and Duckles, 1991), and NA (Kawasaki et al., 1990a) has been described, strongly indicative of modulatory interactions, or "cross-talk", between different populations of perivascular nerves.

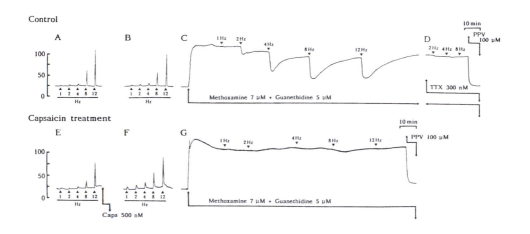

Figure 5.6 Typical records of the effect of treatment with (lower) and without (upper) 500 nM capsaicin (Caps) on pressor response and neurogenic vasodilation to periarterial nerve stimulation (PNS) (1–12 Hz) in the perfused mesenteric vascular bed of rats. (A) Control pressor response. (B) Pressor responses after treatment not containing Caps. (C) Vasodilator response to PNS in the preparation contracted with 7 μM methoxamine in the presence of 5 μM guanethidine. (D) Effect of 300 nM TTX (tetrodotoxin) on vasodilator response to PNS. (E) Control pressor responses. (F) Pressor responses after treatment with 500 nM Caps. (G) Vasodilator response to PNS in the contracted preparation. PPV, papaverine. (From Kawasaki et al., 1990b).

NADPH-d-positive labelling has been detected in afferent neurons of some dorsal root ganglia (Vizzard, Erdman and deGroat, 1993). Substantial NOS- and NADPH-d-immunopositive nerve fibres were observed in vagal sensory ganglia in guinea-pig airways, with sparse labelling in sympathetic ganglia, while tracheal and peribronchial ganglia were devoid of labelling, suggesting that extrinsic rather than intrinsic neurons are the source of NO release (Fischer et al., 1993; Suzuki et al., 1993).

PERIVASCULAR NERVES ARISING FROM INTRAMURAL NEURONS

While it seems likely that most of the neurons in intrinsic ganglia of heart, airways and bladder are of parasympathetic origin, it is possible that some arise from the neural crest and are not parasympathetic or sympathetic, as is clearly the case in the enteric ganglia. Little is known of the physiological roles or the pharmacology of intrinsic neurons of the heart because of the inherent difficulties in studying these in situ. However, studies of cultured intrinsic neurons from the atria of newborn guinea-pigs have shown that some of these nerves show immunofluorescence for NPY, some for 5-HT, and some for variable proportions of both of these transmitter substances (Hassall and Burnstock, 1984, 1986). Projections of these neurons in situ form perivascular plexuses in small-resistance coronary vessels (Corr et al., 1990). Both NPY and 5-HT are potent vasoconstrictors of coronary vessels and may have synergistic actions.

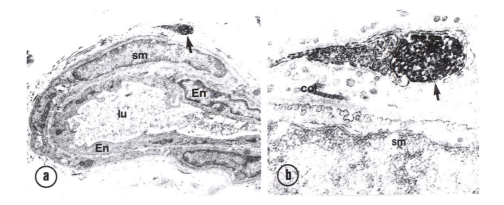

Figure 5.7   Arterioles in guinea-pig atria labelled for NOS. Intensely labelled NOS-positive perivascular nerves fibres (*arrow*); a labelled axonal varicosity containing small clear vesicles is shown at higher magnification in b; *En* endothelium; *sm* smooth muscle; *lu* lumen; *col* collagen fibres a × 6, 250; b × 29, 500. (From Sosunov *et al.*, 1995).

NOS has been shown in cardiac ganglion cells and in nerve fibres of the coronary and pulmonary arteries of the guinea-pig, where it may be of intrinsic parasympathetic or sensory origin (Klimaschewski *et al.*, 1992). NOS has been localized in a subpopulation of intrinsic cardiac neurons of the guinea-pig (Hassall *et al.*, 1992). Figure 5.7 shows NOS-immunopositive perivascular nerves in arterioles of the guinea-pig atria (Sosunov *et al.*, 1995). Sparse NOS reactivity was reported in vessels of the pig heart (Ursell and Mayes, 1993).

NO in nerves in some cerebral, penile and other vessels may be derived from local neurons, although a parasympathetic or sensory origin cannot be excluded. Intrinsic enteric neurons are known to supply some vessels in the gut and mesentery, and it is well known that monoamine-containing neurons in the brain contribute to the innervation of some cerebral vessels (Burnstock and Griffith, 1988). A few NOS-immunopositive fibres have been shown in guinea-pig mesenteric and coeliac arteries, but were absent from the abdominal and thoracic aorta, brachial, carotid, iliac, renal, splenic and skin arteries (Kummer *et al.*, 1992). NOS-positive fibres have been detected in the outer zones of the media and in the adventitia of dog mesenteric and femoral arteries (Yoshida *et al.*, 1993). Neurally-induced relaxation of the monkey mesenteric artery (Toda and Okamura, 1992) was attenuated by inhibitors of NO suggesting a possible role for NO as a transmitter or modulator. Human uterine arteries have also been shown to utilize NO as a vasodilator transmitter (Toda *et al.*, 1994).

NO and ATP have been claimed to be co-mediators of non-adrenergic, non-cholinergic relaxation of the rabbit portal vein (Brizzolara, Crowe and Burnstock, 1993).

ENDOTHELIUM

Endothelial cells form a continuous monolayer at the innermost surface of all blood vessels and are thus uniquely situated to sense and respond to changes in the circulation. The importance of the endothelium as a mediator of vasodilatation stemmed from the pioneering discovery of Furchgott and Zawadzki (1980), which showed that endothelial cells have a crucial role in the vasodilator response of a blood vessel to ACh via the release of a diffusible, non-prostanoid mediator which they termed 'endothelium-derived relaxing factor' (EDRF). An important breakthrough in the study of EDRF was made in 1986 when it was proposed that EDRF was, in fact, NO (Furchgott, Khan and Jothianandan, 1987; Ignarro *et al.*, 1987). To date, the general consensus is that EDRF is NO or a labile nitroso compound, synthesized from L-arginine (Palmer, Ferrige and Moncada, 1987). There is a continuous basal release of NO from most blood vessels, particularly arteries, that contributes to resting vascular tone; inhibition of NO synthesis or endothelial cell damage thus leads to an increase in vessel tone.

Endothelial cells are also sources of endothelium-derived vasoconstrictor factors (EDCF), hyperpolarizing factor (EDHF) and prostaglandins, which, as with EDRF, can be released following stimulation of endothelial cells by a number of vasoactive substances or by other physiological stimuli such as changes in blood flow, pH or pO_2 (Rubanyi, 1991; Ryan and Rubanyi, 1992). The endothelium integrates these signals, which are produced in variable proportions between arteries and veins, and between different vascular beds (Vanhoutte and Miller, 1985).

ENDOTHELIUM-MEDIATED VASODILATATION

Endothelium-dependent vasodilatation has been shown to occur in response to many substances including ACh, ATP, adenosine $5'$-diphosphate (ADP), arachidonic acid, substance P, neurokinin A, 5-HT, bradykinin, histamine, neurotensin, vasopressin (VP), angiotensin II (AgII) and thrombin (Furchgott, 1984; Mione, Ralevic and Burnstock, 1990). EDRF/NO can also be released by receptor-independent stimuli such as the calcium ionophore A23187 (Furchgott, 1984). Activation of endothelial cells stimulates the enzymatic (NOS) production of NO from L-arginine. NO binds to iron in the heme group of cytosolic guanylate cyclase in vascular smooth muscle cells causing an increase in cyclic GMP and subsequent smooth muscle relaxation.

Not all endothelium-dependent vasodilatation can be explained by the release/action of EDRF/NO. Prostaglandin release from endothelial cells has been demonstrated in response to several of those agents which produce EDRF as well as by increased flow or hypoxia (Kalsner, 1977; Roberts, Messina and Kaley, 1981; Busse *et al.*, 1983, 1984; Frangos *et al.*, 1985; Grabowski, Jaffe and Weksler, 1985; Rubanyi, Romero and Vanhoutte, 1986; Bhagyalakshmi and Frangos, 1989). However, its contribution to endothelium-dependent vasodilatation appears to be limited, and confined to certain vessels. EDHF, a diffusible substance shown to be released from endothelial cells by substance P, ACh and ATP (Bolton and Clapp, 1986; Chen, Suzuki and Weston, 1988; Feletou and Vanhoutte, 1988; Taylor and Weston, 1988; Keefe, Pasco and Eckman, 1992), may contribute to smooth muscle relaxation in some vessels.

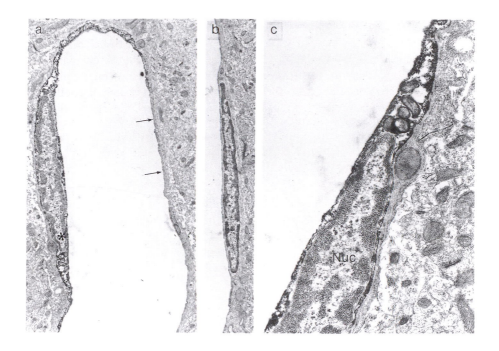

Figure 5.8   Longitudinal section through part of a capillary in the upper layers of the rat visual cortex. The wall of the capillary comprises a ChAT-labelled endothelial cell (*) and a process (arrows) of an unlabelled endothelial cell. (b) Unlabelled endothelial cell from the same capillary. (c) The labelled cell shows a clear nucleus (Nuc) and thin perinuclear cytoplasm containing a few organelles and a cluster of mitochondria. a, b, × 5, 500, c, × 14, 890. (From Parnavelas, Kelly and Burnstock, 1985).

In 1985, Parnavelas, Kelly and Burnstock reported that ChAT, the enzyme responsible for the synthesis of ACh, could be localized in endothelial cells lining capillaries and small vessels in the rat cortex (Figure 5.8). Since then, using the same technique of immunocytochemical staining combined with electron microscopy, ChAT, substance P, 5-HT, VP, AgII, NPY and atrial natriuretic peptide have been localized in endothelial cells in a variety of blood vessels (Burnstock *et al.*, 1988; Loesch and Burnstock, 1988; Lincoln, Loesch and Burnstock, 1990; Milner *et al.*, 1990; Loesch, Bodin and Burnstock, 1991; Loesch, Tomlinson and Burnstock, 1991; Cai *et al.*, 1992) (Figure 5.9). In addition, substance P levels have been measured in endothelial cells isolated from human cerebral arteries and aorta (Linnik and Moskowitz, 1989). Synthesis of AgII and histamine by endothelial cells has also been described (Hollis and Rosen, 1972; Kifor and Dzau, 1987). Questions raised about the possible sources of endothelially-acting vasoactive agents, such as ACh and substance P, contributed to the concept that endothelial cells themselves store and can release these and other vasoactive agents (Parnavelas, Kelly and Burnstock, 1985; Burnstock, 1989; Ralevic, Lincoln and Burnstock, 1992). It was clear that in large blood vessels neurotransmitters, released from perivascular nerves, did not represent endothelially-acting agents because of the presence of degradative enzymes and

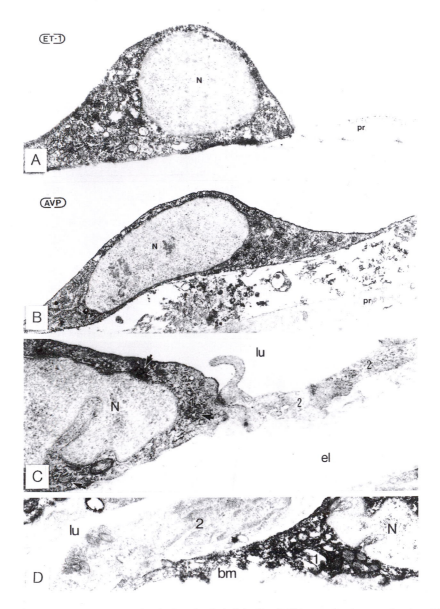

Figure 5.9   A,B. Electron micrographs of cultured endothelial cells of rabbit aorta showing cytoplasmic staining of cells positive for endothelin-1 (ET-1) (A) and arginine-vasopressin (AVP) (B). The labelled cells contain numerous organelles. Note the unlabelled nuclei (N) and also the unlabelled neighbouring endothelial cell processes (pr). A, × 5, 400; B × 5, 400.

C. A fragment of rat femoral artery demonstrates a substance P-positive endothelial cell (1). Note vesicles (*arrows*) dispersed through the labelled cytoplasm. The nucleus of the cell is unlabelled. Profiles of neighbouring endothelial cells are substance P-negative (2). N, nucleus; lu, lumen; el, elastic lamina. × 21, 200.

D. Electron micrograph of rat mesenteric artery. An example of AgII-positive (1) and AgII-negative (2) endothelial cells; *bm* basement membrane. N, nucleus; lu, lumen; bm, basal membrane. × 10, 780.

(Reprinted A,B: from Loesch, Bodin and Burnstock, 1991. C: from Loesch and Burnstock, 1988. D: from Lincoln, Loesch and Burnstock, 1990).

the physical barriers to diffusion presented by the media and basal lamina. The blood itself represents a possible source of vasoactive agents; however, in the case of substance P and ACh, circulating levels are low because of their rapid breakdown.

Studies of the release of vasoactive substances from endothelial cells by various stimuli have contributed to our understanding of their possible physiological roles. 5-HT, ATP, substance P and ACh, all of which are present in coronary endothelial cells, are released coincidentally with hypoxic vasodilatation during hypoxic perfusion of the isolated rat heart (Paddle and Burnstock, 1974; Burnstock *et al.*, 1988; Milner *et al.*, 1989). Since 5-HT, ATP, substance P and ACh elicit endothelium-dependent vasodilatation, and since hypoxic vasodilatation has been shown to be endothelium-dependent, a role for these endothelially-derived vasoactive agents as mediators of hypoxic vasodilatation should be considered.

The response of large arteries and resistance vessels to an increase in blood flow is to vasodilate via a mechanism involving the endothelium (Holtz *et al.*, 1984; Smiesko, Kozik and Dolezel, 1985; Hull *et al.*, 1986; Rubanyi, Romero and Vanhoutte, 1986; Bevan and Joyce, 1988). In the perfused vasculature of the rat hindlimb, an increase in flow stimulates the release of substance P into the effluent (Ralevic *et al.*, 1990). The source of the substance P was determined to be the vascular endothelial cells since, after removal of the endothelium by perfusion with air bubbles (Ralevic *et al.*, 1989), increased flow no longer evoked the release of substance P. Substance P-containing nerves did not contribute to this release since capsaicin-denervation had no effect on the flow-induced release of substance P (Ralevic *et al.*, 1990). Substance P is a potent endothelium-dependent vasodilator and has been localized within endothelial cells of the rat femoral artery (Loesch and Burnstock, 1988). Hence it is likely that a physiological role of substance P released from endothelial cells by increased flow is to contribute to flow-induced endothelium-dependent vasodilatation.

Further support for the concept that endothelial vasoactive substances have a physio-logical role in the local control of vascular tone comes from studies showing flow-evoked release of substance P, ATP and ACh from freshly isolated endothelial cells and endothelial cells in culture (Milner *et al.*, 1990a,b; Bodin *et al.*, 1992; Milner *et al.*, 1992), and endothelium-dependent, flow-induced release of ATP from the isolated perfused rat mesenteric arterial vasculature (Ralevic *et al.*, 1992). More recently, flow-evoked release of substance P has been shown from isolated rat brain microvessels (Milner *et al.*, 1995).

ENDOTHELIUM-MEDIATED VASOCONSTRICTION

Endothelial cells can mediate vasoconstriction via EDCF, a diffusible factor(s) produced in response to various chemical and physical stimuli, such as NA, thrombin, high extracellular potassium, hypoxia, and stretch (De Mey and Vanhoutte, 1983; Rubanyi and Vanhoutte, 1985; Katusic, Shepherd and Vanhoutte, 1987a,b). Divergent findings regarding the identity of EDCF are best explained by the existence of multiple EDCFs, which appear to be different in blood vessels of different anatomical origin, and also to depend on the nature of the stimulus. At least three different classes of endothelial-derived vasoconstrictor substances have been recognized: (1) metabolites of arachidonic acid; (2) the polypeptide endothelin; (3) a still-unidentified diffusible factor released from anoxic/hypoxic endothelial cells (Rubanyi and Vanhoutte, 1985; Lüscher, 1988). Stretch-activated ion channels, permeable to Ca^{2+}, have been demonstrated in endothelial cells and proposed to act as mechanotransducers (Lansman, Hallam and Rink, 1987).

Endothelin-1 is a 21-residue polypeptide (belonging to a family of structurally related endothelins) which is found in endothelial cells and has attracted considerable interest because of its potent and long-lasting constrictor actions in many vessels including porcine coronary arteries (Yanagisawa et al., 1988), rabbit, rat and human skin microvasculature (Brain, Tippins and Williams, 1988; Lawrence and Brain, 1992), isolated human resistance vessels (Sunman et al., 1993), and rat mesenteric arteries and rabbit aorta (Warner, de Nucci and Vane, 1989). Endothelin can also elicit endothelium-dependent vasodilatation in a variety of isolated blood vessels and vascular beds (Warner, de Nucci and Vane, 1989; Baydoun et al., 1990; Fukuda et al., 1990; Hasunuma et al., 1990; Perreault and De Marte, 1991; Namiki et al., 1992) as well as regional vasodilatation in whole animals (Gardiner et al., 1989; Whittle, Lopez-Belmonte and Rees, 1989; Fozard and Part, 1992). Intravenous injection of endothelin in rats produces a biphasic response consisting of a rapid and transient decrease in systemic blood pressure, followed by a profound and long-lasting increase in blood pressure (De Nucci et al., 1988; Miyauchi et al., 1989).

Endothelin and ATP, but not VIP, have been shown to be released from isolated rat (Bodin et al., 1992) (Figure 5.10) and rabbit (Milner et al., 1990a, 1992) aortic endothelial cells exposed to increased flow. Release of endothelin has also been shown from the perfused rat mesenteric arterial bed in response to increased flow (Ralevic, Milner and Burnstock, 1995) and hypoxia (Rakugi et al., 1990). However, there is no strong evidence to suggest that endothelin is a mediator of increased tone in, for example, hypoxic vasoconstriction or hypertension and its physiological and pathophysiological roles are largely unknown. It is possible that endothelin may be involved in the long-term maintenance of vascular tone and/or structure.

INTERACTIONS BETWEEN PERIVASCULAR NERVES AND ENDOTHELIUM

Interactions between perivascular nerves and endothelial cells may be subdivided into short-term dynamic effects or long-term trophic effects. The size of the vessel, and hence the separation between perivascular nerves and endothelial cells, has a crucial influence on the relative importance of these interactions at different levels of the vascular tree. Short-term interactions may be further divided into two types. One type of interaction involves the dynamic balance of independent effects produced by perivascular nerves (predominantly sympathetic constrictor) and endothelial cells (predominantly vasodilator), and is likely to be important throughout the vasculature. The other type of short-term interaction involves pre- and/or postjunctional modulation of neurotransmitter release or action by factors released from the endothelium, and the action of neurotransmitters on endothelial receptors, and is likely to be physiologically relevant particularly in small vessels where neural-endothelial separation is small. By definition, short-term interactions are temporary and therefore are readily reversible. Long-term interactions involve sustained, altered patterns of release of neurotransmitters or endothelial factors, which result in chronic

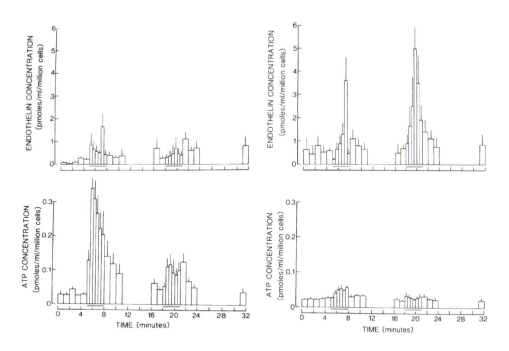

Figure 5.10   (A) Release of (i) endothelin, and (ii) ATP, by freshly isolated endothelial cells from the thoracic aorta of normoxic rats. Cells were perfused at a low flow rate (0.5 ml min^{-1}) and stimulated twice (with an interval of 10 min) by an increased flow rate (3.0 ml min^{-1}) for 3 min (shown by lines under the x-axis); $n = 4$. (B) Release of (i) endothelin, and (ii) ATP, by freshly isolated endothelial cells from the thoracic aorta of chronically hypoxic rats. Cells were perfused at a low flow rate (0.5 ml min^{-1}) and stimulated twice (with an interval of 10 min) by an increased flow rate (3.0 ml min^{-1}) for 3 min (shown by lines under the x-axis); $n = 4$. (Reprinted from Bodin *et al.*, 1992).

changes in the morphology and/or function of endothelial cells and perivascular nerves. Such interactions are likely to be relevant at all levels, but particularly in the micro-vasculature.

A schematic diagram of the neural and endothelial factors involved in control of vascular tone is illustrated in Figure 5.11.

SHORT-TERM PHYSIOLOGICAL INTERACTIONS

There is a continuous basal release of NO in many vessels which contributes importantly to resting tone. Hence, removal of the endothelium or blockade of NO formation with inhibitors of NOS causes a non-specific increase in constrictor responses, for example to electrical field stimulation (EFS), NA and potassium chloride (González *et al.*, 1990; Li and Duckles, 1992; Reid and Rand, 1992; Schwarzacher *et al.*, 1992; Vo, Reid and Rand, 1992). Increased shear stress attenuated sympathetic constriction, and it was suggested that this was due to augmented release of EDRF (Tesfamariam and Cohen, 1988). In the rat tail artery (Bucher *et al.*, 1992) and guinea-pig pulmonary artery

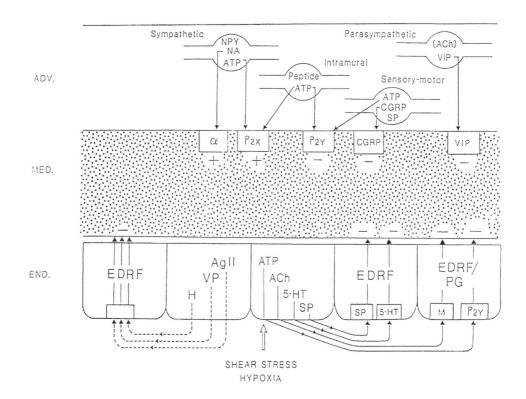

Figure 5.11 Regulation of vascular tone by perivascular nerves and endothelial cells. Neuropeptide Y (NPY), noradrenaline (NA), adenosine 5′-triphosphate (ATP), calcitonin gene-related peptide (CGRP), substance P (SP), and vasoactive intestinal polypeptide (VIP) can be released from nerve varicosities in the adventitia (ADV) to act on receptors in the media (MED), causing vasoconstriction or vasodilatation. ATP, acetylcholine (ACh), 5-hydroxytryptamine (5-HT), and SP, released from endothelial cells (END) by shear stress or hypoxia, act on their receptors on endothelial cells to cause a release of endothelium-derived relaxing factor (EDRF) or prostaglandins (PG), which, in turn, act on the smooth muscle to cause relaxation. Angiotensin II (AgII), vasopressin (VP), and histamine (H) are also contained in, and may be released from, subpopulations of endothelial cells. In areas denuded of endothelial cells, opposite effects may be produced by receptors on the smooth muscle cells; for example, *via* P_{2X}- and P_{2Y}-purinoceptors and muscarinic receptors (M). (Adapted from Burnstock, 1990b).

(Cederqvist *et al.*, 1991; Cederqvist and Gustafsson, 1994) the endothelium-dependent potentiation of responses to EFS and exogenous NA during NO-inhibition was postjunctional, release of [^{3}H]NA being unaffected.

Potentiation of responses to constrictors after removal of the endothelium or inhibition of endothelial-derived vasodilator factors may also be a consequence of the abolition of vasodilator effects mediated at endothelial receptors, for example endothelial α_2-adrenoceptors (Angus and Cocks, 1989). Different subtypes of receptors for vasoactive substances are typically found on the endothelium and on the underlying vascular smooth muscle. This highlights the importance of the endothelium under basal conditions since

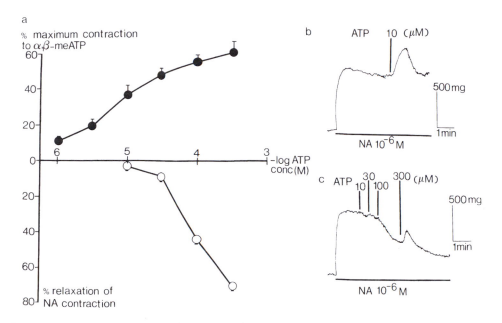

Figure 5.12.   The effect of ATP (10^{-6} to 3×10^{-4} M) on isolated rat femoral artery with tone raised by 10^{-6} M noradrenaline (NA) (a) when endothelium is either intact (o) or removed (•) ($n = 4$). Vertical bars show S.E.M. Upper curve shows ATP-induced contractions in the absence of endothelium. Lower curves show ATP relaxations in the presence of endothelium. (b) Endothelium is removed. Contraction to 10^{-5} M ATP. (c) Endothelium intact. Relaxations to ATP (10^{-5} to 3×10^{-4} M). (From Kennedy, Delbro and Burnstock, 1985).

many of those same vasoactive substances which produce vasodilatation in the presence of the endothelium elicit vasoconstriction when endothelial function or integrity is impaired, with serious implications for vasospasm. For example, in the presence of an intact endothelium, ACh and ATP elicit relaxation via muscarinic and P_{2Y}-purinoceptors on the endothelium, whereas when the endothelium is removed or damaged ACh and ATP may elicit vasoconstriction via muscarinic and P_{2X}-purinoceptors present on the underlying smooth muscle (Furchgott, 1984; **Burnstock and Kennedy, 1985**; **Burnstock, 1988a,b**) (Figure 5.12).

Endothelin-1 has been shown to non-specifically enhance vasoconstrictor responses to EFS, NA, 5-HT, ATP and vasopressin in rabbit arteries (Wong-Dusting, La and Rand, 1990; La and Rand, 1993). Potentiation of rat mesenteric venous, but not arterial, responses to nerve stimulation by endothelin-1 has been reported (Warner, D'Orleans-Juste and Vane, 1990). It is possible that several of the other vasoactive substances described in endothelial cells may also postjunctionally modulate neurotransmitter actions.

Prejunctional neuromodulation by NO, which can readily diffuse across cell membranes, has been reported. NO was suggested to increase [^{3}H]NA outflow in rat mesenteric arteries (Yamamoto et al., 1992) and the endothelium was found to inhibit radiolabelled NA release from adrenergic nerves of the rabbit carotid artery (Cohen and Weisbrod, 1988) and canine pulmonary artery and vein (Greenberg *et al.*, 1989), although this does not necessarily involve NO.

Non-endothelial NO may contribute to inhibition of responses in some vessels since potentiation by N^G-nitro-L-arginine methyl ester (L-NAME) occurs in endothelial-denuded preparations. Endothelium-independent potentiation of constriction to EFS in dog temporal arteries was postjunctional (release of [^{3}H]NA was unaffected) and was suggested to be due to an elimination of the effect of neuronal NO (Toda, Yoshida and Okamura, 1991). Neuronal NO was also suggested to account for the potentiation of constriction to EFS in endothelium-denuded monkey mesenteric arteries (Tsuchiya *et al.*, 1994). However, a non-neuronal non-endothelial source of NO is implicated in the endothelium-independent N^G-momomethyl-L-arginine (L-NMMA) enhancement of contractile responses to exogenous NA in guinea-pig (Cederqvist *et al.*, 1991) and rabbit (MacLean *et al.*, 1993) pulmonary arteries and in the rabbit saphenous vein (Gordon *et al.*, 1992). Endogenous NO has been suggested to prejunctionally inhibit sensory-motor vasodilatation in endothelium-denuded rat mesenteric arteries (Li, Yu and Deng, 1993).

LONG-TERM INTERACTIONS IN AGEING AND DISEASE

Because perivascular nerves and endothelial cells are separated by a layer of vascular smooth muscle, the possibility of trophic interactions between these two systems has received little direct attention. However, direct evidence for long-term trophic interactions is provided by studies where chronic denervation or nerve stimulation has resulted in alterations in endothelial cell morphology and function. The converse, alterations in perivascular nerves after endothelial damage, has also been shown. Such interactions may be particularly relevant in the microvasculature where perivascular nerve varicosities have been demonstrated in close apposition to endothelial cells in capillaries. The following section discusses current evidence for long-term interactions between perivascular nerves and endothelial cells. Also discussed are the age- and disease-related specific changes in perivascular nerves and endothelium, which by implication will trigger chronic changes in endothelial cells and perivascular nerves respectively.

Surgery, trauma, selective denervation and chronic exposure to hormones

Certain neuropeptides may have trophic effects on the vasculature, influencing the growth and development of nerves, smooth muscle and endothelial cells (Burnstock, 1985; Maggi and Meli, 1988), which may account for the fact that some of the peptides identified in perivascular nerves have little direct actions on blood vessels. For instance, positive trophic effects of CGRP on endothelial cells in culture have been shown (Haegerstrand *et al.*, 1990). Whether the peptides that are found in endothelial cells also have trophic effects on components of the blood vessel wall remains to be determined. Adenosine can be formed from the extracellular breakdown of ATP released from nerves and chronic inhibition of adenosine uptake with dipyridamole has been shown to cause proliferation of capillary endothelium and increased capillary density in skeletal muscle and heart (Hudlicka, 1984).

In the rabbit ear artery, endothelium-dependent vasodilatation to methacholine was significantly impaired 2–8 weeks after sympathetic and sensory denervation, while endothelium-independent vasodilatation was unaffected (Mangiarua and Bevan, 1986). In mesenteric arterial preparations from rats treated as neonates with the sensory neurotoxin capsaicin, endothelium-dependent vasodilator responses to ACh were selectively impaired; in contrast, sympathectomy with 6-OHDA had no effect on endothelially-mediated responses (Miller and Scott, 1990). Endothelium-dependent relaxations were selectively inhibited 3 weeks postsympathectomy in rabbit carotid arterial rings (Kars et al., 1993). Long-term sympathetic denervation in rabbits resulted in an increase in the sensitivity of cerebral arteries to hypercapnia, hypoxia, and 5-HT (Aubinea et al., 1989). Although morphological changes in the endothelial cells were not detected after sympathectomy (Dimitriadou et al., 1988), it is possible that changes in endothelial cell mechanisms contributed to the supersensitivity. Surgical sympathectomy or long-term adrenoceptor blockade by propanolol have been claimed to prevent or reduce the induction of atherosclerosis by diet (Lichtor et al., 1987).

Long-term, but not short-term, sympathectomy was associated with a selective increase in the flow-evoked release of endothelin from the isolated perfused rat mesenteric arterial bed (Ralevic, Milner and Burnstock, 1995). Gold-labelling of rat aortic endothelial cells at the electron microscope level showed an increase in particles with positive staining for endothelin and a decrease in particles positive for NOS after long-, but not short-term sympathectomy, suggesting that the endothelial content of endothelin and NO may undergo compensatory changes to maintain vascular tone in the absence of sympathetic constrictor innervation (G. Aliev, V. Ralevic and G. Burnstock, unpublished observations). In isolated brain microvessels an increase in the flow-evoked release of substance P has been shown in rats having undergone long-term sensory denervation with capsaicin (Milner et al., 1995).

It is possible that the changes in endothelial cell mechanisms after selective denervation are a consequence of trophic effects mediated by the remaining populations of perivascular nerves, some of which may undergo marked compensatory changes. Compensatory changes occurring after superior cervical ganglionectomy include increased substance P levels in the ipsilateral iris and ciliary body (Cole et al., 1983), increased CGRP content of pial vessels (Schon et al., 1985), and increased expression of NPY in non-adrenergic VIP-containing nerves in the cerebral vasculature (Gibbins and Morris, 1988). Long-term chemical sympathectomy of developing rats, induced by chronic guanethidine treatment, leads to increased brightness and density of CGRP-positive immunofluorescent nerves innervating blood vessels (Aberdeen et al., 1990).

Chronic stimulation (10 days in vivo) of the rabbit auricular nerve produced marked structural and immunocytochemical changes in the endothelial cells of the central ear artery; a subpopulation of endothelial cells were found to have developed cytoplasmic protrusions of the apical region, which showed positive immunoreactivity for CGRP and NPY (Loesch, Maynard and Burnstock, 1992) (Figure 5.13). In the same model of chronic stimulation, there was selective impairment of contractile responses to ATP mediated via the P_{2X}-purinoceptor while constrictor responses to NA were unaffected (Maynard, Loesch and Burnstock, 1992). Exactly how perivascular nerves influence endothelial cells is not known but may involve alterations in the nerve impulse regulation of activity, a specific involvement of the neurotransmitter, or an unidentified trophic factor (Azevedo and Osswald, 1986; Warren, Brady and Taylor, 1990).

Mechanical injury of the endothelium of the dog coronary artery, without disruption of the elastic lamina, resulted in an increase in the number of neuron-specific enolase-positive

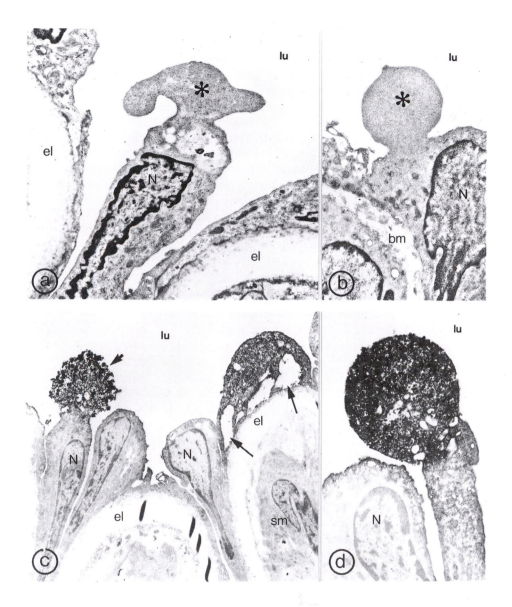

Figure 5.13 Conventional electron microscopy (a, b) and electron-immunocytochemistry (c, d) of rabbit central ear artery following long-term electrical stimulation of perivascular nerves *in vivo*. (a, b) Note the differences in shapes of the endothelium-associated protrusions (asterisks) and the granular nature of the cytoplasm of the protrusions. N, nucleus; el, elastic lamina; bm, basement membrane; lu, lumen of the artery. (c) Note calcitonin gene-related peptide (CGRP)-like immunoreactivity associated with an endothelial cell partially separated from subendothelial cell layer (longer arrows). Protrusion at the apical region of another endothelial cell (short arrow) also shows CGRP-like immunoreactivity; sm, smooth muscle. (d) Note neuropeptide Y (NPY)-like immunoreactivity which is restricted to protrusion at the apical region of endothelial cell.
  Magnifications are (a, b) × 8, 100 (c) × 6, 450; (d) × 8, 900. (From Loesch, Maynard and Burnstock, 1992).

nerve fibres after 1 and 3 months (Taguchi *et al.*, 1986). This is likely to have been a reflection of the increased density of substance P-containing nerve fibres, also observed in the dog coronary artery 3 months after mechanical injury of the endothelium (Taguchi *et al.*, 1986).

Four-week treatment with estrogen, but not progesterone, leads to a marked reduction in the density and varicosity diameters of 5-HT-containing nerves supplying the basilar artery (Dhall *et al.*, 1988). In late pregnancy, sympathetic innervation of guinea-pig uterine blood vessels exhibits a remarkable switch from adrenergic vasoconstrictor to cholinergic vasodilator control (Bell, 1968); ultrastructural studies showed that there was no degeneration of serotonergic or peptidergic (NPY-, VIP-, substance P- and CGRP-containing) nerves (Mione *et al.*, 1988).

Development and ageing

Considerable variations in the density of innervation with age have been described in different vessels (Cowen *et al.*, 1982; Mione *et al.*, 1988). For example, CGRP-like immunoreactivity (-LI) was found earlier than substance P-LI in cerebrovascular nerves, and increased in old age, while the density of substance P-LI nerve fibres did not change (Mione *et al.*, 1988) (Figure 5.14). Similarly, NA and NPY underwent different expression in cerebrovascular nerves during development (Dhital *et al.*, 1988; Mione *et al.*, 1988).

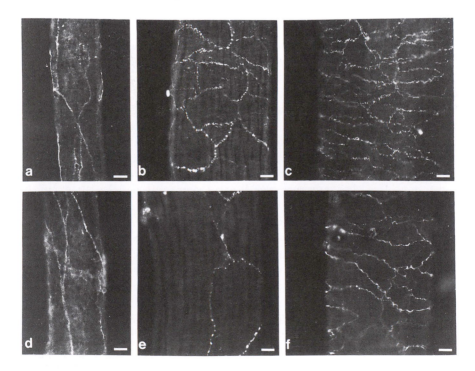

Figure 5.14 Photomicrographs of stretch preparations of cerebral arteries showing perivascular nerve fibres at various age stages. VIP-containing nerves in the middle cerebral artery at 1 day (a), 8 months (b) and 27 months (c). CGRP-containing nerve fibres in the posterior cerebral artery at 1 day (d), 4 months (e) and 27 months (f). Nerve density is increased in old age for both VIP and CGRP. Scale bars = 25 μm. (From Mione *et al.*, 1988).

An interesting observation from these studies was that in ageing the expression of the vasoconstrictor transmitters NA and 5-HT decreased, whereas expression of the vasodilator transmitters VIP and CGRP increased (Mione et al., 1988). In guinea-pig mesenteric and carotid arteries, adrenergic nerve density reached a peak 4 weeks after birth, whereas nerves containing VIP, CGRP and substance P reached a peak at birth and declined with age (Dhall et al., 1986), raising the possibility that perivascular neuropeptides may play a trophic role in early development. This is supported by the finding of an early appearance of CGRP-immunoreactive nerves in human foetal skin (Terenghi et al., 1993).

Functional studies have supported the immunohistochemical findings of changes in peptidergic innervation with increasing age. For instance, there is a decrease in CGRP-LI in mesenteric (and femoral and renal) arteries with age which parallels the age-related decrease in sensory-motor vasodilatation of the rat mesenteric arterial bed (Kawasaki, Saito and Takasaki, 1990a; Li and Duckles, 1993). An age-related decrease in axon reflexes and in repair processes is also suggestive of a reduction in sensory innervation with age (Helme and McKernan, 1985; Parkhouse and LeQuesne, 1988).

Impaired (Shimizu and Toda, 1986; Toda, Bian and Inoue, 1987; Miyata et al., 1992), unchanged (Mayhan et al., 1990) and increased (Hynes and Duckles, 1987) endothelium-dependent relaxation has been reported in different vessels with age.

Hypertension

The sympathetic nervous system has been implicated in the development and maintenance of hypertension in various models of hypertension, as well as in humans. Hyperinnervation of various arteries and increased sympathetic activity has been shown (Westfall and Meldrum, 1985; Dhital et al., 1988; Esler et al., 1988; Head, 1989; Mangiarua and Lee, 1989). Increased sympathetic innervation and significantly higher levels of the sympathetic transmitters NA and NPY were shown in cerebral vessels of the spontaneously hypertensive rat (SHR) (Dhital et al., 1988; Mangiarua and Lee, 1989). A reduction of NPY levels has been reported in the kidney and renal arteries in experimental hypertension (Ballesta et al., 1987). In stroke-prone SHR there was an increase in NPY and VIP nerve density, but no change in substance P nerve density in peripheral vessels, and a decrease in substance P nerve density in cerebral vessels (Lee et al., 1988). In mesenteric arteries of SHR a decrease in CGRP density has been described, and there was a corresponding decrease in (CGRP-mediated) sensory-motor vasodilatation (Kawasaki, Saito and Takasaki, 1990a,b). Attenuated prejunctional inhibition by NPY and augmented postjunctional potentiation by NPY of sympathetic neurotransmission have been suggested to contribute to enhanced sympathetic activity in the mesenteric arterial bed of SHR (Westfall et al., 1990).

In the tail and mesenteric arteries of SHR, the ATP component of sympathetic cotransmission has been claimed to be enhanced to the extent that it comprises the dominant component of the sympathetic response (Vidal, Hicks and Langer, 1986; Woolridge and Van Helden, 1990; Bulloch and McGrath, 1992). Defective prejunctional P_1-purinoceptor-mediated modulation has been claimed to contribute to enhanced sympathetic neurotransmission in hypertension (Kamikawa, Cline and Su, 1980; Kubo and Su, 1983; Illes et al., 1989). Constriction of the isolated kidney to renal nerve stimulation was increased in SHR compared to controls and appeared to be entirely due to ATP released from sympathetic nerves (Rump, Wilde and Schollmeyer, 1990).

Hypertension has been associated with distinct morphological changes in the endothelium, including alterations in cell shape, replication rate and permeability (Luscher, 1988). In extreme cases, intimal lesions may develop (Todd, 1992). Pharmacological studies have generally confirmed that hypertension is associated with impaired endothelial function. For example, endothelium-dependent relaxation of the rat aorta (Van de Voorde and Leusen, 1986) and mesenteric resistance arteries (Carvalho et al., 1987; Dohi et al., 1990) are decreased in hypertension.

Diabetes

In the streptozotocin-diabetic rat, a model of insulin-dependent diabetes, contractile responses of the mesenteric arterial bed (Takiguchi et al., 1988) and tail artery (Hart et al., 1988) to sympathetic nerve stimulation were markedly decreased. Perivascular nerves in penile vessels containing VIP and ACh were shown to be damaged or lost in diabetic impotent men and in streptozotocin-diabetic rats (Crowe et al., 1983; Lincoln et al., 1987; Blanco et al., 1990). A reduction in the expression of VIP and 5-HT, but not NPY and NA, has been demonstrated in perivascular nerves supplying the cerebral blood vessels of streptozotocin-diabetic rats (Lagnado et al., 1987). An increase in the relative number of PGP 9.5- (a general neuronal marker), CGRP- and VIP-immunoreactive fibres has been seen in rat skin in early diabetes (Karanth et al., 1990). In mesenteric arteries from streptozotocin-diabetic rats, impaired sensory-motor vasodilatation, but intact responses to exogenous CGRP, is indicative of diabetic sensory neuropathy (Ralevic, Belai and Burnstock, 1993).

Impaired endothelium-dependent relaxation, but generally unimpaired endothelium-independent relaxation, has been demonstrated in clinical (De Tejada et al., 1989), and experimental diabetes (Oyama et al., 1986; Meraji et al., 1987; Durante, Sen and Sunahara, 1988; Takiguchi et al., 1988; Kamata, Miyata and Kasuya, 1989; Mayhan, 1989; Pieper and Gross, 1989; Kiff et al., 1991; Mayhan, 1992; Taylor et al., 1992). Atherosclerosis is a common cardiovascular complication of diabetes and extreme morphological changes have been observed in the endothelium of some diabetic vessels (Strandness, Preist and Gibbens, 1964; Robertson and Strong, 1968; Jarrett, Keen and Chakrabarti, 1982).

Atherosclerosis

Endothelial cell damage or dysfunction is widely regarded as the critical initiating factor in atherogenesis. In animal models of atherosclerosis or hypercholesterolemia, impairment of endothelium-dependent vasodilatation to ACh, with relative preservation of endothelium-independent vasodilatation, has been reported (Aksulu, Cellek and Turker, 1986; Freiman et al., 1986; Verbeuren et al., 1986; Förstermann et al., 1988; Yamamoto et al., 1988; Guerra et al., 1989; Shimokawa and Vanhoutte, 1989). Since impaired endothelium-dependent relaxations to ACh, thrombin and the calcium ionophore A23187 could be restored by dietary treatment, which did not reverse the thickening of the intima, it was suggested that atherosclerosis does not present a functional barrier to prevent EDRF from reaching the underlying vascular smooth muscle. Bioassays have shown that atherosclerotic vessels release significantly less EDRF than normal vessels in response to both receptor (ACh and 5-HT) and non-receptor (calcium ionophore, A23187) stimuli, and the consensus is that decreased EDRF release is responsible for attenuated endothelium-dependent vascular relaxation in atherosclerosis (Sreeharan *et al.*, 1986; Verbeuren *et al.*, 1986; Harrison *et al.*, 1987; Guerra *et al.*, 1989; Shimokawa and Vanhoutte, 1989). Recently, diet-induced atherosclerosis was shown to inhibit the release of [^{3}H]NA from sympathetic nerves in rabbit arteries (Verbeuren, Simonet and Herman, 1994).

An increase in endothelium-dependent vasodilatation has been observed in mesenteric, femoral, ear, saphenous and hepatic arteries from the Watanabe heritable hyperlipidemic rabbit; in contrast, heavily lesioned vessels from the same animals, namely the aorta and carotid artery, showed seriously attenuated endothelium-mediated relaxation (Burnstock *et al.*, 1991; Brizzolara *et al.*, 1992).

Chronic hypoxia

Chronic hypoxia in man (Surks, Beckwith and Chidsey, 1967) and in animals (Johnson, Young and Landsberg, 1983), is associated with an increase in sympathetic activity. Chronic hypobaric hypoxia causes contraction of the vascular smooth muscle leading to a rise in pressure of the pulmonary vessels and thence to a remodelling of the pulmonary vasculature (Meyrick and Reid, 1978; Rabinovitch *et al.*, 1981; Hung *et al.*, 1986). Profound morphological changes have been observed in the endothelium, including thickening, vacuolation, vesiculation and occasionally detachment of endothelial cells (Meyrick and Reid, 1978; Hung *et al.*, 1986).

The morphological changes in the endothelium in hypoxia-induced pulmonary hypertension are similar to those seen in systemic hypertension, both of which are associated with functional defects in the endothelium. In the rat pulmonary artery, chronic hypoxia caused a decrease in endothelium-dependent relaxation (Rui and Cai, 1991). In a recent study of the effect of chronic hypoxia on the content of endothelial vasoactive substances, it was revealed that, in response to shear stress, endothelial cells isolated from hypoxic rats released less ATP, but more endothelin than cells from normoxic rats (Bodin *et al.*, 1992) (Figure 5.10). It was suggested that, under conditions of reduced oxygen tension, a dynamic balance between ATP and endothelin could regulate the response of vessels to flow.

REFERENCES

Aberdeen, J., Corr, L., Milner, P., Lincoln, J. and Burnstock, G. (1990). Marked increases in calcitonin gene-related peptide-containing nerves in the developing rat following long-term sympathectomy with guanethidine. *Neuroscience*, **35**, 175–184.

Aksulu, H.E., Cellek, S. and Turker, R.K. (1986). Cholesterol feeding attenuates endothelium-dependent relaxation response to acetylcholine in the main pulmonary artery of chickens. *Eur J Pharmacol*, **129**, 397–400.

Anderson, C.R. (1992). NADPH diaphorase-positive neurons in the rat spinal cord include a subpopulation of autonomic preganglionic neurons. *Neurosci Lett*, **139**, 280–284.

Anderson, C.R., Edwards, S.L., Furness, J.B., Bredt, D.S. and Snyder, S.H. (1993). The distribution of nitric-oxide synthase-containing autonomic preganglionic terminals in the rat. *Brain Res*, **614**, 78–85.

Angus, J.A. and Cocks, T.M. (1989). Endothelium-derived relaxing factor. *Pharmacol Ther*, **41**, 303–351.

Aubinea, P., Pearce, W., Reynier-Rebuffel, A.M., Cuevas, J. and Issertial, O. (1989). Long-term sympathetic denervation increases sensitivity of cerebral arteries to CO_2 and 5-HT *in vitro. J Cereb Blood Flow Metab*, **9**, (Suppl. 1), S506–510.

Ayajiki, K., Okamura, T. and Toda, N. (1993). Nitric oxide mediates, and acetylcholine modulates, neurally induced relaxation of bovine cerebral arteries. *Neuroscience*, **54**, 819–825.

Ayajiki, K., Okamura, T. and Toda, N. (1994). Neurogenic relaxation caused by nicotine in isolated cat middle cerebral arteries. *J Pharmacol Exp Ther*, **270**, 795–801.

Azevedo, I. and Osswald, W. (1986). Trophic role of the sympathetic nervous system. *J Pharmacol*, **17**, 30–43.

Ballesta, J., Lawson, J.A., Pals, D.T., Ludens, J.H., Lee, Y.C., Bloom, S.R., *et al.* (1987). Significant depletion of NPY in the innervation of the rat mesenteric, renal arteries and kidneys in experimentally (aorta coarction) induced hypertension. *Hypertension*, **87**, 273–278.

Bao, J.X., Eriksson, I.E. and Stjärne, L. (1989). On pre- and/or postjunctional roles of ATP and an unknown "substance X" as sympathetic co-transmitters in rat tail artery. *Acta Physiol Scand*, **135**, 65–66.

Barja, F., Mathison, R. and Huggel, M. (1983). Substance P-containing nerve fibres in large peripheral blood vessels of the rat. *Cell Tissue Res*, **229**, 411–422.

Bartfai, T., Iverfeldt, K. and Fisone, G. (1988). Regulation of the release of coexisting neurotransmitters. *Annu Rev Pharmacol Toxicol*, **28**, 285–310.

Baydoun, A.R., Peers, S.H., Cirino, G. and Woodward, B. (1990). Vasodilator action of endothelin-1 in the perfused rat heart. *J Cardiovasc Pharmacol*, **15**, 759–763.

Bell, C. (1968). Dual vasoconstrictor and vasodilator innervation of the uterine arterial supply in guinea-pig. *Circ Res*, **23**, 279–289.

Bevan, J.A. and Joyce, E.H. (1988). Flow-dependent dilation in myograph-mounted resistance artery segments. *Blood Vessels*, **25**, 101–104.

Bhagyalakshmi, A. and Frangos, J.A. (1989). Mechanism of shear-induced prostacyclin production in endothelial cells. *Biochem Biophys Res Commun*, **158**, 31–37.

Blanco, R., de Tejada, I.S., Goldstein, I., Krane, R.J., Wotiz, H.H. and Cohen, R.A. (1990). Dysfunctional penile cholinergic nerves in diabetic impotent men. *J Urol*, **144**, 278–280.

Bloom, S.R. and Edwards, A.V. (1980). Vasoactive intestinal polypeptide in relation to atropine resistant vasodilatation in the sub-maxillary gland of the cat. *J Physiol*, **300**, 41–53.

Bodin, P., Milner, P., Winter, R. and Burnstock, G. (1992). Chronic hypoxia changes the ratio of endothelin to ATP release from rat aortic endothelial cells exposed to high flow. *Proc Roy Soc Lond Ser B*, **247**, 131–135.

Bolton, T.B. and Clapp, L.H. (1986). Endothelial-dependent relaxant actions of carbachol and substance P in the arterial smooth muscle. *Br J Pharmacol*, **87**, 713–723.

Brain, S.D., Tippins, J.R. and Williams, T.J. (1988). Endothelin induces potent microvascular constriction. *Br J Pharmacol*, **95**, 1005–1007.

Brain, S.D. and Williams, T.J. (1988). Substance P regulates the vasodilator activity of calcitonin gene-related peptide. *Nature*, **355**, 73–75.

Bredt, D.S. and Snyder, S.H. (1992). Nitric oxide, a novel neuronal messenger. *Neuron*, **8**, 3–11.

Brizzolara, A.L. and Burnstock, G. (1990). Evidence for noradrenergic-purinergic cotransmission in the hepatic artery of the rabbit. *Br J Pharmacol*, **99**, 835–839.

Brizzolara, A.L., Crowe, R. and Burnstock, G. (1993). Evidence for the involvement of both ATP and nitric oxide in non-adrenergic, non-cholinergic inhibitory neurotransmission in the rabbit portal vein. *Br J Pharmacol*, **109**, 606–608.

Brizzolara, A.L., Tomlinson, A., Aberdeen, J., Gourdie, R.G. and Burnstock, G. (1992). Sex and age as factors influencing the vascular reactivity in Watanabe heritable hyperlipideamic (WHHL) rabbits: A pharmacological and morphological study of the hepatic artery. *J Cardiovasc Pharmacol*, **19**, 86–95.

Bucher, B., Ouedraogo, S., Tschopl, M., Paya, D. and Stoclet, J.C. (1992). Role of the L-arginine pathway and of cyclic GMP in electrical field-induced noradrenaline release and vasoconstriction in the rat tail artery. *Br J Pharmacol*, **107**, 976–982.

Bulloch, J.M. and McGrath, J.C. (1988). Blockade of vasopressor and vas deferens responses by α,β-methylene ATP in the pithed rat. *Br J Pharmacol*, **94**, 103–108.

Bulloch, J.M. and McGrath, J.C. (1992). Evidence for increased purinergic contribution in hypertensive blood vessels exhibiting co-transmission. *Br J Pharmacol*, **107**, (Suppl.), 145P.

Burnett, A.L., Lowenstein, C.J., Bredt, D.S., Chang, T.S.K. and Snyder, S.H. (1992). A physiologic mediator of penile erection. *Science*, **257**, 401–403.

Burnstock, G. (1976). Do some nerve cells release more than one transmitter? *Neuroscience*, **1**, 239–248.

Burnstock, G. (1977). Autonomic neuroeffector junctions — reflex vasodilatation of the skin. *J Invest Dermatol*, **69**, 47–57.

Burnstock, G. (1983). Recent concepts of chemical communication between excitable cells. In Dale's Principle and Communication between Neurones, edited by N.N. Osborne, pp. 7–35. Oxford: Pergamon Press.

Burnstock, G. (1985). Neurohumoral control of blood vessels: some future directions. *J Cardiovasc Pharmacol*, **7**, (Suppl. 3), S137–146.

Burnstock, G. (1986a). Autonomic neuromuscular junctions: current developments and future directions. The Third Anatomical Society Review Lecture. *J Anat*, **146**, 1–30.

Burnstock, G. (1986b). Purines as cotransmitters in adrenergic and cholinergic neurones. Coexistence of Neuronal Messengers: A New Principle in Chemical Transmission. Progress in Brain Research, Vol. 68, edited by T. Hökfelt, K. Fuxe, and B. Pernow, pp. 193–203. Amsterdam: Elsevier, pp. 193–203.

Burnstock, G. (1987). Mechanisms of interaction of peptide and nonpeptide vascular neurotransmitter systems. *J Cardiovasc Pharmacol*, **10**, (Suppl. 12), S74–S81.

Burnstock, G. (1988a). Local purinergic regulation of blood pressure. (The First John T. Shepherd Lecture), Vasodilatation: Vascular Smooth Muscle, Peptides, Autonomic Nerves, and Endothelium, edited by P.M. Vanhoutte, pp. 1–14. New York: Raven Press.

Burnstock, G. (1988b). Regulation of local blood flow by neurohumoral substances released from perivascular nerves and endothelial cells. *Acta Physiol Scand*, **133**, (Suppl. 571), 53–59.

Burnstock, G. (1989). Vascular control by purines with emphasis on the coronary system. *Eur Heart J*, **10**, 15–21.

Burnstock, G. (1990a). The Fifth Heymans Lecture, Ghent. Co-transmission. *Arch Int Pharmacodyn Ther*, **304**, 7–33.

Burnstock, G. (1990b). Local mechanisms of blood flow control by perivascular nerves and endothelium. *J Hypertens*, **8**, (Suppl. 7), S95–S106.

Burnstock, G. and Griffith, S.G. (eds.) (1988). Noradrenergic Innervation of Blood Vessels. Vol. I: pp. 1–49, Vol II: pp. 1–233. Boca Raton, FL: CRC Press.

Burnstock, G. and Kennedy, C. (1985). Is there a basis for distinguishing two types of P_2-purinoceptor? *Gen Pharmacol*, **16**, 433–440.

Burnstock, G., Lincoln, J., Fehér, E., Hopwood, A.M., Kirkpatrick, K., Milner, P., *et al.* (1988). Serotonin is localized in endothelial cells of coronary arteries and released during hypoxia: a possible new mechanism for hypoxia-induced vasodilatation of the rat heart. *Experientia*, **44**, 705–707.

Burnstock, G., Stewart-Lee, A.L., Brizzolara, A.L., Tomlinson, A. and Corr, L. (1991). Dual control by nerves and endothelial cells of arterial blood flow in atherosclerosis. Atherosclerotic Plaques, edited by R.W. Wissler, M.G. Bond, M. Mercuri and P. Tanganelli, pp. 285–92. New York: Plenum Press.

Burnstock, G. and Warland, J.J.I. (1987). A pharmacological study of the rabbit saphenous artery *in vitro*: a vessel with a large purinergic contractile response to sympathetic nerve stimulation. *Br J Pharmacol*, **90**, 111–120.

Busse, R., Förstermann, U., Matsuda, H. and Pohl, U. (1984). The role of prostaglandins in the endothelium-mediated vasodilatory response to hypoxia. *Pflügers Arch*, **401**, 77–83.

Busse, R., Pohl, U., Keller, C. and Klemm, U. (1983). Endothelial cells are involved in the vasodilatory response to hypoxia. *Pflügers Arch*, **397**, 78–80.

Cai, W.Q., Bodin, P., Sexton, A., Loesch, A. and Burnstock, G. (1992). Localization of neuropeptide Y and atrial natriuretic peptide in the endothelial cells of human umbilical vessels. *Cell Tissue Res*, **272**, 175–181.

Carvalho, M.H.C., Scivoletto, R., Fortes, Z.B., Nigro, D. and Cordellini, S. (1987). Reactivity of aorta and mesenteric microvessels to drugs in spontaneously hypertensive rats: role of the endothelium. *J Hypertens*, **5**, 377–382.

Cederqvist, B. and Gustafsson, L.E. (1994). Modulation of neuroeffector transmission in guinea-pig pulmonary artery and vas deferens by exogenous nitric oxide. *Acta Physiol Scand*, **150**, 75–81.

Cederqvist, B., Wiklund, N.P., Persson, M.G. and Gustafsson, L.E. (1991). Modulation of neuroeffector transmission in the guinea pig pulmonary artery by endogenous nitric oxide. *Neurosci Lett*, **127**, 67–69.

Chan-Palay, V. and Palay, S.L. (eds.) (1984). Co-existence of Neuroactive Substances in Neurones, pp. 433. New York: Wiley.

Chen, F.Y. and Lee, T.J. (1993). Role of nitric oxide in neurogenic vasodilation of porcine cerebral artery. *J Pharmacol Exp Ther*, **265**, 339–345.

Chen, G., Suzuki, H. and Weston, A.H. (1988). Acetylcholine releases endothelium-derived hyperpolarizing factor and EDRF from rat blood vessels. *Br J Pharmacol*, **95**, 1165–1174.

Cheung, D.W. and Fujioka, M. (1986). Inhibition of the excitatory junction potential in the guinea-pig saphenous artery by ANAPP₃. *Br J Pharmacol*, **89**, 3–5.

Cole, D.F., Bloom, S.R., Burnstock, G., Butler, J.M., McGregor, G.P., Saffrey, M.J., *et al.* (1983). Increase in SP-like immunoreactivity in nerve fibres of rabbit iris and ciliary body one to four months following sympathetic denervation. *Exp Eye Res*, **37**, 191–197.

Corr, L.A., Aberdeen, J.A., Milner, P., Lincoln, J. and Burnstock, G. (1990). Sympathetic and nonsympathetic neuropeptide Y-containing nerves in the rat myocardium and coronary arteries. *Circ Res*, **66**, 1602–1609.

Cowen, T., Haven, A.J., Wen-Qin, C., Gallen, D.D., Franc, F. and Burnstock, G. (1982). Development and ageing of perivascular adrenergic nerves in the rabbit. A quantitative fluorescence histochemical study using image analysis. *J Auton Nerv Syst*, **5**, 317–336.

Crowe, R., Lincoln, J., Blacklay, P.F., Pryor, J.P., Lumley, J.S.P. and Burnstock, G. (1983). Vasoactive intestinal polypeptide-like immunoreactive nerves in diabetic penis. A comparison between streptozotocin-treated rats and man. *Diabetes*, **32**, 1075–1077.

Cuello, A.C. (ed.) (1982). Co-transmission. Proc Symp 50th Anniversary Meet. Brit Pharmacol Soc, Oxford, edited by A.C. Cuello. pp. 264. London: Macmillan Press.

De Mey, J.G. and Vanhoutte, P.M. (1983). Anoxia and endothelium-dependent reactivity of the canine femoral artery. *J Physiol (Lond)*, **335**, 65–74.

De Nucci, G., Thomas, R., D'Orleans-Juste, P., Autunes, E., Walder, C., Warner, T.D., *et al.* (1988). Pressor effects of circulating endothelin are limited by its removal in the pulmonary circulation and by the release of prostacyclin and endothelium-derived relaxing factor. *Proc Natl Acad Sci USA*, **85**, 9797–9800.

De Tejada, I.S., Goldstein, I., Azadzoi, K., Krane, R.J. and Cohen, R.A. (1989). Impaired neurogenic and endothelium-mediated relaxation of penile smooth muscle from diabetic men with impotence. *N Engl J Med*, **320**, 1025–1030.

Dhall, U., Cowen, T., Haven, A.J. and Burnstock, G. (1988). Effect of oestrogen and progesterone on noradrenergic nerves and on nerves showing serotonin-like immunoreactivity in the basilar artery of the rabbit. *Brain Res*, **442**, 335–339.

Dhall, U., Cowen, T., Haven, A.J. and Burnstock, G. (1986). Perivascular noradrenergic and peptide-containing nerves show different patterns of changes during development and ageing in the guinea-pig. *J Auton Nerv Syst*, **16**, 109–126.

Dhital, K.K. and Burnstock, G. (1989). Adrenergic and non-adrenergic neural control of the arterial wall. Diseases of the Arterial Wall, edited by J.-P. Camilleri, C.L. Berry, J.-N. Fiessinger, J. Bariéty, pp. 97–126. London: Springer.

Dhital, K.K., Gerli, R., Lincoln, J., Milner, P., Tanganelli, P., Weber, G., *et al.* (1988). Increased density of perivascular nerves to the major cerebral vessels of the spontaneously hypertensive rat: differential changes in noradrenaline and neuropeptide Y during development. *Brain Res*, **444**, 33–45.

Dimitriadou, V., Aubineau, P., Taxi, J. and Seylaz, J. (1988). Ultrastructural changes in the cerebral artery wall induced by long-term sympathetic denervation. *Blood Vessels*, **25**, 122–143.

Dohi, Y., Thiel, M.A., Buhler, F.R. and Luscher, T.F. (1990). Activation of endothelial L-arginine pathway in resistance arteries. Effect of age and hypertension. *Hypertension*, **15**, 170–179.

Duckles, S.P. and Buck, S.M. (1982). Substance P in the cerebral vasculature: depletion by capsaicin suggests a sensory role. *Brain Res*, **245**, 171–174.

Dun, N.J., Dun, S.L., Wu, S.Y. and Förstermann, U. (1993). Nitric oxide synthase in rat superior cervical ganglia and adrenal glands. *Neurosci Lett*, **158**, 51–54.

Durante, W., Sen, A.K. and Sunahara, F.A. (1988). Impairment of endothelium-dependent relaxation in aortae from spontaneously diabetic rats. *Br J Pharmacol*, **94**, 463–468.

Esler, M., Jennings, G., Korner, P., Willett, I., Dudley, F., Hasking, G., *et al.* (1988). Assessment of human sympathetic nervous system activity from measurements of norepinephrine turnover. *Hypertension*, **11**, 3–20.

Estrada, C., Mengual, E., Gonzalez, C. (1993). Local NADPH-diaphorase neurons innervate pial arteries and lie close or project to intracerebral blood vessels: a possible role for nitric oxide in the regulation of cerebral blood flow. *J Cereb Blood Flow Metab*, **13**, 978–984.

Evans, R.J. and Surprenant, A. (1992). Vasoconstriction of guinea-pig submucosal arterioles following sympathetic nerve stimulation is mediated by the release of ATP. *Br J Pharmacol*, **106**, 242–249.

Feletou, M. and Vanhoutte, P.M. (1988). Endothelium-dependent hyperpolarization of canine coronary smooth muscle. *Br J Pharmacol*, **93**, 515–524.

Fischer, A., Mundel, P., Mayer, B., Preissler, U., Philippin, B. and Kummer, W. (1993). Nitric oxide synthase in guinea pig lower airway innervation. *Neuroscience*, **149**, 157–160.

Flavahan, N.A. and Vanhoutte, P. (1986). Sympathetic purinergic vasoconstriction and thermosensitivity in a canine cutaneous vein. *J Pharmacol Exp Ther*, **239**, 784–789.

Flugel, C., Tamm, E.R., Mayer, B. and Lutjen-Drecoll, E. (1994). Species differences in choroidal vasoactive innervation: evidence for specific intrinsic nitrergic and VIP-positive neurons in the human eye. *Invest Ophthalmol Vis Sci*, **35**, 592–599.

Förstermann, U., Mugge, A., Alheid, U., Haverich, A. and Frolich, J.C. (1988). Selective attenuation of endothelium-mediated vasodilation in atherosclerotic human coronary arteries. *Circ Res*, **62**, 185–190.

Fozard, J.R. and Part, M.-L. (1992). The role of nitric oxide in the regional vasodilator effects of endothelin-1 in the rat. *Br J Pharmacol*, **105**, 744–750.

Franco-Cereceda, A., Henke, H., Lundberg, J.M., Petermann, J.B., Hökfelt, T. and Fischer, J.A. (1987). Calcitonin gene-related peptide (CGRP) in capsaicin-sensitive substance P-immunoreactive sensory neurons in animals and man: Distribution and release by capsaicin. *Peptides*, **8**, 399–410.

Frangos, J.A., Eskin, S.G., McIntire, L.V. and Ives, C.L. (1985). Flow effects on prostacyclin production by cultured human endothelial cells. *Science*, **227**, 1477–1479.

Freiman, P.C., Mitchell, G.C., Heistad, D.D., Armstrong, M.L. and Harrison, D.G. (1986). Atherosclerosis impairs endothelium-dependent vascular relaxation to acetylcholine and thrombin in primates. *Circ Res*, **58**, 783–789.

Fukuda, N., Izumi, Y., Soma, M., Watanabe, Y., Watanabe, M., Hatano, M., *et al.* (1990). L-N^G-Monomethyl arginine inhibits the vasodilating effects of low dose of endothelin-3 on rat mesenteric arteries. *Biochem Biophys Res Commun*, **167**, 739–745.

Furchgott, R.F., Khan, M.T. and Jothianandan, D. (1987). Comparison of endothelium dependent relaxation and nitric oxide induced relaxation in rabbit aorta. *Fed Proc* (Abstr), **46**, 385.

Furchgott, R.F. and Zawadzki, J.V. (1980). The obligatory role of endothelial cells in the relaxation of arterial smooth muscle by acetylcholine. *Nature*, **288**, 373–376.

Furchgott, R.F. (1984). Role of endothelium in responses of vascular smooth muscle. Frontiers in Physiological Research, edited by D.G. Garlick and P.I. Korner, pp. 116–133. Cambridge: Cambridge University Press.

Furness, J.B. and Costa, M. (1987). The Enteric Nervous System. Edinburgh: Churchill Livingstone.

Furness, J.B., Papka, R.E., Della, N.G., Costa, M. and Eskay, R.L. (1982). Substance P-like immunoreactivity in nerves associated with the vascular system of guinea-pigs. *Neuroscience*, **7**, 447–459.

Fyffe, R.E.W. and Perl, E.R. (1984). Is ATP a central synaptic mediator for certain primary afferent fibres from mammalian skin? *Proc Natl Acad Sci USA*, **81**, 6890–6893.

Gamse, R. and Saria, A. (1985). Potentiation of tachykinin-induced protein extravasation by calcitonin gene-related peptide. *Eur J Pharmacol*, **114**, 61–66 .

Gardiner, S.M., Compton, A.M., Bennett, T., Palmer, R.M. and Moncada, S. (1989). N^G-monomethyl-L-arginine does not inhibit the hindquarters vasodilator action of endothelin-1 in conscious rats. *Eur J Pharmacol*, **171**, 237–240.

Gibbins, I.L., Furness, J.B., Costa, M., MacIntyre, I., Hillyard, C.J. and Girgis, S. (1985). Co-localization of calcitonin gene-related peptide-like immunoreactivity with substance P in cutaneous, vascular and visceral sensory neurons of guinea-pigs. *Neurosci Lett*, **57**, 125–130.

Gibbins, I.L., Furness, J.B. and Costa, M. (1987). Pathway-specific patterns of coexistence of substance P, calcitonin gene-related peptide, cholecystokinin and dynorphin in neurons of the dorsal root ganglia of the guinea-pig. *Cell Tissue Res*, **248**, 417–437.

Gibbins, I.L. and Morris, J.L. (1988). Co-existence of immunoreactivity to neuropeptide Y and vasoactive intestinal polypeptide in non-adrenergic axons innervating guinea-pig cerebral arteries after sympathectomy. *Brain Res*, **444**, 402–406.

Gibbins, I.L. and Morris, J.L. (1990). Sympathetic noradrenergic neurons containing dynorphin but not neuropeptide Y innervate small cutaneous blood vessels of guinea-pigs. *J Auton Nerv Syst*, **29**, 137–150.

Gonzalez, C. and Estrada, C. (1991). Nitric oxide mediates the neurogenic vasodilation of bovine cerebral arteries. *J Cereb Blood Flow Metab*, **11**, 366–370.

González, C., Martin, C., Hamel, E., Galea, E., Gómez, B., Lluch, S., *et al.* (1990). Endothelial cells inhibit the vascular response to adrenergic nerve stimulation by a receptor-mediated mechanism. *Can J Physiol Pharmacol*, **68**, 104–109.

Gordon, J.F., Baird, M., Daly, C.J. and McGrath, J.C. (1992). Endogenous nitric oxide modulates sympathetic neuroeffector transmission in the isolated rabbit lateral saphenous vein. *J Cardiovasc Pharmacol*, **20**, S68–S71.

Grabowski, E.F., Jaffe, E.F. and Weksler, B.B. (1985). Prostacyclin production by cultured endothelial cell monolayers exposed to step increases in shear stress. *J Lab Clin Med*, **105**, 36–43.

Greenberg, S., Diecke, F.P.J., Peevy, K. and Tanaka, T.P. (1989). The endothelium modulates adrenergic neurotransmission to canine pulmonary arteries and veins. *Eur J Pharmacol*, **162**, 67–80.

Griffith, S.G. and Burnstock, G. (1983). Immunohistochemical demonstration of serotonin in nerves supplying human cerebral and mesenteric blood vessels: some speculations about their involvement in vascular disorders. *Lancet*, **i**, 561–562.

Guerra, R., Brotherton, A.F.A., Goodwin, P.J., Clark, C.R., Armstrong, M.L. and Harrison, D.G. (1989). Mechanisms of abnormal endothelium-dependent vascular relaxation in atherosclerosis: Implications for altered autocrine and paracrine functions of EDRF. *Blood Vessels*, **26**, 300–314.

Gulbenkian, S., Merighi, A., Wharton, J., Varndell, I.M. and Polak, J.M. (1986). Ultrastructural evidence for the coexistence of calcitonin gene-related peptide and substance P in secretory vesicles of peripheral nerves in the guinea pig. *J Neurocytol*, **15**, 535–542.

Haegerstrand, A., Dalsgaard, C.-J., Jonzon, B., Larsson, O. and Nilsson, J. (1990). Calcitonin gene-related peptide stimulates proliferation of human endothelial cells. *Proc Natl Acad Sci USA*, **87**, 3299–3303.

Harrison, D.G., Armstrong, M.L., Freiman, P.C. and Heistad, D.D. (1987). Restoration of endothelium-dependent relaxation by dietary lipid treatment of atherosclerosis. *J Clin Invest*, **80**, 1808–1811.

Hart, J.L., Freas, W., McKenzie, J.E. and Muldoon, S.M. (1988). Adrenergic nerve function and contractile activity of the caudal artery of the streptozotocin diabetic rat. *J Auton Nerv Syst*, **25**, 49–57.

Hassall, C.J.S. and Burnstock, G. (1986). Intrinsic neurones and associated cells of the guinea-pig heart in culture. *Brain Res*, **364**, 102–113.

Hassall, C.J.S. and Burnstock, G. (1984). Neuropeptide Y-like immunoreactivity in cultured intrinsic neurones of the heart. *Neurosci Lett*, **52**, 111–115.

Hassall, C.J.S., Saffrey, M.J., Belai, A., Hoyle, C.H.V., Moules, E.W., Moss, J., *et al.* (1992). Nitric oxide synthase immunoreactivity and NADPH-diaphorase activity in a subpopulation of intrinsic neurones of the guinea pig heart. *Neurosci Lett*, **143**, 65–68.

Hasunuma, K., Rodman, D.M., O'Brien, R.F. and McMurtry, I.F. (1990). Endothelin-1 causes pulmonary vasodilation in rats. *Am J Physiol*, **259**, H48–H54.

Head, R.J. (1989). Hypernoradrenergic innervation: its relationship to functional and hyperplastic changes in the vasculature of the spontaneously hypertensive rat. *Blood Vessels*, **26**, 1–20.

Helme, R.D. and McKernan, S. (1985). Neurogenic responses following topical application of capsaicin in man. *Ann Neurol*, **18**, 505–509.

Hollis, T.M. and Rosen, R.A. (1972). Histidine decarboxylase activities of bovine aortic endothelium and intima-media. *Proc Soc Exp Biol Med*, **141**, 978–981.

Holtz, J., Förstermann, U., Pohl, U., Giesler, M. and Bassenge, E. (1984). Flow-dependent, endothelium-mediated dilation of epicardial coronary arteries in conscious dogs: effects of cyclo-oxygenase inhibition. *J Cardiovasc Pharmacol*, **6**, 1161–1169.

Hökfelt, T., Fuxe, K. and Pernow, B. (eds.) (1986). Coexistence of Neuronal Messengers: A New Principle in Chemical Transmission. Progress in Brain Research, Vol 68, Amsterdam: Elsevier.

Hudlická, O. (1984). Development of microcirculation: capillary growth and adaptation. In Handbook of Physiology — The Cardiovascular System, Vol IV, 165th Ed, pp. 165–216. Bethesda: American Physiological Society.

Hull, S.S. Jr, Kaiser, L., Jaffe, M.D. and Sparks, H.V. (1986). Endothelium-dependent flow-induced dilation of canine femoral and saphenous arteries. *Blood Vessels*, **23**, 183–198.

Hung, K.-S., McKenzie, J.C., Mattioli, L., Klein, R.M., Menon, C.D. and Poulose, A.K. (1986). Scanning electron microscopy of pulmonary vascular endothelium in rats with hypoxia-induced hypertension. *Acta Anat*, **126**, 13–20.

Hynes, M.R. and Duckles, S.P. (1987). Effect of age on the endothelium-mediated relaxation of rat blood vessels *in vitro*. *J Pharmacol Exp Ther*, **241**, 387–392.

Iadecola, C., Beitz, A.J., Renno, W., Xu, X., Mayer, B. and Zhang, F. (1993). Nitric oxide synthase-containing neural processes on large cerebral arteries and cerebral microvessels. *Brain Res*, **606**, 148–155.

Ignarro, L.J., Bush, P.A., Buga, G.M., Wood, K.S., Fukoto, J.M. and Rajfer, J. (1990). Nitric oxide and cyclic GMP formation upon electrical field stimulation cause relaxation of corpus cavernosum smooth muscle. *Biochem Biophys Res Commun*, **170**, 843–850.

Ignarro, L.J., Byrns, R.E., Buga, G.M. and Wood, K.S. (1987). Endothelium-derived relaxing factor from pulmonary artery and vein possess pharmacologic and chemical properties identical to those of nitric oxide radical. *Circ Res*, **61**, 866–879.

Illes, P., Rickmann, H., Brod, I., Bucher, I. and Stoclet, J.-C. (1989). Subsensitivity of presynaptic adenosine A_1-receptors in caudal arteries of spontaneously hypertensive rats. *Eur J Pharmacol*, **174**, 237–251.

Ishikawa, S. (1985). Actions of ATP and α,β-methylene ATP on neuromuscular transmission and smooth muscle membrane of the rabbit and guinea-pig mesenteric arteries. *Br J Pharmacol*, **86**, 777–787.

Jackowski, A., Crockard, A. and Burnstock, G. (1989). 5-Hydroxytryptamine demonstrated immunohistochemically in rat cerebrovascular nerves largely represents 5-hydroxytryptamine uptake into sympathetic nerve fibres. *Neuroscience*, **29**, 453–462.

Jahr, C.E. and Jessel, T.M. (1983). ATP excites a subpopulation of rat dorsal horn neurones. *Nature*, **304**, 730–733.

Jarrett, R.J., Keen, H. and Chakrabarti, R. (1982). Diabetes, hyperglycemia and arterial disease. Complications of Diabetes, edited by H. Keen and R.J. Jarrett, pp. 179–204. London: Arnold.

Johnson, T.S., Young, J.B. and Landsberg, L. (1983). Sympathoadrenal responses to acute and chronic hypoxia in the rat. *J Clin Invest*, **71**, 1263–1272.

Kalsner, S. (1977). The effect of hypoxia on prostaglandin output and on tone in isolated coronary arteries. *Can J Physiol Pharmacol*, **55**, 882–887.

Kamata, K., Miyata, N. and Kasuya, Y. (1989). Impairment of endothelium-dependent relaxation and changes in levels of cyclic GMP in aorta from streptozotocin-induced diabetic rats. *Br J Pharmacol*, **97**, 614–618.

Kamikawa, Y., Cline, W.H. and Su, C. (1980). Diminished purinergic modulation of the vascular adrenergic neurotransmission in spontaneously hypertensive rats. *Eur J Pharmacol*, **66**, 347–353.

Karanth, S.S., Springall, D.R., Francavilla, S., Mirrlees, D.J. and Polak, J.M. (1990). Early increase in CGRP- and VIP-immunoreactive nerves in the skin of streptozotocin-induced diabetic rats. *Histochemistry*, **94**, 659–666.

Kars, H.Z., Utkan, T., Sarioglu, Y. and Yaradanakul, V. (1993). Selective inhibition of endothelium-dependent relaxation by sympathectomy in rabbit carotid artery rings *in vitro*. *Methods Find Exp Clin Pharmacol*, **15**, 35–40.

Katsuragi, T. and Su, C. (1982). Augmentation by theophylline of [^{3}H]purine release from vascular adrenergic nerves: evidence for presynaptic autoinhibition. *J Pharmacol Exp Ther*, **220**, 152–156.

Katusic, Z.S., Shepherd, J.T. and Vanhoutte, P.M. (1987a). Potassium-induced endothelium-dependent rhythmic activity in the canine basilar artery. *J Cardiovasc Pharmacol*, **12**, 37–41.

Katusic, Z.S., Shepherd, J.T. and Vanhoutte, P.M. (1987b). Endothelium-dependent contraction to stretch in canine basilar arteries. *Am J Physiol*, **252**, H671–673.

Kawasaki, H., Takasaki, K., Saito, A. and Goto, K. (1988). Calcitonin gene-related peptide acts as a novel vasodilator transmitter in mesenteric resistance vessels of the rat. *Nature*, **335**, 164–167.

Kawasaki, H., Chikako, N., Saito, A. and Takasaki, K. (1991). NPY modulates neurotransmission of CGRP-containing vasodilator nerves in rat mesenteric arteries. *Am J Physiol*, **261**, H683–690.

Kawasaki, H., Nuki, C., Saito, A. and Takasaki, K. (1990a). Adrenergic modulation of calcitonin gene-related peptide (CGRP)-containing nerve-mediated vasodilation in the rat mesenteric resistance vessel. *Brain Res*, **506**, 287–290.

Kawasaki, H., Nuki, C., Saito, A., and Takasaki, K. (1990b). Role of calcitonin gene-related peptide-containing nerves in the vascular adrenergic transmission. *J Pharmacol Exp Ther*, **252**, 403–409.

Kawasaki, H., Saito, A. and Takasaki, K. (1990a). Age-related decrease of calcitonin gene-related peptide-containing vasodilator innervation in the mesenteric resistance vessel of the spontaneously hypertensive rat. *Circ Res*, **67**, 733–743.

Kawasaki, H., Saito, A. and Takasaki, K. (1990b). Changes in calcitonin gene-related peptide (CGRP)-containing vasodilator nerve activity in hypertension. *Brain Res*, **518**, 303–307.

Keast, J.R. (1992). A possible source of nitric oxide in the penis. *Neurosci Lett*, **143**, 69–73.

Keefe, K.D., Pasco, J.S. and Eckman, D.M. (1992). Purinergic relaxation and hyperpolarization in guinea pig and rabbit coronary artery: role of the endothelium. *J Pharmacol Exp Ther*, **260**, 592–600.

Kennedy, C. and Burnstock, G. (1986). ATP causes postjunctional potentiation of noradrenergic contractions in the portal vein of guinea pig and rat. *J Pharm Pharmacol*, **38**, 307–309.

Kennedy, C. and Burnstock, G. (1985). ATP produces vasodilation via P_1 purinoceptors and vasoconstriction via P_2 purinoceptors in the isolated rabbit central ear artery. *Blood Vessels*, **22**, 145–155.

Kennedy, C., Delbro, D. and Burnstock, G. (1985). P_2-purinoceptors mediate both vasodilatation (via the endothelium) and vasoconstriction of the isolated rat femoral artery. *Eur J Pharmacol*, **107**, 161–168.

Kennedy, C., Saville, V.L. and Burnstock, G. (1986). The contributions of noradrenaline and ATP to the responses of the rabbit central ear artery to sympathetic nerve stimulation depend on the parameters of stimulation. *Eur J Pharmacol*, **122**, 291–300.

Kiff, R.J., Gardiner, S.M., Compton, A.M. and Bennett, T. (1991). Selective impairment of hindquarters vasodilator responses to bradykinin in conscious Wistar rats with streptozotocin-induced diabetes mellitus. *Br J Pharmacol*, **103**, 1357–1362.

Kifor, I. and Dzau, V.J. (1987). Endothelial renin-angiotensin pathway: evidence for intracellular synthesis and secretion of angiotensin. *Circ Res*, **60**, 422–428.

Kim, N., Azadzoi, K.M., Goldstein, I. and de Tejada, I.S. (1991). A nitric oxide-like factor mediates non-adrenergic non-cholinergic relaxation of penile corpus cavernosum smooth muscle. *J Clin Invest*, **88**, 112–118.

Klimaschewski, L., Kummer, W., Mayer, B., Couraud, J.Y., Preissler, U., Philippin, B., *et al.* (1992). Nitric oxide synthase in cardiac nerve fibers and neurons of rat and guinea pig heart. *Circ Res*, **71**, 1533–1537.

Krishtal, O.A., Marchenko, S.M. and Obukhov, A.G. (1988). Cationic channels activated by extracellular ATP in rat sensory neurons. *Neuroscience*, **27**, 995–1000.

Kubo, T. and Su, C. (1983). Effects of adenosine on [^{3}H]norepinephrine release from perfused mesenteric arteries of SHR and renal hypertensive rats. *Eur J Pharmacol*, **87**, 349–352.

Kummer, W., Fischer, A., Mundel, P., Mayer, B., Hoba, B., Philippin, B., *et al.* (1992). Nitric oxide synthase in VIP-containing vasodilator nerve fibres in the guinea-pig. *Neuroreport*, **3**, 653–655.

Kupfermann, I. (1991). Functional studies of cotransmission. *Physiol Rev*, **71**, 683–732.

La, M. and Rand, M.J. (1993). Endothelin-1 enhances vasoconstrictor responses to exogenously administered and neurogenically released ATP in rabbit isolated perfused arteries. *Eur J Pharmacol*, **249**, 133–139.

Lagnado, M.L.J., Crowe, R., Lincoln, J. and Burnstock, G. (1987). Reduction of nerves containing vasoactive intestinal polypeptide and serotonin, but not neuropeptide Y and catecholamine, in cerebral blood vessels of the 8-week streptozotocin-induced diabetic rat. *Blood Vessels*, **24**, 169–180.

Lansman, J.B., Hallam, T.J. and Rink, T.J. (1987). Single stretch-activated ion channels in vascular endothelial cells as mechanotransducers? *Nature*, **325**, 811–813.

Lawrence, E. and Brain, S.D. (1992). Responses to endothelins in the rat cutaneous microvasculature: a modulatory role of locally-produced nitric oxide. *Br J Pharmacol*, **106**, 733–738.

Leblanc, G.C., Trimmer, B.A. and Landis, S.C. (1987). Neuropeptide Y-like immunoreactivity in rat cranial parasympathetic neurons: coexistence with vasoactive intestinal peptide and choline acetyltransferase. *Proc Natl Acad Sci USA*, **84**, 3511–3515.

Leblanc, G.G. and Landis, S.C. (1988). Target specificity of neuropeptide Y-immunoreactive cranial parasympathetic neurones. *J Neurosci*, **8**, 146–155.

Lee, T.J.-F. and Sarwinski, S.J. (1991). Nitric oxidergic neurogenic vasodilation in the porcine basilar artery. *Blood Vessels*, **28**, 407–412.

Lee, R.M.K.W., Nagahama, M., McKenzie, R. and Daniel, E.E. (1988). Peptide-containing nerves around blood vessels of stroke-prone spontaneously hypertensive rats. *Hypertension*, **11**, I117–120.

Lee, Y., Takami, K., Kawai, Y., Girgis, S., Hillyard, C.J., MacIntyre, I., *et al.* (1985). Distribution of calcitonin gene-related peptide in the rat peripheral nervous system with special reference to coexistence with substance P. *Neuroscience*, **15**, 1227–1237.

Li, Y. and Duckles, S.P. (1991). Differential effects of neuropeptide Y and opioids on neurogenic responses of the perfused rat mesentery. *Eur J Pharmacol*, **195**, 365–372.

Li, Y.J. and Duckles, S.P. (1992). Effect of endothelium on the actions of sympathetic and sensory nerves in the perfused rat mesentery. *Eur J Pharmacol*, **210**, 23–30.

Li, Y. and Duckles, S.P. (1993). Effect of age on vascular content of calcitonin gene-related peptide and mesenteric vasodilator nerve activity in the rat. *Eur J Pharmacol*, **236**, 373–378.

Li, Y.J., Yu, X.J. and Deng, H.W. (1993). Nitric oxide modulates responses to sensory nerve activation of the perfused rat mesentery. *Eur J Pharmacol*, **239**, 127–132.

Lichtor, T., Davis, H.R., Johns, L., Vesselinovitch, D., Wisler, R.W. and Mullan, S. (1987). The sympathetic nervous system and atherosclerosis. *J Neurosurg*, **67**, 906–914.

Lincoln, J., Crowe, R., Blacklay, P.F., Pryor, J.P., Lumley, J.S.P. and Burnstock, G. (1987). Changes in the VIPergic, cholinergic and adrenergic innervation of human penile tissue in diabetic and non-diabetic impotent males. *J Urol*, **137**, 1053–1059.

Lincoln, J., Loesch, A. and Burnstock, G. (1990). Localization of vasopressin, serotonin and angiotensin II in endothelial cells of the renal and mesenteric arteries of the rat. *Cell Tissue Res*, **259**, 341–344.

Linnik, M.D. and Moskowitz, M.A. (1989). Identification of immunoreactive substance P in human and other mammalian endothelial cells. *Peptides*, **10**, 957–962 .

Liu, X., Gillespie, J.S. and Martin, W. (1991). Effects of N^G-substituted analogues of L-arginine on NANC relaxation of the rat anococcygeus and bovine retractor penis muscles and the bovine penile artery. *Br J Pharmacol*, **104**, 53–58.

Loesch, A., Bodin, P. and Burnstock, G. (1991). Colocalization of endothelin, vasopressin and serotonin in cultured endothelial cells of rabbit aorta. *Peptides*, **12**, 1095–1103.

Loesch, A. and Burnstock, G. (1988). Ultrastructural localisation of serotonin and substance P in vascular endothelial cells of rat femoral and mesenteric arteries. *Anat Embryol*, **178**, 137–142.

Loesch, A., Maynard, K.I. and Burnstock, G. (1992). CGRP- and NPY-like immunoreactivity in endothelial cells after long-term stimulation of perivascular nerves. *Neuroscience*, **48**, 723–736.

Loesch, A., Tomlinson, A. and Burnstock, G. (1991). Localization of arginine-vasopressin in endothelial cells of rat pulmonary artery. *Anat Embryol*, **183**, 129–134.

Lundberg, J.M., Rudehill, A., Sollevi, A., Theodorsson-Norheim, E. and Hamberger, B. (1986). Frequency- and reserpine-dependent chemical coding of sympathetic transmission. Differential release of noradrenaline and neuropeptide Y from pig spleen. *Neurosci Lett*, **63**, 96–100.

Lundberg, J.M., Ånggård, A., Theodorsson-Norheim, E. and Pernow, J. (1984a). Guanethidine-sensitive release of neuropeptide Y-like immunoreactivity in the cat spleen by sympathetic nerve stimulation. *Neurosci Lett*, **52**, 175–180.

Lundberg, J.M., Fahrenkrug, J., Larsson, O. and Ånggård, A. (1984b). Corelease of vasoactive intestinal polypeptide and peptide histidine isoleucine in relation to atropine resistant vasodilatation in cat submandibular salivary gland. *Neurosci Lett*, **52**, 37–45.

Lundberg, J.M., Franco-Cereceda, A., Hua, X., Hökfelt, T. and Fischer, J.A. (1985). Coexistence of substance P and calcitonin gene-related peptide-like immunoreactivities in sensory nerves in relation to cardiovascular and bronchoconstrictor effects of capsaicin. *Eur J Pharmacol*, **108**, 315–319.

Lundberg, J.M., Terenius, L., Hökfelt, T. and Goldstein, M. (1983). High levels of neuropeptide Y in peripheral noradrenergic neurons in various mammals including man. *Neurosci Lett*, **42**, 167–172.

Lundberg, J.M. (1981). Evidence for coexistence of vasoactive intestinal polypeptide (VIP) and acetylcholine in neurons of cat exocrine glands. Morphological, biochemical and functional studies. *Acta Physiol Scand*, **112**, (Suppl. 496), 1–57.

Lüscher, T.F. (1988). Endothelial Vasoactive Substances and Cardiovascular Disease. Basel: Karger.

Machalay, M., Dalziel, H.H. and Sneddon, P. (1988). Evidence for ATP as a cotransmitter in dog mesenteric artery. *Eur J Pharmacol*, **147**, 83–91.

MacKenzie, I., Manzini, S. and Burnstock, G. (1988). Regulation of voltage-dependent excitatory responses to α,β-methylene ATP, ATP and non-adrenergic nerve stimulation by dihydropyridines in the guinea-pig vas deferens. *Neuroscience*, **27**, 317–332.

MacLean, M.R., McCulloch, K.M., MacMillan, J.B. and McGrath, J.C. (1993). Influences of the endothelium and hypoxia on neurogenic transmission in the isolated pulmonary artery of the rabbit. *Br J Pharmacol*, **108**, 150–154.

Maggi, C.A. and Meli, A. (1988). The sensory-efferent function of capsaicin-sensitive sensory nerves. *Gen Pharmacol*, **19**, 1–43.

Mangiarua, E.I. and Bevan, R.D. (1986). Altered endothelium-mediated relaxation after denervation of growing rabbit ear artery. *Eur J Pharmacol*, **122**, 149–152.

Mangiarua, E.I. and Lee, R.M.K.W. (1989). Increased sympathetic innervation in the cerebral and mesenteric arteries of hypertensive rats. *Can J Physiol Pharmacol*, **68**, 492–499.

Mayhan, W.G. (1989). Impairment of endothelium-dependent dilatation of cerebral arterioles during diabetes mellitus. *Am J Physiol*, **256**, H621–H625.

Mayhan, W.G. (1992). Impairment of endothelium-dependent dilatation of the basilar artery during diabetes mellitus. *Brain Res*, **580**, 297–302.

Mayhan, W.G., Faraci, F.M., Baumbach, G.L. and Heistad, D.D. (1990). Effects of aging on responses of cerebral arterioles. *Am J Physiol*, **258**, H1138–H1143.

Maynard, K.I., Loesch, A. and Burnstock, G. (1992). Changes in purinergic responses of the rabbit isolated central ear artery after chronic electrical stimulation *in vivo*. *Br J Pharmacol*, **107**, 833–836.

Meraji, S., Jayakody, L., Senaratne, M.P.J., Thompson, A.B.R. and Kappadoga, T. (1987). Endothelium-dependent relaxation in aorta of BB rat. *Diabetes*, **36**, 978–981.

Meyrick, B. and Reid, L. (1978). The effect of continued hypoxia on rat pulmonary arterial circulation. An ultrastructural study. *Lab Invest*, **38**, 188–200.

Miller, M.E. and Scott, T.M. (1990). The effect of perivascular denervation on endothelium-dependent relaxation to acetylcholine. *Artery*, **17**, 233–247.

Milner, P., Bodin, P., Loesch, A. and Burnstock, G. (1992). Increased shear stress leads to differential release of endothelin and ATP from isolated endothelial cells from 4- and 12-month-old male rabbit aorta. *J Vasc Res*, **29**, 420–425.

Milner, P., Bodin, P., Loesch, A. and Burnstock, G. (1990a). Endothelin and ATP but not vasopressin are released from isolated aortic endothelial cells exposed to increased flow. *Biochem Biophys Res Commun*, **170**, 649–656.

Milner, P., Bodin, P., Loesch, A. and Burnstock, G. (1995). Interactions between sensory perivascular nerves and the endothelium in brain microvessels. *Int J Microcirc*, **15**, 1–9.

Milner, P., Kirkpatrick, K., Ralevic, V., Toothill, V., Pearson, J.D. and Burnstock, G. (1990b). Endothelial cells cultured from human umbilical vein release ATP, Substance P and acetylcholine in response to altered shear stress. *Proc R Soc Lond B*, **241**, 245–248.

Milner, P., Ralevic, V., Hopwood, A.M., Fehér, E., Lincoln, J., Kirkpatrick, K.A., *et al.* (1989). Ultrastructural localisation of substance P and choline acetyltransferase in endothelial cells of rat coronary artery and release of substance P and acetylcholine during hypoxia. *Experientia*, **45**, 121–125.

Minami, Y., Kimura, H., Aimi, Y. and Vincent, S.R. (1994). Projections of nitric oxide synthase-containing fibers from the sphenopalatine ganglion to cerebral arteries in the rat. *Neuroscience*, **60**, 745–759.

Mione, M.C., Cavallotti, C., Burnstock, G. and Amenta, F. (1988). The peptidergic innervation of the guinea pig uterine artery in pregnancy. *Basic Appl Histochem*, **32**, 153–159.

Mione, M.C., Dhital, K.K., Amenta, F. and Burnstock, G. (1988). An increase in the expression of neuropeptidergic vasodilator, but not vasoconstrictor, cerebrovascular nerves in aging rats. *Brain Res*, **460**, 103–113.

Mione, M.C., Ralevic, V. and Burnstock, G. (1990). Peptides and vasomotor mechanisms. *Pharmacol Ther*, **46**, 429–468.

Miyata, N., Tsuchida, K., Okuyama, S., Otomo, S., Kamata, K. and Kasuya, Y. (1992). Age-related changes in endothelium-dependent relaxation in aorta from genetically diabetic WBN/Kob rats. *Am J Physiol*, **262**, H1104–H1109.

Miyauchi, T., Ishikawa, T., Tomobe, Y., Yanagisawa, M., Kimura, S., Sugishita, Y., *et al.* (1989). Characteristics of pressor response to endothelin in spontaneously hypertensive and Wistar Kyoto rats. *Hypertension*, **14**, 427–434.

Modin, A. (1994). Non-adrenergic, non-cholinergic vascular control with reference to neuropeptide Y, vasoactive intestinal polypeptide and nitric oxide. *Acta Physiol Scand Suppl*, **622**, 1–74.

Morita-Tsuzuki, Y., Hardebo, J.E. and Bouskela, E. (1993). Inhibition of nitric oxide synthase attenuates the cerebral blood flow response to stimulation of postganglionic parasympathetic nerves in the rat. *J Cereb Blood Flow Metab*, **13**, 993–997.

Morris, J.L. (1993). Co-transmission from autonomic vasodilator neurons supplying the guinea-pig uterine artery. *J Auton Nerv Syst*, **42**, 11–21.

Morris, R., Southam, E., Gittins, S.R. and Garthwaite, J. (1993). NADPH-diaphorase staining in autonomic and somatic cranial ganglia of the rat. *Neuroreport*, **4**, 62–64.

Muir, T.C. and Wardle, K.A. (1988). The electrical and mechanical basis of co-transmission in some vascular and non-vascular smooth muscles. *J Auton Pharmacol*, **8**, 203–218.

Muramatsu, I. and Kigoshi, S. (1987). Purinergic and non-purinergic innervation in the cerebral arteries of the dog. *Br J Pharmacol*, **92**, 901–908.

Muramatsu, I. (1992). Evidence for sympathetic, purinergic transmission in the mesenteric artery of the dog. *Br J Pharmacol*, **87**, 478–480.

Namiki, A., Hirata, Y., Ishikawa, M., Moroi, M., Aikawa, J. and Machii, K. (1992). Endothelin-1- and endothelin-3-induced vasorelaxation via common generation of endothelium-derived nitric oxide. *Life Sci*, **50**, 677–682.

Nozaki, K., Moskowitz, M.A., Maynard, K.I., Koketsu, N., Dawson, T.M., Bredt, D.S., *et al.* (1993). Possible origins and distribution of immunoreactive nitric oxide synthase-containing nerve fibres in cerebral arteries. *J Cereb Blood Flow Metab*, **13**, 70–79.

Osborne, N.N. (1983). Dale's Principle and Communication between Neurones, pp. 204. Oxford: Pergamon Press.

Oyama, Y., Kawasaki, H., Hattori, Y. and Kanno, M. (1986). Attenuation of endothelium-dependent relaxation in aorta from diabetic rats. *Eur J Pharmacol*, **131**, 75–78.

Paddle, B.M. and Burnstock, G. (1974). Release of ATP from perfused heart during coronary vasodilatation. *Blood Vessels*, **11**, 110–119.

Palmer, R.M.J., Ferrige, A.G. and Moncada, S. (1987). Nitric oxide release accounts for the biological activity of endothelium-derived relaxing factor. *Nature*, **327**, 524–526.

Parkhouse, N. and LeQuesne, P.M. (1988). Impaired neurogenic vascular response in patients with diabetes and neuropathic foot lesions. *New Engl J Med*, **318**, 1306–1309.

Parnavelas, J.G., Kelly, W. and Burnstock, G. (1985). Ultrastructural localization of choline acetyltransferase in vascular endothelial cells in rat brain. *Nature*, **316**, 724–725.

Pernow, J., Saria, A. and Lundberg, J.M. (1986). Mechanisms underlying pre- and postjunctional effects of neuropeptide Y in sympathetic vascular control. *Acta Physiol Scand*, **126**, 239–249.

Perreault, T. and De Marte, J. (1991). Endothelin-1 has a dilator effect on neonatal pig pulmonary vasculature. *J Cardiovasc Pharmacol*, **18**, 45–50.

Pickard, R.S., Powell, P.H. and Zar, M.A. (1991). The effect of inhibitors of nitric oxide biosynthesis and cyclic GMP formation on nerve-evoked relaxation of human cavernosal smooth muscle. *Br J Pharmacol*, **104**, 755–759.

Pieper, G.M. and Gross, G.J. (1989). Selective impairment of endothelium-dependent relaxation by oxygen-derived free radicals. *Blood Vessels*, **26**, 44–47.

Rabinovitch, M., Gamble, W.J., Miettinen, O.S. and Reid, L. (1981). Age and sex influence on pulmonary hypertension of chronic hypoxia and on recovery. *Am J Physiol*, **240**, H62–72.

Rajfer, J., Aronson, W.J., Bush, P.A., Dorey, F.F.J. and Ignarro, L.J. (1992). Nitric oxide as a mediator of nonadrenergic, noncholinergic neurotransmission. *N Engl J Med*, **326**, 90–94.

Rakugi, H., Tabuchi, Y., Nakamaru, M., Nagano, M., Higashimori, K., Mikami, H., *et al.* (1990). Evidence for endothelin-1 release from resistance vessels of rats in response to hypoxia. *Biochem Biophys Res Commun*, **29**, 973–977.

Ralevic, V., Milner, P. and Burnstock, G. (1995). Augmented flow-induced endothelin release from the rat mesenteric arterial bed after long-term sympathectomy. *Endothelium*, **3**, 67–73.

Ralevic, V., Belai, A. and Burnstock, G. (1993). Impaired sensory-motor nerve function in the isolated mesenteric arterial bed of streptozotocin-diabetic and ganglioside-treated streptozotocin-diabetic rats. *Br J Pharmacol*, **110**, 1105–1111.

Ralevic, V. and Burnstock, G. (1990). Postjunctional synergism of noradrenaline and adenosine 5′-triphosphate in the mesenteric arterial bed of the rat. *Eur J Pharmacol*, **175**, 291–299.

Ralevic, V., Kristek, F., Hudlická, O. and Burnstock, G. (1989). A new protocol for removal of the endothelium from the perfused rat hindlimb preparation. *Circ Res*, **64**, 1190–1196.

Ralevic, V., Lincoln, J. and Burnstock, G. (1992). Release of vasoactive substances from endothelial cells. Endothelial Regulation of Vascular Tone, edited by U. Ryan and G.M. Rubanyi, pp. 297–328. New York: Marcel Dekker.

Ralevic, V., Milner, P., Hudlická, O., Kristek, F. and Burnstock, G. (1990). Substance P is released from the endothelium of normal and capsaicin-treated rat hindlimb vasculature, in vivo, by increased flow. Circ Res, 66, 1178–1183.

Ralevic, V., Milner, P., Kirkpatrick, K.A. and Burnstock, G. (1992). Flow-induced release of adenosine 5'-triphosphate from endothelial cells of the rat mesenteric arterial bed. Experientia, 48, 31–34.

Ralevic, V., Rubino, A. and Burnstock, G. (1994). Prejunctional modulation of sensory-motor nerve-mediated vasodilatation of the rat mesenteric arterial bed by opioid peptides. J Pharmacol Exp Ther, 268, 772–778.

Ramme, D., Regenold, J.T., Starke, K., Busse, R. and Illes, P. (1987). Identification of the neuroeffector transmitter in jejunal branches of the rabbit mesenteric artery. Naunyn Schmiedeberg's Arch Pharmacol, 336, 267–273.

Reid, J.J. and Rand, M.J. (1992). Renal vasoconstriction is modulated by nitric oxide. Clin Exp Pharmacol Physiol, 19, 376–379.

Roberts, A.M., Messina, E.J. and Kaley, G. (1981). Prostacyclin (PGI$_2$) mediates hypoxic relaxation of bovine coronary artery strips. Prostaglandins, 21, 555–569.

Robertson, W.B. and Strong, J.P. (1968). Atherosclerosis in persons with hypertension and diabetes mellitus. Lab Invest, 18, 538–551.

Rubanyi, G.M., Romero, J.C. and Vanhoutte, P.M. (1986). Flow-induced release of endothelium-derived relaxing factor. Am J Physiol, 250, H1145–H1149.

Rubanyi, G.M. and Vanhoutte, P.M. (1985). Hypoxia releases a vasoconstrictor substance from the canine vascular endothelium. J Physiol (Lond), 249, H95–H101.

Rubanyi, G.M. (ed.) (1991). Cardiovascular Significance of Endothelium-Derived Vasoactive Factors. New York: Futura.

Rubino, A., Ralevic, V. and Burnstock, G. (1993). The P$_1$-purinoceptors that mediate the prejunctional effect of adenosine on capsaicin-sensitive non-adrenergic non-cholinergic neurotransmission in the rat mesenteric arterial bed are of the A$_1$ subtype. J Pharmacol Exp Ther, 267, 1100–1104.

Rui, L. and Cai, Y. (1991). Effect of chronic hypoxia on endothelium-dependent relaxation and cGMP content in rat pulmonary artery. Chin Med Sci J, 6, 145–147.

Rump, L.C., Wilde, K. and Schollmeyer, P. (1990). Prostaglandin E$_2$ inhibits noradrenaline release and purinergic pressor responses to renal nerve stimulation at 1 Hz in isolated kidneys of young spontaneously hypertensive rats. J Hypertens, 8, 897–908.

Ryan, U.S. and Rubanyi, G.M. (eds.) (1992). Endothelial Regulation of Vascular Tone. New York: Marcel Dekker.

Salt, T.E. and Hill, R.G. (1983). Excitation of single sensory neurones in the rat caudal trigeminal nucleus by iontophoretically applied adenosine 5'-triphosphate. Neurosci Lett, 35, 53–57.

Saville, V.L. and Burnstock, G. (1988). Use of reserpine and 6-hydroxydopamine supports evidence for purinergic cotransmission in the rabbit ear artery. Eur J Pharmacol, 155, 271–277.

Saville, V.L., Maynard, K.I. and Burnstock, G. (1990). Neuropeptide Y potentiates purinergic as well as adrenergic responses of the rabbit ear artery. Eur J Pharmacol, 176, 117–126.

Schlicker, E., Urbanek, E. and Göthert, M. (1989). ATP, α,β-methylene ATP and suramin as tools for characterization of vascular P$_{2X}$ receptors in the pithed rat. J Auton Pharmacol, 9, 371–380.

Schon, F., Ghatei, M., Allen, J.M., Mulderry, P.K., Kelly, J.S. and Bloom, S.R. (1985). The effect of sympathectomy on calcitonin gene-related peptide levels in the rat trigemino-vascular system. Brain Res, 348, 197–200.

Schwartz, D.D. and Malik, K.U. (1989). Renal periarterial nerve stimulation-induced vasoconstriction at low frequencies is primarily due to release of a purinergic transmitter in the rat. J Pharmacol Exp Ther, 250, 764–771.

Schwarzacher, S., Weidinger, F., Schemper, M. and Raberger, G. (1992). Blockade of endothelium-derived relaxing factor synthesis with N^G-nitro-L-arginine methyl ester leads to enhanced venous reactivity in vivo. Eur J Pharmacol, 229, 253–258.

Sheng, H., Gagne, G.D., Matsumoto, T., Miller, M.F., Förstermann, U. and Murad, F. (1993). Nitric oxide synthase in bovine superior cervical ganglion. J Neurochem, 61, 1120–1126.

Shimada, S.G. and Stitt, J.T. (1984). An analysis of the purinergic component of active muscle vasodilatation obtained by electrical stimulation of the hypothalamus in rabbits. Br J Pharmacol, 83, 577–589.

Shimizu, I. and Toda, N. (1986). Alterations with age of the response to vasodilator agents in isolated mesenteric arteries of the beagle. Br J Pharmacol, 89, 769–778.

Shimokawa, H. and Vanhoutte, P.M. (1989). Impaired endothelium-dependent relaxation to aggregating platelets and related vasoactive substances in porcine coronary arteries in hypercholesterolemia and atherosclerosis. Circ Res, 64, 900–914.

Sjöblom-Widfeldt, N. (1990). Neuromuscular transmission in blood vessels: phasic and tonic components: An *in vitro* study of mesenteric arteries of the rat. *Acta Physiol Scand Suppl*, **138**, 1–52.

Smiesko, V., Kozik, J. and Dolezel, S. (1985). Role of endothelium in the control of arterial diameter by blood flow. *Blood Vessels*, **22**, 247–251.

Sneddon, P. and Burnstock, G. (1984). ATP as a co-transmitter in rat tail artery. *Eur J Pharmacol*, **106**, 149–152.

Sosunov, A.A., Hassall, C.J.S., Loesch, A., Turmaine, M. and Burnstock, G. (1995). Ultrastructural investigation of nitric oxide synthase-immunoreactive nerves associated with coronary blood vessels of rat and guinea-pig. *Cell Tissue Res*, **280**, 575–582.

Sreeharan, N., Jayacody, R.L., Senaratne, M.P.J., Thompson, A.B.R. and Kappagoda, C.T. (1986). Endothelium-dependent relaxation and experimental atherosclerosis in the rabbit aorta. *Can J Physiol Pharmacol*, **64**, 1451–1453.

Stjärne, L., Lundberg, J.M. and Åstrand, P. (1986). Neuropeptide Y — a cotransmitter with noradrenaline and adenosine 5′-triphosphate in the sympathetic nerves of the mouse vas deferens? A biochemical, physiological and electropharmacological study. *Neuroscience*, **18**, 151–166.

Stjärne, L. (1989). Basic mechanisms and local modulation of nerve-impulse-induced secretion of neurotransmitters from individual sympathetic nerve varicosities. *Rev Physiol Biochem Pharmacol*, **112**, 1–137.

Stone, T.W. (1981). Differential blockade of ATP, noradrenaline and electrically evoked contractions of the rat vas deferens by nifedipine. *Eur J Pharmacol*, **74**, 373–376.

Strandness, J.W., Preist, R.W. and Gibbens, G.E. (1964). Combined clinical and pathological study of peripheral arterial disease. *Diabetes*, **13**, 336–372.

Sunman, W., Martin, G., Hair, W.M., Sever, P.S. and Hughes, A.D. (1993). Effect of calcium antagonists on endothelin-induced contraction of isolated human resistance arteries: differences related to site of origin. *J Hum Hypertens*, **7**, 189–191.

Surks, M.I., Beckwith, H.J. and Chidsey, C.A. (1967). Changes in plasma thyroxine concentration and metabolism, catecholamine excretion and basal O_2 consumption in man during acute exposure to high altitude. *J Clin Endocrinol*, **27**, 789–799.

Suzuki, H. (1985). Electrical responses of smooth muscle cells of the rabbit ear artery to adenosine triphosphate. *J Physiol (Lond)*, **359**, 401–415.

Suzuki, N., Fukuuchi, Y., Koto, A., Naganuma, Y., Isozumi, K., Matsuoka, S., *et al.* (1993). Cerebrovascular NADPH diaphorase-containing nerve fibres in the rat. *Neurosci Lett*, **151**, 1–3.

Szolcsanyi, J. (1988). Antidromic vasodilatation and neurogenic inflammation. *Agents Actions*, **23**, 4–11.

Taguchi, T., Ishii, Y., Matsubara, F. and Tenaka, K. (1986). Intimal thickening and the distribution of vasomotor nerves in the mechanically injured dog coronary artery. *Exp Mol Pathol*, **444**, 138–146.

Takiguchi, Y., Satoh, N., Hashimoto, H. and Nakashima, M. (1988). Changes in vascular reactivity in experimental diabetic rats: Comparison with hypothyroid rats. *Blood Vessels*, **25**, 250–260.

Taylor, E.M. and Parsons, M.E. (1989). Adrenergic and purinergic neurotransmission in arterial resistance vessels of the cat intestinal circulation. *Eur J Pharmacol*, **164**, 23–33.

Taylor, P.D., McCarthy, A.L., Thomas, C.R. and Poston, L. (1992). Endothelium-dependent relaxation and noradrenaline sensitivity in mesenteric resistance arteries of streptozotocin-induced diabetic rats. *Br J Pharmacol*, **107**, 393–399.

Taylor, S.G. and Weston, A.H. (1988). Endothelium-derived hyperpolarizing factor: a new endogenous inhibitor from the vascular endothelium. *Trends Pharmacol Sci*, **9**, 272–274.

Terenghi, G., Sundaresan, M., Moscoso, G. and Polak, J.M. (1993). Neuropeptides and a neuronal marker in cutaneous innervation during human foetal development. *J Comp Neurol*, **328**, 595–603.

Terenghi, G., Polak, J.M., Rodrigo, J., Mulderry, P.K. and Bloom, S.R. (1986). Calcitonin gene-related peptide-immunoreactive nerves in the tongue, epiglottis and pharynx of the rat: Occurrence, distribution and origin. *Brain Res*, **365**, 1–14.

Tesfamariam, B. and Cohen, R.A. (1988). Inhibition of adrenergic vasoconstriction by endothelial cell shear stress. *Circ Res*, **63**, 720–725.

Toda, N. (1993). Mediation by nitric oxide of neurally-induced human cerebral artery relaxation. *Experientia*, **49**, 51–53.

Toda, N., Ayajiki, K., Yoshida, K., Kimura, H. and Okamura, T. (1993). Impairment by damage of the pterygopalatine ganglion of nitroxidergic vasodilator nerve function in canine cerebral and retinal arteries. *Circ Res*, **72**, 206–213.

Toda, N., Ayajiki, K. and Okamura, T. (1993). Cerebroarterial relaxations mediated by nitric oxide derived from endothelium and vasodilator nerve. *J Vasc Res*, **30**, 61–67.

Toda, N., Bian, K. and Inoue, S. (1987). Age-related changes in the response to vasoconstrictor and dilator agents in isolated beagle coronary arteries. *Naunyn-Schmiedeberg's Arch Pharmacol*, **336**, 359–364.

Toda, N., Kimura, T., Yoshida, K., Bredt, D.S., Snyder, S.H., Yoshida, Y., *et al.* (1994). Human uterine arterial relaxation induced by nitroxidergic nerve stimulation. *Am J Physiol*, **266**, H1446–H1450 .

Toda, N., Kitamura, Y. and Okamura, T. (1994). Role of nitroxidergic nerve in dog retinal arterioles *in vivo* and arteries *in vitro*. *Am J Physiol*, **266**, H1985–H1992.

Toda, N. and Okamura, T. (1992). Mechanism of neurally induced monkey mesenteric artery relaxation and contraction. *Hypertension*, **19**, 161–166.

Toda, N., Yoshida, K. and Okamura, T. (1991). Analysis of the potentiating action of N^G-nitro-L-arginine on the contraction of the dog temporal artery elicited by transmural stimulation of noradrenergic nerves. *Naunyn-Schmiedeberg's Arch Pharmacol*, **343**, 221–224.

Todd, M.E. (1992). Hypertensive structural changes in blood vessels: Do endothelial cells hold the key? *Can J Physiol Pharmacol*, **70**, 536–551.

Tomimoto, H., Nishimura, M., Suenaga, T., Nakamura, S., Akiguchi, T., Wakita, H., *et al.* (1994). Distribution of nitric oxide synthase in the human cerebral blood vessels and brain tissues. *J Cereb Blood Flow Metab*, **14**, 930–938.

Tsuchiya, K., Urabe, M., Yamamoto, R., Asada, Y. and Lee, T.J. (1994). Effects of N^ω-nitro-L-arginine and capsaicin on neurogenic vasomotor responses in isolated mesenteric arteries of the monkey. *J Pharm Pharmacol*, **46**, 155–157.

Uddman, R., Edvinsson, L., Ekman, R., Kingman, T. and McCulloch, J. (1985). Innervation of the feline cerebral vasculature by nerve fibres containing calcitonin gene-related peptide: trigeminal origin and co-existence with substance P. *Neurosci Lett*, **62**, 131–136.

Ursell, P.C. and Mayes, M. (1993). The majority of nitric oxide synthase in pig heart is vascular and not neural. *Cardiovasc Res*, **27**, 1920–1924.

Van de Voorde, J. and Leusen, I. (1986). Endothelium-dependent and independent relaxation of aortic rings from hypertensive rats. *Am J Physiol*, **250**, H711–H717.

Vanhoutte, P.M. and Miller, V.M. (1985). Heterogeneity of endothelium-dependent responses in mammalian blood vessels. *J Cardiovasc Pharmacol*, **7**, (Suppl. 3), S12–S23.

Vanhoutte, P.M. and Rimele, T.J. (1983). Role of endothelium in the control of vascular smooth muscle function. *J Physiol (Paris)*, **78**, 681–686.

Verbeuren, T.J., Jordaens, F.H., Zonnekeyn, L.L., Van Hove, C.E., Coene, M.-C. and Herman, A.G. (1986). Effect of hypercholesterolemia on vascular reactivity in the rabbit. I. Endothelium-dependent and endothelium-independent contractions and relaxations in isolated arteries of control and hypercholesterolemic rabbits. *Circ Res*, **58**, 552–564.

Verbeuren, T.J., Simonet, S. and Herman, A.G. (1994). Diet-induced atherosclerosis inhibits release of nor-adrenaline from sympathetic nerves in rabbit arteries. *Eur J Pharmacol*, **270**, 27–34.

Vidal, M., Hicks, P.E. and Langer, S.Z. (1986). Differential effects of α,β-methylene ATP on responses to nerve stimulation in SHR and WKY tail arteries. *Naunyn Schmiedeberg's Arch Pharmacol*, **332**, 384–390.

Vizzard, M.A., Erdman, S.L. and deGroat, W.C. (1993). Localization of NADPH diaphorase in bladder afferent and postganglionic efferent neurones of the rat. *J Auton Nerv Syst*, **44**, 85–90.

Vo, P.A., Reid, J.J. and Rand, M.J. (1992). Attenuation of vasoconstriction by endogenous nitric oxide in rat caudal artery. *Br J Pharmacol*, **107**, 1121–1128.

Von Kügelgen, I. and Starke, K. (1985). Noradrenaline and adenosine triphosphate as co-transmitters of neurogenic vasoconstriction in rabbit mesenteric artery. *J Physiol (Lond)*, **367**, 435–455.

Wahlestedt, C., Yanaihara, N., Håkanson, R. (1986). Evidence for different pre- and postjunctional receptors for neuropeptide Y and related peptides. *Regul Pept*, **13**, 307–318.

Warland, J.J.I. and Burnstock, G. (1987). Effects of reserpine and 6-hydroxydopamine on the adrenergic and purinergic components of sympathetic nerve responses of the rabbit saphenous artery. *Br J Pharmacol*, **92**, 871–880.

Warner, T.D., D'Orleans-Juste, P. and Vane, J.R. (1990). Endothelin-1 and U46619 potentiate selectively the venous responses to nerve stimulation within the perfused superior mesenteric vascular bed of the rat. *Biochem Biophys Res Commun*, **172**, 745–750.

Warner, T.D., de Nucci, G. and Vane, J.R. (1989). Rat endothelin is a vasodilator in the isolated perfused mesentery of the rat. *Eur J Pharmacol*, **159**, 325–326.

Warren, J.B., Brady, A.J. and Taylor, A.J. (1990). Vascular smooth muscle influences the release of endothelium-derived relaxing factor. *Proc R Soc Lond B*, **241**, 127–131.

Westfall, T.C., Han, S.-P., Kneupfer, M., Martin, J., Chen, X., Del Valle, K., *et al.* (1990). Neuropeptides in hypertension: role of neuropeptide Y and calcitonin gene related peptide. *Br J Clin Pharmacol*, **30**, 75S–82S.

Westfall, T.C. and Meldrum, M.J. (1985). Alterations in the release of norepinephrine at the vascular neuroeffector junction in hypertension. *Ann Rev Pharmacol Toxicol*, **25**, 621–641.

Wharton, J. and Gulbenkian, S. (1987). Peptides in the mammalian cardiovascular system. *Experientia*, **43**, 821–832.

Whittle, B.J.R., Lopez-Belmonte, J. and Rees, D.D. (1989). Modulation of the vasodepressor actions of acetylcholine, bradykinin, substance P and endothelin in the rat by a specific inhibitor of nitric oxide formation. *Br J Pharmacol*, **98**, 646–652.

Wiencke, A.K., Nilsson, H., Nielsen, P.J. and Nyborg, N.C. (1994). Nonadrenergic noncholinergic vasodilation in bovine ciliary artery involves CGRP and neurogenic nitric oxide. *Invest Ophthalmol Vis Sci*, **35**, 3268–3277.

Wong-Dusting, H.K., La, M. and Rand, M.J. (1990). Mechanisms of the effects of endothelin on responses to noradrenaline and sympathetic nerve stimulation. *Clin Exp Pharmacol Physiol*, **17**, 269–273.

Woollridge, S.M. and Van Helden, D.F. (1990). Enhanced excitatory junction potentials in arteries of the spontaneously hypertensive rat. *Proc Austral Physiol Pharmacol Soc*, **21**, 60P.

Yamamoto, H., Bossaller, C., Cartwright, J. Jr. and Henry, P.D. (1988). Videomicroscopic demonstration of defective cholinergic arteriolar vasodilation in atherosclerotic rabbit. *J Clin Invest*, **81**, 1752–1758.

Yamamoto, R., Bredt, D.S., Snyder, S.H. and Stone, R.A. (1993). The localization of nitric oxide synthase in the rat eye and related cranial ganglia. *Neuroscience*, **54**, 189–200.

Yamamoto, R., Wada, A., Asada, Y., Niina, H. and Sumiyoshi, A. (1993). N^{ω}-nitro-L-arginine, an inhibitor of nitric oxide synthesis, decreases noradrenaline outflow in rat isolated perfused mesenteric vasculature. *Naunyn-Schmiedeberg's Arch Pharmacol*, **347**, 238–240.

Yanagisawa, M., Kurihara, H., Kimura, S., Tomobe, Y., Kobayashi, M., Mitsui, Y., et al. (1988). A novel potent vasoconstrictor peptide produced by vascular endothelial cells. *Nature*, **332**, 411–415.

Yoshida, K., Okamura, T., Kimura, H., Bredt, D.S., Snyder, S.H. and Toda, N. (1993). Nitric oxide synthase-immunoreactive nerve fibers in dog cerebral and peripheral arteries. *Brain Res*, **629**, 67–72.

6 Nervous Control of the Cerebral Circulation

David W. Busija

Department of Physiology and Pharmacology,
Bowman Gray School of Medicine, Wake Forest University,
Winston-Salem, NC 27157–1083, USA

The cerebral circulation receives several types of traditional peripheral innervation, including sympathetic, parasympathetic, and sensory nerve fibers. In addition, cerebral resistance vessels may be innervated via pathways that exist entirely within the central nervous system. Cerebral blood vessels are also exposed to neurotransmitters that escape into the extracellular fluid from synapses. Sympathetic nerves appear to limit cerebrovascular dilatation during arterial hypertension, hypoxia, and hypercapnia, to attenuate disruption of the blood-brain barrier during arterial hypertension, and to contribute to development and maintenance of vascular morphology. Less is known about the role of parasympathetic innervation, but these fibers appear to contribute to cerebrovascular dilatation during several conditions, including ischaemia/reperfusion. Sensory fibers appear to participate in cerebrovascular dilation during post-ischaemia reperfusion, cortical spreading depression, and arterial hypotension. While not conclusive as yet, there is good evidence that some central nervous system pathways such as the fastigial nucleus could contribute to cerebrovascular control. However, this issue is not fully resolved at this time. Synaptic escape of neurotransmitters may affect cerebrovascular tone, especially during pathological conditions, and the final vascular effects of these neurotransmitters may depend on interactions with prostanoids, nitric oxide, or other vasoactive agents released by cerebral blood vessels and tissues. Neural stimuli appear to play a major role in regulation of the cerebral circulation.

KEY WORDS: cerebral circulation; neurotransmitters; sympathetic innervation; parasympathetic innervation; trigeminal nerve; prostanoids; nitric oxide; endothelium-derived relaxing factor.

INTRODUCTION

Vascular resistance in regional circulatory beds is regulated by metabolic factors, chemical stimuli, perfusion pressure, and nerves. There always has been general agreement among investigators that the first three factors are important in regulation of the cerebral circulation (Busija and Heistad, 1984a). However, the contribution of neural stimuli to cerebrovascular control has been controversial (Busija *et al.*, 1982a; Busija and Heistad, 1984a; Busija 1993), and it has only been in the last decade and a half that the importance of this mode of control has been fully appreciated. A unique feature of the cerebral circulation is that neural stimuli have access to cerebral blood vessels via several different routes (Figure 6.1).

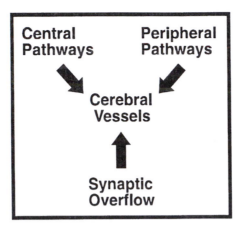

Figure 6.1   Routes of access of neurotransmitters to the cerebral circulation.

I will review recent studies concerning the functional importance of neural stimuli on the cerebral circulation. The most impressive, recent findings, in my opinion, are the continued documentation of important sympathetic effects on the cerebral circulation, the elucidation of sources and functional significance of parasympathetic and peptidergic innervations, the documentation of the presence of nitric oxide synthase (NOS)-containing nerves in cerebral vessels, the demonstration that central pathways could play a role in regulation of cerebral hemodynamics, and the evidence that synaptic overflow could be an important source of neurotransmitters to cerebral blood vessels.

SYMPATHETIC INNERVATION

Cerebral vessels are supplied by sympathetic nerves that originate predominantly from the superior cervical ganglia, and these postganglionic fibers form a well developed plexus in cerebral arteries and arterioles in the adventia, and the nerve fibers end in the adventia-medial border (Nielsen and Owman, 1967; Edvinsson et al., 1972b; Mueller, Heistad, and Marcus, 1977; Purdy and Bevan, 1977). In general, density of innervation of resistance vessels is extensive, being similar to mesenteric and femoral vascular beds (Rosenblum, 1976a,b) where sympathetic activation has major effects on vascular resistance. Noradrenaline is located in granular, electron dense vesicles 25–100 nm in diameter (Nielsen, Owman and Sporrong, 1971; Cervos-Navarro and Matakas, 1974; Lee and Saito, 1984) (Figure 6.2). An unusual aspect of the sympathetic innervation is that in some vessels there is a relatively wide synaptic cleft (Lee, 1977; Lee and Saito, 1984). Density of innervation of veins generally is less than precapillary vessels (Nielsen and Owman, 1967), but not in all cases (Asada and Lee, 1992). Capillaries apparently are not innervated by peripheral sympathetic fibers (Nielsen and Owman, 1967). Origins of sympathetic innervation were first to be well-documented, due to early availability of suitable immunohistochemical approaches for demonstrating the presence of catecholamines in nerves and to the surgical accessibility of the ganglia in the neck. Innervation, while predominantly ipsilateral especially in distal vessels, overlaps in vessels in basal and medial areas of the brain, such as the circle of Willis, anterior cerebral artery, and basilar artery (Nielsen and Owman, 1967; Peerless and Yasargi, 1971). In some species, cerebral vessels in caudal areas of the brain are supplied to a limited extent by fibers originating from sympathetic ganglia other than the superior cervical ganglia (Edvinsson et al., 1975). In addition, innervation is very heterogeneous. Innervation of arteries arising from the internal carotid system is denser than in vessels of the vertebral system. Approximately 60–90% of the arterioles in the medial geniculate body, parietal and temporal cortices, caudate nucleus, inferior colliculus, thalamus, and hypothalamus are innervated, in contrast to 10–30% of arterioles in the medulla, occipital cortex, and cerebellum (Edvinsson and Owman, 1977). Variation in the density of innervation is suggestive of preferential sympathetic effects in certain areas of the brain.

An interesting finding is that neuropeptide Y is co-localization with noradrenaline in sympathetic nerve endings in the cerebral as well as other circulations (Edvinsson et al., 1983a; Allen et al., 1984; Edvinsson et al., 1984b; Uddman et al., 1985; Edvinsson et al., 1987a,b; Nakakita, 1990). Co-release of NPY could be involved in presynaptic or postsynaptic activities, such as control of neurotransmitter release or modulation of degree of constriction. Although most of the NPY seems to be located in sympathetic nerve endings, it appears that NPY is also located to a limited extent in nerve endings of parasympathetic fibers (Gibbins and Morris, 1988; Suzuki et al., 1990a).

Topical application of noradrenaline or electrical stimulation of sympathetic nerves have been used to simulate reflex activation and these interventions presumably produce near-maximal effects on cerebral vessels. During baseline conditions in anaesthetized animals, topical application of noradrenaline is a potent constrictor agent in cats, mice, piglets, lambs, (Kuschinsky and Wahl, 1975; Wei et al., 1975; Busija, Marcus and Heistad, 1982; Busija, Leffler and Wagerle, 1985; Wagerle, Kumar and Delivoria-Papadopoulos, 1986); these effects are blocked with typical α-adrenoceptor antagonists (Kuschinsky and Wahl, 1975; Busija and Leffler, 1987b) (Figure 6.2). In addition, responses are pH sensitive and are inhibited by alkalosis (Navari et al., 1978). Finally, a number of dilator factors can counteract constrictor effects of noradrenaline. Thus, prostanoids, nitric oxide and histamine buffer cerebrovascular effects of noradrenaline (Gross, Harper and Teasdale, 1983; Busija and Leffler, 1987a; Bauknight, Faraci and Heistad, 1992).

During normotension, electrical stimulation of sympathetic pathways causes constriction of cerebral arterioles in piglets, cats and lambs and reduces CBF in piglets, rabbits, lambs and monkeys, but not in sheep, dogs and cats (Kuschinsky and Wahl, 1975; Wei et al., 1975; Heistad, Marcus and Gross, 1978; Sercombe et al., 1979; Busija, Marcus and Heistad, 1982a; Gross, Harper and Teasdale, 1983; Busija, 1985a; Busija, Leffler and Wagerle, 1985; Wagerle, Kumar and Delivoria-Papadopoulos, 1986; Busija and Leffler, 1987b; Wagerle, Kurth and Roth, 1990). Thus, species differences exist in cerebrovascular responsiveness to sympathetic nerve stimulation. In cats sympathetic stimulation constricts pial arterioles, but CBF fails to fall because of compensatory downstream dilatation (Busija, Marcus and Heistad, 1982; Baumbach and Heistad, 1983).

Effects are greatest on rostral structures, such as cerebral cortex, where blood flow may decrease by up to 30%. Veins also constrict to sympathetic stimulation (Gross, Harper and Teasdale, 1983), but it is unclear whether this response is a direct one, or whether it occurs secondarily to a drop in intravascular pressure as precapillary vessels constrict (Baumbach and Heistad, 1983). Since the animals used in these experiments were anaesthetized, and CBF was reduced because of an anaesthetic agent-induced depression of metabolic rate, it seems likely that effects of sympathetic stimulation on the cerebral circulation are underestimated. At the same time cerebral vessels are constricted and CBF is reduced by sympathetic stimulation, blood flow to other cranial structures supplied by the same nerves, such as skeletal muscle, blood flow decreases to near zero (Marcus et al., 1982; Busija, 1985a,b; Busija, 1986). Although there is some evidence that the cerebral circulation escapes from the sympathetic stimulation over a 5–7 min period (Sercombe et al., 1979; Marcus et al., 1982), electrical or reflex activation of sympathetic nerves maintains pial arteriolar constriction in cats and pigs, and reduces CBF in piglets and lambs and rabbits for as long as stimulation lasts (at least 10 minutes) (Busija, 1985a; Busija, Leffler and Wagerle, 1985; Wagerle, Kumar and Delivoria-Papadopoulos, 1986; Kurth, Wagerle and Delivoria-Papadopoulos, 1988). This finding supports that concept that sympathetic nerves are important in regulation of CBF.

Although ipsilateral sympathetic stimulation has been widely used to examine effects on the cerebral circulation, the normal mode of reflex activation would be bilateral. Results indicate that bilateral effects on cerebral arteries reduce CBF more than ipsilateral stimulation (MacKenzie et al., 1979; Busija and Heistad, 1984b; Busija, 1986), and that even with this greater reduction in CBF there is little evidence of escape except perhaps in caudate nucleus (Busija, 1985a, 1986).

Sympathetic effects are more pronounced during elevations in blood pressure and perturbations of blood gases than during normal conditions. The common factor in experiments of that type are that the vessels are dilated either by distending pressure (Busija, Heistad and Marcus, 1980, 1981) or by arterial blood hypercapnia or hypoxia (Busija, Heistad and Marcus, 1981; Wagerle et al., 1983; Busija and Heistad, 1984b). During acute, moderate, sustained increases in arterial blood pressure within the autoregulatory range, CBF transiently increases before returning to baseline values. Pial arterioles initially dilate, but eventually constrict to or below baseline values (Busija, Heistad and Marcus, 1980). Electrical stimulation of sympathetic nerves under these conditions attenuates the transient increase in CBF (Busija, Heistad and Marcus, 1981). During more severe arterial hypertension, when the autoregulatory capacity of cerebral vessels would normally be exceeded and the blood-brain barrier disrupted, sympathetic stimulation attenuates both increased blood flow and barrier disruption (Bill and Linder, 1976; Edvinsson, Owman and Siesjö, 1976; MacKenzie et al., 1976; Heistad and Marcus, 1979; Waldemar et al., 1989). There are several possibilities to explain why sympathetic stimulation has larger effects during arterial hypertension compared to normotensive conditions. First, the initial vascular stretch that occurs at the onset of hypertension may potentiate responsiveness to constrictor stimuli such as sympathetic nerves (Toda, Hatano and Hayaski, 1978). Second, increased resistance of large vessels, due to sympathetic stimulation, may protect downstream vessels from forced dilatation during sudden increases in arterial pressure (Baumbach and Heistad, 1983). Third, sympathetic stimulation may reduce compliance of cerebral vessels and attenuate passive dilatation. Fourth, as suggested by Bauknight, Faraci and Heistad, (1992), superoxide anion generated in response to acute hypertension (Wei *et al.*, 1985), could inactivate NO and accentuate cerebrovascular effects of sympathetic nerves. Since large increases can occur in arterial pressure during stressful conditions such as weight lifting, it is easy to see why a protective role of sympathetic nerves can be so important to prevent inappropriate cerebral hyperaemia and damage to the blood-brain barrier.

Effects of electrical activation of sympathetic nerves are also potentiated during arterial hypercapnia (Harper *et al.*, 1972; Busija and Heistad, 1984b) and hypoxia (Wagerle *et al.*, 1983). The reason for enhanced sympathetic effects is that downstream resistance vessels are already dilated by these stimuli, so that compensation in distal vascular segments cannot occur when larger arteries and arterioles constrict (Harper *et al.*, 1972; Busija, Marcus and Heistad, 1982).

Resting sympathetic tone is minimal in the cerebral circulation. Section of sympathetic nerves has little or no effect on CBF in anaesthetized dogs, cats, monkeys, rabbits, lambs, or piglets, or awake dogs, cats and rabbits (Mueller, Heistad and Marcus, 1977; Heistad *et al.*, 1977; Heistad, Marcus and Gross, 1978; Marcus and Heistad, 1979; Sadoshima, Busija and Heistad, 1983; Busija, 1984; Kurth, Wagerle and Delivoria-Papadopoulos, 1988). In addition, administration of α-adrenoceptor antagonists does not alter pial arteriolar diameter in anaesthetized cats, piglets or lambs (Kuschinsky and Wahl, 1975; Busija and Leffler, 1987b; Wagerle, Kurth and Roth, 1990). Thus, apparently there is little or no resting sympathetic tone to cerebral vessels while sympathetic tone is present in other vascular beds.

Animals have been exposed to several physiological stresses to examine reflex mechanisms. During systemic hypotension, sympathetic nerves have no detectable effect on CBF in anaesthetized cats and dogs, or in awake cats, piglets or rabbits (Fitch, MacKenzie and Harper, 1975; Mueller, Heistad and Marcus, 1977; Gross *et al.*, 1979; Busija, 1984; Armstead *et al.*, 1988b). However, sympathetic nerves reduce CBF modestly in awake monkeys and dogs at pressures between 40–60 mmHg (Fitch, MacKenzie and Harper, 1975; Marcus and Heistad, 1979). Sympathetic nerves are but one type of competing perivascular innervation activated by hypotension (see below). Consequently, it is not surprising that sympathetic effects vary according to species and condition.

On the other hand, sympathetic nerves attenuate increases in CBF that occur during arterial hypertension. Sino-aortic deafferentation, which results in intense sympathetic discharge and doubling of arterial blood pressure, increases CBF several-fold. However, intact sympathetic pathways attenuate this increase in CBF (Gross *et al.*, 1979). Similarly, stimulation of carotid chemoreceptors with nicotine in awake, but paralyzed and ventilated dogs, evoked arterial hypertension that was associated with a 40% increase in CBF in animals in which the sympathetic nerves supplying cerebral vessels were sectioned (Vatner *et al.*, 1980). In contrast, in dogs with intact sympathetic nerves, CBF did not increase.

Sympathetic nerves are also activated during other conditions and attenuate increases in CBF. During bicuculline-induced seizures, where CBF increases several-fold, due to both increases in cerebral metabolic rate as well as arterial hypertension, intact sympathetic nerves limit increases in CBF in dogs, cats and lambs (Gross *et al.*, 1979; Mueller, Heistad and Marcus, 1979; Lacombe, Miller and Seylez, 1985; Kurth, Wagerle and

Delivoria-Papadopoulos, 1988). Sympathetic nerves also limit CBF responses in puppies and piglets during asphyxia (Hernandez, Brennan and Hawkins, 1980; Goplerud, Wagerle and Delivoria-Papadopoulous, 1991). Similarly, sympathetic nerves limit increases in CBF or decreases in cerebrovascular resistance during arterial hypercapnia and hypoxia in anaesthetized and awake cats and rabbits (Busija, 1984; Busija and Heistad, 1984b; Neubauer and Edelman, 1984), but not in lambs (Wagerle et al., 1983). Lastly, an inappropriate constrictor role of sympathetic nerves may occur during middle cerebral artery occlusion, which would limit perfused capillary volume (Anwar, Buckweitz-Milton and Weiss, 1988).

In addition to these findings, it also seems that there are developmental changes in cerebrovascular responsiveness to α-adrenoreceptor-mediated stimuli in some species. In sheep, pigs and baboons, there is a decrease in sensitivity to noradrenaline with advancing developmental stage. In baboons and lambs, cerebral arteries are more responsive to exogenous noradrenaline in preterm, compared to term, animals (Hayashi, Park and Kuehl, 1984; Wagerle, Kurth and Roth, 1990). In addition, while exogenous noradrenaline and sympathetic nerve stimulation both constrict pial arterioles in lambs, neither constricts pial arterioles in adult sheep (Wagerle, Kurth and Roth, 1990). Further, while exogenous noradrenaline and sympathetic stimulation constrict cerebral resistance vessels in piglets (Wagerle, Kumar and Delivoria-Papadopoulos, 1986; Busija and Leffler, 1987a,b), these agents fail to do so in adult pigs (Lee, Kinkhead and Sarwinski, 1982). The reasons for developmental changes in responsiveness to α-adrenoreceptor-mediated stimuli are presently unclear. However, it is interesting that such mechanisms are present in the cerebral circulation of most animals at birth, in contrast to other regional circulations where these mechanisms may not yet be functional (Buckley, Brazeau and Gootman, 1983; Buckley, 1986). While decreases in responsiveness to sympathetic stimuli occur with development in several species, substantial sympathetic constrictor effects occur in adults of many species.

In addition to direct effects on cerebral vascular tone, sympathetic nerves also appear to exert important trophic effects on cerebral vessels. Intact sympathetic nerves result in greater vessel mass and wall thickness in normotensive and hypertensive animals (Hart, Heistad and Brody, 1980; Sadoshima et al., 1981; Bevan, Tsuru and Bevan, 1983; Sadoshima, Busija and Heistad, 1983; Werber and Heistad, 1984), and protect genetically hypertensive animals from cerebral haemorrhages and infarcts (Sadoshima et al., 1981).

Even though the degree of sympathetic innervation appears to be similar among species, there do appear to be differences in α-adrenoreceptor subtypes in cerebral vessels. For example, postjunctional and extrajunctional noradrenergic receptors appear to be predominantly of the α_1-adrenoceptor-subtype in cerebral arteries and arterioles of lambs (Wagerle, Kurth and Roth, 1990), rabbits (Busija, 1985a; Bevan, 1987), nonhuman primates (Toda, 1983; Hayashi, Park and Kuehl, 1985), rats (Hogestatt and Andersson, 1984) and humans (Toda, 1983; Skärby and Andersson, 1984), but of the α_2-adrenoceptor-subtype in dogs (Sakakibara, Fujiwara and Muramatsu, 1982; Toda, 1983), cats (Skärby, Andersson and Edvinsson, 1981; Medgett and Langer, 1983; Skärby, 1984), and cows (Tsukahara et al., 1983). Cerebral resistance arteries appear to have both α_1- and α_2-adrenoceptor-subtypes in the piglet (Wagerle, Kumar and Delivoria-Papadopoulos, 1986; Busija and Leffler, 1987c), with the latter subtype predominating for both postjunctional and extrajunctional receptors in the pial arterioles (Busija and Leffler, 1987c). Noradrenaline also constricts porcine pial veins predominantly via α_2-adrenoceptors (Asada and Lee, 1992).

As described earlier, neuropeptide Y often is co-localized and co-released from sympathetic nerve endings together with noradrenaline. NPY constricts surface cerebral arteries and arterioles and parenchymal arterioles, and decreases CBF in several species (Edvinsson et al., 1983a, 1984a, 1987a,b; Dacey, Bassett and Takayasu, 1988; Suzuki et al., 1989; Tuor et al., 1990). NPY also appears to potentiate effects of electrical stimulation and exogenous noradrenaline on blood vessels (Ekblad et al., 1984).

Sympathetic nerve terminals can also take up serotonin from the extracellular fluid, store it, and release serotonin when depolarized (Verbeuren, Jordaens and Herman, 1983; Saito and Lee, 1987; Chang et al., 1989). Thus, serotonin can act as a "false neurotransmitter", associated with sympathetic nerve terminals in the cerebral circulation. Neurally-released serotonin can interact with the sympathetic fibers by either limiting release of noradrenaline from nerve terminals (McGrath, 1977; Feniuk, Humphrey and Watts, 1979) or by potentiating vasoconstrictor effects of noradrenaline (Lande, Cannell and Waterson, 1966; Van Nueten and Janssens, 1986). Serotonin also has direct constriction effects (Figure 6.2). Presently, it is unclear whether cerebral vessels receive independent serotonergic innervation (see below).

PARASYMPATHETIC INNERVATION

Cerebral blood vessels receive innervation from nerves containing vasoactive intestinal polypeptide (VIP), acetylcholine and NOS (Figure 6.2). These two neurotransmitters and NOS are included together in this section because there is extensive evidence that their fibers share final common neuronal pathways to cerebral blood vessels. Acetylcholine and VIP are standard neurotransmitters and are stored in vesicles associated with nerve endings, while NO is produced and released immediately upon depolarization and activation of NOS.

Cholinergic innervation is documented by the following observations in cerebral blood vessels: (1) the presence of the acetylcholine synthesizing enzyme, choline acetyl-transferase (ChAT) (Hardebo et al., 1977; Florence and Bevan, 1979; Duckles, 1981; Bevan et al., 1982; Estrada, Hamel and Krause, 1983; Saito, Wu and Lee, 1985); (2) measurable levels of acetylcholine (Duckles, 1981); (3) evoked release of acetylcholine from cerebral arteries (Duckles, 1981); and (4) the presence of a high-affinity choline uptake system (Florence and Bevan, 1979; Duckles, 1981). ChAT is localized in the adventitia of cerebral vessels.

VIP, a 28-amino acid polypeptide, has also been localized at the adventitia-medial border using immunohistochemical approaches (Larsson et al., 1976; Edvinsson et al., 1980; Lee, Saito and Berezin, 1981; Gibbins, Brayden and Bevan, 1984). VIP can be released from cerebral blood vessels (Bevan et al., 1984).

Importance of nerves that can release NO is shown by the extensive network of NOS-containing fibers in cerebral arteries (Bredt, Hwang and Snyder, 1990; Nozaki et al., 1993; Suzuki et al., 1993; Toda et al., 1993). NOS-innervation is most dense in proximal and middle cerebral arteries, and less prevalent in caudal circle of Willis and small pial arterioles. Nitric oxide synthase also is located in endothelial cells (Furchgott, 1984).

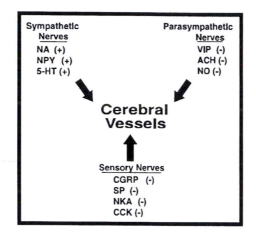

Figure 6.2 Predominant actions of neurotransmitters released by peripheral nerves. (+) constriction, (–) dilation. NA = noradrenaline, NPY = neuropeptide Y, 5-HT = serotonin, CGRP = calcitonin gene-related peptide, SP = substance P, NKA = neurokinin A, CCK = cholecystokinin, VIP = vasoactive intestinal polypeptide, ACH = acetylcholine, NO = nitric oxide.

The similarity in anatomical pathways for VIP- and acetylcholine-containing fibers in the adventia of and the superimposition of acetylcholinesterase activity and VIP immuno-reactivity (Itakura et al., 1984; Hara, Hamill and Jacobowitz, 1985; Hara et al., 1989) have led to the suggestion that VIP and acetylcholine are co-localized in the same nerve endings, as appears to happen in exocrine glands (Lundberg et al., 1980, 1982). However, other findings comparing localization of ChAT and VIP immunoreactivity discount this possibility (Suzuki, Hardebo and Owman, 1988; Miao and Lee, 1990). On the other hand, it appears that VIP is often contained in NOS-containing nerves (Nozaki et al., 1993).

The close spatial approximation (within 25 nm) between non-adrenergic, possibly cholinergic, terminals with noradrenergic nerve endings (Edvinsson et al., 1972), suggests that the cholinergic nerves could act on presynaptic noradrenergic terminals and modify neurotransmitter release. Edvinsson, Falck and Owman, (1977) reported that activation of nicotinic receptors on sympathetic nerves attenuated the induced release of noradrenaline in cats. In addition, Aubineau, Sercombe and Seylaz (1980) showed that a nicotinic agonist reduced the constrictor effects of sympathetic stimulation on cerebral vessels in caudate nucleus in rabbits. Finally, Duckles (1981) has found that activation of muscarinic, but not nicotinic, receptors reduces noradrenaline release by cerebral vessels, a mode of cholinergic inhibition reported to operate in non-cerebral vascular beds (Shepherd and Vanhoutte, 1981). Thus, although there are minor discrepancies in results among investigators, it appears that cholinergic nerves have the potential to interact with sympathetic nerve terminals near cerebrovascular smooth muscle.

The parasympathetic innervation arises from several sources in cats and rats and probably other species as well (Gibbins, Brayden and Bevan, 1984; Walters, Gillespie and Moskowitz, 1986; Suzuki, Hardebo and Owman, 1988; Hara et al., 1989; Suzuki, Hardebo and Owman,

1990): (1) from the sphenopalatine ganglion to innervate the circle of Willis and its branches; (2) from the internal carotid mini-ganglion to innervate the internal carotid and its intracranial branches; and (3) from the otic ganglion supplying the internal carotid artery and the posterior part of the circle of Willis through the lesser superficial petrosal nerve. The major source of NOS innervation is via the sphenopalatine ganglia (Nozaki *et al.*, 1993). The innervation appears to exhibit some bilateral distribution, and to be more dense in blood vessels in rostral areas of the brain. Innervation seems to be heaviest in arteries and larger arterioles, and somewhat sparse, but present at least for VIP, in parenchymal vessels.

VIP causes cerebral arterial and arteriolar dilatation and increases CBF (Larsson *et al.*, 1976; McCulloch and Edvinsson, 1980; Wei, Kontos and Said, 1980; Lee, Saito and Berezin, 1981; Yaksh *et al.*, 1987; Dacey, Bassett and Takayasu, 1988). Unfortunately, there are at present no extremely selective and specific receptor antagonist for VIP, which has hindered research on its role in cerebrovascular control. VIP appears to cause vasodilatation via a prostanoid-dependent mechanism (Wei, Kontos and Said, 1980).

Acetylcholine application may cause dilatation or constriction, depending upon vascular segment and species studied (Kuschinsky, Wahl and Neiss, 1974; Busija and Heistad, 1982, 1983; Usui *et al.*, 1983; Wei *et al.*, 1985; Rosenblum, 1986; Armstead *et al.*, 1988a; Katusic, Shepherd and Vanhoutte, 1988; Tsuiji and Cook, 1988; Armstead *et al.*, 1989a; Wagerle and Busija, 1989, 1990). Dilatation probably reflects activation of muscarinic receptors on endothelium and subsequent synthesis and release of NO (Furchgott, 1984) whereas the normal response of direct activation of muscarinic receptors on vascular smooth muscle is vasoconstriction (Lee, 1985). When exogenous acetylcholine comes into contact with blood vessels and the muscarinic receptor-linked NO mechanism is present, the overall response is dilatation. It seems unlikely that the normal response to neural release of acetylcholine would be dilatation due to a NO mechanism, considering the distance and environment that acetylcholine would need to traverse in order to reach the endothelium (Lee, 1985).

In some species, such as the pig and dog, the normal response to acetylcholine is cerebrovascular constriction, which is mediated via a prostanoid-dependent mechanism (Usui *et al.*, 1983; Armstead *et al.*, 1988a; Busija *et al.*, 1988; Katusic, Shepherd and Vanhoutte, 1988; Tsuiji and Cook, 1988; Armstead *et al.*, 1989a; Wagerle and Busija, 1989, 1990). Thus, in the dog basilar artery and porcine cerebral circulation, acetylcholine-induced constriction is blocked by quinacrine, indomethacin, or a thromboxane A_2/prostaglandin H_2 receptor antagonist. Prostanoids do not appear to directly mediate the vascular response. Rather, only low concentrations of prostanoids appear to be necessary for acetylcholine to cause constriction (Armstead *et al.*, 1989a). It is unclear where the prostanoids exert their permissive influence, but it could be at the level of the muscarinic receptor, or at sites associated with activation and expression of second messenger systems. A similar permissive role seems to occur in at least one other system. The N-methyl-D-aspartate receptor has a binding site for glycine, and it is difficult to activate intracellular events unless glycine as well as glutamate are available for the receptor (Snell, Morter and Johnson, 1982; Johnson and Ascher, 1987). Although the vascular response associated with acetylcholine is usually thought to be dilatation, acetylcholine-induced constriction is found to be prevalent in many vascular beds in most species under normal conditions, and also to be prominent in cerebral and non-cerebral vascular beds following vascular damage or disease (Kalsner, 1989; Mayhan, Simmons and Sharpe, 1991; Nelson *et al.*, 1992).

Nitric oxide is a potent dilator agent of cerebral arteries and arterioles (Marshall, Wei and Kontos, 1988; Busija, Leffler and Wagerle, 1990; Colonna *et al.*, 1994; Faraci and Brian, 1994) and its effects can be blunted or eliminated by oxygen radicals (Nelson *et al.*, 1992) and inhibition of guanylyl cyclase (Kontos and Wei, 1993). Nitric oxide is an atypical neurotransmitter, being a gas, and can reach cerebrovascular smooth muscle from endothelium, perivascular nerves and parenchyma (Faraci and Brian, 1994). Several studies have shown that transmural electrical stimulation releases NO in cerebral arteries (González and Estrada, 1991; Lee and Sarwinski, 1991; Chen and Lee, 1993; Toda, Ayajiki and Okamura, 1993; Toda *et al.*, 1993). The major source of NOS innervation is via the sphenopalatine ganglia (Nozaki *et al.*, 1993).

Electrical stimulation of the sphenopalatine ganglion or post-ganglionic fibers increases CBF up to 40% in rat and cat (Seylaz *et al.*, 1988; Goadsby, 1990; Suzuki *et al.*, 1990b; Morita-Tsuzuki, Harbedo and Bonskela, 1993). Increases in blood flow are predominantly to rostral areas of the brain. Failure to block dilation with muscarinic antagonists but with a NOS-inhibitor may suggest that NO rather than acetylcholine is the neurotransmitter responsible for cerebrovascular responses (Suzuki *et al.*, 1990b; Morita-Tsuzuki, Hardebo and Bonskela, 1993). Section of postganglionic fibers of this pathway have been reported to impair auto-regulatory responses during haemorrhagic hypotension (Koketsu *et al.*, 1992) and to increase infarct size following middle cerebral artery occlusion, (Kano, Moskowitz and Yokota, 1991; Koketsu *et al.*, 1992), probably by interrupting a vasodilator response.

Activation of parasympathetic pathways at other sites may lead either to increases or no changes in CBF. Several studies have reported that electrical stimulation of the greater superficial petrosal nerve (GSPN) or facial nerve dilates pial arterioles (Cobb and Finesinger, 1932) or increases CBF (D'Alecy and Rose, 1979; Pinard *et al.*, 1979; Goadsby, 1991). Chemical activation of facial nerve pathways resulted in only a modest change in cerebrovascular resistance which were blocked by pentolinium but not scopolamine (Nakai *et al.*, 1993). On the other hand, two studies (Busija and Heistad, 1981; Linder, 1981) have reported that stimulation of the greater superficial petrosal nerve or facial nerve has little effect on CBF. In contrast to the other studies, in one of those studies effectiveness of GSPN stimulation was demonstrated by showing lacrimal blood flow to increase dramatically during stimulation (Busija and Heistad, 1981). Section of pathways does not alter responses to arterial hypercapnia or hypoxia (Hoff, MacKenzie and Harper, 1977; Pinard *et al.*, 1979; Busija and Heistad, 1981), and atropine does not alter the response to hypercapnia (Busija and Heistad, 1982).

TRIGEMINAL INNERVATION

Sensory fibers, arising from the first (ophthalmic) division of the trigeminal ganglia, supply cerebral arterioles (Liu-Chen, Han and Moskowitz, 1983; Liu-Chen, Mayberg and Moskowitz, 1983; Liu-Chen *et al.*, 1984a, 1984b; Mayberg, Zerras and Moskowitz, 1984). Heaviest innervation is to the distal internal carotid artery, circle of Willis, and pial arterioles. Arterioles supplying deep grey matter such as the thalamus and caudate receive sparse innervation. Innervation is primarily ipsilateral, except to medial structures such as circle of Willis and sagittal sinus. These unmyelinated fibers contain several peptides which appear to be co-localized in some but not all nerve terminals, including Substance P (Liu-Chen, Han and Moskowitz, 1983; Liu-Chen *et al.*, 1984a), calcitonin-gene related peptide (CGRP) (McCulloch *et al.*, 1986), neurokinin A (Saito, Greenberg and Moskowitz, 1987), and cholecystokinin-8 (Liu-Chen *et al.*, 1984b) (Figure 6.2). Exposure of cerebral arteries and arterioles to high potassium ion concentrations, capsaicin, or electrical field stimulation results in augmented release of at least Substance P (Duckles and Buck, 1982; Edvinsson, Rosendal-Helgesen and Uddman, 1983; Moskowitz, Brody and Liu-Chen, 1983). In addition, exposure to blood *in vivo* results in release of CGRP and Substance P into cerebrospinal fluid or cerebral venous blood (Juul *et al.*, 1990). The pattern of innervation for various types of trigeminal nerve fibers types is different (Nakakita, 1990). First, Substance P fibers form a meshwork around cerebral arterioles, while CGRP fibers form both meshwork and spiral patterns. Second, Substance P-immunoreactive nerve terminals exist apart from the arterial smooth muscle cells, while CGRP exists both near, and apart from smooth muscle cells and in the adventia. Lastly, Substance P provides abundant innervation to veins of many sizes, while CGRP does not. Thus, based upon distribution patterns, it appears that these two types of innervation would have different effects on the cerebral circulation.

Substance P (Edvinsson, McCulloch and Uddman, 1981; Edvinsson and Uddman, 1982; Moskowitz *et al.*, 1987; Busija and Chen, 1992), CGRP (McCulloch *et al.*, 1986; Busija and Chen, 1992; Colonna *et al.*, 1994), and neurokinin A (Moskowitz *et al.*, 1987) are potent dilators of pial arterioles. Effects of Substance P and neurokinin A seem to be endothelium-dependent and involve release of NO and activation of guanylate cyclase, while those of CGRP are not endothelium-dependent and involve activation of smooth muscle adenylate cyclase (Edvinsson *et al.*, 1985; Moskowitz *et al.*, 1987; Edwards, Stack and Trizna, 1991; Busija and Chen, 1992), except perhaps in small arterioles (Kontos and Wei, 1993; Rosenblum, Shimizu and Nelson, 1993). Substance P application leads to desensitization of receptors and reduced responsiveness to subsequent application (Moskowitz *et al.*, 1987). There is evidence for (Wei *et al.*, 1992) and against (Kitazono, Heistad and Faraci, 1993) the view that nitric oxide donors are able to cause cerebral arteriolar dilation, in part, via activation of sensory fibers and release of CGRP. Antidromic stimulation leads to vasodilatation and extravasation due to disruption of the blood-brain barrier (Lembeck and Holzer, 1979; Markowitz, Saito and Moskowitz, 1987; Moskowitz *et al.*, 1989). In contrast with other neurotransmitters, such as noradrenaline and acetylcholine, prostanoids do not seem to play an important role in cerebrovascular responses to these peptides (Table 6.1).

The pattern of trigeminal projections to pial and to cerebral and dura blood vessels, the dilator effects of Substance P on cerebral blood vessels, and increases in blood-brain barrier permeability due to Substance P application, as well as extensive clinical evidence, provide strong evidence that this trigeminal innervation may be linked to migraine headaches and pain associated with intracranial haemorrhage (Mayberg *et al.*, 1981; Norregaard and Moskowitz, 1985).

Several intriguing studies indicate that the trigeminal nerves are able to affect cerebral blood vessels during various experimental conditions and that the predominant effects are in vessels served by the anterior, middle, and posterior cerebral arteries. For example, cerebral arteriolar dilation during cortical spreading depression is partially mediated by

TABLE 6.1

Functional interactions between exogenous neurotransmitters and the endogenous prostanoid system relating to changes in vascular tone in newborn pigs

Neurotransmitter constrictor stimuli	Vascular* effect	CSF levels of prostanoids	Effects of indomethacin	References
1. Noradrenaline	constricts	increases	potentiates	Busija and Leffler, 1987a
2. Dopamine	constricts	no change	none	Busija and Leffler, 1989b
3. Vasopressin**	constricts	increases	potentiates	Armstead et al., 1989b
4. Dynorphin**	constricts	increases	potentiates	Armstead et al., 1991
5. β-endorphin	constricts	increases	potentiates	Armstead et al., 1991
6. Acetylcholine	constricts	increases	abolishes	Busija et al., 1988; Armstead et al., 1989a; Wagerle and Busija, 1989
Dilator Stimuli				
1. Glutamate	dilates	no change	none	Busija and Leffler, 1989a
2. Asparate	dilates	no change	none	Busija and Leffler, 1989a
3. Isoprenaline	dilates	no change	none	Busija and Leffler, 1987a
4. Substance P	dilates	no change	none	Busija and Chen, 1992
5. CGRP	dilates	no change	none	Busija and Chen, 1992
6. Vasopressin**	dilates	increase	none	Armstead et al., 1989b
7. Dynorphin**	dilates	increase	attenuates	Armstead et al., 1991
8. Leu-enkephalin	dilates	increase	attenuates	Armstead et al., 1991
9. Met-enkephalin	dilates	increase	attenuates	Armstead et al., 1991
10. Histamine	dilates	increase	attenuates	Mirro et al., 1988
11. Angiotensin II	dilates	not measured	attenuates	Meng and Busija, 1993
12. Oxytocin	dilates	increase	allows constriction	Busija, Khries and Chen, 1992

*Vascular effects represent direction of change of pial arteriolar diameter after topical application of neurotransmitter.

**Vasoactive responses of these substances are tone-dependent (Armstead et al., 1989a, 1991); application results in dilatation in arterioles under baseline conditions and constriction in arterioles previously dilated with other interventions.

CGRP (Figure 6.3) (Colonna et al., 1994; Wahl et al., 1994). In addition, sensory nerves appear to participate in cerebrovascular dilation during arterial hypotension (Hong et al., 1994). Further, trigeminal ganglionectomy has been reported to potentiate vasoconstriction to noradrenaline (Moskowitz et al., 1988), attenuate increases in CBF during severe arterial hypertension and seizures (Moskowitz et al., 1988; Sakas et al., 1989), decrease extravasation of albumin during severe arterial hypertension (Moskowitz et al., 1988), and to attenuate post-occlusive cerebral hyperaemia (Moskowitz et al., 1989; Macfarlane et al., 1991; Moskowitz et al., 1991). The sensory innervation may affect the cerebral circulation via a mechanism which operates similar to a peripheral axon-reflex-like mechanism. An analogous system exists in birds for control of choroidal blood flow (these animals lack direct blood flow to the retina). Shining light onto the retina increases choroidal blood flow via the Edinger-Westphal nucleus and ciliary ganglion (Fitzgerald, Vana and Reiner, 1990a, 1990b). The direction and magnitude of trigeminal nerve effects indicate that activation of these fibers could be beneficial during several stresses.

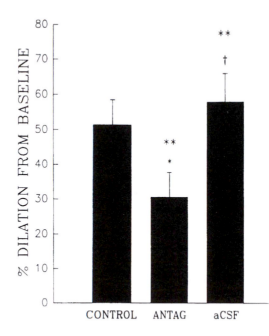

Figure 6.3 Reduction of arterior dilation to cortical spreading depression by application of calcitonin gene-related peptide receptor antagonist (ANTAG). aCSF represents response following removal of antagonist. Values are means ± SEM for 6 animals. *p < 0.05, compared to CONTROL; $^2 p$ < 0.05, compared to ANTAG. From Colonna *et al.*, 1994. Reprinted by permission of American Physiological Society.

CENTRAL INNERVATION

In addition to innervation of via traditional, peripheral pathways, it has been suggested that cerebral blood vessels also receive innervation via pathways through the central nervous system. These putative pathways originate at the locus coeruleus, raphé nucleus, dorsal medullary reticular formation, rostral ventrolateral medulla and fastigial nucleus. Many of these areas are interconnected. In contrast to the peripheral pathways, it has proved difficult to demonstrate that these pathways innervate cerebral vessels in a traditional manner (i.e., fibers ending in the adventio-medial border). There is always a basement membrane, associated with glial cells, between resistance vessels and nerve endings, and diffusion distances for neurotransmitters are relatively greater than in conventional neuromuscular mechanisms (Rennels *et al.*, 1977). However, it is possible that cerebral capillaries could be innervated by central noradrenergic neurons (Rennels *et al.*, 1977). An unproved possibility is that the primary targets of central innervation are astroglia (Stone and Ariano, 1989), and that vascular effects are dependent upon activation of astroglia or release of astroglia-derived vasoactive substances (Murphy *et al.*, 1990; Thore, Nam and Busija, 1994).

It has been suggested that noradrenergic fibers that originate in the locus coeruleus and adjacent areas innervate cerebral vessels (Hartman, Zide and Udenfriend, 1972; Edvinsson et al., 1973). Several investigators have reported that electrical stimulation of the locus coeruleus decreases CBF and increases capillary permeability (Raichle et al., 1975; Hartman et al., 1980; Goadsby, Lambert and Lance, 1985). However, since locus coeruleus stimulation decreases the firing rate of distant neurons (Abraham et al., 1979; Katayama et al., 1981), which would reduce metabolic rate, a probable explanation is that decreased CBF is secondary to decreased metabolic rate (Buchweitz, Edelman and Weiss, 1985). In addition, lesions of the locus coeruleus have no effect on cerebral blood flow or metabolic rate during several conditions, and do not alter brain capillary permeability to water (Dahlgren et al., 1981; McCulloch, Savaki and Angersen, 1982). Stimulation of another brainstem structure, namely the parabrachial nucleus, also decreases cerebral metabolic rate and blood flow (Mraovitch et al., 1985).

Stimulation of the fastigial nucleus of the cerebellum activates cholinergic dilator pathways to the brain that involve a synapse in the basal forebrain. The blood flow response occurs in virtually every area of the brain, with the largest increases (about 100%) in cerebral cortex and the smallest increases (about 50%) in brainstem (Doba and Reis, 1972; Nakai, Iadecola and Reis, 1982; Nakai et al., 1983; Mraovitch, Pinard and Seylaz, 1986; Iadecola and Reis, 1990). Nitric oxide appears to participate in cerebrovascular dilation elicited by fastigial nucleus stimulation (Iadecola, 1992; Iadecola, Zhang and Xu, 1993). Studies using ^{14}C-deoxyglucose indicate that local glucose utilization does not change during fastigial nucleus stimulation (Nakai et al., 1983). Stimulation of the fastigial nucleus reduces infarct size following middle cerebral artery occlusion (Reis et al., 1991; Zhang and Iadecola, 1992, 1993). Cerebrovascular dilatation during fastigial nucleus stimulation is abolished by lesions of the basal forebrain (Iadecola et al., 1983a) and by administration of atropine (Iadecola, Underwood and Reis, 1986; Arneric et al., 1987), but not by lesions of sphenopalatine ganglia (Iadecola, Zhang and Xu, 1993). In addition, stimulation of the basal forebrain increases CBF via a NO-dependent mechanism (Adachi, Inanami and Sato, 1992; Raszkiewicz et al., 1992). Involvement of local neurons is suggested by experiments involving cortical application of ibotenic acid, which destroys local neurons but not cholinergic innervation, and abolishes increases in CBF with fastigial nucleus stimulation (Iadecola et al., 1987a). However, there is evidence to the contrary that suggests caution in accepting the importance of fastigial nucleus projections to cerebral vessels. First, chronic lesions of basal forebrain have been reported to decrease metabolic rate in cerebral cortex (Orzi et al., 1988), indicating that this area supplies neurons and astroglia as well as possibly blood vessels. However, it is possible that a pool of fibers originating from this area directly innervate cerebral vessels. Second, two studies from the same laboratory have shown that fastigial nucleus does not change CBF in cats (Williams et al., 1989, 1990). In response to that study, Iadecola, Springston and Reis (1990), have presented evidence which indicates that α-chloralose, the anaesthetic agent used in the latter studies, prevents the increase in CBF during fastigial nucleus stimulation. Third, as mentioned previously, there has been no documentation of central pathways directly innervating cerebral resistance vessels, although the possibility exists that astroglial are innervated (Stone and Ariano, 1989) and participate in vascular responses. In contrast to the fastigial nucleus, stimulation of another caudal area of the brain, namely the dorsal medullary reticular formation, has been reported to similarly increase both cerebral metabolic rate and blood flow (Iadecola *et al.*, 1983b). Although the increased metabolic rate should be sufficient to account for the increased CBF, it appears that adrenal medullary-derived catecholamines, acting on β-adrenoreceptors, also play a role in blood flow changes during stimulation of the dorsal medullary reticular formation (Iadecola *et al.*, 1987b; Lacombe *et al.*, 1990).

The rostral ventrolateral medulla has been suggested as a site for central control of CBF. Stimulation of this area increases CBF in rats without increasing metabolic rate (Saeki *et al.*, 1989; Underwood *et al.*, 1992a; Golanov and Reis, 1994). However, contrary findings have been reported (Maeda *et al.*, 1991). A unique feature of the increase in CBF is its slow onset and persistence after cessation of stimulation. Both prostanoids and nitric oxide appear to be involved in cerebrovascular dilation to rostral ventrolateral medulla stimulation (Golanov and Reis, 1994).

Early evidence (Chan-Palay, 1976) had indicated that serotonergic fibers, possibly originating from the raphé nucleus, innervate the cerebral vasculature. Biochemical and immunohistological approaches demonstrated the presence of serotonin around cerebral arteries in rat, mice, guinea pig, cat, rabbit, and human (Griffith, Lincoln and Burnstock, 1982; Edvinsson *et al.*, 1983b; Griffith and Burnstock, 1983; Edvinsson *et al.*, 1984b). In addition, a possible connection between the raphé nucleus and cerebral arteries was suggested by retrograde tracing experiments (Tsai *et al.*, 1985). Further, tryptophan hydroxylase activity is reported to be associated with large arteries in rat, and amount of enzyme is reduced following lesions of the dorsal but not median raphé nucleus (Moreno, López de Pablo and Marco, 1994). Also, destruction of the raphé nucleus abolished presence of serotonin in cerebral blood vessels (Reinhard *et al.*, 1979; Edvinsson *et al.*, 1983b; Scatton *et al.*, 1985). Lastly, electrical stimulation of the raphé nucleus decreased CBF Bonvento, Lacombe and Seylaz, 1989) without corresponding changes in metabolic rate (Cudennec *et al.*, 1988), although increases in CBF with raphé nucleus stimulation have also been reported (Underwood *et al.*, 1992b). Bonvento *et al.* (1991) have suggested that small pial arterioles but not large cerebral arteries receive central serotonergic innervation. However, recent evidence do not support the concept that cerebral vessels have direct serotonergic innervation. Sympathetic nerve endings are avid scavengers of serotonin via a high affinity uptake system, and once loaded, release serotonin as well as noradrenaline with depolarization (Levitt and Duckles, 1986; Saito and Lee, 1987; Chang, Owman and Steinbusch, 1988). Potential pools for serotonin include mast cells, blood, and neuronal release (Reinhard *et al.*, 1979; Edvinsson *et al.*, 1983b; Scatton *et al.*, 1985). In addition, careful flushing of vessels to remove blood prior to dissection and preparation prevents significant accumulation of serotonin in cerebral blood vessels (Saito and Lee, 1987; Yu and Lee, 1989). Also, removal of the superior cervical ganglia eliminates serotonin in pial and parenchymal blood vessels (Alafaci *et al.*, 1986; Cowen *et al.*, 1986; Saito and Lee, 1987; Chang, Owman and Steinbusch, 1988; Yu and Lee, 1989). Further Mathiau *et al.* (1993) do not find trytophan hydroxylase activity in cerebral vessels. Lastly, changes in CBF during raphé stimulation do not correspond on a regional basis with distribution of serotonergic projections (Cudennec *et al.*, 1988; Bonvento, Lacombe and Seylaz, 1989). Thus, although the issue is not yet closed (Moreno *et al.*, 1994), the weight of current evidence indicates that at least large and perhaps small cerebral arteries are not innervated by serotonergic fibers.

SYNAPTIC ESCAPE OF NEUROTRANSMITTERS

In peripheral circulations, neurotransmitters originating from perivascular nerves and blood have access to vascular smooth muscle. In the cerebral circulation, many neurotransmitters have access to cerebrovascular smooth muscle after escaping into the extracellular fluid from neuron-neuronal or neuron-glial synapses (Figure 6.1). Thus, under baseline conditions, but more commonly under stressed conditions, neurotransmitter levels near cerebral resistance vessels may reach or exceed threshold values in extracellular fluid for vascular effects. For example, levels in brain extracellular fluid increase into the vasoactive range for: (1) opioids during haemorrhic hypotension (Armstead *et al.*, 1991); (2) dopamine (Bentue-Ferrer *et al.*, 1986; Harik *et al.*, 1986; Slivka *et al.*, 1988) and excitatory amino acid neurotransmitters (Hagberg *et al.*, 1987; Nakakita, Hiroyuki and Kogure, 1993) during ischaemia or arterial hypoxia; (3) excitatory amino acid neurotransmitters during sensory stimulation (Kendrick *et al.*, 1988; Skilling *et al.*, 1988; Graham *et al.*, 1993) and during cortical spreading depression (Van Harreveld and Fifkova, 1970); and (4) acetylcholine during fastigial nucleus or magnocellular nucleus electrical stimulation (Arneríc *et al.*, 1987; Kurosana, Sato and Sato, 1989). In addition, accumulation of serotonin into perivascular noradrenergic nerve terminals, possibly from neurons arising from the raphé nucleus (Reinhard *et al.*, 1979; Edvinsson *et al.*, 1983b; Scatton *et al.*, 1985), indicates that considerable amounts of serotonin, as well as other neurotransmitters, normally have access to the cerebral extracellular space. Thus, the likelihood exists that neurotransmitters, derived from non-perivascular nerves, can exert effect upon cerebral vessels under baseline conditions, when these neurons are physiologically activated, and during pathophysiological conditions. As with noradrenaline or other factors released by sympathetic nerves, these neurotransmitters may have trophic effects on cerebral vessels at doses below vasoactive threshold.

Since neurotransmitters in the extracellular fluid have access not only to vascular smooth muscle but to other cells as well, the potential exists for these neurotransmitters to cause release of other vasoactive substances. Studies conducted over the past decade in newborn pigs indicate that neurotransmitters, once released into the extracellular fluid, can affect vascular tone, not only by themselves, but also could induce synthesis and release of prostanoids from neurons, astroglia and vascular cells which will determine the final vascular response (Table 6.1). The evidence for this interaction comes from two independent sources. First, whether application of a neurotransmitter under a closed cranial window would increase levels of prostanoids in cerebrospinal fluid sampled from under this window. Second, whether vascular responses to a neurotransmitter before and after inhibition of prostanoid production with indomethacin. Our results indicate this interaction between neurotransmitters and prostanoids occurs at several different levels (Table 6.1). First, many constrictor and dilator neurotransmitters, such as dopamine, excitatory amino acids, isoprenaline, vasopressin (normal tone), CGRP and Substance P, exert cerebrovascular effects independently of the prostanoid system. Second, dilator prostanoids appear to mediate effects on cerebral arterioles of histamine, leu-enkephalin, met-enkaphalin, and oxytocin in piglets, and vasoactive intestinal polypeptide in adult cats (Wei, Kontos and Said, 1980). Third, dilator prostanoids can counteract constrictor effects on cerebral arterioles of noradrenaline, vasopressin (decreased tone), dynorphin (decreased tone), and β-endorphin.

Lastly, prostanoids, probably working at a thromboxane A_2/prostaglandin H_2 receptor, could play a permissive role and allow cerebrovascular constriction due to acetylcholine. As mentioned earlier, histamine and nitric oxide also can modulate noradrenaline effects on cerebrovascular tone.

SUMMARY AND CONCLUSIONS

Cerebral vessels are innervated by sympathetic, parasympathetic, and trigeminal fibers and possibly central pathways, and consequently are exposed to many different neurotransmitters from these sources as well as synaptic overflow from neurons and/or astroglia. Sympathetic nerves are reflexively activated during conditions in which cerebral arteries and arterioles are dilated, and serve to attenuate this dilatation. In addition, sympathetic nerves exert a trophic role in development and possibly maintenance of cerebral vessel wall morphology. Less is known about the role of parasympathetic fibers, but they appear to exert a dilator role on cerebral arterioles, especially following occlusion of upstream vessels. Trigeminal fibers appear to convey pain impulses from the meninges and pial to the brain, to modify constriction due to topical noradrenaline and arterial hypertension, and to promote dilatation during cortical spreading depression, arterial hypotension, and reperfusion after ischaemia. Central pathways such as the fastigial nucleus might provide important dilator influences to cerebral resistance vessels. Lastly, neurotransmitters accumulating in extracellular fluid via synaptic overflow may be an important source of vasoactive agents to cerebral vessels, and endogenous prostanoids and other substances released by adjacent cells may influence the final vascular response.

ACKNOWLEDGEMENTS

Supported by grants HL-30260 and HL-46558 from the Heart, Lung and Blood Institute, National Institutes of Health, Bethesda, MD.

REFERENCES

Abraham, W.C., Delanay, R.L., Dunn, A.J. and Zornetzer, S.F. (1979). Locus coeruleus stimulation decreases deoxyglucose uptake in ipsilateral mouse cerebral cortex. *Brain Research*, **172**, 387–392.

Adachi, T., Inanami, O. and Sato, A. (1992). Nitric oxide (NO) is involved in increased cerebral cortical blood flow following stimulation of the nucleus basalis of Meynert in anaesthetized rats. *Neuroscience Letters*, **1939**, 201–204.

Alafaci, C., Cowen, T., Crockard, H.A. and Burnstock, G. (1986). Cerebral perivascular serotonergic fibers have a peripheral origin in the gerbil. *Brain Research Bulletin*, **16**, 303–304.

Allen, J.M., Schon, F., Todd, N., Yeats, J.C., Crockard, H.A. and Bloom, S.R. (1984). Presence of neuropeptide Y in human circle of Willis and its possible role in cerebral vasospasm. *Lancet*, **1**, 550–552.

Anwar, M., Buckweitz-Milton, E. and Weiss, H.R. (1988). Effect of prazosin on microvascular perfusion during middle cerebral artery ligation in the rat. *Circulation Research*, **63**, 27–34.

Armstead, W.M., Mirro, R.C., Leffler, W. and Busija, D.W. (1988a). Acetylcholine produces cerebrovascular constriction through activation of muscarinic-1 receptors in the newborn pig. *Journal of Pharmacology and Experimental Therapeutics*, **247**, 926–933.

Armstead, W.M., Mirro, R., Busija, D.W. and Leffler, C.W. (1989a). Permissive role of prostanoids in acetylcholine-induced cerebral vasoconstriction. *Journal of Pharmacology and Experimental Therapeutics*, **251**, 1012–1019.

Armstead, W.M., Mirro, R., Busija, D.W. and Leffler C.W. (1989b). Vascular responses to vasopressin are tone-dependent in the cerebral circulation of the newborn pig. *Circulation Research*, **64**, 136–144.

Armstead, W.M., Mirro, R., Busija, D.W., Desiderio, D.M. and Leffler C.W. (1991). Opioids in cerebrospinal fluid in hypotensive newborn pigs. *Circulation Research*, **68**, 922–929.

Armstead, W.M., Leffler, C.W., Busija, D.W., Beasley, D.G. and Mirro, R. (1988b). Adrenergic and prostanoid mechanisms in the control of cerebral blood flow in hypotensive newborn pigs. *American Journal of Physiology*, **23**, H671–H677.

Arneríc, S.P., Iadecola, C., Underwood, M.D. and Reis, D.J. (1987). Local cholinergic mechanisms participate in the increase in cortical cerebral blood flow elicited by electrical stimulation of the fastigial nucleus in rat. *Brain Research*, **411**, 212–225.

Asada, Y. and Lee, T.S.-F. (1992). α_2-adrenoceptor mediates norepinephrine constriction of porcine pial veins. *American Journal of Physiology*, **263**, H1907–H1910.

Aubineau, P., Sercombe, R. and Seylaz, J. (1980). Parasympathetic influence of carbachol on local cerebral blood flow in the rabbit by a direct vasodilator action and an inhibition of the sympathetic mediated vasoconstriction. *British Journal of Pharmacology*, **68**, 449–459.

Bauknight, G.C.Jr., Faraci, F.M. and Heistad, D.D (1992). Endothelium-derived relaxing factor modulates noradrenergic constriction of cerebral arterioles in rabbits. *Stroke*, **23**, 1522–1526.

Baumbach, G.L. and Heistad, D.D. (1983). Effects of sympathetic stimulation and changes in arterial pressure on segmental resistance of cerebral vessels in rabbits and cats. *Circulation Research*, **52**, 527–533.

Bentue-Ferrer, D., Reymann, J.M., Bagot, H., Van den Driessche, J., de Certaines, J. and Allain, H. (1986). Aminergic neurotransmitter and water content changes in rats after transient forebrain ischaemia. *Journal of Neurochemistry*, **47**, 1672–1677.

Bevan, J.A. (1987). Comparison of the contractile response of the rabbit basilar and pulmonary arteries to sympathomimetic agonists. Further evidence for variation in vascular adrenoceptor characteristics. *Journal of Pharmacology and Experimental Therapeutics*, **216**, 83–89.

Bevan, R.D., Tsuru, H. and Bevan, J.A. (1983). Cerebral artery mass in the rabbit is reduced by chronic sympathetic denervation. *Stroke*, **14**, 393–396.

Bevan, J.A., Moskowitz, M., Said, S.I. and Buga, G. (1984). Evidence that vasoactive intestinal polypeptide is a dilator transmitter to some cerebral and extracerebral cranial arteries. *Peptides*, **5**, 385–388.

Bevan, J.A., Buga, G.M., Florence, V.M., Gonsalves, A. and Snowden, A. (1982). Distribution of choline acetyltransferase in cerebral and extracerebral arteries of the cat. *Circulation Research*, **50**, 470–476.

Bill, A. and Linder, J. (1976). Sympathetic control of cerebral blood flow in acute arterial hypertension. *Acta Physiologica Scandinavica*, **96**, 114–121.

Bonvento, G., Lacombe, P. and Seylaz, J. (1989). Effects of electrical stimulation of the dorsal raphé nucleus on local cerebral blood flow in the rat. *Journal of Cerebral Blood Flow and Metabolism*, **9**, 251–255.

Bonvento, G., Lacombe, P., Mackenzie, E.T., Fage, D., Benavides, J., Rouquier, L., *et al.* (1991). Evidence for differing origins of the serotonergic innervation of major cerebral arteries and small pial vessels in the rat. *Journal of Neurochemistry*, **56**, 681–689.

Bredt, D.S., Hwang, P.M. and Snyder, S.H. (1990). Localization of nitric oxide synthase indicating a neural role for nitric oxide. *Nature*, **347**, 768–770.

Buchweitz, E., Edelman, N.H. and Weiss, H.R. (1985). Effect of locus coeruleus stimulation on regional cerebral oxygen consumption in the cat. *Brain Research*, **325**, 107–114.

Buckley, N. (1986). Maturation of cardiovascular system in three mammalian models of human development. *Comparative Biochemistry and Physiology. A: Comparative Physiology*, **83**, 1–7.

Buckley, N., Brazeau, P. and Gootman, P.M. (1983). Maturation of circulatory responses to adrenergic stimuli. *Federation Proceedings*, **42**, 1643–1647.

Busija, D.W. (1984). Sympathetic nerves reduce cerebral blood flow during hypoxia in awake rabbits. *American Journal of Physiology*, **247**, H446–H451.

Busija, D.W. (1985a). Sustained cerebral vasoconstriction during bilateral sympathetic stimulation in anaesthetized rabbits. *Brain Research*, **345**, 341–344.

Busija, D.W. (1985b). Role of prostaglandins in modulating sympathetic vasoconstriction in the cerebral circulation in anaesthetized rabbits. *Journal of Cerebral Blood Flow and Metabolism*, **5**, 17–25.

Busija, D.W. (1986). Unilateral and bilateral sympathetic effects on cerebral blood flow during normocapnia. *American Journal of Physiology*, **19**, H498–H502.

Busija, D.W. (1993). The role of central neural pathways in the regulation of cerebral blood flow. *The regulation of cerebral blood flow*, edited by S.W. Phillis, pp. 65–77, Boca Raton: CRC Press.

Busija, D.W. and Chen, J. (1992). Effects of trigeminal neurotransmitters on piglet pial arterioles. *Journal of Developmental Physiology*, **263**, H1455–H1459.

Busija, D.W. and Heistad, D.D. (1981). Effects of cholinergic nerves on cerebral blood flow in cats. *Circulation Research*, **48**, 62–69.

Busija, D.W. and Heistad, D.D. (1982). Atropine does not attenuate cerebral vasodilatation during hypercapnia. *American Journal of Physiology*, **242**, H683–H687.

Busija, D.W. and Heistad, D.D. (1983). Effects of indomethacin on cerebral blood flow during hypercapnia in cats. *American Journal of Physiology*, **244**, H519–H524.

Busija, D.W. and Heistad, D.D. (1984a). Factors involved in physiological regulation of cerebral blood flow. *Reviews of Physiology, Biochemistry and Pharmacology*, **101**, 161–211.

Busija, D.W. and Heistad, D.D. (1984b). Effects of activation of sympathetic nerves on cerebral blood flow during hypercapnia in cats and rabbits. *Journal of Physiology (London)*, **347**, 35–45.

Busija, D.W. and Leffler, C.W. (1987a). Eicosanoid synthesis elicited by norepinephrine in piglet parietal cortex. *Brain Research*, **403**, 243–248.

Busija, D.W. and Leffler, C.W. (1987b). Postjunctional α_2-adrenoceptors in pial arteries of anaesthetized newborn pigs. *Developmental Pharmacology and Therapeutics*, **10**, 36–46.

Busija, D.W. and Leffler, C.W. (1987c). Exogenous norepinephrine constricts cerebral arterioles via α_2-adrenoceptors in newborn pigs. *Journal of Cerebral Blood Flow and Metabolism*, **7**, 184–188.

Busija, D.W. and Leffler, C.W. (1989a). Dilator effects of amino acid neurotransmitters on piglet pial arterioles. *American Journal of Physiology*, **26**, H1200–1203.

Busija, D.W. and Leffler, C.W. (1989b). Effects of dopamine on pial arteriolar diameter and CSF prostanoid levels in piglets. *Journal of Cerebral Blood Flow and Metabolism*, **9**, 264–267.

Busija, D.W., Heistad, D.D. and Marcus, M.L. (1980). Effects of sympathetic nerves on cerebral vessels during acute, moderate increases in arterial pressure in dogs and cats. *Circulation Research*, **46**, 696–702.

Busija, D.W., Heistad, D.D. and Marcus, M.L. (1981). Continuous measurement of cerebral blood flow in anaesthetized cats and dogs. *American Journal of Physiology*, **10**, H228–H234.

Busija, D.W., Khries, I. and Chen, J. (1992). Prostanoids promote pial arteriolar dilation and mask constriction to oxytocin in piglets. *American Journal of Physiology*, **264**, H1023–H1027.

Busija, D.W., Leffler, C.W. and Wagerle, L.C. (1985). Responses of newborn pig pial arteries to sympathetic nervous stimulation and exogenous noradrenaline. *Pediatric Research*, **19**, 1210–1214.

Busija, D.W., Leffler, C.W. and Wagerle, L.C. (1990). Mono-L-arginine-containing compounds dilate piglet pial arterioles via an endothelium-derived relaxing factor-like substance. *Circulation Research*, **67**, 1374–1380.

Busija, D.W., Marcus, M.L. and Heistad, D.D. (1982). Pial artery diameter and blood flow velocity during sympathetic stimulation in cats. *Journal of Cerebral Blood Flow and Metabolism*, **2**, 363–367.

Busija, D.W., Sadoshima, S., Marcus, M.L. and Heistad, D.D. (1982). Functional significance of sympathetic innervation of cerebral vessels. Can the issue now be resolved? *Trends in Autonomic Pharmacology*, edited by S. Kalsner, pp. 187–204, Baltimore: Urban and Schwarzenberg.

Busija, D.W., Wagerle, L.C., Pourcyrous, M.P. and Leffler, C.W. (1988). Acetylcholine dramatically increases prostanoid synthesis in piglet parietal cortex. *Brain Research*, **439**, 122–126.

Cervos-Navarro, J. and Matakas, F. (1974). Electron microscopic evidence for innervation of intracerebral arterioles in the cat. *Neurology*, **24**, 282–286.

Chan-Palay, V. (1976). Serotonin axons in the supra- and sub-ependymal plexuses and in the leptomeninges; their roles in local alterations of cerebrospinal and vasomotor activity. *Brain Research*, **102**, 103–130.

Chang, J.-Y., Owman, C. and Steinbusch, H.W.M. (1988). Evidence for coexistence of serotonin and noradrenaline in sympathetic nerves supplying brain vessels of guinea pig. *Brain Research*, **438**, 237–246.

Chang, J.-Y., Ekblad, E., Kannisto, P. and Owman, C. (1989). Serotonin uptake into cerebrovascular nerve fibers of rat, visualization by immunohistochemistry, disappearance following sympathectomy and release during electrical stimulation. *Brain Research*, **492**, 79–88.

Chen, F.-Y. and Lee, T.J.-F. (1993). Role of nitric oxide in neurogenic vasodilation of porcine cerebral artery. *Journal of Pharmacology and Experimental Therapeutics*, **265**, 339–345.

Cobb, S. and Finesinger, J.E. (1932). Cerebral Circulation XIX. The vagal pathway of the vasodilator impulse. *Archives of Neurological Psychiatry*, **28**, 1234–1256.

Colonna, D.M., Meng, W., Deal, D.D. and Busija, D.W. (1994). Calcitonin gene-related peptide promotes cerebrovascular dilation during cortical spreading depression in rabbits. *American Journal of Physiology*, **266**, H1095–H1102.

Cowen, T., Alafaci, C., Crockard, H.A. and Burnstock, G. (1986). 5-HT-containing nerves to major cerebral arteries of the gerbil originate in the superior cervical ganglia. *Brain Research*, **384**, 51–59.

Cudennec, A., Duverger, D., Serrano, A., Scatton, B. and MacKenzie, E.T. (1988). Influence of ascending serotonergic pathways on glucose use in the conscious rat brain. II. Effects of electrical stimulation of the rostral raphé nuclei. *Brain Research*, **444**, 227–246.

D'Alecy, L.G. and Rose, C.J. (1979). Parasympathetic cholinergic control of cerebral blood flow in dogs. *Circulation Research*, **41**, 324–331.

Dacey, R.G., Bassett, J.E. and Takayasu, M. (1988). Vasomotor responses of rat intracerebral arterioles to vasoactive intestinal peptide, substance P, neuropeptide Y and bradykinin. *Journal of Cerebral Blood Flow and Metabolism*, **8**, 254–261.

Dahlgren, N., Lindvall, O., Sakabe, T., Steneni, U. and Siesjö, B.K. (1981). Cerebral blood flow and oxygen consumption in the rat brain after lesions of the noradrenergic locus coeruleus system. *Brain Research*, **209**, 11–23.

Doba, N. and Reis, D.J. (1972). Changes in regional blood flow and cardiodynamics evoked by electrical stimulation of the fastigial nucleus in cat and their similarity to orthostatic reflexes. *Journal of Physiology (London)*, **227**, 729–747.

Duckles, S.P. (1981). Evidence for a functional cholinergic innervation of cerebral arteries. *Journal of Pharmacology and Experimental Therapeutics*, **217**, 544–548.

Duckles, S.P. and Buck, S.H. (1982). Substance P in the cerebral vasculature: depletion by capsaicin suggests a sensory role. *Brain Research*, **245**, 171–174.

Edvinsson, L. and Owman, C. (1977). Sympathetic innervations and adrenergic receptors in intraparenchymal cerebral arteries of baboon. In *Proceedings of the 8th international symposium on cerebral function, metabolism and circulation*, edited by D.H. Ingvar and N.A. Lassen, pp. 403–405, Copenhagen: Munksgaarde.

Edvinsson, L. and Uddman, R. (1982). Immunohistochemical localization and dilatatory effect of Substance P on human cerebral vessels. *Brain Research*, **232**, 466–471.

Edvinsson, L., Owman, C. and Siesjö, B. (1976). Physiological role of cerebrovascular sympathetic nerves in the autoregulation of cerebral blood flow. *Brain Research*, **117**, 518–523.

Edvinsson, L., Falck, B. and Owman, C. (1977). Possibilities for a cholinergic action on smooth musculature and on sympathetic axons in brain vessels mediated by muscarinic and nicotinic receptors. *Journal of Pharmacology and Experimental Therapeutics*, **200**, 117–126.

Edvinsson, L., McCulloch, J. and Uddman, R. (1981). Substance P: immunohistochemical localization and effect upon cat pial arteries *in vitro* and *in situ*. *Journal of Physiology (London)*, **318**, 251–258.

Edvinsson, L., Rosendal-Helgesen, S. and Uddman, R. (1983). Substance P: Localization, concentration and release in cerebral arteries, choroid plexus, and dura mater. *Cell Tissue Research*, **234**, 1–7.

Edvinsson, L., Lindvall, M., Nielsen, K.C. and Owman, C. (1973). Are brain vessels innervated also by central (non-sympathetic) adrenergic neurones? *Brain Research*, **63**, 396–399.

Edvinsson, L., Nielsen, K.C., Owman, C. and Sporrong, B. (1972). Cholinergic mechanisms in pial vessels. *Zeitschrift fumar Zellforschang und mikroskopische Anatomie*, **134**, 311–325.

Edvinsson, L., Copeland, J.R., Emson, P.C., McCulloch J. and Uddman, R. (1987a). Nerve fibers containing neuropeptide Y in the cerebrovascular bed: immunocytochemistry, radioimmunoassay and vasomotor effects. *Journal of Cerebral Blood Flow and Metabolism*, **7**, 45–57.

Edvinsson, L., Degueurce, A., Duverger, D., MacKenzie, E.R. and Scatton, B. (1983b). Central serotonergic nerves project to the pial vessels of the brain. *Nature (London)*, **306**, 55–57.

Edvinsson, L., Ekman, R., Jansen, I., Ottosson, A. and Uddman, R. (1987b). Peptide-containing nerve fibers in human cerebral arteries: immunocytochemistry, radioimmunoassay and *in vitro* pharmacology. *Annals of Neurology*, **21**, 432–437.

Edvinsson, L., Emson, P., McCulloch, J., Tatemoto, K. and Uddman, R. (1983a). Neuropeptide Y: cerebrovascular innervation and vasomotor effects in the cat. *Neuroscience Letters*, **43**, 79–84.

Edvinsson, L., Emson, P., McCulloch, J., Tatemoto, K. and Uddman, R. (1984a). Neuropeptide Y: immunocytochemical localization to and effect upon feline pial arteries and veins *in vitro* and *in situ*. *Acta Physiologica Scandinavica*, **122**, 155–163.

Edvinsson, L., Kakanson, M., Lindvall, M., Owman, Ch. and Svensson, K.G. (1975). Ultrastructural and biochemical evidence for a sympathetic neural influence on the choroid plexus. *Experimental Neurology*, **48**, 241–251.

Edvinsson, L., Birath, E., Uddman, R., Lee, T.J.-F., Duverger, D., MacKenzie, E.T., et al. (1984b). Indoleaminergic mechanisms in brain vessels: localization, concentration, uptake and *in vitro* response of 5-hydroxytryptamine. *Acta Physiologica Scandinavica*, **121**, 291–299.

Edvinsson, L., Fahrenkrug, J., Hanko, J., Owman, Ch., Sundler, F. and Uddman, R. (1980). VIP (vasoactive intestinal polypeptide)-containing nerves of intracranial arteries in mammals. *Cell Tissue Research*, **208**, 135–142.

Edvinsson, L., Fredholm, B.B., Hamel, E., Jansen, I. and Verrecchi, C. (1985). Perivascular peptides relax cerebral arteries concomitant with stimulation of cyclic adenosine monophosphate accumulation of release of an endothelium-derived relaxing factor in the cat. *Neuroscience Letters*, **58**, 213–217.

Edwards, R.M., Stack, E.J. and Trizna, W. (1991). Calcitonin-gene related peptide stimulates adenylate cyclase and relaxes intracerebral arterioles. *Journal of Pharmacology and Experimental Therapeutics*, **257**, 1020–1024.

Ekblad, E., Edvinsson, L., Wahlestedt, C., Uddman, R., Hakanson, R. and Sundler, F. (1984). Neuropeptide Y co-exists and co-operates with noradrenaline in perivascular nerve fibers. *Regulatory Peptides*, **8**, 225–235.

Estrada, C., Hamel, E. and Krause, D.N. (1983). Biochemical evidence for cholinergic innervation of intracerebral blood vessels. *Brain Research*, **266**, 261–270.

Faraci, F.M. and Brian, J.E. (1994). Nitric oxide and the cerebral circulation. *Stroke*, **25**, 692–703.

Faraci, F.M., Heistad, D.D. and Mayhan, W.G. (1987). Role of large arteries in regulation of blood flow to brain stem in cats. *Journal of Physiology (London)*, **387**, 115–123.

Feniuk, E., Humphrey, P.P.A. and Watts, A.D. (1979). Presynaptic inhibitory action of 5-hydroxytryptamine in dog isolated saphenous vein. *British Journal of Pharmacology*, **67**, 247–254.

Fitch, W., MacKenzie, E.T. and Harper, A.M. (1975). Effects of decreasing arterial blood pressure in cerebral blood flow in the baboon. *Circulation Research*, **37**, 550–557.

Fitzgerald, M.E.C., Vana, B.A. and Reiner, A. (1990a). Control of choroidal blood flow by the nucleus of Edinger-Westphal in pigeons: A laser doppler study. *Investigative Ophthalmology and Visual Science*, **31**, 2483–2492.

Fitzgerald, M.E.C., Vana, B.A. and Reiner, A. (1990b). Evidence for retinal pathology following interruption of neural regulation of choroidal blood flow: Muller cell express GFAP following lesions of the nucleus of Edinger-Westphal in pigeons. *Current Eye Research*, **9**, 583–589.

Florence, V.M. and Bevan, J.A. (1979). Biochemical determinations of cholinergic innervation in cerebral arteries. *Circulation Research*, **45**, 212–218.

Furchgott, R.F. (1984). The role of endothelium in the responses of vascular smooth muscle to drugs. *Annual Review of Pharmacology and Toxicology*, **24**, 175–197.

Gibbins, I.L. and Morris, J.L. (1988). Co-existence of immunoreactivity to neuropeptide Y and vasoactive intestinal peptide in non-noradrenergic axons innervating guinea-pig cerebral arteries after sympathectomy. *Brain Research*, **444**, 402–406.

Gibbins, I.L., Brayden, J.E. and Bevan, J.A. (1984). Perivascular nerves with immunoreactivity to vasoactive intestinal polypeptide in cephalic arteries of the cat: distribution, possible origins and functional implications. *Neuroscience*, **13**, 1327–1346.

Goadsby, P.J. (1990). Sphenopalatine ganglion stimulation increases regional cerebral blood flow independent of glucose utilization in the cat. *Brain Research*, **506**, 145–148.

Goadsby, P.J. (1991). Characteristics of facial nerve-elicited cerebral vasodilation determined using laser Doppler flowmetry. *American Journal of Physiology*, **260**, R255–262.

Goadsby, P.J., Lambert, G.A. and Lance, J.W. (1985). The mechanism of cerebrovascular vasoconstriction in response to locus coeruleus stimulation. *Brain Research*, **326**, 213–217.

Golanov, E.V. and Reis, D.J. (1994). Nitric oxide and prostanoids participate in cerebral vasodilation elicited by electrical stimulation of the rostral ventrolateral medulla. *Journal of Cerebral Blood Flow and Metabolism*, **14**, 492–502.

González, C. and Estrada, C. (1991). Nitric oxide mediates the neurogenic vasodilation of bovine cerebral arteries. *Journal of Cerebral Blood Flow and Metabolism*, **11**, 366–370.

Goplerud, J.M., Wagerle, J.C. and Delivoria-Papadopoulos, M. (1991). Sympathetic nerve modulation of regional cerebral blood flow during asphyxia in newborn pigs. *American Journal of Physiology*, **29**, H1575–1580.

Graham, S.H., Chen, J., Sharp, F.R. and Simon, R.P. (1993). Limiting ischemic injury by inhibition of excitatory amino acid release. *Journal of Cerebral Blood Flow and Metabolism*, **13**, 88–97.

Griffith, S.G. and Burnstock, G. (1983). Immunohistochemical demonstration of serotonin in nerves supplying human cerebral and mesenteric blood vessels. *Lancet*, **1** , 561–562.

Griffith, S.G., Lincoln, J. and Burnstock, G. (1982). Serotonin as a neurotransmitter in cerebral arteries. *Brain Research*, **247**, 388–392.

Gross, P.M., Harper, A.M. and Teasdale, G.M. (1983). Interaction of histamine with noradrenergic constrictory mechanisms in cat cerebral arteries and veins. *Canadian Journal of Physiology and Pharmacology*, **61**, 756–763.

Gross, P.M., Heistad, D.D., Strait, M.R., Marcus, M.L. and Brody, M.J. (1979). Cerebral vascular responses to physiological stimulation of sympathetic pathways in cats. *Circulation Research*, **44**, 288–294.

Hagberg, H., Andersson, P., Kjellmer, I., Thiringer, K. and Thordstein, M. (1987). Extracellular overflow of glutamate, aspartate, GABA and taurine in the cortex and basal ganglia of fetal lambs during hypoxia-ischaemia. *Neuroscience Letters*, **78**, 311–317.

Hara, H., Hamill, G.S. and Jacobowitz, D.M. (1985). Origin of cholinergic nerves to the rat major cerebral arteries: coexistence with vasoactive intestinal polypeptide. *Brain Research Bulletin*, **4**, 179–188.

Hara, H., Jansen, I., Ekman, R., Hamel, E., MacKenzie, E.T., Uddman, R., *et al.* (1989). Acetylcholine and vasoactive intestinal peptide in cerebral blood vessels: Effect of extirpation of the sphenoplatine ganglion. *Journal of Cerebral Blood Flow and Metabolism*, **9**, 204–211.

Hardebo, J.E., Edvinsson, L., Emson, P.G. and Owman, C. (1977). Isolated brain microvessels: enzymes related to adrenergic and cholinergic functions. In *Neurogenic Control of the Brain Circulation*, edited by C. Owman and L. Edvinsson, pp. 105–113, Oxford: Pergamon Press.

Harik, S.I., Yoshida, S., Busto, R. and Ginsberg, M.D. (1986). Monoamine neurotransmitters in diffuse reversible forebrain ischaemia and early recirculation: increased dopaminergic activity. *Neurology*, **36**, 971–976.

Harper, A.M., Deshmukh, V.D., Rowman, J.O. and Jennett, W.B. (1972). The influence of sympathetic nervous activity on cerebral blood flow. *Archives of Neurology*, **27**, 1–6.

Hart, M., Heistad, D.D. and Brody, M.J. (1980). Effect of chronic hypertension and sympathetic denervation on wall-lumen ratio of cerebral arteries. *Hypertension*, **2**, 419–423.

Hartman, B.K., Swanson, L.W., Raichle, M.E., Preskorn, S.H. and Clark, H.B. (1980). Central adrenergic regulation of cerebral microvascular permeability and blood flow; anatomic and physiologic evidence. *Advances in Experimental Medicine and Biology*, **131**, 113–126.

Hartman, B.K., Zide, D. and Udenfriend, D. (1972). The use of dopamine β hydroxylase as a marker for the central noradrenergic nervous system in rat brain. *Proceedings of the National Academy of Sciences of the USA*, **69**, 2722–2726.

Hayashi, S., Park, M.K. and Kuehl, T.J. (1984). Higher sensitivity of cerebral arteries isolated from premature and newborn baboons to adrenergic and cholinergic stimulation. *Life Sciences*, **35**, 253–260.

Hayashi, S., Park, M.K. and Kuehl, T.J. (1985). Post-synaptic α-adrenoceptors in baboon cerebral and mesenteric arteries. *Journal of Pharmacology and Experimental Therapeutics*, **235**, 113–121.

Heistad, D.D. and Marcus, M.L. (1979). Effect of sympathetic stimulation on permeability of the blood-brain barrier to albumin during acute hypertension in cats. *Circulation Research*, **45**, 331–338.

Heistad, D.D., Marcus, M.L. and Gross, P.M. (1978). Effects of sympathetic nerves on cerebral vessels in dog, cat and monkey. *American Journal of Physiology*, **235**, H544–H552.

Heistad, D.D., Marcus, M.L., Sandberg, S. and Abbouod, F.M. (1977). Effect of sympathetic nerve stimulation on cerebral blood flow and on large cerebral arteries of dog. *Circulation Research*, **41**, 342–350.

Hernandez, M.J., Brennan, R.W. and Hawkins, R.A. (1980). Regional cerebral blood flow during neonatal asphyxia. In *Cerebral Metabolism and Neural Function*, edited by J.V. Passonneau, R.A. Hawkins, W.D. Lust and F.A. Welsh, pp. 196–201. Baltimore: MD Williams and Wilkins.

Hoff, J.T., MacKenzie, E.T. and Harper, A.M. (1977). Responses of the cerebral circulation to hypercapnia and hypoxia after 7th cranial nerve transection in baboons. *Circulation Research*, **40**, 258–262.

Hogestatt, E.D. and Andersson, K.-E. (1984). On the postjunctional α-adrenoceptors in rat cerebral and mesenteric arteries. *Journal of Autonomic Pharmacology*, **4**, 166–173.

Hong, K.W., Pyo, K.M., Lee, W.S., Yu, S.S. and Rhim, B.Y. (1994). Pharmacological evidence that calcitonin gene-related peptide is implicated in cerebral autoregulation. *American Journal of Physiology*, **266**, H11–H16.

Iadecola, C. (1992). Nitric oxide participates in the cerebrovasodilation elicited from cerebellar fastigial nucleus. *American Journal of Physiology*, **263**, R1156–1161.

Iadecola, C. and Reis, D.J. (1990). Continuous monitoring of cerebrocortical blood flow during stimulation of the cerebellar fastigial nucleus: a study by laser-doppler flowmetry. *Journal of Cerebral Blood Flow and Metabolism*, **10**, 608–617.

Iadecola, C., Springston, M.E. and Reis, D.J. (1990). Dissociation by chloralose of the cardiovascular and cerebrovascular responses evoked from the cerebellar fastigial nucleus. *Journal of Cerebral Blood Flow and Metabolism*, **10**, 375–382.

Iadecola, C., Underwood, M.D. and Reis, D.J. (1986). Muscarinic cholinergic receptors mediate the cerebrovasodilation elicited by stimulation of the cerebellar fastigial nucleus in the rat. *Brain Research*, **368**, 375–379.

Iadecola, C., Zhang, F. and Xu, X. (1993). Role of nitric oxide synthase-containing vascular nerves in cerebrovasodilation elicited from cerebellum. *American Journal of Physiology*, **264**, R738–746.

Iadecola, C., Mraovitch, S., Meeley, M.P. and Reis, D.J. (1983a). Lesions of the basal forebrain in rat selectively impair the cortical vasodilatation elicited from cerebellar fastigial nucleus. *Brain Research*, **279**, 41–52.

Iadecola, C., Arnerić, S.P., Baker, H.D., Tucker, L.W. and Reis, D.J. (1987a). Role of local neurons in cerebrocortical vasodilatation elicited from cerebellum. *American Journal of Physiology*, **252**, R1082–R1091.

Iadecola, C., Lacombe, P.M., Underwood, M.D., Ishitsuka, T. and Reis, D.J. (1987b). Role of adrenal catecholamines in cerebrovasodilation evoked from brain stem. *American Journal of Physiology*, **21**, H1183–H1191.

Iadecola, C., Nakai, M., Mraovitch, S., Ruggiero, D.A., Tucker, L.W. and Reis, D.J. (1983b). Global increase in cerebral metabolism and blood flow produced by focal electrical stimulation of dorsal medullar reticular formation in rat. *Brain Research*, **272**, 101–114.

Itakura, T., Okuno, T., Nakakita, K., Kamei, I., Naka, Y., Nakai, K., *et al.* (1984). A light and electron microscopic immunohistochemical study of vasoactive intestinal polypeptide and Substance P-containing nerve fibers along the cerebral blood vessels: Comparison with aminergic and cholinergic nerve fibers. *Journal of Cerebral Blood Flow and Metabolism*, **4**, 407–414.

Johnson, J.W. and Ascher, P. (1987). Glycine potentiates the NMDA response in cultured mouse brain neurons. *Nature*, **325**, 529–531.

Juul, R., Edvinsson, L., Ekman, R., Brubrak, D. and Fredriksen, T.A. (1990). Calcitonin gene-related peptide-LI in subarachnoid haemorrhage in man: signs of activation of the trigeminal cerebrovascular system? *British Journal of Neurosurgery*, **4**, 171–180.

Kalsner, S. (1989). Cholinergic constriction in the general circulation and its role in coronary artery spasms. *Circulation Research*, **65**, 237–257.

Kano, M., Moskowitz, M.A. and Yokota, M. (1991). Parasympathetic denervation of rat pial vessels significantly increases infarction volume following middle cerebral artery occlusion. *Journal of Cerebral Blood Flow and Metabolism*, **11**, 628–637.

Katayama, Y., Aeno, Y., Tsukiyama, T. and Tsubakawa, T. (1981). Long lasting suppression of firing of cortical neurons and decrease in cortical blood flow following train pulse stimulation of the locus coeruleus in the cat. *Brain Research*, **216**, 173–179.

Katusic, Z.S., Shepherd, J.T. and Vanhoutte, P.M. (1988). Endothelium-dependent contractions to calcium ionophore A23187, arachidonic acid and acetylcholine in canine basilar arteries. *Stroke*, **19**, 476–479.

Kendrick, K.M, Keverne, E.B., Chapman, C. and Baldwin, B.A. (1988). Microdialysis measurement of oxytocin, aspartate, δ-amino butyric acid and glutamate release from the olfactory bulb of the sheep during vaginocervical stimulation. *Brain Research*, **442**, 171–174.

Kitazono, T., Heistad, D.D. and Faraci, F.M. (1993). Role of ATP-sensitive K^+ channels in CGRP-induced dilation of basilar artery *in vivo*. *American Journal of Physiology*, **265**, H581–585.

Kontos, H.A. and Wei, E.P. (1993). Hydroxyl radical-dependent inactivation of guanylate cyclase in cerebral arterioles by methylene blue and by LY83583. *Stroke*, **24**, 427–434.

Koketsu, N., Moskowitz, M.A., Kontos, H.A., Yokota, M. and Shimizu, T. (1992). Chronic parasympathetic sectioning decreases regional cerebral blood flow during haemorrhagic hypotension and increases infarct size after middle cerebral artery occlusion in spontaneously hypertensive rats. *Journal of Cerebral Blood Flow and Metabolism*, **23**, 613–620.

Kurosana, M., Sato, A. and Sato, Y. (1989). Well-maintained responses of acetylcholine release and blood flow in the cerebral cortex to local electrical stimulation of the nucleus basalis of Megnert in aged rats. *Neuroscience Letters*, **100**, 198–202.

Kurth, C.D., Wagerle L.C. and Delivoria-Papadopoulos, M. (1988). Sympathetic regulation of cerebral blood flow during seizures in newborn lambs. *American Journal of Physiology*, **24**, H563–H568.

Kuschinsky, W. and Wahl, M. (1975). α-receptor stimulation by endogenous and exogenous noradrenaline and blockade by phentolamine in pial arteries in cats. A microapplicaton study. *Circulation Research*, **37**, 168–174.

Kuschinsky, W., Wahl, M. and Neiss, A. (1974). Evidence for cholinergic dilatory receptors in pial arteries of cats. *Pflügers Archives*, **347**, 199–208.

Lacombe, P.M., Iadecola, C., Underwood, M.D., Sved, A.F. and Reis, D.J. (1990). Plasma epinephrine modulates the cerebrovasodilation evoked by electrical stimulation of the dorsal medulla. *Brain Research*, **506**, 93–100.

Lacombe, P., Miller, M.C. and Seylaz, J. (1985). Effect of sympathetic nerves on cerebral vessels during seizures. *American Journal of Physiology*, **17**, H672–H680.

Lande, I.S., Cannell, V.A. and Waterson, J.G. (1966). The interaction of serotonin and noradrenaline on the perfused artery. *British Journal of Pharmacology*, **28**, 255–272.

Larsson, L.I., Edvinsson, L., Fahrenkrug, J., Hakanson R., Owman, Ch., Schaffalitzky de Muckadel, O.B., *et al.* (1976). Immunohistochemical localization of a vasodilatory polypeptide (VIP) in cerebrovascular nerves. *Brain Research*, **113**, 400–404.

Lee, T.J.-F. (1985). Cholinergic interactions and vascular smooth muscle tone. In *Calcium and Contractility*, edited by A.K. Grover and E.E. Daniel, pp. 351–383, Bethesda, MD: The Humana Press.

Lee, T.J.-F. (1977). Sympathetic innervation of rabbit basilar artery: neuromuscular relationship. *Federation Proceedings*, **36**, 1036, abstract.

Lee, T.J.-F. and Saito, A. (1984). Altered cerebral vessels innervation in the spontaneously hypertensive rat. *Circulation Research*, **55**, 392–403.

Lee, T.J.-F. and Sarwinski, S. (1991). Nitric oxidergic neurogenic vasodilation in porcine basilar artery. *Blood Vessels*, **28**, 407–412.

Lee, T.J., Kinkhead, L.R. and Sarwinski, S. (1982). Noradrenaline and acetylcholine transmitter mechanism in large cerebral arteries of the pig. *Journal of Cerebral Blood Flow and Metabolism*, 2, 439–450.

Lee, R.J.-F., Saito, A. and Berezin, I. (1981) Vasoactive intestinal polypeptide-like substance: the potential transmitter for cerebral vasodilatation. *Science*, 224, 898–901.

Lembeck, F. and Holzer, P. (1979). Substance P as neurogenic mediator of antidromic vasodilatation and neurogenic plasma extravasation. *Naunyn-Schmiedeberg's Archives of Pharmacology*, 310, 175–183.

Levitt, B. and Duckles, S.P. (1986). Evidence against serotonin as a vasoconstrictor neurotransmitter in the rabbit basilar artery. *Journal of Pharmacology and Experimental Therapeutics*, 238, 880–885.

Linder, J. (1981). Effects of facial nerve stimulation on cerebral and ocular blood flow in haemorrhagic hypotension. *Acta Physiologica Scandinavica*, 112, 185–193.

Liu-Chen, L.-Y., Han, D.H. and Moskowitz, M.A. (1983). Pial arachnoid contains substance P originating from trigeminal neurons. *Neuroscience*, 9, 803–838.

Liu-Chen, L.-Y., Mayberg, M.R. and Moskowitz, M.A. (1983). Immunohistochemical evidence for a substance P-containing trigeminovascular pathway to pial arteries in cats. *Brain Research*, 268, 162–166.

Liu-Chen, L.-Y., Gillespie, S.A., Norregaard, T.V. and Moskowitz, M.A. (1984a). Co-localization of retrogradely transported wheat germ agglutinin and the putative neurotransmitter substance P within trigeminal ganglion cells projecting to cat middle cerebral artery. *Journal of Comparative Neurology*, 225, 187–192.

Liu-Chen, L.-Y., Gillespie, S.A., Norregaard, T.V., Go, V.L.W. and Moskowitz, M.A. (1984b). Cholecystokinin-8 (CCK8) immunoreactivity in cerebral arteries and pial arachnoid and the effect of unilateral trigeminal ganglionectomy. *Federation Proceedings*, 43, 304, abstract.

Lundberg, J.M., Anggard, A., Fahrenkrug, J., Lundgren, G. and Holmstedt, B. (1982). Corelease of VIP and acetylcholine in relation to blood flow and salivary secretion in cat submandibular salivary gland. *Acta Physiologica Scandinavica*, 115, 525–528.

Lundberg, J.M., Anggard, A., Fahrenkrug, J., Hokfelt, T. and Mutt, V. (1980). Vasoactive intestinal polypeptide (VIP) in cholinergic neurons of exocrine glands: functional significance of coexisting transmitters for vasodilatation and secretion. *Proceedings of the National Academy of Sciences USA*, 77, 1651–1655.

Macfarlane, R., Tasdemiroglu, E., Moskowitz, M.A., Uemura, Y., Wei, E.P. and Kontos, H.A. (1991). Chronic trigeminal ganglionectomy or topical capsaicin application to pial vessels attenuates post-occlusive cortical hyperemia but does not influence post-ischemic hypoperfusion. *Journal of Cerebral Blood Flow and Metabolism*, 11, 261–271.

MacKenzie, E.T., McGeorge, A.P., Graham, D.I., Fitch, W., Edvinsson, L. and Harper, A.M. (1979). Effects of increasing arterial pressure of cerebral blood flow in the baboon: influence of the sympathetic nervous system. *Pflügers Archives*, 378, 189–195.

MacKenzie, E.T., Strandgaard, S, Graham, D.I., Jones, J.V., Harper, A.M. and Farar, J.K. (1976). Effects of acutely induced hypertension in cats on pial arteriolar caliber, local cerebral blood flow and the blood-brain barrier. *Circulation Research*, 39, 33–41.

Maeda, M., Krieger, A.J., Nakai, M. and Sapru, H.N. (1991). Chemical stimulation of the rostral ventrolateral medullary pressor area decreases cerebral blood flow in anaesthetized rats. *Brain Research*, 563, 261–269.

Marcus, M.L. and Heistad, D.D. (1979). Effects of sympathetic nerves on cerebral blood flow in awake dogs. *American Journal of Physiology*, 5, H549–H553.

Marcus, M.L., Busija, D.W., Gross, P.M., Brooks, L.A. and Heistad, D.D. (1982). Sympathetic escape in the cerebral circulation during normotension and acute severe hypertension. In *Cerebral Blood Flow: Effect of Nerves and Neurotransmitters*, edited by D.D. Heistad and M.L. Marcus, pp. 281–289. New York: Elsevier.

Markowitz, S., Saito, K. and Moskowitz, M.A. (1987). Neurogenically-mediated leakage of plasma protein occurs from blood vessels in dura mater but not brain. *Journal of Neuroscience*, 7, 4129–4136.

Markowitz, S., Saito, K., Buzzi, M.G. and Moskowitz, M.A. (1989). The development of neurogenic plasma extravasation in the rat dura mater does not depend upon the degranulation of mast cells. *Brain Research*, 477, 157–165.

Marshall, J.J., Wei, E.P. and Kontos, H.A. (1988). Independent blockade of cerebral vasodilation from acetylcholine and nitric oxide. *American Journal of Physiology*, 255, H847–H854.

Mathiau, P., Reynier-Rebuffel, A.-M., Issertal, O., Callebert, J., Decreme, C. and Aubineau, P. (1993). Absence of serotonergic innervation from raphé nuclei in rat cerebral blood vessels. II: lack of tryptophan hydroxylase activity *in vitro*. *Neuroscience*, 52, 657–665.

Mayberg, M.R., Zervas, N.T. and Moskowitz, M.T. (1984). Trigeminal projections to supratentorial pial and dural blood vessels in cats demonstrated by horseradish peroxidase histochemistry. *Journal of Comparative Neurology*, 223, 46–56.

Mayberg, M.R., Langer, R.S., Zervas, N.T. and Moskowitz, M.A. (1981). Perivascular meningeal projections from cat trigeminal ganglia: possible pathway for vascular headaches in man. *Science*, 213, 228–230.

Mayhan, W.G., Simmons, L.K. and Sharpe, G.M. (1991). Mechanism of impaired responses of cerebral arterioles during diabetes mellitus. *American Journal of Physiology*, **29**, H319–H326.

McCulloch, J., Savaki, H.E. and Angersen, W. (1982). Regional water permeability in the CNS of conscious rats: Effects of hypercapnia and locus coeruleus lesions. In *Cerebral Blood Flow: Effects of Nerves and Neurotransmitters*, edited by D.D. Heistad and M.L. Marcus, pp. 509–516. North Holland, New York: Elsevier.

McCulloch, J., Uddman, R., Kingman, T. and Edvinsson, L. (1986). Calcitonin gene-related peptide: Function role in cerebrovascular regulation. *Proceedings of the National Academy of Sciences USA*, **83**, 5731–5735.

McCulloch, J. and Edvinsson, L. (1980). Cerebral circulatory and metabolic effects of vasoactive intestinal polypeptide. *American Journal of Physiology*, **238**, H449–H456.

McGrath, M.A. (1977). 5-Hydroxytryptamine and neurotransmitter release in canine blood vessels. *Circulation Research*, **41**, 428–435.

Medgett, I.C. and Langer, S.Z. (1983). Characterization of smooth muscle α-adrenoreceptors and of response to electrical stimulation in the cat isolated perfused middle cerebral artery. *Naunyn-Schmiedeberg's Archives of Pharmacology*, **323**, 24–32.

Meng, W. and Busija, D.W. (1993). Comparative effects of angiotensin-(1–17) and Angiotensin II on piglet pial arterioles. *Stroke*, **24**, 2041–2045.

Miao, F.J.-P. and Lee, T.J.-F. (1990). Cholinergic and VIPergic innervation in cerebral arteries: A sequential double-labeling immunohistochemical study. *Journal of Cerebral Blood Flow and Metabolism*, **10**, 32–37.

Mirro, R., Busija, D.W., Armstead, W.M. and Leffler, C.W. (1988). Histamine dilates the pial arterioles of newborn pigs through prostanoid production. *American Journal of Physiology*, **23**, H1023–H1026.

Moreno, M.J., López de Pablo, A.L. and Marco, E.J. (1994). Tryptophan hydroxylase activity in rat brain base arteries related to innervation originating from the dorsal raphé nucleus. *Stroke*, **25**, 1046–1049.

Morita-Tsuzuki, Y., Hardebo, J.E. and Bouskela, E. (1993). Inhibition of nitric oxide synthase attenuates cerebral blood flow response to stimulation of postganglionic parasympathetic nerves in the rat. *Journal of Cerebral Blood Flow and Metabolism*, **13**, 993–997.

Moskowitz, M.A., Brody, M. and Liu-Chen, L.-Y. (1983). *In vitro* release of immunoreactive substance P from putative afferent nerve endings in bovine pial arachnoid. *Neuroscience*, **9**, 809–814.

Moskowitz, M.A., Wei, E.P., Saito, K. and Kontos, H.M. (1988). Trigeminalectomy modifies pial arteriolar responses to hypertension and noradrenaline. *American Journal of Physiology*, **24**, H1–H6.

Moskowitz, M.A., Kuo, C., Leeman, S.E., Jessen, M.E. and Derian, C.K. (1987). Desensitization to substance P-induced vasodilatation *in vitro* is not shared by endogenous tachykinin neurokinin A. *Journal of Neuroscience*, **7**, 2344–2351.

Moskowitz, M.A., Sakas, D.E., Wei, E.P., Kano, M., Buzzi, M.G., Ogilvy, C., *et al.* (1989). Postocclusive cerebral hyperaemia is markedly attenuated by chronic trigeminal ganglionectomy. *American Journal of Physiology*, **26**, H1736–H1739.

Moskowitz, M.A., Macfarlane, R., Tasdemiroglu, E., Wei, E.P. and Kontos, H.A. (1991). Neuroeffector functions of sensory nerves in the cerebral circulation after global cerebral ischemia. *Arzneimittel-Forschung*, **41**, 315–318.

Mraovitch, S., Pinard, E. and Seylaz, J. (1986). Two neural mechanisms in rat fastigial nucleus regulating systemic and cerebral circulation. *American Journal of Physiology*, **251**, H153–H163.

Mraovitch, S., Iadecola, C., Ruggiero, D.A. and Reis, D.J. (1985). Widespread reductions in cerebral blood flow and metabolism elicited by electrical stimulation of the parabrachial nucleus in rat. *Brain Research*, **341**, 283–296.

Mueller, S.M., Heistad, D.D. and Marcus, M.L. (1977). Total and regional cerebral blood flow during hypotension, hypertension and hypocapnia: Effect of sympathetic denervation in dogs. *Circulation Research*, **41**, 350–356.

Mueller, S.M., Heistad, D.D. and Marcus, M.L. (1979). Effect of sympathetic nerves on cerebral vessels during seizures. *American Journal of Physiology*, **6**, H178–H184.

Murphy, S., Minor, R.L., Welk, G. and Harrison, D.G. (1990). Evidence from an astrocyte-derived vasorelaxing factor with properties similar to nitric oxide. *Journal of Neurochemistry*, **55**, 349–351.

Nakai, M., Iadecola, C. and Reis, D.J. (1982). Global cerebral vasodilatation by stimulation of rat fastigial cerebellar nucleus. *American Journal of Physiology*, **243**, H226–H235.

Nakai, M., Iadecola, C., Ruggiero, D.A., Tucker, L.W. and Reis, D.J. (1983). Electrical stimulation of cerebellar fastigial nucleus increases cerebrocortical blood flow without change in local metabolism: evidence for an intrinsic system in brain for primary vasodilatation. *Brain Research*, **260**, 35–49.

Nakai, M., Tamaki, K., Ogato, J, Matsui, Y. and Maeda, M. (1993). Parasympathetic cerebrovasodilator center of the facial nerve. *Circulation Research*, **72**, 470–475.

Nakakita, K. (1990). Peptidergic innervation in the cerebral blood vessels of the guinea pig: an immunohistochemical study. *Journal of Cerebral Blood Flow and Metabolism*, **10**, 819–826.

Nakakita, N., Hiroyuki, K. and Kogure, K. (1993). Effects of repeated cerebral ischemia on extracellular amino acid concentrations measured with intracerebral microdialysis in the gerbil hippocampus. *Stroke*, **24**, 458–464.

Navari, R., Wei, E.P., Kontos, H.A. and Patterson, J.L. Jr. (1978). Comparison of the open skull and cranial window preparations in the study of the cerebral microcirculation. *Microvascular Research*, **16**, 304–315.

Nelson, C.W., Wei, E.P., Povlishock, J.T., Kontos, H.A. and Moskowitz, M.A. (1992). Oxygen radicals in cerebral ischemia. *American Journal of Physiology*, **263**, H1356–H1362.

Neubauer, J.A. and Edelman, N.H. (1984). Nonuniform brain blood flow response to hypoxia in unanaesthetized cats. *Journal of Applied Physiology*, **57**, 1803–1808.

Nielsen, K.C. and Owman, C. (1967). Adrenergic innervation of pial arteries related to the circle of Willis in the cat. *Brain Research*, **6**, 773–776.

Nielsen, K.C., Owman, C. and Sporrong, B. (1971). Ultrastructure and the autonomic innervation apparatus in the main pial arteries of rats and cats. *Brain Research*, **27**, 25–32.

Norregaard, T. and Moskowitz, M.A. (1985). Substance P and the sensory innervation of intracranial and extracranial feline cephalic arteries. *Brain*, **108**, 517–533.

Nozaki, K., Moskowitz, M.A., Maynard, K.I., Koketsu, N., Dawson, T.M., Bredt, D.S., *et al.* (1993). Possible origins and distribution of immunoreactive nitric oxide synthase-containing nerve fibers in cerebral arteries. *Journal of Cerebral Blood Flow and Metabolism*, **13**, 70–79.

Orzi, F., Diana, G., Casamenti, F., Palombo, E. and Fieschi, C. (1988) Local cerebral glucose utilization following unilateral and bilateral lesions of the nucleus basalis magnocellularis in the rat. *Brain Research*, **462**, 99–103.

Peerless, S.J. and Yasargi, M.G. (1971). Adrenergic innervation of the cerebral blood vessels in the rabbit. *Journal of Neurosurgery*, **35**, 148–154.

Pinard, E., Purves, M.J., Seylaz, J. and Vasquez, J.V. (1979). The cholinergic pathway to cerebral blood vessels. II. Physiological studies. *Pflügers Archives*, **379**, 165–172.

Purdy, R.E. and Bevan, J.A. (1977). Adrenergic innervation of large cerebral blood vessels of the rabbit studied by fluorescence microscopy: Absence of features that might contribute to non-uniform change in cerebral blood flow. *Stroke*, **8**, 82–87.

Raichle, M.E., Hartman, B.K., Eichling, J.O. and Sharpe, L.G. (1975). Central noradrenergic regulation of cerebral blood flow and vascular permeability. *Proceedings of the National Academy of Sciences USA*, **72**, 3726–3730.

Raszkiewicz, J.L., Linville, D.G., Kerwin, J.F., Wagengar, J. and Aneric, S.P. (1992). Nitric oxide synthases is critical in mediating basal forebrain regulation of cortical cerebral circulation. *Journal of Neuroscience Research*, **33**, 129–135.

Reinhard, J.F. Jr., Liebmann, J.E., Schlosberg, A.J. and Moskowitz, M.A. (1979). Serotonin neurons project to small blood vessels in the brain. *Science*, **206**, 85–87.

Reis, D.J., Berger, S.B., Underwood, M.D. and Khayata, M. (1991). Electrical stimulation of cerebellar fastigial nucleus reduces ischemic infarction elicited by middle cerebral artery occlusion in rat. *Journal of Cerebral Blood Flow and Metabolism*, **11**, 810–818.

Rennels, M.G., Forbes, M.S., Anders, J.J. and Nelson, E. (1977). Innervation of the microcirculation in the central nervous system and other tissues. In *Neurogenic Control of the Brain Circulation*, edited by C. Owman and L. Edvinsson, pp. 91–104. Oxford: Pergamon.

Rosenblum, W.I. (1976a). Some physiologic properties of nerves in the adventitia of cerebral blood vessels as revealed by fluorescence microscopy. In *The Cerebral Vessel Wall*, edited by J. Cervos-Navarro, E. Betz, F. Matakas and R. Wullenweber, pp. 183–189. New York: Raven.

Rosenblum, W.I. (1976b). The "richness" of sympathetic innervation. A comparison of cerebral blood vessels. *Stroke*, **7**, 270–271.

Rosenblum, W.I. (1986). Endothelium dependent relaxation demonstrated *in vivo* in cerebral arterioles. *Stroke*, **17**, 494–497.

Rosenblum W.I., Shimizu, T. and Nelson, G.H. (1993). Endothelium-dependent effects of substance P and calcitonin gene-related peptide on mouse pial arterioles. *Stroke*, **24**, 1043–1048.

Sadoshima, S., Busija, D.W. and Heistad, D.D. (1983). Mechanisms of protection against stroke in stroke-prone spontaneously hypertensive rats. *American Journal of Physiology*, **244**, H406–H412.

Sadoshima, S., Busija, D.W., Brody, M.J. and Heistad, D.D. (1981). Sympathetic nerves protect against stroke in stroke-prone hypertensive rats. A preliminary study. *Hypertension*, **3**, 1124–1127.

Saeki, Y., Sato, A., Sato, Y. and Trzebski, A. (1989). Stimulation of rostral ventrolateral medullary neurons increases cortical cerebral blood flow via activation of the intracerebral neuronal pathway. *Neuroscience Letters*, **107**, 26–32.

Saito, A. and Lee, T.J.-F. (1987). Serotonin as an alternative transmitter in sympathetic nerves of large cerebral arteries of the rabbit. *Circulation Research*, **60**, 220–228.

Saito, A., Wu, J.-Y. and Lee, T.J.-F. (1985). Evidence for the presence of cholinergic nerves in cerebral arteries: an immunohistochemical demonstration of choline acetyltransferase. *Journal of Cerebral Blood Flow and Metabolism*, **5**, 327–334.

Saito, K., Greenberg, S. and Moskowitz, M.A. (1987). Trigeminal origin of β-preprotachykinin projects in feline pial blood vessels. *Neuroscience Letters*, **76**, 69–73.

Sakakibara, Y., Fujiwara, M. and Muramatsu, I. (1982). In: Pharmacological characterization in the α adrenoreceptors of the dog basilar artery. *Naunyn-Schmiedeberg's Archives of Pharmacology*, **319**, 1–7.

Sakas, D.E., Moskowitz, M.A., Wei, E.P., Kontos, H.A., Kano, M. and Ogilvy, C.S. (1989). Trigeminovascular fibers increase blood flow in cortical grey matter by axon reflex-like mechanisms during acute severe hypertension or seizures. *Proceedings of the National Academy of Sciences USA*, **86**, 1401–1405.

Scatton, B., Duverger, D., L'Heureux, R., Serrano, A., Fage, D., Nowicki, J.-P., *et al.* (1985). Neurochemical studies on the existence, origin and characteristics of the serotonergic innervation of small pial vessels. *Brain Research*, **345**, 219–229.

Sercombe, R., Lacombe, P., Aubineau, P., Mamo, H., Pinard, E., Reynier-Rebuffel, A.M., *et al.* (1979). Is there an active mechanism limiting the influence of the sympathetic system on the cerebral vascular bed? Evidence for vasomotor escape from sympathetic stimulation in the rabbit. *Brain Research*, **164**, 81–102.

Seylaz, J., Hara, H., Pinard, E., Mraovitch, S., MacKenzie, E.T. and Edvinsson, L. (1988). Effect of stimulation of the sphenopalatine ganglion on cortical blood flow in the rat. *Journal of Cerebral Blood Flow and Metabolism*, **8**, 875–878.

Shepherd, J.T. and Vanhoutte, P.M. (1981). Local modulation of adrenergic neurotransmission. *Circulation*, **64**, 655–666.

Skärby, T. (1984). Pharmacological properties of prejunctional α-adrenoceptors in isolated feline middle cerebral arteries; comparison with the post-junctional α-adrenoceptors. *Acta Physiologica Scandinavica*, **122**, 165–174.

Skärby, T. and Andersson, K.-E. (1984). Contraction-mediating α-adrenoreceptors in isolated human omental, temporal and pial arteries. *Journal of Autonomic Pharmacology*, **4**, 219–229.

Skärby, T., Andersson, K.-E. and Edvinsson, L. (1981). Characterization of the post-synaptic α-adrenoreceptor in isolated feline cerebral arteries. *Acta Physiologica Scandinavica*, **112**, 105–107.

Skilling, S.R., Smullin, D.H., Beitz, A.J. and Larson, A.A. (1988). Extracellular amino acid concentrations in the dorsal spinal cord of freely moving rats following verotridine and nociceptive stimuli. *Journal of Neurochemistry*, **51**, 127–132.

Slivka, A., Brannan, T.S., Weinberger, J., Knott, P.J. and Cohen, G. (1988). Increase in extracellular dopamine in the striatum during cerebral ischaemia: as study utilizing cerebral microdialysis. *Journal of Neurochemistry*, **50**, 1714–1718.

Snell, L.D., Morter, R.S. and Johnson, K.M. (1982). Glycine potentiates, N-methyl-D-aspartate-induced [^{3}H] TCP binding to rat cortical membranes. *Neuroscience Letters*, **83**, 313–317.

Stone, E.A. and Ariano, M.A. (1989). Are glial cells targets of the central noradrenergic system? A review of the evidence. *Brain Research Reviews*, **14**, 297–309.

Suzuki, N., Hardebo, J.E. and Owman, C. (1988). Origins and pathways of cerebrovascular vasoactive intestinal polypeptide-positive nerves in rats. *Journal of Cerebral Blood Flow and Metabolism*, **8**, 697–712.

Suzuki, N., Hardebo, J.E. and Owman, C. (1990). Origins and pathways of choline acetyltransferase — positive parasympathetic nerve fibers to cerebral vessels in rats. *Journal of Cerebral Blood Flow and Metabolism*, **10**, 399–408.

Suzuki, N., Hardebo, J.E., Kahrstrom, J. and Owman, J. (1990a). Neuropeptide Y coexists with vasoactive intestingal polypeptide in parasympathetic cerebrovascular nerves originating in the sphenopalatine, otic and internal carotid ganglia of the rat. *Neuroscience*, **36**, 507–519.

Suzuki, N., Hardebo, J.E., Kahrstrom, J. and Owman, C. (1990b). Selective electrical stimulation of postganglionic cerebrovascular parasympathetic nerve fibers originating from the sphenopalatine ganglion enhances cortical blood flow in the rat. *Journal of Cerebral Blood Flow Metabolism*, **10**, 383–391.

Suzuki, N., Fukuuchi, Y., Koto, A., Naganuma, Y., Isozumi, K., Matsuoka, S., *et al.* (1993). Cerebrovascular NADPH Diaphorase-containing nerve fibers in the rat. *Neuroscience Letters*, **151**, 1–3.

Suzuki, Y., Satoh, S.-I., Ikegaki, I., Okada, T., Shibuya, M., Sugita, K., *et al.* (1989). Effects of neuropeptide Y and calcitonin gene-related peptide on local cerebral blood flow in rat striatum. *Journal of Cerebral Blood Flow and Metabolism*, **9**, 268–270.

Thore, C.R., Nam, M. and Busija, D. (1994). Phorbol ester-induced prostaglandin production in piglet cortical astroglia. *American Journal of Physiology*, **267**, R34–R37.

Toda, N. (1983). α-adrenergic receptor subtypes in human, monkey, and dog cerebral arteries. *Journal of Pharmacology and Experimental Therapeutics*, **226**, 861–868.

Toda, N., Hatano, Y. and Hayaski, S. (1978). Modifications by stretches of the mechanical response of isolated cerebral and extra-cerebral arteries to vasoactive agents. *Pflügers Archives*, **374**, 73–77.

Toda, N., Ayajiki, K. and Okamura, T. (1993). Cerebroarterial relaxations mediated by nitric oxide derived from endothelium and vasodilator nerve. *Journal of Vascular Research*, **30**, 61–67.

Toda, N., Ayajiki, K, Yoshida, K., Kimura, H. and Okamura, T. (1993). Impairment by damage of the pterygopalatine ganglion of nitroxidergic vasodilator nerve function in canine cerebral and retinal arteries. *Circulation Research*, **72**, 206–213.

Tsai, S.H., Lin, S.Z., Wang, S.D., Liu, J.C. and Shih, C.J. (1985). Retrograde localization of the innervation of the middle cerebral artery with horseradish peroxidase in cats. *Neurosurgery*, **16**, 463–467.

Tsuiji, T. and Cook, D.A. (1988). Role of endothelium in canine cerebrovascular responses to acetylcholine, adenosine and ATP. *Proceedings of the Western Pharmacology Society*, **31**, 189–192.

Tsukahara, T., Taniguchi, T., Fujiwara, M. and Handa, H. (1983). Characterization of α-adrenoceptors in pial arteries of the bovine brain. *Naunyn-Schmiedeberg's Archives of Pharmacology*, **324**, 88–93.

Tuor, U.I., Kelley, P.A.T., Edvinsson, L. and McCulloch, J. (1990). Neuropeptide Y and the cerebral circulation. *Journal of Cerebral Blood Flow and Metabolism*, **10**, 591–601.

Uddman, R., Ekblad, R., Edvinsson, L., Håkanson, R. and Sundler, F. (1985). Neuropeptide Y-like immunoreactivity in perivascular nerve fibers of guinea-pig. *Regulatory Peptides*, **10**, 243–257.

Underwood, M.D., Iadecola, C., Sved, H.F. and Reis, D.J. (1992a). Stimulation of C1 area neurons globally increases regional cerebral blood flow but not metabolism. *Journal of Cerebral Blood Flow and Metabolism*, **12**, 844–855.

Underwood, M.D., Bakalian, M.J., Arango, V., Smith, R.W. and Mann, J.J. (1992b). Regulation of cortical blood flow by the dorsal raphé nucleus: Topographical organization of cerebrovascular regulatory regions. *Journal of Cerebral Blood Flow and Metabolism*, **12**, 664–673.

Usui, H., Kurahashi, K., Ashida, D. and Fujiwara, M. (1983). Acetylcholine-induced contractile response in canine basilar artery with activation of thromboxane A_2 synthesis sequence. *IRCS Journal of Medical Science*, **11**, 418–419.

Van Harreveld, A. and Fifkova, E. (1970). Glutamate release from the retina during spreading depression. *Journal of Neurobiology*, **2**, 13–29.

Van Nueten, J.M. and Janssens, W.J. (1986). Augmentation of vasoconstrictor responses to serotonin by acute and chronic factors: inhibition by ketanserin. *Journal of Hypertension*, Suppl. 4 (**1**), 55–59.

Vatner, S.F., Priano, L.L., Rutherford, J.D. and Manders, W.T. (1980). Sympathetic regulation of the cerebral circulation by the carotid chemoreceptor reflex. *American Journal of Physiology*, **238**, H594–H598.

Verbeuren, T.J., Jordaens, F.H. and Herman, A.G. (1983). Accumulation and release of (^{3}H)-5-hydroxytryptamine in saphenous veins and cerebral arteries of the dog. *Journal of Pharmacology and Experimental Therapeutics*, **226**, 579–588.

Wagerle, L.C. and Busija, D.W. (1989). Cholinergic mechanisms in the cerebral circulation of the newborn piglet: Effect of inhibitors of arachidonic acid metabolism. *Circulation Research*, **64**, 1030–1036.

Wagerle, L.C. and Busija, D.W. (1990). Effect of thromboxane A_2/endoperoxide antagonist SQ29548 on the contractile response to acetylcholine in newborn piglet cerebral arteries. *Circulation Research*, **66**, 824–831.

Wagerle, L.C., Kumar, S.P. and Delivoria-Papadopoulos, M. (1986). Effect of sympathetic nerve stimulation on cerebral blood flow in newborn pigs. *Pediatric Research*, **20**, 131–135.

Wagerle, L.C., Kurth, C.D. and Roth, R.A. (1990). Sympathetic reactivity of cerebral arteries in developing fetal lamb and adult sheep. *American Journal of Physiology*, **27**, H1432–H1438.

Wagerle, L.C., Heffernan, T.M., Sacks, L.M. and Delivoria-Papadopoulos, M. (1983). Sympathetic effect on cerebral blood flow regulation in hypoxia newborn lambs. *American Journal of Physiology*, **245**, H487–H494.

Wahl, M., Schilling, L., Parsons, A.A. and Kaumann, A. (1994). Involvement of calcitonin gene-related peptide (CGRP) and nitric oxide (NO) in the pial artery dilatation elicited by cortical spreading depression. *Brain Research*, **637**, 204–210.

Waldemar, G., Pauson, O.B., Barry, D.I. and Knudsen, G.M. (1989). Angiotensin converting enzyme inhibition and the upper limit of cerebral blood flow autoregulation: effect of sympathetic stimulation. *Circulation Research*, **64**, 1197–1204.

Walters, B.B., Gillespie, S.A. and Moskowitz, M.A. (1986). Cerebrovascular projections from the sphenopalatine and otic ganglia to the middle cerebral artery of the cat. *Stroke*, **17**, 488–494.

Wei, E.P., Kontos, H.A. and Said, S.I. (1980). Mechanism of action of vasoactive intestinal polypeptide on cerebral arteries. *American Journal of Physiology*, **239**, H765–H768.

Wei, E.P., Raper, R.J., Kontos, H.M. and Patterson, J.L., Jr. (1975). Determinants of response of pial arteries to noradrenaline and sympathetic nerve stimulation. *Stroke*, **6**, 654–658.

Wei, E.P., Kontos, H.A., Christman, C.W., Dewitt, D.S. and Povlishock, J.T. (1985). Superoxide generation and reversal of acetylcholine-induced cerebral arteriolar dilatation after acute hypertension. *Circulation Research*, **57**, 781–787.

Wei, E.P., Moskowitz, M.A., Boccalini, P. and Kontos, H.A. (1992). Calcitonin gene-related peptide mediates nitroglycerin and sodium nitroprusside-induced vasodilation in feline cerebral arterioles. *Circulation Research*, **70**, 1313–1319.

Werber, A.H. and Heistad, D.D. (1984). Effects of chronic hypertension and sympathetic nerves on the cerebral microvasculature of stroke-prone spontaneously hypertensive rats. *Circulation Research*, **55**, 286–294.

Williams, J.L., Heistad, D.D., Siems, J.L. and Talman, W.T. (1989). Effects of stimulation of fastigial nucleus on cerebral blood flow in cats. *American Journal of Physiology*, **26**, H297–H304.

Williams, J.L., Murray, M.A., Schalk, K.A. and Heistad, D.D. (1990). Cerebral blood flow during fatigial pressor response in cats. *American Journal of Physiology*, **27**, H729–H733.

Yaksh, T.L., Wang, J.-Y., Go, V.L.W. and Harty, G.J. (1987). Cortical vasodilatation produced by vasoactive intestinal polypeptide (VIP) and physiological stimuli in the cat. *Journal of Cerebral Blood Flow and Metabolism*, **7**, 315–326.

Yu, J.-G. and Lee, T.J.-F. (1989). 5-hydroxytryptamine-containing fibers in cerebral arteries of the cat, rat and guinea pig. *Blood Vessels*, **26**, 33–34.

Zhang, F. and Iadecola, C. (1992). Stimulation of the fastigial nucleus enhances EEG recovery and reduces tissue damage after focal cerebral ischemia. *Journal of Cerebral Blood Flow and Metabolism*, **12**, 962–970.

Zhang, F. and Iadecola, C. (1993). Fastigial stimulation increases ischemic blood flow and reduces brain damage after focal ischemia. *Journal of Cerebral Blood Flow and Metabolism*, **13**, 1013–1019.

7 Blood Flow Regulation in the Adrenal and Pituitary Glands

Michael J. Breslow, David Wilson, Daniel F. Hanley
and Richard J. Traystman

The Johns Hopkins Medical Institutions,
Department of Anesthesiology/Critical Care Medicine,
Baltimore, Maryland 21287–7294, USA

The pituitary and adrenal glands are neurosecretory structures that depend upon the cardiovascular system not only for nutrient support, but also for the transport of secretory products to target tissues throughout the body. The secretory products produced by these structures are continually secreted in the course of daily activities at low levels. However, in times of stress, such as haemorrhage, oxygen deficiency, or severe disturbances in salt and water balance, the hormonal output of these organs is increased. Until recently it has been difficult to study the role served by the blood vessels of these structures. However, indicator/dilution techniques now allow blood flow levels to be measured several times in the course of an experiment, providing some insight into the relationship between secretory activity and blood flow regulation. A number of studies indicate that both glands have developed unique vascular control systems which enable them to continue to function during these stresses, despite dramatic alterations in arterial blood pressure, oxygen availability or circulating blood volume. These haemodynamic changes are brought about by an ability to dramatically reduce the resistance of their vessels, thus ensuring that their neurosecretory products will be cleared and transported to distant target sites. In this chapter we review the histological structures of these two organs, placing emphasis upon the vasculature and the nerves that innervate these vessels. Vascular and hormonal responses to a variety of stressful challenges are reviewed and data on metabolism-based and neurogenic-based mechanisms of blood flow regulation are presented.

KEY WORDS: adrenal cortex; adrenal medulla; neurohypophysis; vasopressin; catecholamines; peptides; cortisol.

INTRODUCTION

The pituitary and adrenal glands have neural and endocrine tissues that form their working structure. Both serve vital roles in the organism's response to stress and there are many similarities between these two endocrine tissues. Each secretes multiple hormones, and each is comprised of tissues of different embryological origins. Marked differences exist in both the organization and regulation of these tissues. This chapter will examine blood flow regulation in the pituitary and adrenal glands, with particular focus on the neural control of blood flow. Throughout, we will attempt to demonstrate how anatomical and functional constraints have led to unique vascular control mechanisms. In most organs, blood provides nutrients essential for the maintenance of cellular processes and removes waste products. In the pituitary and adrenal glands, blood serves to transport secretory products to their site of action. In all likelihood, this interaction between blood flow and secretory activity accounts for the unique vasoregulatory mechanisms seen in these two tissues.

GENERAL STRUCTURAL ORGANIZATION AND VASCULAR ANATOMY

ADRENAL GLAND

The adrenal glands are located in the retroperitoneum immediately adjacent to the kidneys. Medullary chromaffin cells are derived from neuroectodermal tissue which invaginates into the mesodermal origins of adrenal cortex early in development; the result is an adrenal gland composed of two distinct tissues, the outer cortex and the inner medulla. There is some variability in the ratio of cortical to medullary cells; in dog and human the ratio is approximately 90:10. The cortex is organized centripetally and is composed of three distinct cell populations. The outermost cell layer, the zona glomerulosa, contains glomerulosa cells which secrete primarily aldosterone. Below the zona glomerulosa lie the cells of the zona fasciculata. These cells produce glucocorticoids and are primarily regulated by circulating levels of adrenocorticotrophic hormone (ACTH). The innermost cell layer, the zona reticularis, consists mainly of senescent cells which are hormonally inactive. Recent evidence suggests that these cells have migrated centrally from the zona fasciculata (Zajicek, Ariel and Arber, 1986). The medulla is composed principally of chromaffin cells, although occasional nerve cell bodies are also seen. Chromaffin cells are rich in granules containing catecholamines, adenosine triphosphate (ATP), enkephalins, and other peptides. Release of these contents into the circulation is under sympathetic control.

Separate arteries supply the cortex and medulla. Adrenal arteries are approximately 60–90 μm in diameter (Nakamura and Masuda, 1981), and originate from multiple larger arteries, including the coeliac, superior mesenteric, phrenic, lumboadrenal, renal, and iliac arteries, and the aorta (Bennett and Kilham, 1940; Dobbie and Symington, 1966). There is species variation in the number of arteries supplying the gland; generally this is proportional to the size of the adrenal (Coupland and Selby, 1976). On reaching the adrenal, the arteries either branch in the subcapsular region and supply the cortex, or traverse the cortex without branching, and supply the medulla (Bennett and Kilham, 1940; Nakamura and Masuda, 1981; Kikuta and Murakami, 1982, 1984). Occasional arteries enter deeper cortical regions and then return to the subcapsular area and branch to supply the cortex. The cells of the adrenal cortex are arranged in palisades, and are surrounded by capillary sinusoids. Cortical arteries branch immediately after penetrating the capsule, giving rise to these sinusoids.

Thus, blood flows from outer to inner cortex. The corticomedullary junction is well defined, and cortical capillaries coalesce into venules at this junction.

As described above, blood reaches the medulla via medullary arteries which traverse the cortex without branching. Despite conjecture about a portal system bringing cortical blood rich in glucocorticoids to the medulla (Pohorecky and Wurtman, 1971), multiple vascular casting experiments have demonstrated a separate vascular supply to the medulla, and discounted the existence of a portal system (Bennett and Kilham, 1940; Kikuta and Murakami, 1982, 1984). Immunohistochemical and electron microscopy studies have identified several different populations of chromaffin cells (Kikuta and Murakami, 1984). While it has been postulated that exposure of some chromaffin cells to high concentrations of glucocorticoids results in expression of the enzyme phenylethanolamine-N-methyltransferase (Coupland and MacDougall, 1966; Wurtman and Axelrod, 1966), thus enabling them to synthesize adrenaline, careful studies have failed to provide an anatomical basis for this differentiation (Kikuta and Murakami, 1984). The medullary capillary complex is more loosely structured than in the cortex (Kikuta and Murakami, 1982), and medullary capillary diameters are larger (Nakamura and Masuda, 1981). Chromaffin cells make direct contact with medullary capillaries; at these interfaces the endothelium is thinner and contains fenestrae, and fusion of medullary and endothelial cell basement membranes can be seen (Elfvin, 1965). Blood draining medullary capillaries flows into medullary venules and then small veins. Medullary and cortical venous structures join within the medulla, and all blood exits the adrenal gland via a single central vein. A schematic drawing of the adrenal vasculature is shown in Figure 7.1.

PITUITARY GLAND

The mammalian pituitary regulates a diverse set of tissues: thyroid, adrenal, musculoskeletal (growth), gonads, skin (pigmentation), lactation, renal and uterine/breast. These endocrine functions can be categorized by the site of secretory activity, with the first six being subserved by the endodermally derived anterior portion of the gland, and the last two being subserved by the neuro-ectodermally derived posterior pituitary. Extensive reviews of pituitary anatomy and species variation in the hypothalamic–pituitary axis are available (Green and Harris, 1947; Harris and Cambell, 1966; Daniel and Prichard, 1975; Porter et al., 1978; Page, 1982).

Green and Harris (1947) divided the pituitary into the adenohypophysis and the neurohypophysis. The former is subdivided into the pars tuberalis and the pars distalis, while the latter is a special region of hypothalamus that can be subdivided into infundibulum, infundibular stem and infundibular process. Although several terminologies have been used to subdefine pituitary tissues, Green and Harris's terminology implies a continuity of parts that accurately describes the contiguous nature of the neurohypophysial vascular bed. Other terminologies are firmly entrenched within the literature and are also useful. Some synonyms are: infundibulum = median eminence, infundibular stem = neural stalk, and infundibular process = neural lobe = pars neuralis.

The pars tuberalis is the portion of the adenohypophysis that is immediately adjacent to the median eminence and connected to it by portal vessels. The median eminence is in

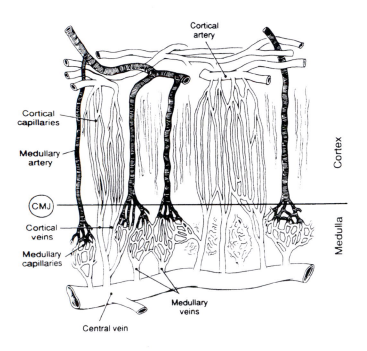

Figure 7.1 Schematic drawing of the adrenal vasculature, showing distinct arteries supplying the medulla and cortex. Note the transition of the cortical capillaries into veins at the corticomedullary junction (CMJ). [Reprinted with permission from Breslow *et al.* (1992).]

continuity with the infundibular stem; the latter being a transition zone between the median eminence and the infundibular process. Microscopically, the median eminence has the most complex vascular and neural organization within the pituitary. It is visible as the caudal extent of the hypothalamus, surrounding the recess of the third ventricle. This portion of the neurohypophysis is composed of five anatomically distinct layers (Kobayashi, Matsui and Ishii, 1970). The innermost layer, abutting on the third ventricle, is the ependymal layer, followed by the subependymal layer, a fibre layer, a reticular layer, and an outermost layer of capillaries (the palisade layer) abutting the pars tuberalis and pars anterior. The vessels of the palisade layer extend through the fibre and reticular layers to the ependymal layer to form large diameter looping vessels that return to this surface zone and converge into portal veins prior to passing into the pars anterior.

Early anatomical descriptions of the pituitary vasculature focused on the portal venous system and its novel neurovascular relationship to the adenohypophysis (Green and Harris, 1947; Green and Harris, 1949; Green, 1951; Porter, Ondo and Cramer, 1974). The superior hypophysial artery was thought to provide blood to the median eminence and adenohypophysis, while a separate supply to the neural lobe was postulated (Daniel and Prichard, 1975). More recent casting and microcinephotographic studies have demonstrated that the entire neurohypophysial vasculature is continuous (Page and Bergland, 1977);

however, blood flow to the median eminence through neural lobe blood vessels has not been demonstrated.

Small (100–300 μm) resistance arteries originate from the intracavernous portion of the internal carotid artery (Hanley *et al.*, 1992). The canine internal carotid artery is 3–5 cm long and enters the cranial cavity caudally through the petrous bone. It traverses the cavernous sinus immediately adjacent to the sella turcica and penetrates the dura at the anterior clinoid process to enter the subarachnoid space. The inferior hypophysial arteries originate as bilateral branches of the intracavernous carotid; they are 10–15 mm in length and 150–300 μm in diameter. At the level of the anterior circle of Willis, a significant, bilateral, intracranial arterial supply, consisting of one to three arterial branches called the superior hypophysial arteries, feeds the neurohypophysial capillary bed. These arteries are 2–4 mm in length and about 100 μm in diameter. They pass directly medially to the median eminence where they turn caudally and pass along the stalk towards the neural lobe. In some species a third hypophysial artery branches from the cavernous sinus to supply blood to capillaries in the infundibular stem and upper infundibular process. It may be either unilateral or bilateral. This artery is called the loral artery (McConnell, 1953), or the trabecular artery (Xuereb, Prichard and Daniel, 1954) in man, and the peduncular artery (Landsmeer, 1951) in rat.

The canine neurohypophysial parenchymal vessels have a relatively short course, passing from the distal aspect of the infundibular process anteriorly and rostrally towards the infundibular stem. They rapidly branch, in a lateral manner, merging into capillaries. With the exception of the entry region, a Virchow–Robin space is not apparent throughout their tissue course. These vessels have not been investigated in any detailed manner. A lobar glandular structure is found in marsupials, such as the opossum. In this situation the individual lobules have an isolated central arterial and venous supply.

The major portion of the portal circulation originates from the median eminence as long portal vessels. A minor portion originates from the neural lobe as the short portal system. These two sets of vessels represent the only source of blood supply to the anterior lobe. This portion of the gland has no direct arterial inflow, with the possible exception of adenomas which appear to develop a separate arterial supply (Gorczyca and Hardy, 1988).

Microcinephotographic studies have demonstrated the importance of the inferior hypophysial route as a major source of neural lobe, infundibular process and median eminence blood flow (Page, 1983). These arterial inputs can supply the entire neural lobe to the level of the infundibular stalk. The median eminence has been investigated extensively. The arterial inputs originate from the superior hypophysial arteries which encircle the median eminence. Small (20–30 μm) branches of the superior hypophysial arteries leave the surface and penetrate the five layers of the median eminence. These vessels form a "loop" that reaches to the ependyma on the ventricular surface, turns 180° and returns to the surface where it joins similar-sized vessels and the surface capillary network to form the long portal vessels. These looping vessels are invested with many nerve terminals that are the source of releasing factors important to the regulation of the anterior pituitary. Within the neural lobe, the capillary bed has a more random character, with vessels forming a network between axon terminals and glia. The relation between these two cellular elements and the capillary basement membrane appears to vary depending on the extent of the neurosecretory stimulation. During periods of sustained arginine vasopressin (AVP) or oxytocin (OT) secretion, axons occupy a greater proportion of the neural lobe capillary surface area than during periods of low, or absent, neurosecretion (Tweedle and Hatton, 1980). Activities such as lactation, parturition, and water retention have been demonstrated to elicit these changes in the capillary bed.

The capillaries of the neurohypophysis are approximately 7–10 μm in diameter. They are accompanied by occasional pericytes and fibrocytes that serve as structural support. The endothelium lacks both tight junctions and glial foot processes. Thus, this area lacks the blood–brain barrier which is characteristic of most central nervous system capillaries. Vesicular transport has been demonstrated to occur. However, given the absence of tight junctions, the importance of this phenomenon is unclear. Nitric oxide synthase (NOS) is present in magnocellular projections to this region, but information about endothelial NOS is not available (Dawson et al., 1991). Similarly, the glucose transporter and factor VII have not been specifically localized to pituitary endothelial cells. The absence of an organized blood–brain barrier suggests that neurohypophysial uptake and secretion relies on concentration gradients between neurons, extracellular space and capillary lumen to carry its neurosecretory products to the peripheral areas. The capillary network within the anterior pituitary has neither a blood–brain barrier nor glial supporting cells. Rather, the capillaries are directly adjacent to the endocrine cells of this lobe.

The venous system is organized to return blood to the surface of the adenohypophysis and the infundibular process separately; these veins then join to form pituitary veins. For the dog, and most mammals that have been investigated, large (approx. 100 μm) surface veins are found on the lateral and dorsal aspects of the respective lobes. These veins join together as a "Y" in the cleft between the anterior and posterior lobes to form the pituitary veins (Page, Munger and Bergland, 1976; Hodde, 1981). These pituitary veins are paired, have a very short course, and leave the gland at the right and left aspects of the sella where they open into the cavernous sinus. While the cavernous sinus has clear connections between sides, some degree of circulatory laterality is preserved since differential concentrations of adenohypophysial hormones are associated with lateralized microadenomas (Miller et al., 1990). When the contents of the long portal veins are selectively sampled, the presence of neurohypophysial hormones in markedly elevated concentrations (compared to peripheral levels) is noted (Porter et al., 1970). This finding suggests a significant release of neurohypophysial hormones in the median eminence, or a retrograde transport of these hormones from the neural lobe to the median eminence capillaries (Oliver, Mical and Porter, 1977; Porter et al., 1978).

SUMMARY

In summary, the blood supply to the adrenal is variable, originates from multiple different large intraabdominal arteries, and arrives via many small vessels. This contrasts with the more predictable, somewhat larger vessels which bring blood to the pituitary. In the adrenal gland, separate arteries supply blood to the cortex and medulla; this parallel blood supply has some similarity to the blood supply of the pituitary, where blood flow to the neurohypophysis arises from vessels different from those supplying blood to adenohypophysis. However, the adenohypophysis receives portal blood draining from the hypothalamus; there is no portal system in the adrenal.

METHODOLOGIES FOR THE MEASUREMENT OF PITUITARY AND ADRENAL BLOOD FLOW

Direct measurement of adrenal and pituitary blood flow is difficult because of the glands' (1) small mass; (2) physical location; (3) small size, number and location of supplying arteries; and (4) complexity of angioarchitecture. No method yet devised allows continuous measurement of total and regional blood flow to these tissues with complete separation of flow into their regional parts.

The preponderance of data on blood flow regulation in the adrenal and pituitary have been generated in the past 10 years as a result of the application of radiolabelled microsphere methodologies. The radiolabelled microsphere technique was first introduced by Rudolph and Heymann (1967). This technique employs radiolabelled latex spheres which are similar in size and density to red blood cells. These radiolabelled spheres are injected into the left cardiac ventricle and are distributed throughout the body in proportion to blood flow. Microspheres are not deformable and are slightly larger than red blood cells, and thus become entrapped in the microcirculation. By using differential spectroscopy to quantify the number of microspheres in each tissue of interest, and comparing tissue counts to counts in a sample of blood withdrawn from the animal at a known rate during the injection period, absolute determination of blood flow can be obtained. While this methodology makes certain assumptions about adequate mixing of microspheres, their flow characteristics and the lack of effect of trapped microspheres, numerous studies have confirmed the validity of the technique in a variety of settings (Neutze, Wyler and Rudolph, 1968; Archie et al., 1973; Hales, 1974; Bassingthwaighte et al., 1987). For both the adrenal (Breslow et al., 1986) and pituitary (Hanley et al., 1988), extensive validation studies have been performed. These validation studies have determined the number of spheres necessary for accurate and reproducible measurement of blood flow in these tissues, confirmed that 15 μm diameter spheres are almost completely entrapped by adrenal and pituitary, and established that repetitive measurements of blood flow have no effect on haemodynamic stability or subsequent measurements of blood flow. These experiments also indicate that significant streaming and/or skimming of microspheres does not occur in these two vascular beds.

Although the vast majority of data on regional adrenal and pituitary blood flow have been obtained using the radiolabelled microsphere technique, other methodologies have been utilized.

ADRENAL GLAND

Few methodologies have been employed to measure adrenal blood flow. For many years, investigators have collected and quantified whole gland venous outflow to study adrenal secretory activity and determine whole adrenal blood flow (Bülbring, Burn and De Elio, 1948; Kovach and Koltay, 1965; Kovach et al., 1970; Raff, Tzankoff and Fitzgerald, 1981; Dempsher and Gann, 1983; Bruhn et al., 1987; Engeland and Gann, 1989). Collection of adrenal outflow is usually accomplished by cannulating an adjacent large vein into which the adrenal vein drains (often the lumboadrenal vein) and using ligatures above and below the adrenal to prevent entry of blood from other structures (Hume and Nelson, 1955; Schapiro and Stjarne, 1958; Sibley et al., 1981). The venous outflow technique has been used widely in a variety of species, and in both conscious and anaesthetized animals. Since the cortex comprises 90% of the gland by weight, these whole gland blood flow data provide some insight into cortical (but not medullary) blood flow regulation. However, because blood flow to the medulla increases several fold under a variety of circumstances, such that blood flow to medulla can represent up to 50% of whole gland flow, changes in whole gland blood flow data cannot be used reliably to reflect behaviour of the cortical vasculature.

Monos et al. (1969a, b) attempted to measure regional adrenal blood flow in dogs using a hydrogen washout technique; however, their measures of medullary and cortical blood flows, when added together, equalled only 10% of the whole gland blood flow that was measured by collecting the venous outflow, suggesting that their technique was not accurate. Kramer and Sapirstein (1967) used a ^{86}Rb-fractionation technique to separately assess blood flow to the medulla and cortex in rats. They reported a slightly higher basal blood flow (by weight) to the medulla and an increased blood flow to both regions during carotid ligation. However, the validity of this technique has not been determined, and no additional studies were reported.

As noted at the beginning of this section, the vast majority of data on adrenal medullary and cortical blood flow have been obtained using radiolabelled microspheres. This methodology is relatively uncomplicated and has been extensively validated in the dog. The major drawbacks of the radiolabelled microsphere technique are: (1) it has been validated in only one animal species; (2) it does not provide continuous blood flow data; and (3) it is expensive, particularly as disposal of radioactive waste becomes more difficult and costly. More recently, Hamaji et al. (1986) measured adrenal medullary and cortical blood flow by visually counting non-radiolabelled microspheres in tissue slices. The limitation of this technique is that it is time consuming and permits only a single determination of blood flow. However, Jasper et al. (1990), by using coloured microspheres, were able to increase the number of measurements per animal. Adaptation of newer spectrophotometric techniques for quantifying coloured spheres could possibly simplify this latter technique and make it an attractive alternative method for determining regional adrenal blood flow.

PITUITARY GLAND

A variety of techniques have been used to study the pituitary vasculature and its blood flow regulating properties. Microscopic visual observation of the vessels supplying the adenohypophysial and neurohypophysial portions of the gland were employed by early investigators because techniques suitable for blood flow measurement in other organs were not applicable to the pituitary. Visual observation has since been replaced by indicator-dilution methods which can provide quantitative measures of neurohypophysial blood flow. A listing of the baseline blood flow levels obtained using these techniques, and the anaesthetic agents used, is provided in Table 7.1.

While the assumptions underlying indicator-dilution theory are sound for application in most brain tissues, the neurohypophysis is a high-flow tissue and as such presents special problems with regards to vessel size and vascular transit time. In this review, we discuss all the techniques of potential use for the measurement of regional pituitary blood flow. Most methods still require validation for use in the pituitary. Thus, in considering the pituitary's vascular responses and baseline blood flow, methodology remains an

TABLE 7.1

Regional pituitary blood flows obtained by differing techniques, species differences, and effects of anaesthesia

Technique	Pituitary region	Species	Anaesthesia	Flow ml/min/100 g	Reference
[131]Iodide clearance	Adenohypophysis	Rat	Pentobarbital	44	Yates, Kirschman and Olshen (1966)
Hydrogen clearance	Adenohypophysis	Rat	None	64 ± 8	Porter et al. (1967)
	Adenohypophysis	Rat	Urethane	90 ± 22	Kemeny et al. (1985)
[86]Rubidium	Adenohypophysis	Rat	None	46 ± 3	Goldman (1963)
	Median eminence			150 ± 12	
	Neural lobe			350 ± 25	
	Adenohypophysis	Rat	None	62 ± 6	Kapitola et al. (1977)
	Neurohypophysis			455 ± 35	
Microspheres	Median eminence	Sheep	Pentobarbital	506 ± 117	Page et al. (1981)
	Neural lobe			347 ± 93	
	Median eminence	Sheep	None	300 ± 43	Ziedonis et al. (1986)
	Neural lobe			203 ± 50	
	Median eminence	Dog	Pentobarbital	243 ± 90	Vella et al. (1989)
	Neural lobe			822 ± 115	
	Neural lobe	Dog	Isoflurane	1268 ± 294	McPherson, R. (personal communication)
	Neural lobe	Dog	None	365 ± 11	Dorman, T. (personal communication)
[125]I-antipyrin	Neurohypophysis	Rat	None	236 ± 26	Lichardus et al. (1977)
	Neural lobe	Rat	None	581 ± 68	Bryan et al. (1987)
[14]C-isopropyliodo-amphetamine	Median eminence	Rat	Halothane	568 ± 63	Williams et al. (1991)
	Neurohypophysis			1036 ± 42	
	Median eminence	Rat	None	577 ± 33	Bryan, Myers and Page (1988)
	Neural lobe			886 ± 11	

important consideration. In some instances, there is reason to suspect that the blood flow is underestimated. For example, indicators such as ^{86}Rb are partially taken up in the capillary bed of the median eminence. Adenohypophysial blood flow measured with ^{86}Rb will be higher than calculated. In other instances, high blood flow rates through neurohypophysial vessels may limit the time required for some indicators to come into equilibrium with the tissue. This condition would cause blood flow to be underestimated. The ^{125}I-antipyrine method demonstrates this clearly. In this section we discuss the strengths and weaknesses of each technique as applied to the pituitary.

In vivo observation of pituitary vessels

Direct observation techniques do not provide a measure of pituitary blood flow. Historically, these techniques have been used to address specific questions regarding either the direction of blood flow within the pituitary (Page, 1983), the nature of the vascular territories served by particular arteries or portal veins (Wislocki and King, 1936; Worthington, 1963; Porter *et al.*, 1970; Baertschi, 1980), or vascular reactivity (Wilson, Traystman and Rapela, 1985; Bergland, Davis and Page, 1977).

Two surgical approaches have been employed. The parapharyngeal, or ventral, approach visualizes the supplying arteries of the median eminence, the ventral surface of the infundibular stalk capillary network and the long portal vessels on the ventral surface of the adenohypophysis (Porter *et al.*, 1970; Porter, 1975). Because the pars distalis enfolds the neural lobe, the short portal vessels connecting these two tissues remain hidden when approached ventrally. These vessels can be visualized using a subtemporal approach (Page, 1983). In piglets [the only species known in which the diaphragm sella does not obscure the view of the pituitary (Page, 1983)], the subtemporal approach visualizes the posterior aspect of the median eminence region, the posterior surface of the infundibular stalk and the dorsal aspect of the neural lobe. Portions of the lateral surface of the pars distalis are seen also. The parapharyngeal approach is suitable for study in rats, whereas the subtemporal approach is better suited to piglet and dog studies.

The principal disadvantages of all techniques requiring surgical exposure are the unphysiological conditions that the operative procedures impose upon the tissues studied. Undoubtedly, the trauma induced by surgical manipulation of the surrounding tissues effects changes in the hormone output, and there is evidence to suggest that changes in the neurosecretory rate affect the baseline blood flow (Ziedonis *et al.*, 1986; Diringer *et al.*, 1992). Moreover, there is no assurance that the vessels observed in such preparations react anything like those in the normal unanaesthetized intact animal (Worthington, 1955). The potential advantages of direct observation techniques are, however, many. They offer a means for studying the interaction between the two arterial supplies to the neurohypophysial capillary bed. Additionally, tissue exposure is required by some techniques such as laser Doppler flowmetry, which has been successfully used to differentiate between neurohypophysial and adenohypophysial tissues in humans undergoing hypophysectomy (Steinmeier *et al.*, 1991).

Techniques based upon indicator delivery

[86]**Rubidium**: Rubidium competes with potassium for entrance into cells through potassium channels. [86]Rb was first used to measure regional pituitary blood flow in 1958, and provided the first qualitative methodology (Goldman and Sapirstein, 1958; Sapirstein, 1958). A detailed rationale for the method can be found in Goldman and Saperstein (1973). The technique requires a single injection of isotope administered through a tail vein of the animal. The tissue is removed within 40 s to prevent any recirculation artifact. [86]Rb has the advantage that it can be used in both anaesthetized and unanaesthetized animals.

The blood flow levels this technique yields have not been verified. Its most notable shortcoming is that a portion of the indicator is extracted from the blood entering into the adenohypophysial vascular bed. Thus, adenohypophysial flow may be underestimated; however, the inability to account for the amount of tracer extracted could be corrected for by employing the ^{86}Rb technique in combination with another isotope technique that is extracted 100% by the median eminence. This would allow the extracted fraction to be quantified.

[125]I-antipyrine: To quantify the neurohypophysial blood flow response in rats undergoing dehydration, Lichardus *et al.* (1977) employed the ^{125}I-antipyrine technique. This technique is well established for blood flow measurement in other brain regions and is relatively simple to perform. However, the technique has since been shown to be in error in high-flow vascular beds, because the diffusion of ^{125}I-antipyrine is not sufficiently fast to allow blood and tissue concentrations to establish equilibrium during their passage through the vasculature (Bryan, Myers and Page, 1988).

[14]C-isopropyliodoamphetamine: As pointed out by Bryan, Myers and Page, (1988), most diffusible markers are very effective for measuring blood flow at lower flow rates, but are less than ideal for measuring high-flow rates. At high rates, diffusible tracers become diffusion limited. Accordingly, the initial assumption of the methods (the tissue concentration of tracer reflects the amount of tracer delivered to the tissue by blood) is invalidated unless a complex equilibrium constant is incorporated into the method. Isopropyliodoamphetamine is extracted 100% by the neurohypophysis in a single pass through capillaries. For this reason, inclusion of a tracer equilibrium constant becomes unnecessary, as flow and tissue tracer concentration are linearly related. However, the isopropyliodoamphetamine technique does have disadvantages. The most important of these is that only one radiolabel is available. Because between-animal variability of pituitary blood flow is relatively large, significant changes may be difficult to detect unless relatively large sample sizes are employed. Moreover, blood flow measurement in larger animal species is prohibitively expensive.

Microspheres: Microsphere techniques have been used in several animal species in an attempt to overcome many of the disadvantages associated with the techniques discussed previously. Microspheres with a diameter of 15 μm are nearly 100% extracted by the tissues of the neurohypophysis, yielding reproducible regional measures of median eminence and neural lobe blood flow (Hanley *et al.*, 1988). The ready availability of several radiolabels allows for multiple measurements within the same animal. Statistical comparisons can be made using control data obtained from the same animal, thereby adding to the certainty of the observations. Like other indicator techniques based upon delivery, microspheres cannot be used to measure adenohypophysial blood flow.

Techniques based upon indicator clearance

[131]Iodide: To measure adenohypophysial blood flow, Yates, Kirschman and Olshen, (1966) injected small quantities of [131]Iodide directly into the adenohypophysis of rat and recorded its clearance. Blood flow was computed from the derived rate constant. The utility of the [131]Iodide clearance technique is uncertain, given that it is invasive and requires surgical exposure and placement of an injection cannula into the adenohypophysis.

Hydrogen gas desaturation: The hydrogen clearance technique has been used successfully by two groups to measure adenohypophysial blood flow (Porter *et al.*, 1967; Kemeny *et al.*, 1985). The hydrogen technique is advantageous over radiolabelled diffusible indicator techniques, because it allows for multiple blood flow measurements and can be employed in both anaesthetized and unanaesthetized animals.

Two approaches have been employed. Using stereotaxic procedures in rats, a specially constructed hydrogen electrode is implanted in the adenohypophysis through the cerebrum. The animal is then allowed to recover. Later, hydrogen gas is administered via the breathing mixture. The accumulation of hydrogen within the pituitary is recorded as an increase in the current passing through the electrode. Upon achieving steady-state conditions, breathing room air is resumed and the clearance of gas from tissues surrounding the probe is recorded. Using curve-fitting procedures, the hydrogen clearance curve is fitted to either a single or double compartment model, and the equations solved to derive the rate constants. Flow is computed as the product of the rate constant and the partition coefficient for hydrogen between blood and tissue phases. The blood flow values derived by hydrogen clearance agree with values obtained by the ^{86}Rb technique (Goldman, 1963), and are slightly higher than values measured by ^{131}I clearance (Yates, Kirschman amd Olshen, 1966).

In their studies, Kemeny et al. (1985) utilized a parapharyngeal approach. Their technique incorporated parallel measurements made in cortical and subcortical tissues so that comparisons between cerebral and pituitary structures could be made. The adenohypophysial blood flow values reported were higher than those recorded by Porter et al. (1967). It is unclear whether this was due to the differing methods of slope analysis, or an effect of the anaesthetic agent.

Thermal clearance: Kopaniky and Gann (1975) developed a miniature thermoelectric probe to continuously record tissue perfusion in the anterior pituitary of dogs. A zero blood flow level could be established at the end of each experiment, which permitted the data to be expressed as a ratio of the control value. The probe has been tested in thyroid tissue and found to be linear over the perfusion range, but it has not been validated in pituitary. The thermal technique is advantageous, in that its output is continuous. Since the probe is placed in contact with, rather than in, the pituitary tissue, it is relatively atraumatic. However, because the thermal diffusion coefficient is not known with certainty, only relative changes in flow are measured. Potentially, this technique could be calibrated *in situ* using other techniques.

Other methodologies

Blood volume: Sooriyamoorthy and Livingston (1972) measured regional blood volume changes in adeno- and neurohypophysial tissues by means of radiolabelled tracers. Inferences regarding the effects of various pharmacological agents on blood flow were drawn from the observed volume changes. However, blood flow and blood volume are interdependent upon vascular transit time and thus not directly related in all conditions (Ferrari et al., 1992). Until this method has been properly validated, the results obtained should be viewed as tentative.

Laser Doppler: With the recent development of laser-Doppler flowmetry, very small probes capable of monitoring perfusion through pituitary tissues have been devised (Steinmeier et al., 1991). Theoretically, laser-Doppler flowmetry provides two real-time signal outputs that correspond to the average velocity of blood flowing through a tissue and the volume of blood within the probe's field of illumination. Although controversial, the product of these two variables appears to be linearly related to blood flow. Laser-Doppler flowmetry offers several advantages over other techniques. It provides continuous measures of microflow, velocity and volume. Since it uses haemoglobin as its intravascular marker, it would appear to offer a means of measuring adenohypophysial blood flow that is independent of artifact induced by changes in the primary capillary bed of the median eminence. Since laser-Doppler flowmetry does not employ radioactive tracers it is suitable for use in humans, and has been used successfully to differentiate between neurohypophysial and adenohypophysial tissues during surgical procedures requiring this information. Of note is the observation that the relative blood flow level measured in neurohypophysial tissue is approximately six times higher than that measured in adenohypophysial tissue (Steinmeier et al., 1991).

SUMMARY

The radiolabelled microsphere technique has been used extensively for the measurement of adrenal medullary, adrenal cortical and neurohypophysial blood flow. This methodology appears to be valid for quantification of blood flow to these tissues. Non-radiolabelled microsphere techniques are also valid, but are more labour intensive and provide fewer measurements. The venous outflow technique yields accurate data on whole adrenal blood flow and permits the direct measurement of glandular secretion; this technique provides little insight into intraglandular blood flow distribution. Recent advances in our understanding of relationships between blood flow and pituitary function have resulted from methodological advances which utilize isopropyliodoamphetamine and other indicators. These techniques are non-destructive to the tissues being studied and meet the criteria for accurate blood flow measurement in high-flow vascular beds, but are limited in the number of measurements that can be made. Questions arise regarding the error induced by loss of indicator to the infundibulum when indicators such as ^{86}Rb are used. Unfortunately, no technique is currently suited for blood flow measurement in the tissues of the adenohypophysis because of the portal nature of the vasculature supplying this structure. New developments in instrumentation, such as laser-Doppler flowmetry, and the use of double indicator techniques may overcome these problems and contribute a new understanding of the role blood vessels play in endocrine and neuroendocrine function.

PHYSIOLOGICAL STUDIES OF ADRENAL AND PITUITARY BLOOD FLOW REGULATION

Extensive studies of adrenal and pituitary blood flow responses to a variety of physiological stimuli have provided considerable insight into the regulation of blood flow in these vascular beds. Data for adrenal and pituitary are presented separately since these tissues differ in important areas.

ADRENAL GLAND

Basal blood flow

Basal blood flow to the adrenal is high compared to most organs; medullary and cortical blood flow were approximately 200 ml/min/100 g in unstressed pentobarbital-anaesthetized

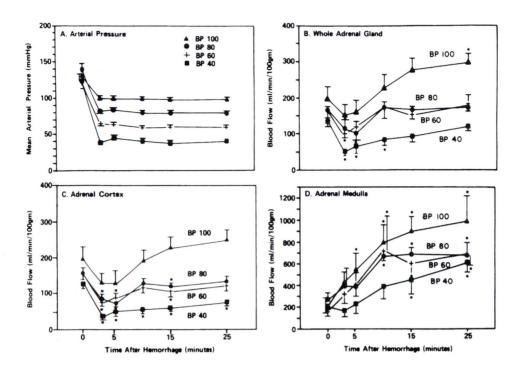

Figure 7.2   Changes in arterial blood pressure (BP) and adrenal blood flow during graded haemorrhage. A: mean arterial BP at control and 3, 5, 10 and 25 min after haemorrhage. *Group 1*, 100 mmHg; *Group 2*, 80 mmHg, *Group 3*, 60 mmHg; *Group 4*, 40 mmHg; n = 5 for each group. B: whole adrenal blood flow with haemorrhage. C: blood flow to the adrenal cortex with haemorrhage. D: blood flow to the adrenal medulla with haemorrhage. *P<0.05 compared with control. Data are means ± SE of five animals. [Reprinted with permission from Breslow *et al.* (1986).]

dogs (Breslow *et al.*, 1986, 1991; Nishijima *et al.*, 1989; Sakima *et al.*, 1991). In conscious dogs, blood flow to the medulla exceeded 1000 ml/min/100 g (Faraci *et al.*, 1989). Cortical blood flow was similar in conscious and pentobarbital-anaesthetized dogs, suggesting a selective effect of barbiturates on blood flow to medulla.

Response to alteration of perfusion pressure

There were large increases in blood flow to the adrenal medulla following a reduction of arterial blood pressure (Breslow *et al.*, 1986). Pentobarbital-anaesthetized dogs, subjected to controlled haemorrhage into a pressurized bottle system to reduce mean arterial blood pressure to 100, 80, 60 and 40 mmHg, increased blood flow by three to four fold (Figure 7.2) (Breslow *et al.*, 1986). In contrast, blood flow to the cortex decreased in proportion to the perfusion pressure, with some late recovery at 25 min (Breslow *et al.*, 1986).

Increases in adrenal medullary blood flow do not appear to be due to intrinsic characteristics of medullary vessels. Reduction of adrenal perfusion pressure by means of an aortic occluder does not result in increases in medullary blood flow (Breslow *et al.*,

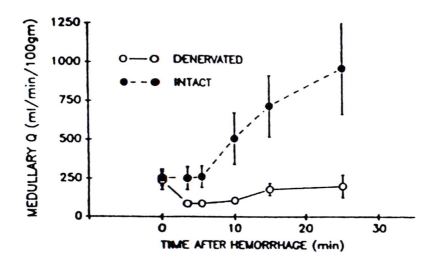

Figure 7.3   Effect of denervation on changes in the medullary blood flow following haemorrhage to 60 mmHg
(n = 4). Data are means ± SE. [Adapted from Breslow *et al.* (1987), reprinted with permission from Breslow
et al. (1992).]

1991). Rather, proportional decreases in medullary blood flow were observed, suggesting
that this vascular bed does not autoregulate. Subsequent studies have demonstrated that
systemic hypotension, by increasing sympathetic outflow and adrenal nerve activity, elicited
a neurally mediated vasodilatation in the medulla. Splanchnic nerve section blocked
hypotension-induced medullary vasodilatation in the denervated adrenal, while increased
blood flow was observed in the contralateral, innervated gland (Figure 7.3) (Breslow *et al.*,
1987). In addition, reductions in medullary blood flow were observed when arterial blood
pressure was reduced by administration of the ganglion blocking agent, hexamethonium
(Kennedy *et al.*, 1980). Splanchnic nerve section had no effect on the cortical blood
flow response to haemorrhage. To summarize, neither the medulla nor cortex demonstrate
autoregulation of blood flow with alteration of perfusion pressure. Systemic reflexes
activated by hypotension elicit marked vasodilatation in the medulla, which is dependent
on an intact innervation of the adrenal.

Oxygen and the control of regional adrenal blood flow

The adrenal medulla and cortex both vasodilate in response to hypoxic hypoxia; however, the
magnitude of the vascular response and the mechanisms differ in the two regions (Breslow,
1992). Reduction of the arterial oxygen tension to 8 vol%, by the addition of nitrogen to the
inspired gas of pentobarbital-anaesthetized, paralyzed, ventilated dogs, resulted in a 100%
increase in blood flow to the adrenal cortex and a two to three fold increase in the blood
flow to the medulla (Nishijima *et al.*, 1989). Increases in cortical blood flow during hypoxia
appeared to be the result of the direct effects of hypoxic hypoxia on the cortical vasculature.

This conclusion is supported by the following observations: (1) cortical vasodilatation with reduction of the partial pressure of oxygen persisted when hypoxia-induced increases in ACTH and corticosteroid secretion were prevented by pretreating dogs with dexamethasone (Breslow et al., 1989); (2) hypoxia-induced cortical vasodilatation was unaffected by adrenal denervation (Breslow et al., 1989); and (3) prevention of hypoxia-induced increases in arterial blood pressure by controlled haemorrhage into a pressurized bottle system had no effect on the blood flow response to hypoxic hypoxia (Nishijima et al., 1989). Thus, increases in cortical blood flow during hypoxia do not appear to be due to alterations in secretory activity or metabolism, nor to changes in nerve traffic. Furthermore, when the arterial oxygen content was reduced to 8 vol% by the addition of carbon monoxide to the inspired gas, the cortical blood flow did not increase (Nishijima et al., 1989). This latter observation further supports the hypothesis that arterial oxygen tension, and not oxygen content, is important in the control of the cortical vasculature.

Hypoxia alters the adrenal medullary blood flow both by direct effects on the vasculature and by indirect effects on the sympathetic outflow. Hypoxic hypoxia increased adrenal catecholamine secretion, an effect which was blocked by adrenal denervation (Breslow et al., 1989). When pentobarbital-anaesthetized dogs were subjected to unilateral adrenal denervation prior to reduction of the partial pressure of oxygen, the adrenal medullary blood flow increased only slightly during hypoxia (Breslow et al., 1989). Medullary blood flow in the contralateral, innervated gland, however, increased by 400%. These data suggest that the direct effects of hypoxia on the medullary vasculature are quite small. In contrast, chemoreceptor-mediated increases in splanchnic nerve activity produce large increases in medullary blood flow during hypoxic hypoxia. Of interest, carbon monoxide-induced hypoxia elicited increases in medullary blood flow and catecholamine secretion which were similar to those observed during hypoxic hypoxia (Nishijima et al., 1989).

Metabolic activity and the control of adrenal blood flow

Secretion of both catecholamines and cortisol are energy-dependent processes. In vascular beds such as the heart and brain, blood flow is tightly coupled to metabolic activity; however, the available data suggest no such relationship between metabolism and blood flow in the adrenal. We measured adrenal medullary oxygen utilization during catecholamine secretion elicited by splanchnic nerve stimulation (Breslow et al., 1990). Dogs were pretreated with the selective adrenocorticolytic agent, o,p′ DDD [1,1-dichloro-2-(0-chlorophenyl)-2-(-p-chlorophenyl)ethane, Bristol-Meyers, Evansville, IN] (Nelson and Woodard, 1949; Cueto, Brown and Richardson, 1958), which destroyed 95% of the cortex. This was done to minimize contamination of medullary venous drainage by blood from the much larger cortex, and to ablate corticosteroid secretion, thus ensuring basal cortical O_2 consumption. Animals received supplemental glucocorticoids and mineralocorticoids to prevent adrenal insufficiency. The adrenal medullary structure and function were unaffected by this pretreatment regimen. O_2 consumption did not increase during nerve stimulation-induced catecholamine secretion. O_2 extraction by the adrenal was 2.7% at rest and decreased to 0.8% during splanchnic nerve stimulation.

Metabolic activity does not appear to be a major regulator of cortical blood flow either. Sakima et al. (1991) measured adrenal O_2 consumption *in vivo* during stimulation of cortisol secretion by exogenous ACTH. Animals were pretreated with dexamethasone for 48 h and were anaesthetized with a fentanyl-based anaesthetic to ensure basal cortisol secretion prior to infusion of ACTH (see Raff, Norton and Flemma (1987)), and the adrenal was denervated to ensure constant medullary activity. With infusion of ACTH at 10 ng/kg/ min, plasma ACTH concentrations of 500 pg/ml were achieved and cortisol secretion increased from < 0.1 to 5.1 μg/min/g cortex (Figure 7.4). O_2 consumption increased by almost 100%, while cortical blood flow did not change; the increase in O_2 consumption was met by augmenting oxygen extraction from 6 to 13%. Thus, increases in cortical metabolic activity do not result in increases in cortical blood flow.

Relationship between blood flow and secretion

Parallel changes in medullary blood flow and adrenal catecholamine secretion during haemorrhage and hypoxia suggest an important relationship between these two events. In addition, splanchnic nerve section prevented hypotension- and hypoxia-induced cat-echolamine secretion and medullary vasodilatation (Breslow *et al.*, 1987, 1989), while electrical stimulation of the greater splanchnic nerve resulted in a tremendous outpouring of catecholamines and a large increase in medullary blood flow (Figure 7.5) (Breslow *et al.*, 1987). Both the medullary blood flow and the catecholamine secretory responses to nerve stimulation have similar frequency-response characteristics and both demonstrate fatigue over time (Silver, 1960; Marley and Paton, 1961; Breslow *et al.*, 1987). These parallel changes in secretion and vasodilatation suggest that changes in secretory activity may account for alterations in medullary vascular tone. One possible mechanism by which secretory activity could affect vascular tone is by diffusion of vasoactive chromaffin granule secretory products to adjacent resistance vessels. This hypothesis requires medullary resistance vessels and chromaffin cells to be in close proximity, otherwise perivascular concentrations of released vasoactive chromaffin granule products would not be sufficient to affect vascular tone. Based on anatomical studies demonstrating no branching of medullary arteries until they enter the medulla (Kikuta and Murakami, 1984), medullary resistance vessels (i.e. small arteries, arterioles) may be sufficiently close to chromaffin cells to be affected by their products. However, physiological data confirming a role for chromaffin granule constituents in medullary vasoregulation are not available. Select chromaffin granule products cause medullary vasodilatation when administered intravascularly (Faraci *et al.*, 1989); yet it is unknown whether perivascular concentrations during physiological conditions are sufficient to produce this effect. Jordan *et al.* (1989) described attenuation of nerve stimulation-induced vasodilatation by the β-adrenoceptor antagonist, pindolol, a finding consistent with released catecholamines stimulating β-adrenoceptors on medullary vessels. However, β-adrenoceptor blockade could also attenuate neurotransmitter release or alter membrane stability; therefore, these findings are not conclusive.

An alternative explanation for the apparent coupling of medullary blood flow and catecholamine secretion is that both events are under direct sympathetic neural control, with nerve traffic to chromaffin cells and medullary resistance vessels changing in parallel under most physiological conditions. In support of the direct neural control of blood flow, nerves have been described in close proximity to medullary blood vessels (Hollinshead, 1936; Swinyard, 1937; Hökfelt *et al.*, 1981; Bruhn *et al.*, 1987). Tomlinson and

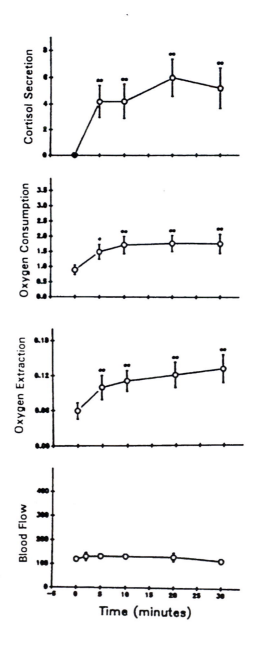

Figure 7.4 Cortisol secretion ($\mu g \cdot min^{-1} \cdot g$ cortex^{-1}), adrenal O_2 consumption (ml·min^{-1}·100 g cortex^{-1} before *(time 0)* and during ACTH infusion at 10 ng·kg^{-1}·min^{-1}). *P < 0.05 compared with *time 0*. Data are means ± SE of seven animals. [Adapted from Sakima *et al.* (1991), reprinted with permission from Breslow (1992).]

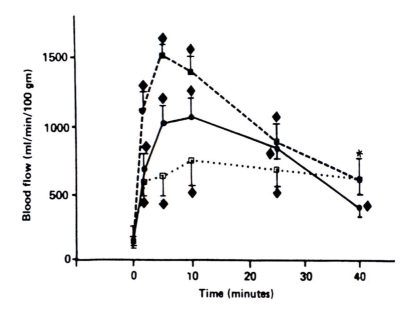

Figure 7.5 Changes in adrenal medullary blood flow during splanchnic nerve stimulation. *$P < 0.05$ compared with the control (0 min). ♦$P < 0.01$ compared with the control. Data are expressed as means ± SE of four animals. [Adapted from Breslow *et al.* (1987), reprinted with permission from Breslow (1992).]

Coupland (1990), however, in a detailed electron microscopic examination of adrenal medullary nerves in the rat, could find no nerve terminals (or synaptic vesicles) associated with medullary vessels. While this study raises questions concerning whether medullary vessels are truly innervated, two recently published studies have been able to dissociate the secretory and vascular responses to nerve stimulation *in vivo* (see Figure 7.6). Hexamethonium, a nicotinic receptor antagonist, reduced nerve stimulation-induced catecholamine secretion by 95% without affecting the vasodilator response (Kennedy *et al.*, 1980). In the second study, N^G-nitro-L-arginine, a potent inhibitor of NOS, blocked nerve stimulation-induced vasodilatation without affecting secretion (Breslow *et al.*, 1992). These data suggest that increases in medullary blood flow are not the direct result of changes in catecholamine secretion; rather, parallel changes in the two reflects parallel changes in nerve activity.

There are conflicting data concerning the relationship between cortical blood flow and adrenal cortical secretory activity. Both increase during hypoxic hypoxia (Breslow *et al.*, 1989; Nishijima *et al.*, 1989), but this response does not require an increase in ACTH or cortisol secretion; rather, it appears to be a direct effect of low PaO_2 on the cortical vasculature. Increases in cortisol secretion induced by carbon monoxide-induced hypoxia (Nishijima *et al.*, 1989) and haemorrhagic hypotension (Breslow *et al.*, 1986) were not associated with increased cortical blood flow or significant changes in cortical vascular resistance. Infusion of physiological doses of ACTH (2 and 10 ng/kg/min) into adult dogs

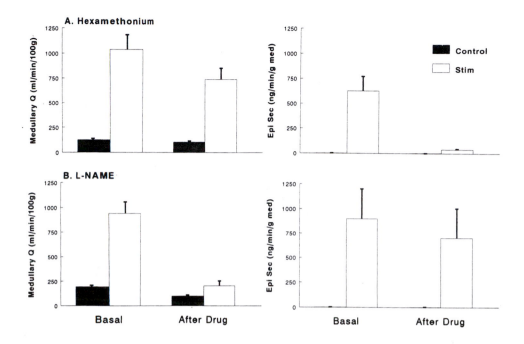

Figure 7.6 Medullary blood flow (Q) and adrenaline secretion (Epi Sec) before (Control) and during (Stim) splanchnic nerve stimulation. Measurements made in the absence of drug (basal) and after administration of (A) 20 mg/kg, Hexamethonium or (B) 40 mg/kg N^G-nitro-L-arginine methylester (L-NAME). Data are means ± SE of six and five animals, respectively. [Adapted from (Kennedy *et al.*, 1991) and (Breslow *et al.*, 1993).]

had no effect on cortical blood flow (Sakima *et al.*, 1991). Edwards, Hardy and Malinowska, (1975) noted increases in whole gland blood flow (75 and 300%, respectively) with the infusion of ACTH at 5 and 50 ng/kg/min in conscious calves. Upon cessation of ACTH administration, the adrenal blood flow returned to control levels despite ongoing high levels of cortisol secretion, suggesting a direct vascular action of ACTH unrelated to secretory effects. Carter *et al.* (1993) noted a two to three fold increase in cortical blood flow when ACTH was infused into fetal sheep. This vasodilator response was not seen until 24 h of ACTH administration. The delayed blood flow response was associated with a 10–15 fold increase in cortisol secretion. Whether the vasodilator response to ACTH observed in this study was due to extremely low baseline cortisol secretion in the fetus or reflects a response to prolonged ACTH stimulation is not known. Long-term studies in adult animals are needed to determine if a similar delayed increase occurs in the adult animal.

It is important to recognize that although blood flow to the medulla and cortex are not directly affected by changes in secretion, there is likely an important relationship between these two events (Breslow, 1992). Both medulla and cortex receive high levels of blood flow compared to most other organs, and the vasculature is the portal of entry by which these hormones gain access to distant sites and elicit physiological effects. It is attractive to hypothesize that high levels of blood flow serve to ensure rapid delivery of these compounds into the systemic circulation. Studies by Urquhart (1965), Porter and Klaiber (1965) and L'Age, Gonzalez-Luque and Yates (1970), suggest that changes in blood flow may affect corticosteroid secretion. Urquart employed an infusion pump to alter perfusion pressure in an isolated arterial segment in dogs, and noted parallel changes in cortisol secretion and adrenal blood flow. This relationship was seen only with ACTH concentrations between 1 and 30 μU/ml; at higher ACTH concentrations, or in the absence of ACTH, cortisol secretion was unaffected by alterations in blood flow. Similar results were reported by Porter and Klaiber (1965) in anaesthetized rats in which blood flow was manipulated by altering the withdrawal rate of venous blood, and by L'Age, Gonzalez-Luque and Yates (1970) in conscious dogs which received infusions of histamine and methacholine to increase adrenal blood flow. The mechanism responsible for this interaction is unclear. Several authors have hypothesized that the rate of delivery of ACTH to the adrenal may be more important than the ACTH concentration. However, Engeland and Gann (1989) reported that increases in cortisol secretion preceded increases in adrenal blood flow following splanchnic nerve stimulation, suggesting that other mechanisms may be involved. Furthermore, Hinson, Vinson and Whitehouse (1986) observed flow-related changes in corticosterone secretion in the rat in the absence of ACTH. The physiological importance of blood flow modulation of cortisol secretion is unclear. Corticosteroid secretion clearly increases during hypotension (Bereiter, Zaid and Gann, 1986), even though levels of cortical blood flow decrease (Breslow *et al.*, 1986). While some investigators report impaired secretion when hypotension is severe (Frank *et al.*, 1955), others find no such reduction (Walker *et al.*, 1959).

Increases in adrenal medullary blood flow during catecholamine secretion may also be an important component of the secretory response, especially during hypotension. Recent data indicate that the adrenal medulla functions normally during profound hypotension; nerve stimulation-induced catecholamine secretion was unaffected by reduction of the adrenal perfusion pressure to 24 mmHg (Breslow *et al.*, 1991). Even at this markedly reduced perfusion pressure, active vasodilator mechanisms increased medullary blood flow five-fold during nerve stimulation. This active vasodilatation is of particular importance, since there are no intrinsic mechanisms to maintain blood flow during hypotension; following adrenal denervation, blood flow falls passively with blood pressure (Breslow *et al.*, 1991). Thus, without active vasodilatation, medullary blood flow would decrease to levels below 50 ml/min/100 g during profound hypotension, and it is unlikely that catecholamine secretion could be maintained.

Increases in medullary blood flow may also contribute to the secretory response in other ways. First, high levels of blood flow may help to avoid catecholamine reuptake by the chromaffin cell. Chromaffin cells resemble postganglionic sympathetic nerves in many ways, and both have an active catecholamine reuptake system (Kenigsberg and Trifara, 1980). In sympathetic nerves, this system acts to terminate the impulse and conserve catecholamines (Bevan, Bevan and Duckles, 1980). Adrenal catecholamines, however, must enter the systemic circulation in order to have an effect. Thus, the rationale for an adrenal reuptake system is unclear. Perhaps high levels of blood flow circumvent reuptake and increase net secretion. Along similar lines, high levels of blood flow may decrease intramedullary concentrations of secreted chromaffin granule constituents, and thus prevent feedback inhibition of secretion. *In vitro* catecholamine secretion is inhibited by catecholamines with α_2-adrenoceptor activity (Greenberg and Zinder, 1982), by opiates

(Saiani and Guidotti, 1982), and by other peptides released during degranulation (Costa et al., 1981). Recent data suggest that some of these are capable of inhibiting secretion in vivo (Jarry et al., 1989). The extent to which this inhibition is affected by levels of blood flow in medulla is unknown.

High levels of blood flow to the adrenal may also help to ensure adequate O_2 delivery. This high level of blood flow is not required to meet metabolic demands; oxygen extraction by both tissues is remarkably low under normal conditions (Breslow et al., 1990; Sakima et al., 1991). However, low basal O_2 extraction may be of some physiological value; a large extraction reserve could help to maintain O_2 consumption during periods of reduced blood flow. It is also possible that a limited capacity to extract oxygen requires basal blood flow to be quite high. Harrison and Seaton (1965) reported no oxygen consumption by the adrenal when the arterial partial pressure of oxygen was decreased to 30 mmHg.

Cortical blood flow regulation may also be important in aldosterone secretion. Aldosterone secretion in vivo has been shown to be impaired by mild degrees of hypoxia (Raff and Chadwick, 1986; Raff and Levy, 1986; Raff, Sandri and Segerson, 1986). In vitro studies suggest that certain cytochromes involved in the synthesis of aldosterone are O_2 sensitive (Raff, Ball and Goodfriend, 1988). The sinusoidal character of the cortical capillary network results in zona glomerulosa cells receiving arterial blood prior to the rest of the cortex. This anatomical arrangement appears to be well suited to maintaining O_2 tensions in the zona glomerulosa at levels adequate for aldosterone synthesis. The need to maintain high O_2 tensions in the zona glomerulosa may provide a physiological role for increases in cortical blood flow during hypoxic hypoxia (Nishijima et al., 1989). Further studies are required to determine whether intra-adrenal O_2 tension is a major determinant of cortical blood flow.

The physiological responses of the adrenal vasculature can be summarized as follows: (1) basal blood flow to the medulla and cortex during anaesthesia is high, and in conscious animals medullary blood flow is higher still; (2) neither the medulla nor cortex autoregulate blood flow in response to changes in perfusion pressure; in the medulla, neurally mediated vasodilatation results in increased blood flow during systemic hypotension; (3) hypoxaemia causes direct vasodilatation in the cortex, while increases in medullary blood flow are neurally mediated; (4) adrenal blood flow does not appear to be coupled to the metabolic activity of the gland; oxygen extraction is sufficiently low that considerable increases in oxygen consumption are possible without increasing blood flow; and (5) blood flow changes parallel secretory changes in medulla but these two responses can be dissociated, suggesting that they are independently mediated. In the cortex, secretory changes are not associated with increased blood flow, but some data suggest that alterations in blood flow can affect cortisol secretion. While it is attractive to postulate that increases in medullary blood flow serve to speed delivery of catecholamines into the systemic circulation during stress, this relationship remains conjectural at this time.

PITUITARY GLAND

Retrograde versus antegrade flow

Historically, Wislocki and King (1936) predicted on the basis of anatomical data that blood flows in the direction of the hypothalamus to the anterior pituitary. Their prediction was confirmed by direct observation of portal vessels (Green and Harris, 1949; Worthington, 1960; Porter, Ondo and Cramer, 1974). The contiguous nature of the neurohypophysial vascular bed continues to generate intriguing questions regarding the influence of the pituitary on brain and hypothalamic function. Blood in some vessels of the hypophysis has been observed to flow in the direction of the hypothalamus (Szentagothai et al., 1962; Torok, 1962). Jazdowska and Dobrowolski (1965), on the basis of anatomical studies in sheep, concluded that blood flows down the infundibular stem in hypophysial vessels, but can flow up the infundibular stem in a plexus of small vessels. Oliver, Mical and Porter (1977) provided additional support for the retrograde flow hypothesis by showing that, in rat, the concentrations of pituitary hormones in the blood reaching the infundibulum by way of the retrograde vasculature was 100–500 times that measured in arterial blood. Similar findings have been reported for sheep (Bergland, Davis and Page, 1977). In addition to hypothalamic releasing factors, neurohypophysial hormones are present in portal blood (Zimmerman et al., 1973; Porter et al., 1977), and labelled pituitary analogues injected into the adenohypophysis appear in the hypothalamus (Mezey et al., 1978). A detailed phenomenological description of the processes involved can be found in Bergland and Page (1979).

In an elegant series of anatomical studies, Page and coworkers (1976, 1977, 1978) showed that the neurohypophysial capillary bed is continuous and supplied both rostrally and caudally by the superior and inferior hypophysial arteries, respectively. Page (1983) found no evidence of blood flow into the median eminence from neural lobe or adenohypophysis. Likewise, blood entering the median eminence did not flow into the neural lobe via the stalk. These two vascular territories appear to be functionally separate. Despite these findings, the issue of blood flow direction will remain controversial until alternative explanations for these earlier observations are found. Blood flow direction in any organ or vasculature is determined primarily by pressure gradients. Thus, in order for retrograde blood flow to occur within the infundibular stalk, vascular resistance between the branching site of the inferior hypophysial arteries (or trabecular arteries) and the capillaries of the median eminence along the carotid artery route must exceed the sum of the vascular resistances of the inferior hypophysial arteries (or trabecular arteries) and the infundibular stem. This seems unlikely, as the latter route is mostly continuously linked capillaries. Percolation of hormone may occur between the anterior and posterior vasculatures, thus accounting for the presence of adenohypophysial hormone in posterior pituitary vessels and neurohypophysial hormones in portal vessels. For now, the only evidence strongly arguing against the occurrence of retrograde blood flow is Page's (1983) microcinephotographic study.

Determinants of baseline regional pituitary blood flow

Baseline regional pituitary blood flow is dependent upon animal species and the type of anaesthesia used. Halothane- (Williams et al., 1991) and isoflurane- (McPherson, 1993) anaesthetized animals have higher baseline blood flow levels than do pentobarbital-anaesthetized or unanaesthetized animals (Table 7.1). These effects appear to be preferentially expressed within the neural lobe. Whether this is a direct effect of anaesthesia on vessels or an effect associated with different rates of release of hormone is unclear. Interestingly, anaesthesia appears to elevate neurohypophysial blood flow, rather than reduce it as is observed in other brain regions. This elevation may reflect "endocrine stress" and an altered hormonal state induced by anaesthetics.

Baseline neural lobe blood flow in anaesthetized dog (Hanley, Wilson and Traystman, 1986; Hanley *et al.*, 1988; Vella *et al.*, 1989; Diringer *et al.*, 1992; Hurn *et al.*, 1993; Saito *et al.*, 1994) and anaesthetized and unanaesthetized rat (Goldman, 1963; Bryan, Myers and Page, 1988; Williams *et al.*, 1991) is greater than median eminence blood flow (Table 7.1). In anaesthetized (Page *et al.*, 1981, 1990) and unanaesthetized sheep (Ziedonis *et al.*, 1986), median eminence blood flow is greater than neural lobe blood flow. It is unclear at this time whether this represents a true species difference or whether it is due to some other unaccounted for difference between study groups.

Recent studies indicate that the high baseline blood flow observed in neuroendocrine organs is dependent upon a high endogenous nitric oxide (NO) synthesis rate (Saito *et al.*, 1994; Wilson, Hanley and Traystman, 1992, 1993). Intravenous administration of N^α-L-arginine methyl ester (L-NAME), an NOS antagonist, reduced baseline neurohypophysial blood flow to levels comparable to that found in other brain regions. In L-NAME-treated dogs, neural lobe blood flow was reduced to only 13% of its control level (Figure 7.7). This reduction was unaccompanied by significant changes in baseline plasma arginine vasopressin (pAVP), suggesting that neurosecretory function was independent of the blood flow level. While this may be true for normal levels of AVP neurosecretion, it is not known if flow is important when AVP release is enhanced.

Response to alteration of perfusion pressure

Autoregulation is a phenomenon whereby the measured blood flow through an organ or tissue is observed to remain constant when the perfusion pressure across the organ is increased or decreased from its baseline value. The presence or absence of autoregulation is established by evaluating the slope of the pressure/flow relationship. If no relationship is found, then the flow is said to be autoregulated. The use of pressure/flow relationships in determining the characteristics of autoregulation assumes that the needs of the tissue remain constant at each of the measured pressure/flow points. Whereas this is probably true for pressure/flow relationships measured in most brain regions, it is unclear whether this assumption is valid for the pituitary, considering arterial pressure and central blood volume are determinants of the AVP neurosecretory rate.

To study pituitary pressure/flow relationships, Page *et al.* (1981) used progressive haemorrhage to reduce arterial pressure, and metaraminol to elevate it. They found that the neurohypophysial autoregulatory relationship was without slope over an extensive range of perfusion pressure. In fact, with the 20–180 mmHg range, the upper and lower limits of regulation were not evident. In blood–brain barrier-intact brain regions, the barrier mechanism prevents these vasoconstrictor substances from penetrating into smooth muscle and biasing the effect of pressure. However, in the light of several recent studies, showing that neurohypophysial arteries constricted in response to topically applied α-adrenoceptor agonists (Hanley *et al.*, 1992), and that intra-arterial catecholamine infusion was accompanied by vasoconstriction of select portions of the neurohypophysial vasculature (Wilson *et al.*, 1983), it appears that the results obtained using pharmacological agents to elevate perfusion pressure should be viewed with caution.

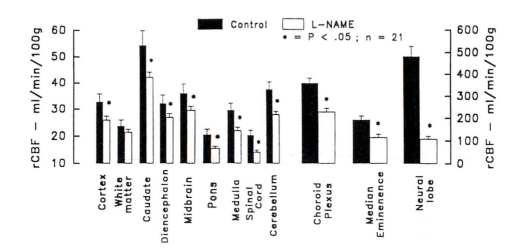

Figure 7.7   NOS blockade by L-NAME (40 mg/kg, i.v.) reduces baseline cerebral blood flow with the largest changes occurring within the neurohypophysis and other high flow vasculatures. Values represent means ± SE of 21 dogs. rCBF, regional cerebral blood flow.

We measured neurohypophysial blood flow in dogs made hypotensive (Vella *et al.*, 1989) to avoid pharmacological manipulations. Because the time course of vascular adjustments was unknown, a group of dogs was studied to obtain this information before proceeding to evaluate steady-state autoregulatory relationships. When arterial pressure was rapidly reduced to 80 mmHg from normotensive levels (~120 mmHg), we found the neurohypophysis exhibited a unique autoregulatory response in which neurohypophysial blood flow increased transiently (228% of control) before re-establishing the control blood flow level (Figure 7.8). During the "hyperaemic" phase, the time course of the flow transient correlated with an increased pAVP neurosecretory transient. However, unlike pAVP, blood flow did not remain elevated. The transient nature of the flow response lead us to further evaluate the hypothesis that peripheral baroreceptor activity may participate in the hyperaemic phase. Bilateral vagotomy and carotid sinus denervation were shown to attenuate the increase in neurohypophysial blood flow (126 and 125% of control, respectively). The pAVP response was enhanced both by vagotomy and carotid sinus denervation. Combined denervation abolished both pAVP and neurohypophysial blood flow responses. The absence of effects of exogenous AVP, and the inability of V_1-receptor antagonists to alter this response, argued against an active involvement of AVP in mediating the vascular component of the response (Hurn *et al.*, 1993). NOS blockade did not prevent the hyperaemic component of the blood flow response (Saito *et al.*, 1994), although baseline level was reduced (Saito *et al.*, 1994). In this circumstance, the ability of the vasculature to maintain blood flow levels constant was actually enhanced (Figure 7.9). Neither AVP

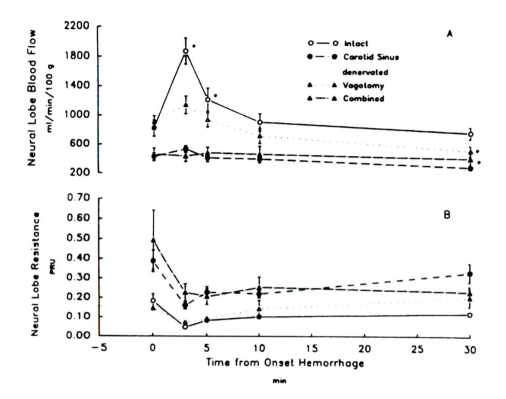

Figure 7.8 Time course of neural lobe blood flow (A) and vascular resistance (B) changes induced by rapid onset haemorrhage. Dogs with intact baroreceptors responded by decreasing the neural lobe vascular resistance proportionately more than was necessary to maintain blood flow constancy at a lower arterial blood pressure. Bilateral vagus nerve section attenuated the hypotensive response. Animals with denervated carotid sinus regions had a higher regional vascular resistance, a lower initial blood flow, and showed no hyperaemic trends. Values are means ± SE of (n = 10) dogs with intact baroreceptors, (n = 8) carotid sinus-denervated dogs, (n = 9) vagotomized dogs and (n = 6) dogs with combined procedures. [Reprinted with permission from Vella et al. (1989).]

nor NO appeared to play important roles in mediating either the rapid or stable vascular resistance changes necessary to bring this regulation about. The peripheral baroreceptors influence neurohypophysial blood flow primarily during periods of changing blood pressure. When blood pressure is stable, local mechanisms appear to be dominant. In the untreated, anaesthetized dog (Saito et al., 1994), the autoregulatory range is narrower than that previously reported for sheep (Page et al., 1981). This phenomenon appears to be explained by differences in baseline blood flow levels found in the two preparations.

Respiratory gases and the control of pituitary blood flow

Oxygen: The vasodilator response of cerebral vessels to hypoxia is well known (Traystman, Fitzgerald and Loscutoff, 1978). Carbon monoxide and hypoxic hypoxia have both been

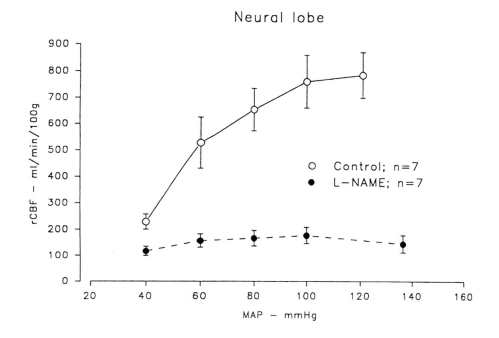

Figure 7.9   Effect of NOS blockade on the neurohypophysial blood flow autoregulatory relationship. Unblocked dogs demonstrated a passive pressure/flow relationship. NOS blockade by L-NAME (40 mg/kg, i.v.) reduced the baseline blood flow. In the presence of NOS block, no relationship between pressure and flow was observed. The absence of a significant relationship between these two variables suggests NOS activity either masks or modulates autoregulatory phenomenon in the neurohypophysis. rCBF, regional cerebral blood flow. MAP, mean arterial pressure.

shown to be potent cerebral vasodilators, and in most brain regions, vasodilatation occurs independent of peripheral chemoreceptor stimulation (Traystman, Fitzgerald and Loscutoff, 1978). In most brain regions, hypoxic hypoxia ($PaO_2 = 30\pm2$ mmHg; $CaO_2 = 8\pm1$ vol%) and carbon monoxide hypoxia ($PaO_2 = 97\pm9$ mmHg; $CaO_2 = 9\pm1$ vol%) result in similar increases in total cerebral blood flow. In contrast, neurohypophysial blood flow increases only when PaO_2 is lowered (Hanley, Wilson and Traystman, 1986) (Figure 7.10). Since hypoxic hypoxia is a strong stimulus for peripheral chemoreceptor activity, these data suggested that hypoxia-induced increase in neurohypophysial blood flow were mediated by either a neural pathway activated by chemoreceptor stimulation or by local mechanisms responsive to PaO_2. In a follow-up study, neurohypophysial blood flow responses to hypoxic hypoxia were studied under conditions of vagotomy, carotid sinus denervation, and combined vagotomy and carotid sinus denervation to determine the role of the chemoreceptors (Hanley *et al.*, 1988). In dogs, arterial O_2 tension was lowered from 128 ± 3 to 31 ± 1 mmHg. Denervation of either the carotid sinus or the aortic arch chemoreceptors alone did not attenuate hypoxic vasodilatation. Combined denervation, however, completely blocked the response for the neurohypophysis but not for other brain

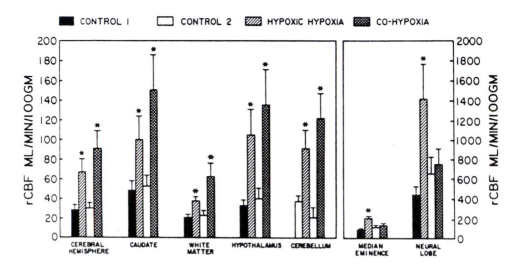

Figure 7.10   Effect of hypoxic hypoxia and carbon monoxide (CO) hypoxia on neurohypophysial and regional cerebral blood flow (rCBF). Each bar represents mean ± SE of five dogs. Both types of hypoxia (diagonal and cross-hatched bars) produced significant increases from control (open and dark bars) in blood flow to all brain regions except the neurohypophysis. Both parts of the neurohypophysis, the median eminence and the neural lobe, showed no change from control with CO hypoxia, but did have significant flow responses to hypoxic hypoxia. Note the change in the vertical axis on the right for the median eminence and neural lobe blood flow. [Reprinted with permission from Hanley, Wilson and Traystman (1986).]

regions. Hypoxic hypoxia resulted in an increase in pAVP from ~8 to ~40 pg/ml. The increase occurred in intact, vagotomized and carotid sinus denervation conditions, but was completely inhibited by combined denervation. These data indicate that peripheral chemoreceptors are a necessary component of the neurohypophysial dilator response. Since vasodilatation was not observed after complete chemodenervation, local PaO_2 changes cannot account for the response.

Carbon dioxide: Hypercapnia is a potent vasodilator of cerebral blood vessels (Kontos, Raper and Patterson, 1977; Wilson, Traystman and Rapela, 1985). The effect is mediated by extracellular $[H^+]$, since HCO_3^- and CO_2 alone do not affect pial vessels (Kontos, Raper and Patterson, 1977). In fact, hypercapnia-induced vasorelaxation appears to be a common property of all smooth muscle cells, but peripheral vasodilatation during hypercapnia is offset by enhanced constrictor tone through activation of central chemoreceptors. Thus, it is remarkable that little effect of hypercapnia on median eminence and neural lobe blood flow has been observed in the rat (Bryan, Myers and Page, 1988), sheep (Page *et al.*, 1981) or dog (Hanley, Wilson and Traystman, 1986) (Figure 7.11). Hypocarbia, which constricts other cerebral vessels, is accompanied by a 20% reduction in neurohypophysial blood flow in sheep (Hanley, Wilson and Traystman, 1986) and dogs (unpublished observations). Recently, Bryan, Myers and Page, (1988) showed that attenuated neurohypophysial hypercapnic reactivity in rats is due to enhanced α-adrenoceptor activity. The stimulus

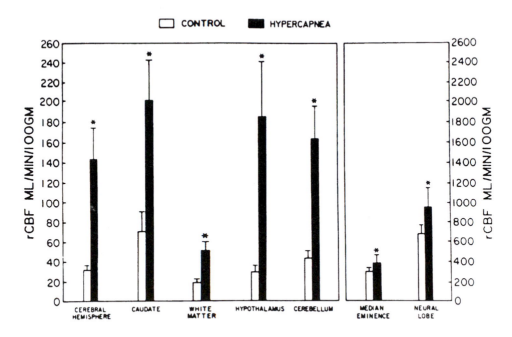

Figure 7.11   Effect of hypercapnia on the neurohypophysial and regional cerebral blood flow (rCBF). Each bar represents mean ± SE of eight dogs. Hypercapnia produces significant increases in all the brain and neurohypophysial regions studied. Note the change in the vertical axis on the right for the median eminence and neural lobe blood flow. [Reprinted with permission from Hanley, Wilson and Traystman (1986).]

for adrenoceptor activation is unclear. Since stimulation of the superior cervical ganglia decreases neurohypophysial blood flow (Wilson *et al.*, 1983), one might speculate that enhanced sympathetic nerve activity during hypercapnia partially accounts for the absence of response seen in the pituitary. This hypothesis remains to be tested.

Osmotic and thirst-related influences

Several lines of evidence strongly suggest that baseline neurohypophysial blood flow is functionally related to the level of osmotic-induced AVP neurosecretory activity. Chronic saline ingestion produced a 140% increase in 2-deoxyglucose uptake in the rat neural lobe (Schwartz *et al.*, 1979). Uptake in hypothalamic regions (paraventricular and supraoptic nuclei, subfornical organ, and septal triangular nucleus), was less affected, but nevertheless, increased (Nikitovitch-Winer and Goldman, 1986). Similar increases occurred during acute disturbances in water intake (Kadekaro, Gross and Sokoloff, 1986), but were most pronounced when water deprivation was induced over longer periods (24 h to 5 days). In these instances, neural lobe glucose metabolism was elevated 367% above its hydrated level (Gross *et al.*, 1985). Studies by Lichardus *et al.* (1977) showed that neural lobe blood flow was elevated during dehydration. This increase was not due to increased AVP neurosecretion, since similar changes have been shown in the Brattleboro rat which does not synthesize AVP (Kapitola *et al.*, 1977; Kadekaro, Gross and Sokoloff, 1986), but may be related to increased RNA synthesis and/or the secretion of other peptides.

Dehydration is a complex stimulus, characterized by increases in plasma osmolality and angiotensin II levels, and decreased central blood volume and afferent baroreceptive activity. Each of these represent pronounced stimuli for increasing pAVP. Any one, or all, of these changes could be responsible for the haemodynamic changes reported by Kapitola *et al.* (1977) and Lichardus *et al.* (1977) and Ziedonis *et al.* (1986) attempted to study hyperosmotic influences selectively by injecting hyperosmotic saline into the common carotid arteries of sheep. They observed a small change in pAVP and an equally small rise in neurohypophysial blood flow. Their data are unconvincing since blood flow measurements were obtained 30 min after injection and only small changes in pAVP were seen at this time.

We studied neurohypophysial blood flow and pAVP responses to three levels of osmotic stimulation in anaesthetized dogs (Malkoff *et al.*, 1990). Plasma osmolalities of 286 ± 3, 309 ± 2 and 343 ± 5 mOsm/kg H_2O were produced with infusion of hypotonic (0.3%), isotonic (0.9%), and hypertonic (5.0%) saline. To minimize confounding influences from volume receptors, infusion rates were controlled to produce similar increments in intravascular volume. Baseline plasma osmolality, pAVP, neurohypophysial blood flow, central venous pressure and pulmonary capillary wedge pressure were similar in all groups. Central venous pressure and pulmonary capillary wedge pressure rose to a similar degree in all three groups. In the 0.9% saline-infused group, the pAVP level and neurohypophysial blood flow were unaltered. In the 0.3% saline group, the pAVP fell from 11 ± 2 to 2 ± 1 pg/ml during the infusion and the neurohypophysial blood flow remained constant. In the group receiving 5% saline, pAVP rose from 11 ± 2 to 21 ± 7 pg/ml and the neurohypophysial blood flow increased by 41%. These findings support the hypothesis that plasma osmolality influences neurohypophysial blood flow, probably via a flow-to-neurosecretory activity coupling mechanism.

Extracellular fluid volume expansion

Neurohypophysial blood flow responses to extracellular fluid volume expansion have been studied in pentobarbital-anaesthetized dogs (Diringer *et al.*, 1992). Measurements were made at baseline and after increasing pulmonary capillary wedge pressure by 10–15 mmHg. pAVP decreased by 70% and neurohypophysial blood flow fell by 40%. Blood flow through the median eminence and other brain regions was unchanged. Vagotomy alone increased pAVP by 126% and did not alter the neurohypophysial blood flow. Vagus nerve section abolished the neurohypophysial blood flow response to extracellular fluid expansion, but not the pAVP response. The contributions of left atrial and pulmonary baroreceptors were tested by inflation of a left atrial balloon to 10–15 mmHg. This resulted in a 20% reduction in the neurohypophysial blood flow, a 35% reduction in pAVP, and a 200–300% increase in plasma atrial natriuretic factor. Atrial natriuretic factor release does not account for the neurohypophysial blood flow changes, since intravenous atrial natriuretic factor infusion has no effect on either neurohypophysial blood flow or pAVP. These data suggest that the neurohypophysial blood flow response to volume expansion is mediated via cardiopulmonary baroreceptor fibres carried within the vagus nerve.

Stress

Among the stresses that have been shown to induce increased pituitary–adrenal activity are acute hypoglycemia and anxiety (Liddle, 1981). These two stresses effect two different pituitary blood flow responses. In female Wistar rats administered ether until the onset of anaesthesia, the anterior pituitary blood flow was elevated 40% above control 2.5 min after exposure (Goldman, 1963). The time course of this increase paralleled similar increases in ACTH (Vernikos-Danellis, 1963). Posterior pituitary blood flow and median eminence blood flow remained unchanged. Bilateral adrenalectomy (performed 30 days prior to study) significantly elevated baseline adenohypophysial blood flow, but did not suppress the blood flow elevation elicited by stress. Likewise, pretreatment with hydrocortisone to block stress-induced ACTH secretion had no effect on stress-induced increases in adenohypophysial blood flow. In no instance was median eminence blood flow affected, although the posterior pituitary blood flow response to stress was enhanced by adrenalectomy. On the basis of these findings, Goldman concluded that adenohypophysial blood flow is partially autoregulated by glandular metabolism.

Insulin-induced hypoglycaemia in the rat was accompanied by significant increases in regional cerebral blood flow in all brain regions except the neural lobe, in which it was decreased (Bryan *et al.*, 1987). Since hypoglycemia increases plasma levels of adrenaline and noradrenaline, it is reasonable to attribute the reduction in neural lobe blood flow to stimulation of adrenoceptors in this blood–brain barrier-deficient region. However, as noted previously, plasma adrenaline and noradrenaline levels also increase during haemorrhagic hypotension, which elicits a transient, 250% increase in neural lobe perfusion. It would appear from these somewhat conflicting observations that the mechanisms of the blood flow changes during stress remain to be elucidated.

Neurohypophysial blood flow — neurosecretory coupling

Regional cerebral blood flow is coupled to brain function by a metabolic link (Heistad and Kontos, 1983). Since the neurohypophysial portion of the pituitary includes axons, glia and vascular elements, it is reasonable to question whether blood flow and neurosecretion are also coupled. Early studies showed that as neurosecretory activity increased, neurohypophysial blood flow also increased (Lichardus *et al.*, 1977). Thus, it has been stated that neurohypophysial blood flow and nerve activity are coupled (Lichardus *et al.*, 1977; Ziedonis *et al.*, 1986). While this may be true during dehydration, changing salt and water balance, and perhaps hypoxia, there are other conditions in which no correlation between blood flow and neurosecretion is found. Moreover, the mechanisms responsible for this coupling, when present, are uncertain. For example, dehydration elevates neurohypophysial blood flow in homozygous, AVP-deficient, Brattleboro rats (Kapitola *et al.*, 1977), indicating that AVP is not responsible for the neurohypophysial blood flow changes. Since the Brattleboro rat does synthesize OT during dehydration, this increase may constitute the stimulus for enhanced neurohypophysial perfusion.

Schwartz *et al.* (1979) suggested that posterior pituitary blood flow–neurosecretory activity coupling may occur via a metabolic link similar to the one coupling cerebral blood flow and brain function. They supported this hypothesis by showing that 2-deoxyglucose uptake by the neurohypophysis was enhanced by water deprivation. However, the significance of enhanced 2-deoxyglucose uptake is unclear. Neurohypophysial energy demands are met by ketone bodies (Hawkins and Biebuyck, 1979) and short-, medium- and long-chain fatty acid metabolism (Vannucci and Hawkins, 1983). Although 2-deoxyglucose is taken up and converted to 2-deoxyglucose-6-phosphate, other glucose labels show that glucose is predominantly metabolized to lactate via the glycolytic pathway (Vina et al., 1984) and to ribose-5-phosphate via the pentose phosphate pathway (Krass and LaBella, 1965, 1967). In the pituitary the metabolic pathways for aerobic metabolism are thought to be non-functional, because carbon label supplied by glucose does not appear in Krebs cycle-associated amino acids. The increased glucose uptake during water deprivation, therefore, may reflect increased glycolysis, increased phospholipid turnover (Redman and Hokin, 1959) or enhanced glutathione/glutathione reductase activity (Spina and Cohen, 1989) via the dependency of the latter on pentose phosphate pathway-generated NADPH (Voet and Voet, 1990). These occurrences are events in which the free energy of metabolite oxidation is used for endergonic reductive biosynthesis rather than for the synthesis of ATP (Voet and Voet, 1990). Furthermore, there is no clear evidence that the pituitary has a large energy demand. Page et al. (1981), in discussing why basal neurohypophysial blood flow is high, implied that it is for reasons other than to provide nutritive support. If the energy demand were large, then the oxygen uptake would, presumably, also be large. Unfortunately, the veins draining the posterior pituitary are difficult to cannulate and neither venous oxygen content nor oxygen uptake has been measured. Vina et al. (1984), however, observed that blood in the draining veins is normally bright red in colour. One is left to conclude that a large amount of oxyhaemoglobin remains in the veins and that the extraction fraction is small.

Hypoxic hypoxia is a potent stimulus for AVP release from the neurohypophysis. During hypoxia, the neurohypophysial blood flow also increases and remains elevated (Hanley, Wilson and Traystman, 1986). However, Page et al. (1981) point out that neurohypophysial blood flow and nerve activity are not coupled in all instances. In sheep, the neurohypophysial blood flow is autoregulated. Thus, the increase in pAVP that occurs at low blood pressure (Page et al., 1981; Vella et al., 1989) is not accompanied by an elevated neurohypophysial blood flow. In fact, when the stimulus for AVP release is hypotension, there is no correlation between neurohypophysial nerve activity and neurohypophysial blood flow in the stable state. Our data in dog (Vella et al., 1989) confirm the observation by Page et al. (1981) but point out that in the early phase of haemorrhage (within the first 3 min) the neurohypophysial blood flow rises dramatically as AVP neurosecretion rises. We also reported that carotid sinus denervation reduced the neurohypophysial blood flow and elevated pAVP. Carotid sinus denervation also abolished the transient increase in the neurohypophysial blood flow elicited by an acute mean arterial blood pressure reduction (Vella et al., 1989). Combined sinoaortic denervation reduced the basal blood flow level and dramatically elevated pAVP. Thus, we concluded that neurohypophysial blood flow–neurosecretory activity coupling is not consistently represented.

SUMMARY

In those instances where neurohypophysial blood flow–neurosecretory coupling is apparent (water deprivation, hyperosmotic states, extracellular fluid volume contracted states and hypoxic hypoxia), it appears to be independent of metabolism and not mediated by direct effects of the secretory products AVP or OT on neurohypophysial vessels (Hurn *et al.*, 1993). Conclusions drawn from studies incorporating stimuli such as hypotension may be inappropriate, as these stimuli also enhance circulating vasoconstrictor substances which may confound interpretation in this blood–brain barrier-deficient brain region.

NEURAL CONTROL OF ADRENAL AND PITUITARY BLOOD FLOW

NEUROANATOMICAL STUDIES

Both the adrenal and the pituitary receive a dense nerve supply. Extensive anatomical studies indicate the existence of a wide variety of nerve fibres in these tissues, with an apparent innervation of both secretory and vascular elements. These data are summarized below.

ADRENAL GLAND

The adrenal gland is densely innervated, particularly the medulla where catecholamine secretion is under sympathetic control. Nerve fibres arrive at the adrenal via the splanchnic nerves (Marley and Prout, 1968). Chromaffin cells are innervated by preganglionic cholinergic fibres which originate in the intermediolateral horn in the lower thoracic and upper lumbar segments of the spinal cord (Haase, Contestabile and Flumerfelt, 1982; Kesse, Parker and Coupland, 1988). More recently, data from retrograde transport studies, utilizing horseradish peroxidase and the dye, Fast Blue, have demonstrated that some adrenal medullary nerves originate in vagal sensory and motor ganglia (Coupland *et al.*, 1989), suggesting a parasympathetic innervation. Similar transport studies have also identified staining of cells in the dorsal root ganglia (Mohamed, Parker and Coupland, 1988), raising the possibility of afferent sensory nerves originating in the adrenal medulla. There are also considerable data suggesting the presence of postganglionic nerves in the adrenal. Morphological studies by Swinyard (in 1937), described ganglia in the splanchnic nerve and within the adrenal parenchyma. Physiological evidence for the existence of postganglionic nerves comes from the studies of Carlsson *et al.* (1990), in which less than half of the adrenal nerve preparations in the rat demonstrated increased firing following ganglionic blockade, the expected response of preganglionic nerves. The remaining nerves demonstrated decreased activity consistent with those fibres being post-ganglionic. Retrograde transport studies in the guinea-pig (Parker, Mohamed and Coupland, 1990) and rat (Kesse, Parker and Coupland, 1988) have demonstrated staining of cell bodies in the paravertebral and suprarenal ganglia. These presumably postganglionic sympathetic nerve bodies represented 10% of the labelled cells in the rat and 30% in the guinea-pig. Morphological studies have demonstrated catecholamine-containing adrenergic fibres in the medulla of the cat (Prentice and Wood, 1974) and the cortex of the rat (Kleitman and Holzwarth, 1985). Many of these adrenergic fibres appeared to be in close proximity to blood vessels, although detailed electron microscopic studies have failed to confirm the presence of nerve terminals (or synaptic vesicles) associated with medullary vessels (Tomlinson and Coupland, 1990). The adrenal also contains a substantial number of peptidergic nerves.

Immunohistochemical studies have identified nerve fibres containing vasoactive intestinal peptide (Hökfelt *et al.*, 1981), substance P (Kuramoto, Kondo and Fujita, 1987), neuropeptide Y (Kuramoto, Kondo and Fujita, 1986), calcitonin gene-related peptide (Kuramoto, Kondo and Fujita, 1987) and corticotropin releasing factor (Bruhn *et al.*, 1987). Also NOS-containing nerve fibres have been described in adrenal medulla (Bredt, Hwang and Snyder, 1990).

These studies demonstrate that the adrenal medulla is densely innervated. In addition to preganglionic sympathetic fibres controlling catecholamine secretion, there are also postganglionic sympathetic and parasympathetic fibres, as well as possible afferent nerves. There are also a multitude of peptidergic nerves and nerve cells containing NOS.

PITUITARY GLAND

Central nervous system

A clear knowledge of the regional neuroanatomy including hypothalamic cells of origin, and their afferent and efferent connections, is important to understanding the interrelations between neuroendocrine secretion and circulatory events. Both the median eminence and the neural lobe represent terminal fields of brain axons. For the neural lobe the predominance of the cell bodies are found in the paraventricular and supraoptic nuclei as magnocellular neurons. These neurons have large cell bodies, significant protein synthetic capabilities and many large, peptide-containing vesicles. For the median eminence, a more diffuse set of cells of origin are present, including the anterior, periventricular and dorsal lateral nuclei of the hypothalamus. These latter cell bodies are smaller, contain a wide variety of neurotransmitters including dopamine, noradrenaline, vasoactive intestinal peptide (Samson, Said and McCann, 1979; Card *et al.*, 1981), substance P, acetylcholine and releasing factors (corticotropin releasing factor, thyrotropic releasing factor, somatostatin, luteinizing hormone releasing factor, follicle stimulating hormone releasing factor).

Within the neural lobe, the tubero-infundibular tract dominates the region, with AVP-containing neurons contributing the major proportion of axons. This is the best studied and the most active portion of the hypothalamic–pituitary axis. The magnocellular neurons receive afferent inputs from rostral and caudal areas. For the release of AVP, these inputs can be grouped as baroreceptive, osmoreceptive or complex behavioural types. The baroreceptive inputs start as pressure signals arising from the atria and ventricles of the heart as well as the aortic and carotid bifurcation regions of the arterial circulation. These baroreceptive inputs enter the brainstem via the IXth and X[th] cranial nerves, project to the dorsal motor nucleus, and then are relayed to the paraventricular and supraoptic magnocellular neurons via the ventral medulla and the retrofacial and locus coeruleus nuclear areas (Li, Gieroba and Blessing, 1992). Additional baroreceptive inputs come via anterior hypothalamic regions such as the subfornicial organ and the organ vasculosum of the lamina terminalis, which respond to circulating angiotensin by increasing the stimulation of the magnocellular neurons. The osmoreceptive pathway involves a central nervous system osmoreceptor, probably located in the AV3V hypothalamic region. This receptor is sensitive to plasma osmolality, so that with increases of osmolality there is an increased stimulation of the magnocellular neurons. The location of this receptor and its connection to the magnocellular neurons remains unknown. The neural system that is associated with behavioural inputs capable of increasing AVP release are the least well understood. Nausea, pain and stress all lead to release via these pathways (Cunningham and Sawchenko, 1991). The anatomical substrate for these reflex-induced secretions probably involve gastric and gustatory afferents to the medulla, and rostral connections to the magnocellular neurons. A second set of connections involves the limbic system with connections from the amygdala to the magnocellular neurons. The physiological nature of this pathway is not well understood.

Release of OT occurs with parturition and lactation. The best studied reflex is the suckling reflex. It is thought that this stimulation occurs by somatosensory and reticular afferents projecting to the nucleus tractus solitarius and then selectively to the OT-containing magnocellular neurons (Dyball and Leng, 1986). Less is known about the genito-urinary pathways of release. Stretch and pressure sensors are likely to increase the release of OT using similar neural pathways. These pathways may be important for the control of the smooth muscle during sexual activities (Cunningham and Sawchenko, 1991).

Other neuronal systems send processes to the neurohypophysis. While control of releasing factor secretion is the major neural process accounted for by these fibres, other activities such as neural–glial and neural–vascular interactions are possibly mediated by these tracts. Immunohistochemical techniques for visualizing the distribution of corticotropin releasing factor, somatostatin, leucine enkephalin, substance P, neurotensin and vasoactive intestinal polypeptide have been used to describe the central nervous system distribution of these peptide neurotransmitters (Hanley et al., 1992). Corticotropin releasing factor, somatostatin and neurotensin localize to the anterior median eminence in a diffuse manner. There is widespread axonal branching of these fibres throughout the subependymal, fibre, and palisade layers. Additionally, these releasing factors have a perivascular distribution, with dense collections of nerve terminals crowding around the looping vessels of the median eminence. Localization of the neuromodulators leucine enkephalin, substance P and vasoactive intestinal peptide has been noted in both the median eminence and infundibular process regions. Within the median eminence region, these peptides have a distribution similar to that of the classical releasing factors. Additionally, substance P appears to have direct contact with blood vessels and cells in the region of the pars intermedia. Within the infundibular process, localization of these three substances is diffuse, with vasoactive intestinal peptide being the most densely distributed peptide. The substance P and vasoactive intestinal peptide systems appear to be distinct from the magnocellular system, while the enkephalinergic system colocalizes with the OT and AVP magnocellular neurons (Martin and Voigt, 1981).

Opiate receptors have been demonstrated in the brain stem (Atweh and Kuhar, 1977a), hypothalamus (Atweh and Kuhar, 1977b), and pituitary (Lightman, Ninkovic and Hunt, 1983). The pituitary has been shown to include glial- or other "non-neuronal" cell-associated enkephalin receptors (Lightman, Ninkovic and Hunt, 1983). The physiological role of neurohypophysial opiate receptors is not presently known. Controversy exists regarding the colocalization of enkephalins with other neurotransmitters (Watson et al., 1982; Van Leeuwen and De Vries, 1983). Most authors suggest that leucine- or methionine-enkephalin and dynorphin coexist in OT or AVP-producing neurons (Mansour et al., 1988). Leucine-enkephalin and dynorphin immunoreactivity have been identified in neurohypophysial-hypothalamic cells containing AVP (Watson *et al.*, 1982; Mansour *et al.*, 1988), while methionine-enkephalin has been found in OT-containing cells (Martin and Voigt, 1981). Detailed studies of the anatomical relations of the neurohypophysis suggest enkephalinergic axons contact glial cells (Van Leeuwen and De Vries, 1983). The effect of enkephalins on glial cell–axon terminal interactions has not been studied, nor has the relationship between these nerve endings and local pituitary blood vessels.

Cell bodies have not been identified for the substance P fibres, however vasoactive intestinal peptide cell bodies projecting towards the median eminence have been described in the region of the suprachiasmatic nucleus. Within the hypothalamic–pituitary axis, the suprachiasmatic nucleus has a very dense concentration of vasoactive intestinal peptide-containing perikarya. These neurons are concentrated in the ventral half of the nucleus, immediately adjacent to the optic chiasm (Card *et al.*, 1981). Besides this region, radioimmunoassay data demonstrate other hypothalamic areas also contain vasoactive intestinal peptide. These include the anterior hypothalamus, the paraventricular nucleus, the dorsomedial and ventromedial nuclei, the premamillary nuclei, and the periventricular regions (Samson, Said and McCann, 1979; Abrams, Nilaver and Zimmerman, 1985). Saito *et al.* (1993) recently were able to show that in the neural lobe, vasoactive intestinal peptide immunoreactivity was closely associated with small arteries.

In the neural lobe, acetylcholinesterase is concentrated around the blood vessels (Holmes, 1961). Palay (1955) described small vesicles (40 μm) within neural lobe nerve endings that Koelle and Geesey (1961) later proposed contain acetylcholine. Lederis and Livingston (1969, 1970) showed that the small vesicles were located in fibres that were distinct from the peptide-secreting fibres. They later showed that the acetylcholine nerve terminals lay adjacent to neurohypophysial blood vessels.

The neural lobe is rich in catecholamines (Bjorklund, 1968; Palkovits *et al.*, 1977, 1980). Noradrenergic and dopaminergic fibres originating from cell groups A1 and A6 (Fuxe and Hökfelt, 1966; Bjorklund and Nobin, 1973; Palkovits *et al.*, 1977, 1980), and the arcuate nucleus (Fuxe and Hökfelt, 1966), supply the majority of the catecholaminergic fibres found in this tissue. However, Bjorklund (1968) showed that the blood vessels of the neural lobe derived their supply from postganglionic fibres originating in the superior cervical ganglion. Recently, radioligand binding studies have shown high concentrations of both α_1- (Kuyatt and DeSouza, 1986) and β_2-adrenoceptors (DeSouza, 1985) within neurohypophysial tissues, but the precise location of these receptors is unclear. It appears that the α_1-adrenoceptor is present only within the posterior lobe, with no evidence of binding either in the anterior or intermediate lobes (Kuyatt and DeSouza, 1986). This α_1-adrenoceptor binding activity decreased after superior cervical ganglionectomy, but was unchanged after stalk section (Kuyatt and DeSouza, 1986). Thus, these receptors appeared to be located on either the blood vessels, the pituicyte, or both.

Peripheral neuroanatomy

The autonomic nervous system sends sympathetic efferent nerves to the pituitary. These project via the superior cervical ganglion to the carotid artery and then follow the artery towards the sella. Tracing studies of these nerves have not been performed to define the location of the cell bodies. Recently, we localized noradrenaline and vasoactive intestinal peptide-containing axon varicosities to these vessels (Hanley *et al.*, 1992). Vasoactive intestinal peptidergic innervation of these vessels probably takes its origin from the carotid miniganglion (Suzuki, Hardebo and Owman, 1988). We are unaware of any attempt to study the peripheral cholinergic innervation of the pituitary.

NEUROPHYSIOLOGICAL STUDIES

Adrenal gland

Physiological data clearly indicate that the adrenal medullary blood flow is regulated by splanchnic nerve activity. Adrenal denervation decreased the medullary blood flow under resting conditions (Sakima *et al.*, 1991), and prevented hypoxia (Breslow *et al.*, 1989) and hypotension-induced medullary vasodilatation (Breslow *et al.*, 1987). Direct stimulation of the splanchnic nerve caused medullary vasodilatation (Breslow *et al.*, 1987, 1990, 1991; Jordan *et al.*, 1989). Although catecholamine secretion also increased, these responses could be dissociated. Thus, the catecholamine secretory and adrenal medullary blood flow responses appear to be under the control of parallel neural mechanisms. In contrast, the role of nerves in the regulation of blood flow to cortex is less clear. Acute adrenal denervation in anaesthetized animals has been reported to result in small increases in cortical blood flow (Kennedy *et al.*, 1980). Similar increases were seen following ganglionic blockade (Kennedy *et al.*, 1980), suggesting a tonic, neurally mediated vasoconstriction. However, in other studies, denervation had no effect on blood flow to the cortex (Sakima *et al.*, 1991). Denervation did not affect cortical blood flow responses to hypoxia and haemorrhage (Breslow *et al.*, 1987, 1989). Splanchnic nerve stimulation normally has no effect on the cortical blood flow (Breslow *et al.*, 1987). However, following inhibition of NOS, nerve stimulation reduced the cortical blood flow (Breslow *et al.*, 1992, 1993). These data suggest the existence of offsetting vasodilator and vasoconstrictor mechanisms.

Pituitary gland

Despite anatomical studies demonstrating the apparent innervation of vessels in the pituitary, and pharmacological studies demonstrating blood flow responses to neurotransmitters present in the gland, direct studies confirming the neural regulation of blood flow are not available. Nerve lesion experiments have established nerve pathways involved in AVP (and adenohypophysial hormone) secretion, but these studies did not examine the effects of specific lesions on blood flow responses.

PHARMACOLOGICAL STUDIES

Despite considerable data demonstrating the neural control of blood flow in the adrenal and pituitary, and extensive attempts to identify neurotransmitters present in these tissues, most information concerning the role of specific nerve systems in blood flow regulation have come from carefully performed pharmacological studies. Relevant data from each tissue are presented separately.

ADRENAL GLAND

The adrenal contains a large number of vasoactive substances which may be important in intra-glandular blood flow regulation (Breslow, 1992). Published data on possible adrenal vascular effects of catecholamines, acetylcholine, adenosine and NO are summarized below. Unfortunately, data are unavailable for the many other compounds contained in the adrenal.

Catecholamines

Intramedullary adrenaline concentrations following chromaffin cell degranulation are extremely high; levels in excess of 10^{-5} M (10,000 times normal plasma levels) have been reported (Jordan *et al.*, 1989). Despite these high concentrations it is not known whether adrenal catecholamines make contact with resistance vessels, nor what their effects on medullary vessels might be. The effects of adrenaline on vascular tone depend upon the population of adrenoceptors present in a given vascular bed. For example, small coronary arteries dilate in response to adrenaline since they possess only β-adrenoceptors (Zuberbuhler and Bohr, 1965), while other vessels constrict as a result of α-adrenoceptor stimulation. *In vitro* studies suggest the presence of α- and β-adrenoceptors on chromaffin cells (Greenberg and Zinder, 1982); however there are no published data on adrenal vascular adrenoceptors.

Initial physiological studies to evaluate the possible role of α- and β-adrenoceptors in control of vascular tone in the adrenal examined effects of specific adrenoceptor antagonists on basal blood flow and on nerve stimulation-induced vasodilatation. β-adrenoceptor antagonists have no effect on regional adrenal vascular resistance in either conscious (Faraci *et al.*, 1989), or anaesthetized (Jordan *et al.*, 1989) animals, suggesting that β-adrenoceptors are not important in the maintenance of resting medullary and cortical blood flow. High levels of medullary blood flow during exercise are also unaffected by propranolol (Faraci *et al.*, 1989), suggesting that β-adrenoceptors do not mediate exercise-induced medullary vasodilatation. In contrast to these studies on basal blood flow, the potent β-adrenoceptor antagonist, pindolol, attenuated the blood flow and catecholamine secretory responses to nerve stimulation by $> 50\%$ (Jordan *et al.*, 1989). To determine whether impaired vasodilatation following pindolol was due to blockade of vascular β-adrenoceptors, or occurred secondary to the effects of pindolol on chromaffin cell degranulation or neurotransmitter release, or was the result of non-specific actions of the drug, pentobarbital-anaesthetized dogs received an intravenous infusion of the β-adrenoceptor agonist, isoproterenol (Ligier *et al.*, 1994). Unilateral denervation was performed to prevent reflex increases in adrenal blood flow or catecholamine secretion. Isoproterenol increased catecholamine secretion but had no effect on vascular tone. These data suggest no direct role of β receptors in the regulation of adrenal blood flow.

Studies examining the possible vascular effects of α-adrenoceptor stimulation noted increases in the medullary blood flow and catecholamine secretory responses to splanchnic nerve stimulation in anaesthetized dogs following administration of the α-adrenoceptor antagonist, prazosin (Jordan *et al.*, 1989). Prazosin also increased medullary blood flow in exercising conscious dogs (Faraci *et al.*, 1989). While these data are consistent with released catecholamines causing vasoconstriction, direct infusion of the α-adrenoceptor agonist, phenylephrine, increased blood flow to the medulla and cortex (Ligier *et al.*,

1994). This vasodilator effect persisted when systemic blood pressure was held constant, and was blocked by prazosin. While phenylephrine-induced vasodilatation is unusual, it is unlikely that catecholamines released during chromaffin cell degranulation have significant effects on adrenal blood flow, since prazosin did not block nerve stimulation-induced vasodilatation.

Acetylcholine

The adrenal receives a dense cholinergic innervation; acetylcholine, acting primarily at nicotinic receptors (Kayaalp and McIsaac, 1969; Wakade and Wakade, 1983), is the major neurotransmitter controlling adrenal catecholamine secretion. Muscarinic cholinoceptors are also present in adrenal medulla (Tobin, Breslow and Traystman, 1992). *In vivo* and *in vitro* studies suggest that chromaffin cell muscarinic receptors can modulate catecholamine secretion (Role and Perlman, 1983; Wakade and Wakade, 1983), although there appears to be significant species variation in their importance. Muscarinic receptors are also present on many blood vessels, where they cause vasodilatation by stimulating the synthesis of potent endothelium-derived relaxing substances (Furchgott and Zawadzki, 1980; Hoeffner *et al.*, 1989). To determine whether vascular muscarinic receptors are important in blood flow regulation in the adrenal, atropine was administered to pentobarbital-anaesthetized dogs prior to splanchnic nerve stimulation (Kennedy *et al.*, 1980). Atropine had no effect on the medullary vascular or catecholamine secretory response to nerve stimulation. In contrast, hexamethonium, a nicotinic receptor antagonist, attenuated the catecholamine secretory response by > 95% without affecting the medullary vascular response. The combined administration of atropine and hexamethonium further reduced the catecholamine response to nerve stimulation and completely blocked the vascular response.

These data demonstrate that *in vivo* chromaffin cell degranulation in the dog is under both nicotinic and muscarinic control, with nicotinic receptor stimulation representing the predominant stimulus. Explaining the blood flow results is more difficult, and several different hypotheses are possible. First, chromaffin granule products may be released in such excess that a 95% reduction still results in sufficient intramedullary concentrations to elicit a maximal vasodilator response. However, studies demonstrating frequency-dependent changes in blood flow and secretion with nerve stimulation suggest this is unlikely. It is also possible that multiple redundant mechanisms cause medullary vasodilatation during splanchnic nerve stimulation, with one mechanism requiring ganglionic transmission or chromaffin cell degranulation (hexamethonium sensitive) and a second involving direct muscarinic receptor-mediated vasodilatation (atropine sensitive). Blockade of either receptor system (i.e. atropine or hexamethonium alone) has no effect on medullary vasodilatation, while blockade of both inhibits the blood flow response. The report of only a single muscarinic receptor subtype in canine adrenal medulla, with binding characteristics consistent with the M-1 subtype (Tobin, Breslow and Traystman, 1992), argues against this hypothesis. The recent reports of NOS-containing nerves in the medulla (Bredt, Hwang and Snyder, 1990) and the blockade of nerve stimulation-induced medullary vasodilatation by inhibitors of NOS (Breslow *et al.*, 1992, 1993) suggest that the splanchnic nerve may contain cholinergic fibres which synapse on NOS-containing nerves (see below). Persistent vasodilatation in the presence of either nicotinic or muscarinic antagonists suggest the presence of both nicotinic and muscarinic receptors in this ganglion. This type of combined cholinergic ganglionic transmission is not without precedent (Flacke and Gillis, 1968; Chinn and Hilton, 1976).

Peptidergic mechanisms

Chromaffin cells and intra-adrenal nerves contain many other vasoactive compounds with the potential to affect medullary vascular tone. These include ATP (Winkler, 1976), neurotensin (Rokaeus, Fried and Lundberg, 1984), vasoactive intestinal peptide (Holzwarth, 1984; Kondo, Kuramoto and Fujita, 1986), corticotropin releasing factor (Bruhn *et al.*, 1987), substance P (Linnoila and Diaugustine, 1980), calcitonin gene-related peptide (Kuramoto, Kondo and Fujita, 1987), neuropeptide Y (De Quidt and Emson, 1986), and enkephalins (Edwards, Hansell and Jones, 1986). Almost no data are available regarding the role of these compounds in the regulation of adrenal blood flow. Although ATP released from chromaffin cells is rapidly degraded to adenosine, a potent vasodilator which produces large increases in the adrenal medullary and cortical blood flow when infused into anaesthetized dogs (Faraci *et al.*, 1989), it is not known whether adenine nucleotides are normally involved in the control of adrenal blood flow.

Other compounds

NO is a potent smooth muscle relaxant which is an important modulator of blood flow in many organs. Initially thought to be produced exclusively by endothelial cells, recent data support the existence of at least three distinct isoforms of the enzyme, NOS (Moncada, Palmer and Higgs, 1991). Endothelial NO is important in the maintenance of resting vascular tone and in mediating the vasodilator effects of a variety of vasoactive compounds, including acetylcholine and adenosine (Gardiner *et al.*, 1990; Chu, Linn and Chambers, 1991; Moncada, Palmer and Higgs, 1991). Neuronal NOS is found in rat brain, intestine, neurohypophysis and adrenal medulla (Bredt, Hwang and Snyder, 1990), and in dog corpus cavernosum (Burnett *et al.*, 1992). NOS-containing nerves in the intestine appear to be important in peristalsis (Shuttleworth, Murphy and Furness, 1991), while NO mediates penile erection by causing vasodilatation in the corpus cavernosum (Burnett *et al.*, 1992). Both the adrenal medulla and the neurohypophysis are neurosecretory organs. Secretory products from these tissues are important in responding to physiological stress, and both organs demonstrate marked vasodilatation during secretory activity. We, therefore, hypothesized that NO may be important in blood flow regulation in the adrenal.

To investigate whether the adrenal is capable of synthesizing NO, homogenates of canine adrenal medulla and cortex were assessed for NOS activity by quantifying the conversion of ^{3}H-arginine to ^{3}H-citrulline (Breslow *et al.*, 1992, 1993). High levels of NOS activity were found in the adrenal medulla and cortex, levels markedly higher than found in other organs (except the brain and the pituitary). These results suggest a major role of NO in the adrenal. To evaluate the role of NO in the maintenance of resting blood flow in the adrenal medulla and cortex, the NOS inhibitor, L-NAME, was administered to pentobarbital-anaesthetized dogs (Breslow *et al.*, 1992, 1993). L-NAME reduced blood flow to both the medulla and the cortex by greater than 50%. These data support the hypothesis that NO is important in the maintenance of high basal levels of blood flow to the medulla and the cortex.

To evaluate the role of NO in medullary vasodilatation during catecholamine secretion, repetitive splanchnic nerve stimulation was performed prior to and following the inhibition of NOS by L-NAME (Breslow *et al.*, 1992, 1993). In the absence of L-NAME, the medullary blood flow increased four to six fold with two repetitive stimuli; following nitroarginine, splanchnic nerve stimulation had no effect on the medullary blood flow. Catecholamine secretion increased similarly with both stimulations. These data suggest a major role for NO in medullary vasodilatation during nerve stimulation-induced catecholamine secretion. Additional studies are required to determine whether nerves are the site of NO production (direct stimulation), or whether an alternate, neurally released vasodilator is acting via stimulation of endothelial NOS (indirect stimulation). Further evidence for medullary NO synthesis comes from the recent report of Moro *et al.* (1993) demonstrating medullary synthesis of cyclic GMP during splanchnic nerve stimulation in the cat. Cyclic GMP accumulation was blocked by L-NAME, which had no effect on catecholamine release.

Few other compounds have been evaluated for adrenal vascular effects (Breslow, 1992). ACTH, in high concentration, increases whole adrenal blood flow (Stark *et al.*, 1965; L'Age, Gonzalez-Luque and Yates, 1970; Edwards, Hardy and Malinowska, 1975). However, more physiological concentrations of ACTH appear to have little effect on cortical blood flow (Sakima *et al.*, 1991). Sakima *et al.* (1991) observed small decreases in the mean arterial blood pressure and the cortical vascular resistance with ACTH levels of 500 pg/ml. Although such levels occur during severe physiological stress (Raff and Fagin, 1984; Bereiter, Zaid and Gann, 1986), the overall effect of ACTH on adrenal blood flow appears to be small. Other investigators have hypothesized that prostaglandins are important in the maintenance of basal blood flow in the adrenal; indomethacin, an inhibitor of prostaglandin synthesis, reportedly decreases whole adrenal gland blood flow (Houck and Lutherer, 1981; Banks *et al.*, 1982). However, Sakima *et al.* (personal communication) noted no effect of indomethacin on the basal cortical or medullary blood flow in anaesthetized dogs. AVP and renin (but not angiotensin II) have been reported to decrease blood flow to adrenal autoplants (Wright, 1963). Finally, based on observations of a substantially higher medullary blood flow in conscious dogs than in pentobarbital-anaesthetized animals (Faraci *et al.*, 1989), it seems likely that pentobarbital anaesthesia decreases adrenal medullary blood flow. Whether this is a direct vascular action or occurs secondary to effects on catecholamine secretion or neural activity is not known.

PITUITARY GLAND

Catecholamines

Radioligand binding studies show high concentrations of both α_1-adrenoceptors (Kuyatt and DeSouza, 1986) and β_2-adrenoceptors (DeSouza, 1985) in neurohypophysial tissues. The α_1-adrenoceptor is present only in the posterior lobe, with no evidence of binding either in the anterior or intermediate lobes (Kuyatt and DeSouza, 1986). α_1-adrenoceptors decrease after superior cervical ganglionectomy, but are unchanged after stalk section (Kuyatt and DeSouza, 1986), suggesting the adrenoceptors are associated with nerves that enter with the blood vessels.

The role adrenoceptors play in neurohypophysial blood flow regulation is unclear. Inferior and superior hypophysial arteries constrict when stimulated pharmacologically with adrenaline (Hanley *et al.*, 1992). The inferior hypophysial artery is more sensitive to adrenaline than is the superior hypophysial artery; a finding that is consistent with the hypothesis that adrenoceptor sensitivity changes as the internal carotid artery passes through the cavernous sinus segment.

Worthington (1960) showed that the arterial vessels supplying the rat pituitary were highly contractile and constricted when catecholamines were applied topically. In the dog it has been shown that neural lobe and median eminence blood flow decrease during intra-arterial phenylephrine infusion (Wilson *et al.*, 1983). For reasons which are unclear, the blood flow reduction was greatest in the median eminence and least in the neural lobe (the dose–response curve for the neural lobe showed a 50% reduction at 68 μg/min, whereas the median eminence flow was reduced by 50% at 27 μg/min). Given that the superior hypophysial artery is relatively unresponsive to noradrenaline *in vitro* (Hanley *et al.*, 1992), greater reductions in neural lobe blood flow might be expected. A potential explanation for the apparent discrepancy between *in vivo* and *in vitro* responses is that infused phenylephrinine acts on adrenoceptors located within the internal zone and in the middle third of the external zone of the median eminence (Bjorklund *et al.*, 1973; Hökfelt *et al.*, 1978) and not on the superior hypophysial artery *per se*. Thus, the reduction in median eminence blood flow seen with intraarterial infusion may reflect the loss of the adenohypophysial component of the flow normally supplied to the anterior lobe via vessels lying within the median eminence.

Sympathetic nerve fibres from the superior cervical ganglia have been described entering with the vasculature connecting the hypothalamus with the hypophysis. These nerves are presumed to be vasomotor nerves (Harris and Cambell, 1966) and a number of investigators have suggested that they play a secondary role in the control of hypophysial function by providing a vasomotor influence on hormone release (Green, 1951; Worthington, 1960; Goldman, 1963). Fendler and Endroczi (1965) attributed inhibition of compensatory adrenal hypersecretion caused by bilateral removal of these ganglia to a modification of resting perfusion within the adenohypophysis. To test this hypothesis, Goldman (1968) used the ^{86}Rb method to measure regional pituitary blood flow in intact, bilaterally cervical sympathetic nerve-sectioned, and bilaterally superior cervical-ganglionectomized rats. No effect of nerve section or ganglionectomy on basal blood flow rate through any pituitary region was observed. Section of the preganglionic fibres supplying the superior cervical ganglion was unaccompanied by significant changes in neural lobe or median eminence blood flow in the dog (Wilson *et al.*, 1982). However, electrical stimulation of the postganglionic fibres reduced the neurohypophysial blood flow by 27%. During hypercarbia, α_1-adrenoceptor stimulation attenuated the neurohypophysial vasodilator response in the rat; pretreatment with phentolamine unmasked CO_2 reactivity (Bryan, Myers and Page, 1988). Pharmacological blockade of α_1-adrenoceptors by phenoxybenzamine reduces resting blood flow through the neural lobe (Table 7.2). However, because the α_1-adrenoceptor is also involved in the regulation of AVP release, it is impossible to differentiate the effects of this agent on blood vessel receptors from receptors associated with AVP release.

We tested the hypothesis that adrenergic activity contributes vasoconstrictor tone to neurohypophysial vessels in baseline conditions in the dog (Diringer *et al.*, 1991). Dogs received a loading dose of 1 mg/kg prazosin over 30–40 min followed by a maintenance

TABLE 7.2
Absence of effects of adrenoreceptor or cholinoreceptor antagonists on the
neurohypophysial blood flow response to rapid hypotension

Treatment	Tissue	Normotension		3' 80 mmHg		30' 80 mmHg	
		flow	% of control	flow	% of control	flow	% of control
Control	Median eminence	240 ± 48	100	300 ± 42	168 ± 29	228 ± 37	110 ± 12
(n = 10)	Neural lobe	822 ± 109	100	1876 ± 168	267 ± 48	714 ± 73	99 ± 11
	CBF	30 ± 4	100	33 ± 3	114 ± 5	39 ± 5	131 ± 6
Phenoxybenzamine	Median eminence	226 ± 53	100	403 ± 115	170 ± 22	247 ± 57	111 ± 9
(1 mg/kg; i.v.)	Neural lobe	580 ± 89	100	1103 ± 144	232 ± 39	613 ± 89	120 ± 18
(n = 10)	CBF	22 ± 3	100	30 ± 3	130 ± 11	29 ± 3	134 ± 12
Atropine	Median eminence	161 ± 42	100	240 ± 58	156 ± 28	149 ± 50	89 ± 14
(1 mg/kg; i.v.)	Neural lobe	678 ± 79	100	1163 ± 48	185 ± 32	623 ± 40	95 ± 8
(n = 4)	CBF	37 ± 5	100	36 ± 3	102 ± 8	40 ± 7	109 ± 14

CBF = cerebral blood flow.

infusion of 0.125 mg/kg/h for 2 h. Control animals were studied without drug infusion. The neurohypophysial blood flow was unchanged immediately after prazosin, but fell to 64 and 49% of control at 1 and 2 h. In contrast, in the control group, the neurohypophysial blood flow was unchanged at 1 h and fell to 75% of control at 2 h. pAVP fell significantly after α_1-adrenoceptor block, but remained unchanged in the controls. Because acute peripheral α_1-adrenoceptor blockade did not alter the neurohypophysial blood flow, but prolonged block produced a delayed fall in the neurohypophysial blood flow, we speculate that α_1-adrenoceptor block does not alter neurohypophysial blood flow by a direct vascular mechanism, but rather by effecting changes in AVP release via action at a central site within the AVP release mechanism. Pretreatment with phenoxybenzamine does not prevent hypotension-induced neurohypophysial hyperperfusion (Table 7.2).

Dopaminergic fibres from the tubero-infundibular tract terminate in the external zone in the perivascular space of the external plexus (Ajika and Hökfelt, 1975; Hökfelt et al., 1978). These fibres secrete dopamine directly into portal blood vessels where concentrations 10-fold higher than peripheral blood concentrations have been measured. The known function of these fibres is to inhibit prolactin secretion. To determine if dopamine and other catecholamines also exert a vascular effect, Page et al. (1990) evaluated the effects of several dopamine agonists and antagonists on neurohypophysial blood flow in sheep. Haloperidol, a dopamine antagonist, significantly elevated serum prolactin and reduced the median eminence and neural lobe blood flow. Neither the D_2-receptor agonist, bromocriptine, nor the D_2-receptor agonist, SKF 38393, nor dopamine, were shown to exert any effects on neurohypophysial blood flow when administered intravenously in amounts sufficient to depress prolactin secretion. By contrast, intra-arterially administered dopamine depressed the prolactin secretory rate and reduced the median eminence and neural lobe blood flow. The effect of intra-arterial dopamine was blocked by pretreatment with phenoxybenzamine, suggesting that at the higher concentrations of dopamine achieved by administration via the arterial route, it was activating α-adrenoceptors. Further support for this hypothesis was provided by showing that the median eminence blood flow in phenoxybenzamine-blocked sheep was significantly higher than in untreated sheep.

Acetylcholine

The characteristics of the cholinergic innervation suggest these fibres may play a more important role in regulating neurohypophysial blood flow than in global cerebral blood flow regulation. Cholinergic innervation is restricted to the larger cerebral arteries (Kobayashi *et al.*, 1981; Sercombe, Lacombe and Seylaz, 1984; Yu, Wu and Lee, 1986). These are the vessels from which the pituitary derives its blood supply. Cholinergic fibres have not been shown to extend as far as the intraparenchymal vessels in brain tissue (Sercombe, Lacombe and Seylaz, 1984; Yu, Wu and Lee, 1986), but this may not be the case in the neurohypophysis where acetylcholine-containing nerve fibres have been shown at the capillary level. Moreover, Baramidze *et al.* (1982) showed there was a higher density of cholinergic innervation at the offshoot branches of the larger cerebral arteries. Changes in the tone of these vessels could have a more pronounced influence on neurohypophysial blood flow than on global cerebral blood flow, since some of these offshoots (superior and inferior hypophysial arteries) directly supply the neurohypophysial vascular bed.

Konstantinova (1967) attempted to confirm these observations using morphological techniques and demonstrated that acetylcholine administered either intraperitoneally or via intracerebroventricular perfusion was associated with the dilatation of neurohypophysial vessels. Evidence supporting a vasomotor role for cholinergic nerves in the neural lobe is both direct and indirect. Acetylcholine, applied topically to the hypothalamic nuclei, caused AVP release (Gosbee and Lederis, 1972). It had no effect on the isolated neural lobe, however (Douglas and Poisner, 1964). *In vivo*, acetylcholine can release AVP (Gosbee and Lederis, 1972). One explanation for these observations is that the *in vivo* neural lobe is perfused, and that acetylcholine somehow acts upon the vasculature to effect release (Sklar and Schrier, 1983). One group has attempted to validate this hypothesis. Sooriyamoorthy and Livingston (1972) showed that the neural lobe blood volume significantly increased in response to saline treatment (drinking water replacement with 2% saline for 120 h), haemorrhage, $CaCl_2$ injection and right vagal nerve stimulation. Atropine (0.5 mg/kg, s.c.) raised the control neural lobe blood volume and attenuated the neural lobe response to these stimuli. Intravenous methacholine was accompanied by vasodilatation, which was blocked by atropine. However, since these authors did not quantify changes in hypothalamo-hypophysial function, it is not possible to differentiate between neurosecretory-linked blood volume change and the direct effects of muscarinic receptor stimulation at the blood vessel level. Pretreatment with atropine does not prevent hypotension-induced neurohypophysial hyperperfusion (Table 7.2).

Peptidergic mechanisms

Vasoactive intestinal peptide: Intraarterially infused vasoactive intestinal peptide increased whole pituitary blood flow (Wilson *et al.*, 1981). To identify the location of the receptors responsible for this rise, we studied vasoactive intestinal peptide and noradrenergic influences on the arterial resistance of the neurohypophysis (Hanley *et al.*, 1992). A dual extracranial and intracranial arterial supply that is differentially sensitive to neurotransmitter substances

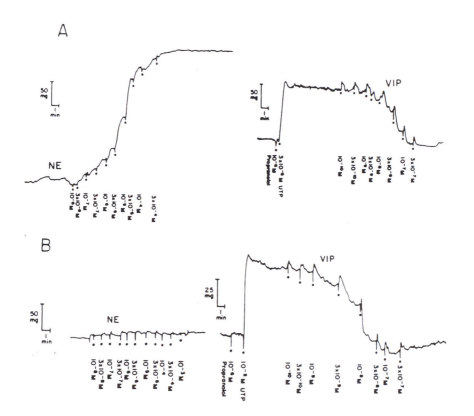

Figure 7.12   Dose–response curves for resistance vessels of the neurohypophysis: inferior hypophysial (A) and superior hypophysial (B). NE, norepinephrine; UTP, uridine 5′-triphosphate; VIP, vasoactive intestinal peptide. [Reprinted with permission from Hanley *et al.* (1992).]

was confirmed (Figure 7.12). Pharmacological sensitivity of the inferior hypophysial artery to vasoactive intestinal peptide ($ED_{50} = 10^{-8.2}$ M) and to noradrenaline ($ED_{50} = 10^{-5.7}$ M) was demonstrated. The superior hypophysial artery reacted only to vasoactive intestinal peptide ($ED_{50} = 10^{-8.6}$ M). The physiological relevance of these findings was tested with transmural nerve stimulation. Frequency-dependent vasodilatation of both the inferior hypophysial artery and the superior hypophysial artery was demonstrated. This dilatation could not be blocked with atropine or propranolol. Frequency-dependent vasoconstriction was identified in extracranial vessels, including the inferior hypophysial artery. This constriction is only partially blocked by prazosin, phentolamine and guanethidine. When compared to other cerebral regions, the neurohypophysis appears to have a regionally unique mechanism for the neural regulation of resistance arteries.

Enkephalin: (D-Ala^2)-Met^5-encephalinamide (AM) and (D-Ala^2)-Leu^5-encephalinamide (AL) were administered into the cisterna magna in anaesthetized dogs to determine whether these opiates affected the neurohypophysial circulation differently than the circulation of other brain areas (Kirsch *et al.*, 1988). Intracisternal radiolabelled AM distributed throughout the brain, with the highest concentration being in the area of the brainstem. Neither AL nor AM altered the cerebral blood flow or the cerebral oxygen uptake, whereas both AL and AM reduced the neurohypophysial blood flow by 43 ± 11 and $46 \pm 8\%$. pAVP was transiently elevated by $\sim 325\%$ with each treatment. Intravenous naloxone administered at the end of the protocol produced a rise toward control neurohypophysial blood flow in both groups. These data suggest that encephalinamides play a role in the regulation of neurohypophysial blood flow through their actions on opiate receptors.

Arginine vasopressin and oxytocin: There are several reasons to speculate that AVP and OT might exert some effect on neurohypophysial blood vessels. In haemorrhagic hypotension, there is an initial, short-lasting increase in the neurohypophysial blood flow, that is followed by a return to the normotensive control blood flow level (Vella *et al.*, 1989). The spike in blood flow is temporally associated with an increase in AVP secretion. A vasodilator influence could also explain the elevation in blood flow that occurs during hypoxic hypoxia (Hanley *et al.*, 1986) and hypertonicity (Ziedonis *et al.*, 1986). OT is also released in response to haemorrhage and hyperosmotic stimuli (Forsling and Brimble, 1985).

We examined the role of AVP as a mediator of neurohypophysial blood flow regulation in anaesthetized dogs (Hurn *et al.*, 1993). First, we evaluated the neurohypophysial hyperaemia that accompanies haemorrhagic hypotension in the presence and absence of the selective $AVPV_1$-receptor antagonist $d(CH_2)_5Tyr(Me)AVP$. AV_1-receptor blockade did not alter neurohypophysial transient or steady-state flow responses to hypotension. We then determined whether exogenous AVP altered neurohypophysial and regional cerebral blood flow. Sequential intra-carotid artery infusions resulted in sagittal sinus blood AVP concentrations ranging from $6.97 \pm 3.3 \times 10^3$ to $2.45 \pm 0.47 \times 10^6$ pg/ml, but no change in the neurohypophysial blood flow was observed. OT was also given by a constant rate intra-carotid artery infusion (1–200 μg/ml). The neurohypophysial blood flow was unchanged at all dosages. Thus, the data suggest that the products of neurohypophysial neurosecretion do not serve as significant mediators of neurohypophysial vasodilatation.

Other compounds

Nitric Oxide: NOS catalyzes the conversion of L-arginine to NO, a potent vasodilator, and L-citrulline (Ignarro, 1990; Luscher and Vanhoutte, 1990; Moncada and Higgs, 1991; Snyder and Bredt, 1991). NOS is concentrated in the pituitary, cerebellum, olfactory bulb, superior and inferior colliculi, dentate gyrus, and bed nucleus of the stria terminalis (Bredt, Hwang and Snyder, 1990). In rat pituitary, the intermediate and anterior lobes do not show immunoreactivity, but intense staining occurs in the posterior lobe. NOS blockade by L-NAME dramatically reduces the neurohypophysial blood flow (417 ± 42 to 58 ± 7 ml/min/100 g), suggesting that NO may be responsible for maintaining the high blood flow level of the neurohypophysis (Saito *et al.*, 1994). Despite the 87% reduction in neurohypophysial blood flow that occurred with NOS block, L-NAME had no effect on the percentage increase in neurohypophysial blood flow induced by hypoxia in dogs with intact chemoreceptors. Two conclusions can be drawn from these results. First, it seems unlikely that increased NO release, resulting from enhanced magnocellular nerve activity, is responsible for hypoxic vasodilatation. Second, increased NO production due to the effects of hypoxia on NOS activity, cannot be the mechanism by which neurohypophysial hypoxic vasodilatation occurs. Other factors, such as enhanced AVP release associated with peripheral chemoreceptor activation, or even local effects of hypoxia on vessels that have been unmasked by eliminating a non-nutrient flow component, cannot be ruled out. Tetrodotoxin, which acts exclusively at voltage-gated sodium channels on nerves to block action potential conduction, mimics the effects of NOS blockade on neural lobe blood flow. This observation, while inferential, suggests that neuronal release of NO is responsible for the maintenance of baseline neurohypophysial blood vessel tone (Diringer *et al.*, 1991).

Potassium: Electrical stimulation of the neurohypophysial stalk releases AVP and K^+ (Baertschi, 1980; Leng and Shibuki, 1987) in large amounts. The increment in extracellular fluid $[K^+]$ during stalk stimulation is the highest observed in any tissue studied. The increment in extracellular fluid $[K^+]$ is thought to facilitate hormone release either by generating additional depolarization or by serving to maintain an elevated $[Ca^{++}]_o$ (Leng and Shibuki, 1987). The effect of potassium on neurohypophysial blood vessels has not been studied. Potentially, changes in potassium ion concentration could serve as a means of coupling pituitary blood flow to neurosecretory activity.

CONCLUSIONS

In attempting to summarize the large amount of data presented in this review, it is important to keep in mind that almost all of the available information on adrenal and pituitary blood flow regulation has been obtained during the past 10 years; technical difficulties in measuring blood flow to these complex endocrine tissues precluded regional blood flow measurements until quite recently. Thus, it is not surprising that many gaps remain in our understanding of vascular control mechanisms in these two organs. The available data demonstrate both similarities and differences in how the adrenal and the pituitary regulate blood flow. Basal blood flow to the adrenal medulla, adrenal cortex and neurohypophysis are high when compared to other organs. This high level of blood flow does not seem to be required to meet metabolic demands. Oxygen extraction in the adrenal medulla and cortex is quite low, and similar observations have been made in the pituitary. While it is attractive to postulate that high levels of blood flow assure a rapid delivery of secreted hormones into the systemic circulation, experimental confirmation of this hypothesis is not available. Blood flow to the adrenal cortex is fairly constant and does not vary with secretory activity. Despite evidence of some neural modulation of cortical blood flow, nerves do not appear to be important in the control of the adrenal cortical vasculature. In contrast to the adrenal cortex, blood flow to the adrenal medulla and the neurohypophysis vary markedly over short periods of time. Increases in blood flow to these two neurosecretory tissues usually parallel increases in secretory activity. In the neurohypophysis, the vasodilator response is transient, and blood flow returns to baseline despite ongoing AVP secretion. In contrast, increases in medullary blood flow are prolonged and seem to parallel secretion. While adrenal catecholamine secretion and medullary vasodilatation are neurally mediated, different nerves regulate these distinct physiological events. Temporal differences in AVP secretion and neurohypophysial vasodilatation suggest similar, distinct innervation of secretory cells and blood vessels in the posterior pituitary. Both adrenal and pituitary have a dense peptidergic innervation, and localization of these nerve fibres in proximity to vessels suggests a possible involvement in blood flow regulation. Of considerable interest, NOS-containing neurons are present in both glands. NO contributes to high basal levels of blood flow in the adrenal medulla, adrenal cortex and neurohypophysis. Current data do not permit conclusions about the source of this tonic NO production. In the adrenal medulla, NO mediates increases in medullary blood flow during catecholamine secretion; the role of NO in vasodilatation during AVP secretion in the neurohypophysis is less clear. Chromaffin granules release large quantities of catecholamines and other vasoactive agents during degranulation. Similarly, high concentrations of vasopressin are present in the neurohypophysis during secretion. These potent vasoconstrictors do not constrict adjacent blood vessels, suggesting a unique adaptation of adrenal and neurohypophysial blood vessels to their local environment.

ACKNOWLEDGEMENTS

We wish to thank Josh Wei and Sherrie Solomon for their assistance in the preparation of this chapter.

REFERENCES

Abrams, G.M., Nilaver, G. and Zimmerman, E.A. (1985). VIP-containing neurons. In *Handbook of Chemical Neuroanatomy, GABA and Neuropeptides in the CNS. Vol. 4*, edited by A. Bjorklund and T. Hökfelt, pp. 335–354. Amsterdam: Elsevier.

Ajika, K. and Hökfelt, T. (1975). Projections to the median eminence and the arcuate nucleus with special reference to monoamine systems: effects of lesions. *Cell and Tissue Research*, **158**, 15–35.

Archie, J.P.J., Fixler, D.E., Ullyot, D.J., Hoffman, J.I.E., Utley, J.R. and Carlson, E.L. (1973). Measurement of cardiac output with and organ trapping of radioactive microspheres. *Journal of Applied Physiology*, **35**, 148–154.

Atweh, S.F. and Kuhar, M.J. (1977a). Autoradiographic localization of opiate receptors in rat brain. I. Spinal cord and lower medulla. *Brain Research*, **124**, 53–67.

Atweh, S.F. and Kuhar, M.J. (1977b). Autoradiographic localization of opiate receptors in rat brain. II. The brain stem. *Brain Research*, **129**, 1–12.

Baertschi, A.J. (1980). Portal vascular route from hypophysial stalk/neural lobe to adenohypophysis. *American Journal of Physiology*, **239**, R463–R469.

Banks, R.A., Beilin, L.J., Soltys, J. and Davidson, L. (1982). Effects of meclofenamate and captopril on adrenal blood flow: contrasts in conscious rabbits at rest and after haemorrhage. *American Journal of Cardiology*, **49**, 1544–1546.

Baramidze, D.G., Reidler, R.M., Gadamski, R. and Mchedlishvili, G.I. (1982). Pattern and innervation of pial microvascular effectors which control blood supply to cerebral cortex. *Blood Vessels*, **19**, 284–291.

Bassingthwaighte, J.B., Malone, M.A., Moffett, T.C., King, R.B., Little, S.E., Link, J.M., *et al.* (1987). Validity of microsphere depositions for regional myocardial flows. *American Journal of Physiology*, **253**, H184–H193.

Bennett, H.S. and Kilham, L. (1940). The blood vessels of the adrenal gland of the adult cat. *Anatomical Record*, **77**, 447–471.

Bereiter, D.A., Zaid, A.M. and Gann, D.S. (1986). Effect of rate of haemorrhage on release of ACTH in cats. *American Journal of Physiology*, **250**, 76–81.

Bergland, R.M. and Page, R.B. (1979). Pituitary-brain vascular relations: a new paradigm. *Science*, **204**, 18–24.

Bergland, R.M., Davis, S.L. and Page, R.B. (1977). Pituitary secretes to brain. Experiments in sheep. *Lancet*, **2**, 276–278.

Bevan, J.A., Bevan, R.D. and Duckles, S.P. (1980). Adrenergic regulation of vascular smooth muscle. In *Handbook of Physiology Section 2: The Cardiovascular System Vol. II Vascular Smooth Muscle*, edited by D.F. Bohr, A.P. Sonlye and H.V. Sparks, Jr., pp. 516–566. Bethesda, MD: American Physiological Society.

Bjorklund, A. (1968). Monoamine-containing fibres in the pituitary neuro-intermediate lobe of the pig and rat. *Zeitschrift für Zellforschung und Mikroskopische Anatomie*, **89**, 573–589.

Bjorklund, A. and Nobin, A. (1973). Fluorescence histochemical and microspectrofluorometric mapping of dopamine and noradrenaline cell groups in the rat diencephalon. *Brain Research*, **51**, 193–205.

Bjorklund, A., Moore, R.Y., Nobin, A. and Stenevi, U. (1973). The organization of tubero-hypophysial and reticulo-infundibular catecholamine neuron systems in the rat brain. *Brain Research*, **51**, 171–191.

Bredt, D.S., Hwang, P.M. and Snyder, S.H. (1990). Localization of nitric oxide synthase indicating a neural role for nitric oxide. *Nature*, **347**, 768–770.

Breslow, M.J. (1992). Regulation of adrenal medullary and cortical blood flow. *American Journal of Physiology*, **262**, H1317–H1330.

Breslow, M.J., Mennen, A., Koehler, R.C. and Traystman, R.J. (1986). Adrenal medullary and cortical blood flow during haemorrhage. *American Journal of Physiology*, **250**, H954–H960.

Breslow, M.J., Jordan, D.A., Thellman, S.T. and Traystman, R.J. (1987). Neural control of adrenal medullary and cortical blood flow during haemorrhage. *American Journal of Physiology*, **252**, 521–528.

Breslow, M.J., Ball, T.D., Miller, C.F., Raff, H. and Traystman, R.J. (1989). Adrenal blood flow and secretory relationships during hypoxia in anaesthetized dogs. *American Journal of Physiology*, **257**, 458–465.

Breslow, M.J., Tobin, J.R., Mandrell, T.D., Racusen, L.C., Raff, H. and Traystman, R.J. (1990). Changes in adrenal oxygen consumption during catecholamine secretion in anaesthetized dogs. *American Journal of Physiology*, **259**, 681–688.

Breslow, M.J., Tobin, J.R., Kubos, K.L., Raff, H. and Traystman, R.J. (1991). Effect of adrenal hypotension on elicited secretory activity in anaesthetized dogs. *American Journal of Physiology*, **260**, 21–26.

Breslow, M.J., Tobin, J.R., Bredt, D.S., Ferris, C.D., Snyder, S.H. and Traystman, R.J. (1992). Role of nitric oxide in adrenal medullary vasodilation during catecholamine secretion. *European Journal of Pharmacology*, **210**, 105–106.

Breslow, M.J., Tobin, J.R., Bredt, D.S., Ferris, C.D., Snyder, S.H. and Traystman, R.J. (1993). Nitric oxide as a regulator of adrenal blood flow. *American Journal of Physiology*, **264**, H464–H469.

Bruhn, T.O., Engeland, W.C., Anthony, E.L.P., Gann, D.S. and Jackson, I.M.D. (1987). Corticotropin-releasing factor in the dog adrenal medulla is secreted in response to haemorrhage. *Endocrinology*, **120**, 25–33.

Bryan, R.M., Jr., Hollinger, B.R., Keefer, K.A. and Page, R.B. (1987). Regional cerebral and neural lobe blood flow during insulin-induced hypoglycemia in unanaesthetized rats. *Journal of Cerebral Blood Flow and Metabolism*, **7**, 96–102.

Bryan, R.M., Jr., Myers, C.L. and Page, R.B. (1988). Regional neurohypophysial and hypothalamic blood flow in rats during hypercapnia. *American Journal of Physiology*, **255**, R295–R302.

Bülbring, E., Burn, J.H. and De Elio, F.J. (1948). The secretion of adrenaline from the perfused suprarenal gland. *Journal of Physiology*, **107**, 222–232.

Burnett, A.L., Lowenstein, C.J., Bredt, D.S., Chang, T.S.K. and Snyder, S.H. (1992). Nitric oxide: a physiologic mediator of penile erection. *Science*, **257**, 401–403.

Card, J.P., Brecha, N., Karten, H.J. and Moore, R.Y. (1981). Immunocytochemical localization of vasoactive intestinal polypeptide-containing cells and processes in the suprachiasmatic nucleus of the rat: light and electron microscopic analysis. *Journal of Neuroscience Research*, **1**, 1289–1303.

Carlsson, S., Skarphedinsson, J.O., Jennische, E., Delle, M. and Thoren, P. (1990). Neurophysiological evidence for and characterization of the post-ganglionic innervation of the adrenal gland in the rat. *Acta Physiologica Scandinavica*, **140**, 491–499.

Carter, A.M., Richardson, B.S., Homan, J., Towstoless, M. and Challis, J.R.G. (1993). Regional adrenal blood flow responses to adrenocorticotropic hormone in fetal sheep. *American Journal of Physiology*, **264**, E264–E269.

Chinn, C. and Hilton, J.G. (1976). Selective activation of nicotinic and muscarinic transmission in cardiac sympathetic ganglia of the dog. *European Journal of Pharmacology*, **40**, 77–82.

Chu, A., Linn, C. and Chambers, D.E. (1991). Effects of inhibition of nitric oxide formation on basal tone and endothelium-dependent responses of the coronary arteries in awake dogs. *Journal of Clinical Investigation*, **84**, 1964–1968.

Costa, E., Guidotti, A., Hanbauer, I., Hexum, T., Saiani, L., Stine, S., *et al.* (1981). Regulation of acetylcholine receptors by endogenous cotransmitters: studies of adrenal medulla. *Federation Proceedings*, **40**, 160–165.

Coupland, R.E. and MacDougall, J.D.B. (1966). Adrenaline formation in noradrenaline-storing chromaffin cells *in vitro* induced by corticosterone. *Journal of Endocrinology*, **36**, 317–324.

Coupland, R.E. and Selby, J.E. (1976). The blood supply of the mammalian adrenal medulla: a comparative study. *Journal of Anatomy*, **122**, 539–551.

Coupland, R.E., Parker, T.L., Kesse, W.K. and Mohamed, A.A. (1989). The innervation of the adrenal gland. III. vagal innervation. *Journal of Anatomy*, **163**, 173–181.

Cueto, C., Brown, J.H.U. and Richardson, A.P.J. (1958). Biological studies on an adrenocorticolytic agent and the isolation of the active components. *Endocrinology*, **62**, 334–339.

Cunningham, E.T., Jr. and Sawchenko, P.E. (1991). Reflex control of magnocellular vasopressin and oxytocin secretion. *Trends in Neurosciences*, **14**, 406–411.

Daniel, P.M. and Prichard, M.M. (1975). Studies of the hypothalamus and the pituitary gland with special reference to the effects of transection of the pituitary stalk. *Acta Endocrinologica Supplementum*, **201**, 1–216.

Dawson, T.M., Bredt, D.S., Fotuhi, M., Hwang, P.M. and Snyder, S.H. (1991). Nitric oxide synthase and neuronal NADPH diaphorase are identical in brain and peripheral tissues. *Proceedings of the National Academy of Sciences of the United States of America*, **88**, 7797–7801.

De Quidt, M.E. and Emson, P.C. (1986). Neuropeptide Y in the adrenal gland; characterization, distribution and drug effects. *Neuroscience*, **19**, 1011–1022.

Dempsher, D.P. and Gann, D.S. (1983). Increased cortisol secretion after small haemorrhage is not attributable to changes in adrenocorticotropin. *Endocrinology*, **113**, 86–93.

DeSouza, E.B. (1985). β_2-adrenergic receptors in pituitary. *Neuroendocrinology*, **41**, 289–296.

Diringer, M.N., Wu, K., Hanley, D.F., Wilson, D.A. and Traystman, R.J. (1991). Prazosin produces a delayed fall in neurohypophysial blood flow. *FASEB Journal*, **5**, A741. (Abstract).

Diringer, M.N., Wilson, D.A., Hanley, D.F., Wu, K.C., Ladenson, P.W. and Traystman, R.J. (1992). Mechanisms regulating neurohypophysial blood flow and function during isotonic volume expansion. *American Journal of Physiology*, **262**, H177–H183.

Dobbie, J.W. and Symington, T. (1966). The human adrenal gland with special reference to the vasculature. *Endocrinology*, **34**, 479–489.

Douglas, W.W. and Poisner, A.M. (1964). Stimulus-secretion coupling in a neurosecretory organ. The role of calcium in the release of vasopressin from the neurohypophysis. *Journal of Physiology*, **172**, 1–18.

Dyball, R.E. and Leng, G. (1986). Regulation of the milk ejection reflex in the rat. *Journal of Physiology*, **380**, 239–256.

Edwards, A.V., Hardy, R.N. and Malinowska, K.W. (1975). The sensitivity of adrenal responses to synthetic adrenocorticotrophin in the conscious unrestrained calf. *Journal of Physiology*, **245**, 639–653.

Edwards, A.V., Hansell, D. and Jones, C.T. (1986). Effects of synthetic adrenocorticotrophin on adrenal medullary responses to splanchnic nerve stimulation in conscious calves. *Journal of Physiology*, **379**, 1–16.

Elfvin, L.-G. (1965). The ultrastructure of the capillary fenestrae in the adrenal medulla of the rat. *Journal of Ultrastructural Research*, **12**, 687–704.

Engeland, W.C. and Gann, D.S. (1989). Splanchnic nerve stimulation modulates steroid secretion in hypophysectomized dogs. *Neuroendocrinology*, **50**, 124–131.

Faraci, F.M., Chilian, W.M., Williams, J.K. and Heistad, D.D. (1989). Effects of reflex stimuli on blood flow to the adrenal medulla. *American Journal of Physiology*, **257**, H590–H596.

Fendler, K. and Endroczi, E. (1965). Changes of adrenal compensatory hypertrophy in the rat after removal of the sympathetic superior cervical ganglia. *Acta Physiologica Hungarica*, **28**, 171–176.

Ferrari, M., Wilson, D.A., Hanley, D.F. and Traystman, R.J. (1992). Effects of graded hypotension on cerebral blood flow, blood volume and mean transit time in dogs. *American Journal of Physiology*, **262**, H1908–H1914.

Flacke, W. and Gillis, R.A. (1968). Impulse transmission via nicotinic and muscarinic pathways in the stellate ganglion of the dog. *Journal of Pharmacology and Experimental Therapeutics*, **163**, 266–276.

Forsling, M.L. and Brimble, M.J. (1985). Role of oxytocin in salt and water balance. In *Oxytocin: Clinical and Laboratory Studies*, edited by J.A. Amico and A.G. Robinson, pp. 167–175. Amsterdam: Excerpta Medica.

Frank, H.A., Frank, E.D., Korman, H., Macchi, I.A. and Hechter, O. (1955). Corticosteroid output and adrenal blood flow during haemorrhagic shock in the dog. *Surgery*, 24–28.

Furchgott, R.F. and Zawadzki, J.V. (1980). The obligatory role of endothelial cells in the relaxation of arterial smooth muscle by acetylcholine. *Nature*, **288**, 373–376.

Fuxe, K. and Hökfelt, T. (1966). Further evidence for the existence of tubero-infundibular dopamine neurons. *Acta Physiologica Scandinavica*, **66**, 245–246.

Gardiner, S.M., Compton, A.M., Bennett, T., Palmer, R.M.J. and Moncada, S. (1990). Control of regional blood flow by endothelium-derived nitric oxide. *Hypertension*, **15**, 486–492.

Goldman, H. (1963). Effect of acute stress on the pituitary gland: Endocrine gland blood flow. *Endocrinology*, **72**, 588–591.

Goldman, H. (1968). Failure of cervical sympathectomy to alter pituitary blood flow. *Endocrinology*, **83**, 603–606.

Goldman, H. and Sapirstein, L.A. (1958). Determination of blood flow to the rat pituitary gland. *American Journal of Physiology*, **194**, 433–435.

Goldman, H. and Sapirstein, L.A. (1973). Brain blood flow in the conscious and anaesthetized rat. *American Journal of Physiology*, **224**, 122–126.

Gorczyca, W. and Hardy, J. (1988). Microadenomas of the human pituitary and their vascularization. *Neurosurgery*, **22**, 1–6.

Gosbee, J.L. and Lederis, K. (1972). *In vivo* release of antidiuretic hormone by direct application of acetylcholine or carbachol to the rat neurohypophysis. *Canadian Journal of Physiology and Pharmacology*, **50**, 618–620.

Green, J.D. (1951). The comparative anatomy of the hypophysis with special reference to its blood supply and innervation. *American Journal of Anatomy*, **88**, 225–312.

Green, J.D. and Harris, G.W. (1947). The neurovascular link between the neurohypophysis and adenohypophysis. *Journal of Endocrinology*, **5**, 136–149.

Green, J.D. and Harris, G.W. (1949). Observation of the hypophysio-portal vessels of the living rat. *Journal of Physiology*, **108**, 359–361.

Greenberg, A. and Zinder, O. (1982). α- and β-receptor control of catecholamine secretion from isolated adrenal medulla cells. *Cell and Tissue Research*, **226**, 655–665.

Gross, P.M., Kadekaro, M., Sokoloff, L., Holcomb, H.H. and Saavedra, J.M. (1985). Alterations of local cerebral glucose utilization during chronic dehydration in rats. *Brain Research*, **330**, 329–336.

Haase, P., Contestabile, A. and Flumerfelt, B.A. (1982). Preganglionic innervation of the adrenal gland of the rat using horseradish peroxidase. *Experimental Neurology*, **78**, 217–221.

Hales, J.R.S. (1974). Radioactive microsphere techniques for studies of the circulation. *Clinical and Experimental Pharmacology and Physiology*, **suppl. 1**, 31–46.

Hamaji, M., Nakamura, M., Izukura, M., Nakaba, H., Hashimoto, T., Tanaka, Y., *et al.* (1986). Autoregulation and regional blood flow of the dog during haemorrhagic shock. *Circulatory Shock*, **19**, 245–255.

Hanley, D.F., Wilson, D.A. and Traystman, R.J. (1986). Effect of hypoxia and hypercapnia on neurohypophysial blood flow. *American Journal of Physiology*, **250**, H7–H15.

Hanley, D.F., Wilson, D.A., Feldman, M.A. and Traystman, R.J. (1988). Peripheral chemoreceptor control of neurohypophysial blood flow. *American Journal of Physiology*, **254**, H742–H750.

Hanley, D.F., Wilson, D.A., Conway, M.A., Traystman, R.J., Bevan, J.A. and Brayden, J.E. (1992). Neural mechanisms regulating neurohypophysial resistance arteries. *American Journal of Physiology*, **263**, H1605–H1615.

Harris, G.W. and Cambell, H.J. (1966). *The Pituitary Gland. Vol. 2*, Berkley: University of California Press.

Harrison, T.S. and Seaton, J. (1965). The relative effects of hypoxia and hypercarbia on adrenal medullary secretion in anaesthetized dogs. *Journal of Surgical Research*, **5**, 560–564.

Hawkins, R.A. and Biebuyck, J.F. (1979). Ketone bodies are selectively used by individual brain regions. *Science*, **205**, 325–327.

Heistad, D.D. and Kontos, H.A. (1983). Cerebral Circulation. In *Handbook of Physiology, Sect 2, Vol 3, Pt 1*, edited by J.T. Shepherd and F.M. Abboud, pp. 137–182. Bethesda, MD: American Physiological Society.

Hinson, J.P., Vinson, G.P. and Whitehouse, B.J. (1986). The relationship between perfusion medium flow rate and steroid secretion in the isolated perfused rat adrenal gland *in situ*. *Journal of Endocrinology*, **111**, 391–396.

Hodde, K.C. (1981). *Cephalic vascular patterns in the rat*, pp. 59–63. Amsterdam, Netherlands: Rodipi.

Hoeffner, U., Feletou, M., Flavahan, N.A. and Vanhoutte, P.M. (1989). Canine arteries release two different endothelium-derived relaxing factors. *American Journal of Physiology*, **257**, H330–H333.

Hökfelt, T., Elde, R., Fuxe, K., Johansson, O., Ljungdahl, A., Goldstein, M., *et al.* (1978). Aminergic and peptidergic pathways in the nervous system with special reference to the hypothalamus. In *The Hypothalamus*, edited by S. Reichlin, R.J. Baldessarini and J.B. Martin, pp. 69–135. New York: Raven Press.

Hökfelt, T., Lundberg, J.M., Schultzberg, M. and Fahrenkrug, J. (1981). Immunohistochemical evidence for a local VIP-ergic neuron system in the adrenal gland of the rat. *Acta Physiologica Scandinavica*, **113**, 575–576.

Hollinshead, W.H. (1936). The innervation of the adrenal glands. *Journal of Comparative Neurology*, **64**, 449–467.

Holmes, R.L. (1961). Phosphatase and cholinesterase in the hypothalamo-hypophysial system of the monkey. *Journal of Endocrinology*, **23**, 63–67.

Holzwarth, M.A. (1984). The distribution of vasoactive intestinal peptide in the rat adrenal cortex and medulla. *Journal of the Autonomic Nervous System*, **11**, 269–283.

Houck, P.C. and Lutherer, L.O. (1981). Regulation of adrenal blood flow: response to haemorrhagic hypotension. *American Journal of Physiology*, **241**, 872–877.

Hume, D.M. and Nelson, D.H. (1955). Adrenal cortical function in surgical shock. *Surgical Forum*, **5**, 568–575.

Hurn, P.D., Wilson, D.A., Hansen, R.B., Hanley, D.F. and Traystman, R.J. (1993). Vasopressin and oxytocin; modulators of neurohypophysial blood flow. *American Journal of Physiology*, **265**, H2027–H2035.

Ignarro, L.J. (1990). Nitric oxide. A novel signal transduction mechanism for transcellular communication. *Hypertension*, **16**, 477–483.

Jarry, H., Dietrich, M., Barthel, A., Giesler, A. and Wuttke, W. (1989). *In vivo* demonstration of a paracrine, inhibitory action of met-enkephalin on adrenomedullary catecholamine release in the rat. *Endocrinology*, **125**, 624–629.

Jasper, M.S., McDermott, P., Gann, D.S. and Engeland, W.C. (1990). Measurement of blood flow to the adrenal capsule, cortex and medulla in dogs after haemorrhage by fluorescent microspheres. *Journal of the Autonomic Nervous System*, **30**, 159–167.

Jazdowska, B. and Dobrowolski, W. (1965). Vascularization of the hypophysis in sheep. *Endokrynologia Polska*, **16**, 269–282.

Jordan, D.A., Breslow, M.J., Kubos, K.L. and Traystman, R.J. (1989). Adrenergic receptors of adrenal medullary vasculature. *American Journal of Physiology*, **256**, H233–H239.

Kadekaro, M., Gross, P.M. and Sokoloff, L. (1986). Local cerebral glucose utilization in Long-Evans and Brattleboro rats during acute dehydration. *Neuroendocrinology*, **42**, 203–210.

Kapitola, J., Dlouha, H., Krecek, J. and Zicha, J. (1977). The effect of dehydration on the neurohypophysial blood flow in rats with hereditary diabetes insipidus. *Experientia*, **33**, 1615–1616.

Kayaalp, S.O. and McIsaac, R.J. (1969). Muscarinic component of splanchnic-adrenal transmission in the dog. *British Journal of Pharmacology*, **36**, 286–293.

Kemeny, A.A., Jakubowski, J.A., Jefferson, A.A. and Pasztor, E. (1985). Blood flow and autoregulation in rat pituitary gland. *Journal of Neurosurgery*, **63**, 116–119.

Kenigsberg, R.L. and Trifara, J.M. (1980). Presence of a high affinity uptake for catecholamines in cultured bovine adrenal chromaffin cells. *Neuroscience*, **5**, 1547–1556.

Kennedy, J.G., Breslow, M.J., Tobin, J.R. and Traystman, R.J. (1980). Cholinergic regulation of adrenal medullary blood flow. *Neuroscience*, **5**, 1547–1556.

Kesse, W.K., Parker, T.L. and Coupland, R.E. (1988). The innervation of the adrenal gland I. The source of pre- and postganglionic nerve fibres to the rat adrenal gland. *Journal of Anatomy*, **157**, 33–41.

Kikuta, A. and Murakami, T. (1982). Microcirculation of the rat adrenal gland: A scanning electron microscope study of vascular casts. *American Journal of Anatomy*, **164**, 19–28.

Kikuta, A. and Murakami, T. (1984). Relationship between chromaffin cells and blood vessels in the rat adrenal medulla: a transmission electron microscopic study combined with blood vessel reconstructions. *American Journal of Anatomy*, **170**, 73–81.

Kirsch, J.R., Hanley, D.F., Wilson, D.A. and Traystman, R.J. (1988). Effect of centrally administered encephalinamides on regional cerebral blood flow in the dog. *Journal of Cerebral Blood Flow and Metabolism*, **8**, 385–394.

Kleitman, N. and Holzwarth, M.A. (1985). Catecholaminergic innervation of the rat adrenal cortex. *Cell and Tissue Research*, **241**, 139–147.

Kobayashi, H.T., Matsui, T. and Ishii, S. (1970). Functional electron microscopy of the median eminence. *International Review of Cytology*, **29**, 281–381.

Kobayashi, S., Tsukahara, S., Sugita, K. and Nagata, T. (1981). Adrenergic and cholinergic innervation of rat cerebral arteries. Consecutive demonstration on whole mount preparations. *Histochemistry*, **70**, 129–138.

Koelle, G.B. and Geesey, C.N. (1961). Localization of acetylcholinesterase in the neurohypophysis and its functional implications. *Proceedings of the Society for Experimental Biology in Medicine*, **106**, 625–628.

Kondo, H., Kuramoto, H. and Fujita, T. (1986). An immuno-electron-microscopic study of the localization of VIP-like immunoreactivity in the adrenal gland of the rat. *Cell and Tissue Research*, **245**, 531–538.

Konstantinova, M. (1967). The effect of adrenaline and acetylcholine on the hypothalamic-hypophysial neurosecretion in the rat. *Zeitschrift für Zellforschung und mikroskopische Anatomie*, **83**, 549–567.

Kontos, H.A., Raper, A.J. and Patterson, J.L. (1977). Analysis of vasoactivity of local pH, pCO_2 and bicarbonate on pial vessels. *Stroke*, **8**, 358–360.

Kopaniky, D.R. and Gann, D.S. (1975). Anterior pituitary vasodilation after haemorrhage in the dog. *Endocrinology*, **97**, 630–635.

Kovach, A.G.B. and Koltay, E. (1965). Adrenal blood flow and corticosteroid secretion: II. The effect of oxytocin on adrenal blood flow and corticoid secretion before and after acute hypophysectomy in the dog. *Acta Physiologica Hungarica*, **28**, 155–161.

Kovach, A.G.B., Monos, E., Koltay, E. and Desrius, A. (1970). Effect of hypothalamic stimulation on adrenal blood flow and glycocorticoid release prior to and after acute hypophysectomy. *Acta Physiologica Academiae Scientiarum Hungaricae*, **38**, 205–216.

Kramer, R.J. and Sapirstein, L.A. (1967). Blood flow to the adrenal cortex and medulla. *Endocrinology*, **81**, 403–405.

Krass, M.E. and LaBella, F.S. (1965). Oxidation of 14-C–1 and 14-C–6-glucose by hormone synthesizing and hormone secreting portions of neurohypophysial neurons. *Molecular Pharmacology*, **1**, 306–311.

Krass, M.E. and LaBella, F.S. (1967). Hexosemonophosphate shunt in endocrine tissues. Quantitative estimation of the pathway in bovine pineal body, anterior pituitary, posterior pituitary and brain. *Biochimica et Biophysica Acta*, **148**, 384–391.

Kuramoto, H., Kondo, H. and Fujita, T. (1986). Neuropeptide tyrosine (NPY)-like immunoreactivity in adrenal chromaffin cells and intraadrenal nerve fibers of rats. *Anatomical Record*, **214**, 321–328.

Kuramoto, H., Kondo, H. and Fujita, T. (1987). Calcitonin gene-related peptide (CGRP)-like immunoreactivity in scattered chromaffin cells and nerve fibers in the adrenal gland of rats. *Cell and Tissue Research*, **247**, 309–315.

Kuyatt, B.L. and DeSouza, E.B. (1986). A1-Adrenergic receptors in the neural lobe of the rat pituitary: Autoradiographic identification and localization. *Society for Neuroscience Abstracts*, **12**, 449.

L'Age, M., Gonzalez-Luque, A. and Yates, F.E. (1970). Adrenal blood flow dependence of cortisol secretion rate in unanaesthetized dogs. *American Journal of Physiology*, **219**, 281–287.

Landsmeer, J.M.F. (1951). Vessels of the rat hypophysis. *Acta Anatomica*, **12**, 89–109.

Lederis, K. and Livingston, A. (1969). Acetylcholine and related enzymes in the neural lobe and anterior hypothalamus of the rabbit. *Journal of Physiology*, **201**, 695–709.

Lederis, K. and Livingston, A. (1970). Neuronal and subcellular localization of acetylcholine in the posterior pituitary of the rabbit. *Journal of Physiology*, **210**, 187–204.

Leng, G. and Shibuki, K. (1987). Extracellular potassium changes in the rat neurohypophysis during activation of the magnocellular neurosecretory system. *Journal of Physiology*, **392**, 97–111.

Li, Y.W., Gieroba, Z.J. and Blessing, W.W. (1992). Chemoreceptor and baroreceptor responses of A1 area neurons projecting to supraoptic nucleus. *American Journal of Physiology*, **263**, R310–R317.

Lichardus, B., Albrecht, I., Ponec, J. and Linhart, L. (1977). Water deprivation for 24 hours increases selectively blood flow in posterior pituitary of conscious rats. *Endocrinologia Experimentalis*, **11**, 99–104.

Liddle, G.W. (1981). *Textbook of Endocrinology*. Philadelphia: W.B. Saunders Company.

Lightman, S.L., Ninkovic, M. and Hunt, S.P. (1983). Neurohypophysial opiate receptors: are they on pituicytes? *Progress in Brain Research*, **60**, 353–356.

Ligier, B., Breslow, M.J., Clarkson, K., Raff, H. and Traystman, R.J. (1993). Adrenal blood flow and secretory effects of adrenergic receptor stimulation. *American Journal of Physiology*, (in press).

Linnoila, R.I. and Diaugustine, R.P. (1980). Distribution of [Met^5]- and [Leu^5]- enkephalin-, vasoactive intestinal polypeptide- and subtance P-like immunoreactivities in human adrenal glands. *Neuroscience*, **5**, 2247–2259.

Luscher, T.F. and Vanhoutte, P.M. (1990). *The endothelium: Modulator of cardiovascular function*. New York: CRC Press.

Malkoff, M., Hanley, D.F., Wilson, D.A. and Traystman, R.J. (1990). Osmotic stimulation increases neurohypophysial blood flow and arginine vasopressin release concurrently. *FASEB Journal*, **4**, A692.

Mansour, A., Khachaturian, H., Lewis, M.E., Akil, H. and Watson, S.J. (1988). Anatomy of CNS opioid receptors. *Trends in Neurosciences*, **11**, 308–314.

Marley, E. and Paton, W.D.M. (1961). The output of sympathetic amines from the cat's adrenal gland in response to splanchnic nerve activity. *Journal of Physiology*, **155**, 1–27.

Marley, E. and Prout, G.I. (1968). Innervation of the cat's adrenal medulla. *Journal of Anatomy*, **102**, 257–273.

Martin, R. and Voigt, K.H. (1981). Enkephalins co-exist with oxytocin and vasopressin in nerve terminals of rat neurohypophysis. *Nature*, **289**, 502–504.

McConnell, E.M. (1953). The arterial supply of the human hypophysis cerebri. *Anatomical Record*, **115**, 175.

McPherson, R. (1993). Personal Communication.

Mezey, E., Palkovits, M., De Kloet, E.R., Verhoef, J. and De Wied, D. (1978). Evidence for pituitary-brain transport of a behaviorally potent ACTH analog. *Life Sciences*, **22**, 831–838.

Miller, D.L., Doppman, J.L., Nieman, L.K., Cutler, G.B., Jr., Chrousos, G., Loriaux, D.L., *et al.* (1990). Petrosal sinus sampling: discordant lateralization of ACTH-secreting pituitary microadenomas before and after stimulation with corticotropin-releasing hormone. *Radiology*, **176**, 429–431.

Mohamed, A.A., Parker, T.L. and Coupland, R.E. (1988). The innervation of the adrenal gland. II. The source of spinal afferent nerve fibres to the guinea-pig adrenal gland. *Journal of Anatomy*, **160**, 51–58.

Moncada, S. and Higgs, E.A. (1991). Endogenous nitric oxide physiology, pathology and clinical relevance. *European Journal of Clinical Investigation*, **21**, 361–374.

Moncada, S., Palmer, R.M.J. and Higgs, E.A. (1991). Nitric oxide: physiology, pathophysiology and pharmacology. *Pharmacological Reviews*, **43**, 109–142.

Monos, E., Biro, A., Sulyok, A. and Kovach, A.G.B. (1969a). Effect of local venous congestion on adrenocortical function III: Adrenal cortical and medullary blood flow. *Acta Physiologica Academiae Scientiarum Hungaricae*, **35**, 321–330.

Monos, E., Biro, Z., Sulyok, A. and Kovach, A.G.B. (1969b). The acute effect of hypophysectomy on tissue blood flow and oxygen consumption of the adrenal cortex and medulla in dogs. *Acta Physiologica Academiae Scientiarum Hungaricae*, **36**, 379–389.

Moro, M.A., Michelena, P., Sanchez-Garcia, P., Palmer, R., Moncada, S. and Garcia, A.G. (1993). Activation of adrenal medullary L-arginine: nitric oxide pathway by stimuli which induce the release of catecholamines. *European Journal of Pharmacology*, **246**, 213–218.

Nakamura, K. and Masuda, T. (1981). Scanning electron microscope of corrosion cast of rat adrenal vasculatures with emphasis on medullary artery under ACTH administration. *Tohoku Journal of Experimental Medicine*, **134**, 203–213.

Nelson, A.A. and Woodard, G. (1949). Severe adrenal cortical atrophy (cytotoxic) and hepatic damage produced in dogs by feeding 2,2-bis(parachlorophenyl)-1,1-dichloroethane (DDD or TDE). *Archives of Pathology*, **48**, 387–394.

Neutze, J., Wyler, F. and Rudolph, A. (1968). Use of radioactive microspheres to assess distribution of cardiac output in rabbits. *American Journal of Physiology*, **215**, 486–495.

Nikitovitch-Winer, M.B. and Goldman, H. (1986). Effect of hypothalamic deafferentation on hypophysial and other endocrine gland blood flows. *Endocrinology*, **118**, 1166–1170.

Nishijima, M.K., Breslow, M.J., Raff, H. and Traystman, R.J. (1989). Regional adrenal blood flow during hypoxia. *American Journal of Physiology*, **256**, H94–H100.

Oliver, C., Mical, R.S. and Porter, J.C. (1977). Hypothalamic-pituitary vasculature: evidence for retrograde blood flow in the pituitary stalk. *Endocrinology*, **101**, 598–604.

Page, R.B. (1982). Pituitary blood flow. *American Journal of Physiology*, **243**, E427–E442.

Page, R.B. (1983). Directional pituitary blood flow: a microcinephotographic study. *Endocrinology*, **112**, 157–165.

Page, R.B. and Bergland, R.M. (1977). The neurohypophysial capillary bed. I. Anatomy and arterial supply. *American Journal of Anatomy*, **148**, 345–357.

Page, R.B., Munger, B.L. and Bergland, R.M. (1976). Scanning microscopy of pituitary vascular casts. *American Journal of Anatomy*, **146**, 273–301.

Page, R.B., Leure duPree, A.E. and Bergland, R.M. (1978). The neurohypophysial capillary bed. II. Specializations within median eminence. *American Journal of Anatomy*, **153**, 33–65.

Page, R.B., Funsch, D.J., Brennan, R.W. and Hernandez, M.J. (1981). Regional neurohypophysial blood flow and its control in adult sheep. *American Journal of Physiology*, **241**, R36–R43.

Page, R.B., Gropper, M., Woodard, E., Townsend, J., Davis, S. and Bryan, R.M. (1990). Role of catecholamines in regulating ovine median eminence blood flow. *American Journal of Physiology*, **258**, R1242–R1249.

Palay, S.L. (1955). An electron microscopy study of the neurohypophysis in normal, hydrated and dehydrated rats. *Anatomical Record*, **121**, 348.

Palkovits, M., Leranth, C., Zaborszky, L. and Brownstein, M.J. (1977). Electron microscopic evidence of direct neuronal connections from the lower brain stem to the median eminence. *Brain Research*, **136**, 339–344.

Palkovits, M., Zaborszky, L., Feminger, A., Mezey, E., Fekete, M.I., Herman, J.P., *et al.* (1980). Noradrenergic innervation of the rat hypothalamus: experimental, biochemical and electron microscopic studies. *Brain Research*, **191**, 161–171.

Parker, T.L., Mohamed, A.A. and Coupland, R.E. (1990). The innervation of the adrenal gland. IV. The source of pre- and postganglionic nerve fibres to the guinea-pig adrenal gland. *Journal of Anatomy*, **172**, 17–24.

Pohorecky, L.A. and Wurtman, R.J. (1971). Adrenocortical control of epinephrine synthesis. *Pharmacological Reviews*, **23**, 1–35.

Porter, J.C. (1975). Methods for studying pituitary-hypothalamic axis *in situ*. *Methods in Enzymology*, **39**, 166–183.

Porter, J.C. and Klaiber, M.S. (1965). Corticosterone secretion in rats as a function of ACTH input and adrenal blood flow. *American Journal of Physiology*, **209**, 811–814.

Porter, J.C., Hines, M.F., Smith, K.R., Repass, R.L. and Smith, A.J. (1967). Quantitative evaluation of local blood flow of the adenohypophysis in rats. *Endocrinology*, **80**, 583–598.

Porter, J.C., Mical, R.S., Kamberi, I.A. and Grazia, Y.R. (1970). A procedure for the cannulation of a pituitary stalk portal vessel and perfusion of the pars distalis in the rat. *Endocrinology*, **87**, 197–201.

Porter, J.C., Ondo, J.G. and Cramer, O.M. (1974). Nervous and vascular supply of the pituitary gland. In *Handbook of Physiology, Endocrinology, Sect IV, Part 1*, edited by E. Knobil and W.H. Sawyer, pp. 33–43. Washington DC: American Physiological Society.

Porter, J.C., Oliver, C., Eskay, R.L., Barnea, A., Park, C.R. and Ben-Jonathan, N. (1977). Hypothalamic-pituitary interaction. In *The Pituitary — A Current Review*, edited by M. Allen and V.B. Mahesh, pp. 215–234. Academic Press.

Porter, J.C., Barnea, A., Cramer, O.M. and Parker, C.R.J. (1978). Hypothalamic peptide and catecholamine secretion: roles for portal and retrograde blood flow in the pituitary stalk in the release of hypothalamic dopamine and pituitary prolactin and LH. *Clinics in Obstetrics and Gynaecology*, **5**, 271–282.

Prentice, F.D. and Wood, J.G. (1974). Adrenergic innervation of cat adrenal medulla. *Anatomical Record*, **181**, 689–704.

Raff, H. and Chadwick, K.J. (1986). Aldosterone responses to ACTH during hypoxia in conscious rats. *Clinical and Experimental Pharmacology and Physiology*, **13**, 827–830.

Raff, H. and Fagin, K.D. (1984). Measurement of hormones and blood gases during hypoxia in conscious cannulated rats. *Journal of Applied Physiology*, **56**, 1426–1430.

Raff, H. and Levy, S.A. (1986). Renin-angiotensin II-aldosterone and ACTH-cortisol control during acute hypoxemia and exercise in patients with chronic obstructive pulmonary disease. *American Review of Respiratory Disease*, **133**, 306–399.

Raff, H., Tzankoff, S.P. and Fitzgerald, R.S. (1981). ACTH and cortisol responses to hypoxia in dogs. *Journal of Applied Physiology*, **51**, 1257–1260.

Raff, H., Sandri, S.B. and Segerson, T.P. (1986). Renin, ACTH and adrenocortical function during hypoxia and haemorrhage in conscious rats. *American Journal of Physiology*, 240–244.

Raff, H., Norton, A.J. and Flemma, R.J. (1987). Inhibition of the adrenocorticotropin response to surgery in humans: interactions between dexamethasone and fentanyl. *Journal of Clinical Endocrinology and Metabolism*, **65**, 295–298.

Raff, H., Ball, D.L. and Goodfriend, T.L. (1988). The effect of hypoxia on aldosterone secretion *in vitro*. *Clinical Research*, **36**, 835.

Redman, C.M. and Hokin, L.E. (1959). Phospholipid turnover in microsomal membranes of the pancreas during enzyme secretion. *Journal of Biophysical and Biochemical Cytology*, **6**, 207–214.

Rokaeus, A., Fried, G. and Lundberg, J.M. (1984). Occurrence, storage and release of neurotensin-like immunoreactivity from the adrenal gland. *Acta Physiologica Scandinavica*, **120**, 373–380.

Role, L.W. and Perlman, R.L. (1983). Both nicotinic and muscarinic receptors mediate catecholamine secretion by isolated guinea-pig chromaffin cells. *Neuroscience*, **10**, 979–985.

Rudolph, A.M. and Heymann, M.A. (1967). The circulation of the fetus *in utero*: methods for studying distribution of blood flow, cardiac output and organ blood flow. *Circulation Research*, **21**, 163–184.

Saiani, L. and Guidotti, A. (1982). Opiate receptor-mediated inhibition of catecholamine release in primary cultures of bovine adrenal chromaffin cells. *Journal of Neurochemistry*, **39**, 1669.

Saito, S., Hanley, D.F., Kidd, G.J., Wilson, D.A., Trapp, B.D. and Traystman, R.J. (1993). Peri-arterial innervation within the neurohypophysis. In *The Neurohypophysis. Window on the Brain. Annals of the New York Academy of Sciences*, **689**, 544–545. New York: New York Academy of Sciences.

Saito, S., Wilson, D.A., Hanley, D.F. and Traystman, R.J. (1994). Nitric oxide synthase does not contribute to cerebral autoregulatory phenomenon in anaesthetized dogs. *Journal of the Autonomic Nervous System*, **49**, 573–576.

Sakima, N.T., Breslow, M.J., Raff, H. and Traystman, R.J. (1991). Lack of coupling between adrenal cortical metabolic activity and blood flow in dogs. *American Journal of Physiology*, **261**, H21–H26.

Samson, W.K., Said, S.I. and McCann, S.M. (1979). Radioimmunologic localization of vasoactive intestinal polypeptide in hypothalamic and extrahypothalamic sites in the rat brain. *Neuroscience Letters*, **12**, 265–269.

Sapirstein, L.A. (1958). Regional blood flow by fractional distribution of indicators. *American Journal of Physiology*, **193**, 161–168.

Schapiro, S. and Stjarne, L. (1958). A method for collection of intermittent samples of adrenal vein blood. *Proceedings of the Society for Experimental Biology and Medicine*, **99**, 414–415.

Schwartz, W.J., Smith, C.B., Davidsen, L., Savaki, H., Sokoloff, L., Mata, M., *et al.* (1979). Metabolic mapping of functional activity in the hypothalamo-neurohypophysial system of the rat. *Science*, **205**, 723–725.

Sercombe, R., Lacombe, P. and Seylaz, J. (1984). Functional significance of the cerebrovascular reactivity to autonomic neurotransmitters. In *Neurotransmitters and the Cerebral Circulation. L.E.R.S. Monograph Series Vol 2*, edited by E.T. MacKenzie, F. Seylaz and A. Bes, pp. 65–89. New York, N.Y.: Raven Press.

Shuttleworth, C.W., Murphy, R. and Furness, J.B. (1991). Evidence that NO participates in nonadrenergic inhibitory transmission to intestinal muscle in the guinea-pig. *Neuroscience Letters*, **130**, 77–80.

Sibley, C.P., Whitehouse, B.J., Vinson, G.P., Goddard, C. and McCredie, E. (1981). Studies on the mechanism of secretion of corticosteroids by the isolated perfused adrenal cortex of the rat. *Journal of Endocrinology*, **91**, 313–323.

Silver, M. (1960). The output of adrenaline and noradrenaline from the adrenal medulla of the calf. *Journal of Physiology*, **152**, 14–29.

Sklar, A.H. and Schrier, R.W. (1983). Central nervous system mediators of vasopressin release. *Physiological Reviews*, **63**, 1243–1280.

Snyder, S.H. and Bredt, D.S. (1991). Nitric oxide as a neuronal messenger. *Trends in Pharmacological Sciences*, **12(4)**, 125–128.

Sooriyamoorthy, T. and Livingston, A. (1972). Variations in the blood volume of the neural and anterior lobes of the pituitary of the rat associated with neurohypophysial hormone-releasing stimuli. *Journal of Endocrinology*, **54**, 407–415.

Spina, M.B. and Cohen, G. (1989). Dopamine turnover and glutathione oxidation: Implications for parkinson disease. *Proceedings of the National Academy of Sciences of the United States of America*, **86**, 1398–1400.

Stark, E., Varga, B., Acs, Z. and Papp, M. (1965). Adrenal blood flow response to adrenocorticotrophic hormone and other stimuli in the dog. *Pflügers Archiv*, **285**, 296–301.

Steinmeier, R., Fahlbusch, R., Powers, A.D., Dotterl, A. and Buchfelder, M. (1991). Pituitary microcirculation: Physiological aspects and clinical implications. A Laser-Doppler flow study during transsphenoidal adenomectomy. *Neurosurgery*, **29**, 47–54.

Suzuki, N., Hardebo, J.E. and Owman, C. (1988). Origins and pathways of cerebrovascular vasoactive intestinal polypeptide-positive nerves in rat. *Journal of Cerebral Blood Flow and Metabolism*, **8**, 697–712.

Swinyard, C.A. (1937). The innervation of the suprarenal glands. *Anatomical Record*, **68**, 417–426.

Szentagothai, J., Flerko, B., Mess, B. and Halasz, B. (1962). Anatomical considerations, hypophysial circulation. In *Hypothalamic Control of the Anterior Pituitary*, 3rd Ed., pp. 81–92. Budapest: Akademiai Kiado.

Tobin, J.R., Breslow, M.J. and Traystman, R.J. (1992). Muscarinic cholinergic receptors in canine adrenal gland. *American Journal of Physiology*, **263**, H1208–H1212.

Tomlinson, A. and Coupland, R.E. (1990). The innervation of the adrenal gland. IV. Innervation of the rat adrenal medulla from birth to old age. A descriptive and quantitative morphometric and biochemical study of the innervation of chromaffin cells and adrenal medullary neurons in Wistar rats. *Journal of Anatomy*, **169**, 209–236.

Torok, B. (1962). Neue Angaben zum Blutkreislauf der Hypophse. *Anatomischer Anzeiger*, **109**, 622–629.

Traystman, R.J., Fitzgerald, R.S. and Loscutoff, S.C. (1978). Cerebral circulatory responses to arterial hypoxia in normal and chemodenervated dogs. *Circulation Research*, **42**, 649–657.

Tweedle, C.D. and Hatton, G.I. (1980). Evidence for dynamic interactions between pituicytes and neurosecretory axons in the rat. *Neuroscience*, **5**, 661–671.

Urquhart, J. (1965). Adrenal blood flow and the adrenocortical response to corticotropin. *American Journal of Physiology*, **209**, 1162–1168.

Van Leeuwen, F.W. and De Vries, G.J. (1983). Enkephalin-glial interaction and its consequence for vasopressin and oxytocin release from the rat neural lobe. *Progress in Brain Research*, **60**, 343–351.

Vannucci, S. and Hawkins, R. (1983). Substrates of energy metabolism of the pituitary and pineal glands. *Journal of Neurochemistry*, **41**, 1718–1725.

Vella, L.M., Hanley, D.F., Wilson, D.A. and Traystman, R.J. (1989). Peripheral baroreceptor control of neurohypophyseal blood flow during haemorrhage. *American Journal of Physiology*, **257**, H1498–H1506.

Vernikos-Danellis, J. (1963). Effect of acute stress on the pituitary gland: changes in blood and pituitary ACTH concentrations. *Endocrinology*, **72**, 574–581.

Vina, J.R., Page, R.B., Davis, D.W. and Hawkins, R.A. (1984). Aerobic glycolysis by the pituitary gland *in vivo*. *Journal of Neurochemistry*, **42**, 1479–1482.

Voet, D. and Voet, J.G. (1990). *Biochemistry*. New York: John Wiley & Sons.

Wakade, A.R. and Wakade, T.D. (1983). Contribution of nicotinic and muscarinic receptors in the secretion of catecholamines evoked by endogenous and exogenous acetylcholine. *Neuroscience*, **10**, 973–978.

Walker, W.F., Shoemaker, W.C., Kaalstad, J. and Moore, F.D. (1959). Influence of blood volume restoration and tissue trauma on corticosteroid secretion in dogs. *American Journal of Physiology*, **197**, 781–785.

Watson, S.J., Akil, H., Fischli, W., Goldstein, A., Zimmerman, E., Nilaver, G., *et al.* (1982). Dynorphin and vasopressin: common localization in magnocellular neurons. *Science*, **216**, 85–87.

Williams, J.L., Page, R.B., Shue, S.G., Jones, S.C. and Bryan, R.M., Jr. (1991). Blood flow to circumventricular organs during infusion of catecholamines. *Physiologist*, **34**, 254. (Abstract).

Wilson, D.A., O'Neill, J.T., Said, S.I. and Traystman, R.J. (1981). Vasoactive intestinal polypeptide and the canine cerebral circulation. *Circulation Research*, **48**, 138–148.

Wilson, D.A., Busija, D., Foster, G. and Traystman, R.J. (1982). Sympathetic vasoconstriction in canine posterior pituitary blood vessels. *Federation Proceedings*, **41**, 7831. (Abstract).

Wilson, D.A., Hanley, D.F., Rogers, M.C. and Traystman, R.J. (1983). Adrenergic vasoconstriction of neurohypophysial blood vessels. *Journal of Cerebral Blood Flow and Metabolism*, **3**(Suppl 1), S166–S167.

Wilson, D.A., Traystman, R.J. and Rapela, C.E. (1985). Transient analysis of the canine cerebrovascular response to carbon dioxide. *Circulation Research*, **56**, 596–605.

Wilson, D.A., Hanley, D.F. and Traystman, R.J. (1992). Nitric oxide synthase contributes to low pituitary blood vessel tone, but does not account for hypoxic vasodilation. *FASEB Journal*, **6**, A1461. (Abstract).

Wilson, D.A., Hanley, D.F. and Traystman, R.J. (1993). Neurally derived nitric oxide sets basal neurohypophysial blood vessel tone. *Journal of Cerebral Blood Flow and Metabolism*, **13**(Suppl 1), S133. (Abstract).

Winkler, H. (1976). The composition of adrenal chromaffin granules: an assessment of controversial results. *Neuroscience*, **1**, 65–80.

Wislocki, G.B. and King, L.S. (1936). The permeability of the hypophysis and hypothalamus to vital dyes, with a study of the hypophysial vascular supply. *American Journal of Anatomy*, **58**, 421–472.

Worthington, W.C. (1955). Some observations on the hypophysial portal system in the living mouse. *Bulletin of the Johns Hopkins Hospital*, **97**, 343–357.

Worthington, W.C. (1960). Vascular responses in the pituitary stalk. *Endocrinology*, **66**, 19–31.

Worthington, W.C. (1963). Functional vascular fields in the pituitary stalk of the mouse. *Nature*, **199**, 461–465.

Wright, R.D. (1963). Blood flow through the adrenal gland. *Endocrinology*, **72**, 418–428.

Wurtman, R.J. and Axelrod, J. (1966). Control of enzymatic synthesis of adrenaline in the adrenal medulla by adrenal cortical steroids. *Journal of Biological Chemistry*, **241**, 2301–2305.

Xuereb, G.P., Prichard, M.M.L. and Daniel, P.M. (1954). The arterial supply and venous drainage of the human hypophysis cerebri. *Quarterly Journal of Experimental Physiology*, **39**, 199–230.

Yates, F.E., Kirschman, R. and Olshen, B. (1966). Analysis of adenohypophysial blood flow in the rat by radioisotope washout: estimate of the vasomotor activity of vasopressin in the anterior pituitary. *Endocrinology*, **79**, 341–351.

Yu, J.G., Wu, J.Y. and Lee, T.J.-F. (1986). Cholinergic innervation of cerebral blood vessels. *Society for Neuroscience Abstracts*, **12(1)**, 440. (Abstract).

Zajicek, G., Ariel, I. and Arber, N. (1986). The streaming adrenal cortex: direct evidence of centripetal migration of adrenocytes by estimation of cell turnover rate. *Journal of Endocrinology*, **111**, 477–482.

Ziedonis, D.M., Severs, W.B., Brennan, R.W. and Page, R.B. (1986). Blood flow and functional responses correlate in the ovine neural lobe. *Brain Research*, **373**, 27–34.

Zimmerman, E.A., Carmel, P.W., Husain, M.K., Ferin, M., Tannenbaum, M., Frantz, A.G., *et al.* (1973). Vasopressin and neurophysin: high concentrations in monkey hypophysial portal blood. *Science*, **182**, 925–927.

Zuberbuhler, R.C. and Bohr, D.F. (1965). Responses of coronary smooth muscle to catecholamines. *Circulation Research*, **16**, 431–440.

8 Neural Control of the Coronary Circulation

David D. Gutterman and Danna Schnoll

Department of Internal Medicine,
University of Iowa College of Medicine,
Iowa City, IA 52242, USA

Coronary blood flow is regulated by products released from myocardial metabolism, extravascular compressive forces, autoregulatory influences, arterial perfusion pressure, and neurohumoral influences. While the principal influence on the coronary circulation is myocardial metabolism, during pathophysiological states or exercise when vasodilator reserve is reduced, the effects of activating sympathetic nerves on coronary flow is augmented. Recent developments in our understanding of neural control of the coronary circulation include identification of brain pathways responsible for sympathetic coronary vasoconstriction and identifying pathophysiological alterations in coronary flow during ischaemia and reperfusion and in specific disease states such as diabetes mellitus.

KEY WORDS: coronary innervation; neural control; brain; diabetes mellitus; ischaemia; noradrenaline; vasodilatation; sympathetic; parasympathetic; myocardial perfusion.

INTRODUCTION

Coronary blood flow is primarily regulated by metabolic products released from the myocardium, although the exact substance(s) which mediate metabolically-induced changes in coronary tone is not known. Other important factors also contribute to coronary flow regulation. *Extravascular compressive forces* from systolic contraction impede coronary inflow. These effects are particularly prominent during conditions where flow reserve is exhausted (Marcus, 1983). *Arterial perfusion pressure* is directly related to coronary flow, but the change in flow with changes in pressure is minimized over physiological ranges of pressure because of prominent *coronary autoregulation*. *Humoral* and locally released products (e.g., prostaglandins) also regulate coronary flow, either directly or through influences on the coronary endothelium. Humoral factors provide more long-term and steady-state adjustments in coronary perfusion, and coupled with autacoid influences, allow for regional changes in coronary resistance to optimize myocardial perfusion. Finally, the coronary circulation receives substantial sympathetic and parasympathetic *innervation*. The functional utility of the coronary innervation has been debated (Shepherd and

Vanhoutte, 1984; Feigl, 1987; Thomas, Jones and Randall, 1988), but the pathophysiological consequences of sympathetic activation can be monumental, as evidenced by precipitation of myocardial ischaemia, left ventricular dysfunction, and angina pectoris during reflex sympathetic activation of the coronary innervation (Buffington and Feigl, 1981; Heusch and Deussen, 1983; Brown *et al.*, 1984; Deussen, Heusch and Thamer, 1985; Thomas, Jones and Randall, 1988).

This review will focus on neural regulation of coronary blood flow, emphasizing central neural control mechanisms. The peripheral anatomy of the coronary innervation will be addressed, reviewing specific receptor and neurotransmitter mechanisms. Functional consequences of peripheral nerve activation will be described. The central nervous system pathways mediating coronary vasoconstriction will also be described, including a discussion of the functionality of these brain tracts. Reflex and behavioral activation of the coronary innervation will be described as well as clinical correlations of CNS regulation of the coronary circulation and the heart.

PERIPHERAL NEURAL CONTROL OF THE CORONARY CIRCULATION

Anatomy of the coronary innervation

Postganglionic, sympathetic, efferent fibres to the heart course along the adventitia of the great vessels, pierce the pericardium and travel on the epicardium along the adventitia of coronary conduit arteries. Anatomical studies show that a broad portion of the coronary tree receives sympathetic innervation, including conduit vessels, resistance arterioles and veins (Hirsch and Borghard-Erdle, 1961; Boucek, Takshita and Fojaco, 1963; Dahlstrom *et al.*, 1965; McKibben and Getty, 1968; Krokhina, 1969; Denn and Stone, 1976). However, the principal physiological influence of the sympathetic nervous system is on the coronary resistance vessels, with a smaller effect on epicardial conduit arteries (Kelley and Feigl, 1978). This is supported by immunochemical data in humans, suggesting denser concentrations of sympathetic neurotransmitters in smaller compared to larger coronary arteries. The response to noradrenergic activation changes across branch points in the coronary arterial tree, consistent with regional heterogeneity of innervations (Cohen, Shepherd and Vanhoutte, 1984).

Preganglionic parasympathetic fibres to the heart terminate in one of several cardiac ganglia located on the posterior base of the heart behind the atria. The course of the postganglionic efferents is not clear. While some studies suggest that they, too, traverse the pericoronary adventitia, the majority of functional studies indicate that after a very brief epicardial course at the base of the heart, vagal efferents descend into the subendocardial region from which they project epicardially and apically (Figure 8.1).

This differential course of parasympathetic and sympathetic fibres has important functional consequences during myocardial ischaemia (Martins and Zipes, 1980; Martins *et al.*, 1987; Yonekura, Watanabe and Downey, 1988). Since cardiac structural damage due to ischaemia progresses in a "wave-front" fashion from endocardium to epicardium (Reimer *et al.*, 1977), subendocardial infarctions may produce heterogeneous autonomic innervation of the overlying viable epicardial layer. In this overlying region, sympathetic

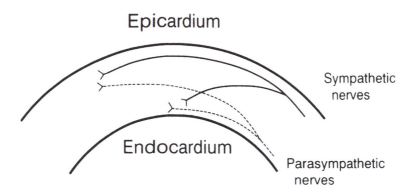

Figure 8.1   Cartoon of the distribution of sympathetic and parasympathetic nerve fibres innervating the transmural myocardium. After traversing the atrioventricular (AV) groove sympathetic efferent fibres course along the epicardial surface with the coronary arteries and descend from there into the inner layers of the myocardium. Vagal efferents, on the other hand, after crossing the atrioventricular (AV) groove on the surface of the heart, dive into the subendocardial region from which they then course along the endocardial surface and project transmurally toward the epicardial surface.

innervation will be intact because of the epicardial course of sympathetic efferents. However, the vagal innervation to this region will be interrupted because the projecting fibres course through the infarcted subendocardial region before projecting epicardially (Martins *et al.*, 1987; Yonekura, Watanabe and Downey, 1988). This observation, first made by Martins and Zipes (1980), may have important implications regarding the genesis of cardiac arrhythmias following myocardial infarction.

A major, unanswered question regarding cardiac innervation is whether efferent fibres selectively innervate one tissue (vascular smooth muscle, cardiac myocyte, SA nodal tissue, conduction system), or whether a single postganglionic neurone innervates multiple tissues through axon branching (Figure 8.2). Functional data have not conclusively resolved this question, and definitive anatomical studies have not been attempted. This question has important bearing on the coronary innervation. The autonomic nervous system has tremendous capacity for heterogeneous, organ-specific responses to accommodate a wide variety of physiological needs. It seems logical that differential control of coronary vasomotion and heart rate, for example, would be useful in certain physiological circumstances. However, this would be difficult to achieve with the cardiac innervation suggested by the ganglion on the right in Figure 8.2, where activation of the preganglionic neuron would stimulate myocardial, coronary and sinoatrial nodal tissue simultaneously. In this situation central activation would produce simultaneous increases in heart rate, contractility, and coronary sympathetic tone. There would be no capacity for tissue specific responses (e.g., increase in heart rate without a direct effect on coronary tone, left side of Figure 8.2) since the innervation does not allow activation of fibres which project selectively to the sinoatrial node. Short of invoking a much more complex innervation, neural control of the heart would become functionally redundant with humoral regulatory mechanisms which produce nonselective activation of tissues.

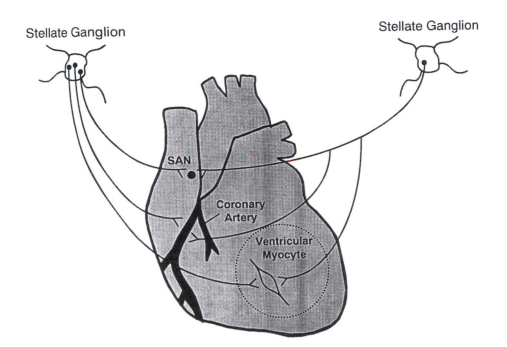

Figure 8.2   Two possible mechanisms by which postganglionic sympathetic fibres innervate the heart. On the left, each cardiac neuron within the stellate ganglion projects to a distinct end organ on the heart (sinoatrial node [SAN] for heart rate control), coronary artery for vasoconstriction, or ventricular myocyte for increases in contractility. This model allows for selective central modulation of specific cardiac structures. In contrast, on the right, activation of neurons in the stellate ganglia produce simultaneous increases in heart rate, coronary vasomotor tone and contractility. In this situation central mechanisms would not be effective in producing selective effects on one or more cardiac elements.

Neurotransmitters and receptors

In addition to classical noradrenergic sympathetic and cholinergic parasympathetic innervation, the coronary circulation is influenced by a variety of neurotransmitters (Figure 8.3). The presence and functional importance of these transmitters varies widely among species. Much of this variation relates to differences in endothelial function and/or the presence of receptors on vascular smooth muscle. For example, in dogs, cats, rats and baboons, cholinergic activation produces coronary vasodilatation (Furchgott, Zawadzki and Cherry, 1981; Cox, Hintze and Vatner, 1983; Van Winkle and Feigl, 1989), while in pigs, cows, and rats, and some primates, only vasoconstriction is demonstrated (Ito, Kitamura and Kuriyama, 1979; Sakai, 1980; Taira *et al.*, 1983; Knight *et al.*, 1987; Matsumoto, Kinoshita and Toda, 1993). In humans, dilatation and constriction are seen (Ginsburg, Bristow and Davis, 1984; Horio *et al.*, 1986; Hodgson and Marshall, 1989; Toda and Okamura, 1989; Yasue *et al.*, 1990).

Sympathetic	Parasympathetic	Other
Noradrenaline	Acetylcholine	Calcitonin/Gene-
Adrenaline	Vasoactive Intestinal	Related Peptide
Neuropeptide Y	Polypeptide	Substance P
Serotonin		
Adenosine		
NO		

Figure 8.3   List of substances for which there is direct or presumptive evidence for a role as neurotransmitters in the coronary circulation.

In addition to species variability, marked differences exist between large and small coronary arteries in response to autonomic activation. This is, in part, due to differential receptor concentrations and density of innervation, but may also relate to different properties of the endothelium in large and small coronary vessels.

Epicardial coronary vessels in dog contain α_1-, α_2-, β_1- and β_2-adrenoceptors. The anatomical and physiological characteristics of these receptors have been reviewed previously (Ross, 1976; Feigl, 1983). As mentioned above, the physiological importance of epicardial coronary innervation is minimal under normal circumstances. However the functional importance becomes evident in pathological states such as coronary atherosclerosis, where even small changes in vascular tone can have a profound effect on stenosis geometry and resistance (Mudge *et al.*, 1976; Brown *et al.*, 1984).

Sympathetic neurotransmitters and receptors in the coronary microcirculation

The majority of studies examining neural control of the coronary circulation have done so indirectly by assessing global or regional parameters of myocardial perfusion or conduit coronary flow. Sympathetic activation can produce a variety of responses depending upon the experimental conditions. The species, presence or absence of anaesthesia, size of vessel being studied, and presence or absence of a stenosis are all factors which contribute to the neurogenic coronary response. In open-chest anaesthetized dogs, stimulation of the stellate ganglia produces α-adrenoceptor-mediated vasoconstriction, which is overwhelmed by a concurrent myocardial metabolic vasodilatation. Following β-adrenoceptor blockade, sympathetic activation results in a transient, but significant, increase in coronary vascular resistance and decrease in coronary flow (Feigl, 1975; Giudicelli *et al.*, 1980). This is due to the attenuated myocardial metabolic stimulus rather than direct blockade of coronary β-adrenoceptors (McRaven *et al.*, 1971; Hamilton and Feigl, 1976). Similarly, during exercise, sympathetic activation produces a modest coronary vasoconstriction which competes with the concurrent metabolic vasodilatation over a wide range of myocardial oxygen consumption (Mohrman and Feigl, 1978). Reflex sympathetic activation in anaesthetized animals, or selective behavioral stimuli in awake animals can produce a sustained neurogenic coronary vasoconstriction (Murray and Vatner, 1981; Billman and Bickerstaff, 1986; Verrier, Hagestad and Lown, 1987). These data, together with the observation by Chilian *et al.* (1981) that, under basal states in the conscious animal, negligible coronary sympathetic tone is present, support a minor role for neural regulation of coronary flow under normal circumstances. However, with reduced vasodilator reserve (e.g., coronary stenosis, exercise), sympathetic coronary vasoconstriction may have profound pathophysiological consequences, even in the absence of β-adrenoceptor blockade (Heusch and Deussen, 1983; Dai *et al.*, 1989).

Both α_1- and α_2- adrenoceptors are present in the coronary microvasculature. In the cat, α_1-adrenoceptors mediate sympathetic coronary constriction (Bonham *et al.*, 1987), while in the dog, coronary constriction is mediated by both α_1- and α_2-adrenoceptors (Heusch *et al.*, 1984; Chen *et al.*, 1988). Although the junctional gap between sympathetic nerve endings and adrenoceptors is relatively large in the canine coronary bed, it appears that functional β (if not α) adrenoceptors are located outside the area of influence of the released neurotransmitter. This is evident from the fact that neurally released noradrenaline produces much less coronary vasodilatation than does infusion of β-adrenoceptor agonists (McRaven *et al.*, 1971; Hamilton and Feigl, 1976). The innervation of α-adrenoceptors is less clear, but differences between sympathetic activation and noradrenaline infusion have been demonstrated in the coronary microcirculation (Chilian *et al.*, 1989).

Sympathetic activation of coronary arterioles is heterogeneous. In a classic study by Chilian *et al.* (1989), stellate stimulation in the presence of β-adrenoceptor blockade produced vasoconstriction in arterioles greater than 100 μm while dilatation was observed in smaller downstream vessels, with no net change in flow. These data support the conclusion that an upstream, adrenoceptor-mediated vasoconstriction is compensated by a downstream autoregulatory vasodilatation.

Interpretation of sympathetic coronary responses is made even more complicated by the presence of additional non-noradrenergic neurotransmitters. Neuropeptide Y (NPY) is co-localized in coronary sympathetic efferent fibres. Exogenous NPY produces prominent coronary vasoconstriction (Hayashi *et al.*, 1986; Maturi *et al.*, 1989). In most organs studied, neuropeptide Y has direct effects through post-junctional receptors, and also potentiates the effects of noradrenaline post-junctionally, and pre-junctionally inhibits release of noradrenaline from sympathetic nerve terminals (Lundberg, Pernow and Lacroix, 1989; Maturi *et al.*, 1989).

The precise role of NPY in regulating coronary flow is not known. Other neurotransmitters may be taken up and subsequently released from sympathetic coronary nerve terminals. For example serotonin is actively transported and subsequently released with noradrenaline from coronary nerve terminals (Cohen, Zitnay and Wiesbrod, 1987). This may be important in disease states such as coronary atherosclerosis, where platelet adhesion and degranulation may induce neuronal uptake of serotonin. Adrenaline is also taken up from the circulation and released with noradrenaline during sympathetic coronary activation (Peronnet *et al.*, 1988). Finally, evidence suggests that nitric oxide, a vasodilator metabolite of arginine is produced in, and released from, sympathetic nerve terminals (Shaffer *et al.*, 1993).

Parasympathetic receptors and neurotransmitters in the coronary circulation

Vagal nerve stimulation produces a frank coronary vasodilatation in most species (Tiedt and Religa, 1979; Reid *et al.*, 1985; Broten *et al.*, 1992). Recent evidence indicates that this dilatation is due to muscarinic activation of the coronary arteriolar endothelium, with subsequent release of nitric oxide (Broten *et al.*, 1992). Although parasympathetic activation releases acetylcholine on the adventitial side of the vessel, the neurotransmitter is able to penetrate the thin walled arteriole to stimulate release of nitric oxide from the endothelium. This mechanism may be less effective in large epicardial vessels where a greater barrier to neurotransmitter diffusion is present. In addition to acetylcholine, calcitonin gene-related peptide (CGRP) is contained within parasympathetic nerve terminals in the coronary vasculature. This peptide produces a direct coronary vasodilatation and may modulate the effects of acetylcholine.

REFLEX CONTROL OF CORONARY VASOMOTION

The coronary circulation is influenced prominently by several cardiovascular reflexes. Carotid sinus hypotension produces a sympathetic mediated coronary vasoconstriction, while activation of the carotid body chemoreceptors produces a more complex response involving the coronary circulation. Activation of cardiopulmonary afferents can reflexly increase coronary flow, while reflex stimuli such as cerebral ischaemia, which produces a potent sympathoexcitation, has little direct effect on coronary flow (De Boel and Gutterman, 1993). Finally, nociceptive stimuli and stimulation of visceral afferents, including those from the heart, can produce increases in sympathetic tone to the coronary circulation. Each of these will be discussed separately.

Baroreflex control of the coronary circulation

A rise in carotid sinus pressure increases activity in the carotid sinus nerve, stimulating neurons with the nucleus of the tractus solitarius (NTS). NTS projections inhibit sympathetic outflow from the medulla. Concurrent with the sympathetic inhibition, baroreflex activation increases efferent parasympathetic outflow from medullary centers.

The effect of carotid sinus nerve activation on the coronary circulation of the dog has been studied. Vatner and colleagues, (1970), directly stimulated the carotid sinus nerve during sleep and during treadmill exercise in conscious dogs. In animals treated with propranolol and atropine, a decrease in arterial pressure and coronary dilatation was observed. This was abolished after α-adrenoceptor blockade, suggesting that withdrawal of sympathetic tone was primarily responsible for the coronary dilatation. A more recent study by Ito and Feigl, (1985), was performed in anaesthetized dogs, carefully controlling changes in blood pressure and heart rate, while closely monitoring coronary sinus blood oxygen tension. In this study, step increases in carotid sinus pressure from 70–150 mmHg resulted in an increase in coronary sinus oxygen tension and coronary blood flow in the presence of β-adrenoceptor blockade. This increase in coronary flow was mostly abolished by atropine, but a small residual vasodilatation was further inhibited with phenoxybenzamine. Unlike the studies in conscious dogs, under conditions of anaesthesia, carotid sinus activation produces a reflex parasympathetic coronary dilatation, with a small dilator component due to withdrawal of α-adrenoceptor-mediated tone.

Reductions in coronary sinus pressure (e.g., following bilateral carotid occlusion) increase heart rate, mean arterial pressure, and coronary flow (DiSalvo et al., 1971). These effects are accompanied by a decrease in coronary vascular resistance, which reflects the myocardial metabolic stimulation during sympathetic activation. Following β-adrenoceptor blockade, brief carotid artery occlusion produces a similar pressor response, but with an increase in coronary vascular resistance which is abolished by sympathectomy (Feigl, 1968). A reflex increase in coronary vascular resistance is also seen in the right coronary circulation of dog and pig in the *absence of propranolol*, since the lower metabolic stimulus during sympathetic activation of the right heart is unable to overcome the reflex coronary vasoconstriction (Ely et al., 1981).

In an elegant study by Murray and Vatner (1981), the effects of bilateral carotid occlusion on the right coronary circulation in conscious dogs was studied. Bilateral carotid occlusion increased coronary vascular resistance in these animals (Figure 8.4). β-adrenoceptor blockade did not further increase the coronary constrictor response, however, the addition of α-adrenoceptor blockade attenuated the increase in right coronary artery resistance. Two additional groups of dogs with right ventricular hypertrophy and with failing right ventricles were studied. In both groups a diminished coronary constriction to bilateral carotid occlusion was observed (Murray and Vatner, 1981).

The effects of the carotid sinus reflex on coronary flow has been examined in humans. Volpe et al. (1985), studied the effect of a reduction in carotid sinus pressure (neck chamber) in 30 patients. Reducing carotid sinus transmural pressure significantly increased mean arterial pressure, cardiac output, heart rate and coronary vascular resistance. In hypertensive patients, coronary vasoconstriction was not seen. Interestingly, this study was performed in patients without coronary artery disease taking no β-adrenoceptor antagonists.

In summary, coronary vasoconstriction is an important component of the cardiovascular response to bilateral carotid occlusion in humans as well as animals. The coronary vasoconstriction is mediated by reflex sympathetic activation. In diseased hearts (e.g., hypertrophy), the magnitude of the reflex coronary response is diminished. Baroreflex coronary constriction is generally overwhelmed by concurrent metabolic dilation but may produce a sustained net constriction in the presence of propranolol which attenuates the cardiac metabolic response.

Chemoreflex effects on the coronary circulation

The coronary vascular response to chemoreflex activation is complex. In a study by Hackett et al. (1972), carotid and aortic injections of nicotine were given to anaesthetized dogs treated with practolol. This stimulus produced decreases in coronary perfusion pressure (constant flow), which were abolished by bilateral vagotomy or atropine, suggesting that chemoreceptor activation produces a vagal cholinergic coronary vasodilatation. Vatner and McRitchie (1975), further examined this phenomenon in conscious dogs.

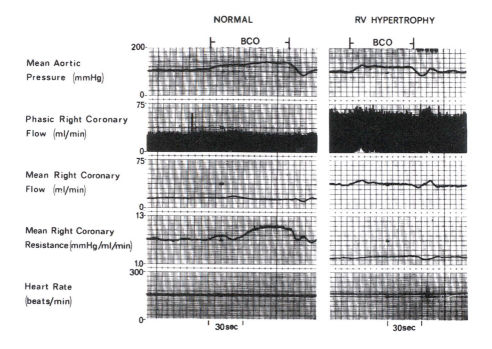

Figure 8.4   Haemodynamic and coronary vascular response to baroreceptor hypotension in conscious dogs (Murray and Vatner, 1981). Carotid sinus hypotension produces increases in mean aortic pressure and sustained and modest increase in resistance was observed. BCO – bilateral carotid occlusion; RV – right ventricular. (Reproduced from *Circulation Research* (1981) **49** p. 1342, Figure 8.1 with permission from authors and The American Heart Association.)

After blockade of β-adrenoceptors and cholinoceptors, coronary dilatation to nicotine occurred *only* when ventilation was not controlled and the respiratory rate increased. When the ventilation rate was controlled, intracarotid nicotine increased coronary resistance in the presence of β-adrenoceptor and cholinoceptor blockade. This constriction was abolished by α-adrenoceptor blockade indicating that an α-adrenoceptor constrictor component to the carotid chemoreflex is present. The mechanism of this constriction was further examined by Murray, Lavallee and Vatner, (1984), who observed an α-adrenoceptor-mediated reduction in coronary flow in conscious dogs during an intracarotid injection of nicotine (Figure 8.5). This vasoconstriction was only seen when heart rate and respiratory rate were held constant; it was observed in the presence or absence of β-adrenoceptor blockade or after combined β-adrenoceptor and cholinoceptor blockade. After the addition of α-noradrenergic blockade, the right coronary resistance no longer increased in response to intracarotid nicotine. The mechanism of the α-adrenoceptor-mediated vasoconstriction involved both activation of

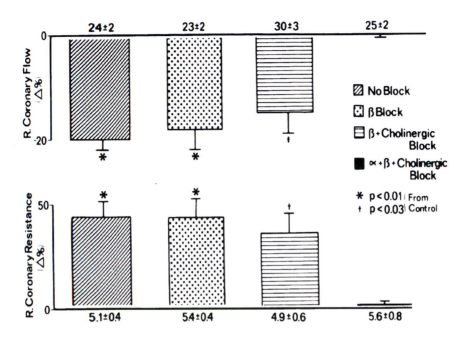

Figure 8.5   Mechanism of chemoreflex-induced changes in right coronary vascular resistance (Murray, Lavallee and Vatner, 1984). Intracarotid nicotine in conscious dogs produced a late increase in right coronary vascular resistance (first bar). Following β-adrenoceptor blockade (second bar) no change in the magnitude of the constriction was observed. Similarly, the addition of cholinoceptor blockade (third bar) had no significant effect on the constriction, however, adding α-adrenoceptor blockade (fourth bar) abolished the increase in coronary resistance demonstrating an α-adrenoceptor–mediated mechanism. (Reproduced from *Circulation Research* (1984) **54** p. 101, Figure 8.3 with permission from The American Heart Association.)

cardiac sympathetic nerves and release of circulating catecholamines (Murray, Lavallee and Vatner, 1984). However, this dual mechanism was not confirmed by Nagata, Pichet and Lavallee, 1988, who showed that, in conscious dogs, cardiac nerves did not contribute significantly to chemoreceptor-induced coronary dilatation.

Thus, the carotid chemoreflex effects on the coronary vasculature are complex. Activation produces a reflex increase in vagal tone to the coronary arteries, reflex sympathetic activation of myocardium and coronary sympathetic fibres, reflex increases in circulating catecholamines, activation of pulmonary stretch receptors, and reflex α-adrenoceptor-mediated coronary vasoconstriction. The composite effect is a decrease in coronary vascular resistance; however, when myocardial metabolic pulmonary inflation and parasympathetic influences are removed, an α-adrenoceptor-mediated coronary vasoconstriction is seen.

Pulmonary inflation reflex

As discussed above (Vatner and McRitchie, 1975), activation of the pulmonary inflation reflex produces a vagally-mediated coronary vasodilatation. Stimulation of pulmonary

C fibres with capsaicin also decreases coronary arteriolar resistance due to combined parasympathetic activation and withdrawal of α-adrenoceptor-mediated tone (Ordway and Pitetti, 1986). Trimarco et al., 1988, demonstrated that cardiopulmonary receptors in humans regulate coronary vascular resistance. Unloading of cardiopulmonary baroreceptors produced an increase in coronary vascular resistance, together with an increase in myocardial oxygen consumption. This response was significantly blunted in hypertensive patients and not altered by treatment with propranolol. Wilson et al., 1984, also showed that the pulmonary inflation reflex produces coronary vasodilatation in humans.

Nociceptive stimuli

The cold-pressor test, initiated by immersing the hand in an ice solution for at least 30 seconds, produces a noxious stimulus associated with a reflex increase in sympathetic tone. In patients without coronary atherosclerosis, the cold-pressor test elicits a reflex tachycardia, pressor response but no significant change in coronary vascular resistance (Feldman et al., 1981; Feldman et al., 1982; Rodger et al., 1984). However, in patients with significant coronary obstructions, regional coronary vascular resistance in the post-stenotic region increases in response to the cold-pressor test (Feldman et al., 1981; Feldman et al., 1982; Rodger et al., 1984). Mudge and colleagues (1976), provided evidence that the cold-pressor test produces reductions in coronary flow in humans, often associated with angina pectoris.

Other nociceptive stimuli have been examined in animal models. For example, in cats, distension of the small intestines produces a coronary vasoconstriction presumably through reflex sympathetic activation (Moore and Parratt, 1977). Similarly, Gilbert, Fenn and LeRoy, 1940, saw reductions in coronary artery flow in response to distension of the stomach in dogs. Thus, mechanical stimulation of remote visceral organs can produce prominent reflex cardiovascular effects including coronary vasoconstriction.

Cardio-coronary reflex

The idea that coronary artery occlusion could reflexly activate sympathetic nerves to produce further constriction in the same or adjacent bed was proposed over 50 years ago (Manning, McEachern and Hall, 1939). Although these original studies were performed using electrocardiographic evidence for changes in coronary flow, confirmation was obtained some twenty-six years later in a study by Joyce and Gregg (1967), where occlusion of the left anterior descending artery of a dog produced reflex changes in the circumflex coronary bed. More recently, Felder and Thames (1981), demonstrated that coronary artery occlusion reflexly increased efferent cardiac sympathetic nerve activity which was inhibited by, but not dependent upon, supraspinal neural elements. Brown and Malliani (1971), demonstrated increased sympathetic nerve activity in the white ramus (efferent fibres) and inferior cardiac nerve in response to several cardiac stimuli (myocardial ischaemia, coronary sinus occlusion). This cardiocardiac excitatory reflex, originally described by Malliani, Schwartz and Zanchetti, 1969, may serve as a mechanism for myocardial ischaemia-induced reflex coronary vasoconstriction.

This hypothesis was tested by Gorman and Sparks (1982), who showed that a prolonged coronary stenosis produced a latent further reduction in coronary flow, which was reversed by α-adrenoceptor blockade. Heusch, Deussen and Thamer (1985), observed reflex coronary vasoconstriction in response to coronary artery occlusion. Interestingly, reflex effects due to increases in efferent cardiac nerve traffic may be greater in remote rather than ischaemic areas. Neely and Hageman (1990), showed that ischaemia reflexly increases sympathetic activity in nerve fibres which innervate distant regions and actually reduce activity in fibres projecting to the ischaemic area.

Parasympathetic cororary dilatation can also be elicited by stimulating cardiac receptors in dog. Feigl (1975), showed that regional injection of veratridine into the anterior descending coronary artery, but not into the circumflex artery, produced reflex coronary dilatation in both beds. The mechanism of this response was shown to be cholinergic and mediated through the efferent vagal nerves. Thus, cholinergic coronary vasodilatation appears to be part of the Bezold-Jarisch reflex.

Somato-coronary reflexes

Simulated hindquarter exercise (spinal ventral nerve root stimulation) in anaesthetized dogs produces reflex sympathoexcitation; in the presence of β-adrenoceptor blockade a significant increase in coronary vascular resistance is seen in both right and left myocardial circulations (Aung-Din, Mitchell and Longhurst, 1981). The observed reduction in coronary flow is sustained and is reversed by α-adrenoceptor blockade.

Cerebral ischaemia reflex

Cerebral ischaemia induces a very potent, reflex sympathoexcitation (Guyton, 1948; Downing, Mitchell and Wallace, 1963; Levy, Ng and Zieske, 1968). However, unlike other sympathoexcitatory reflexes, bradycardia rather than tachycardia is often observed. This suggests a discrepancy between the reflex sympathetic output to the heart and peripheral vasculature, raising the question of whether cerebral ischaemia activates sympathetic fibres to the coronary circulation (as part of a general vascular sympathetic activation) or whether coronary sympathetic fibres are excluded from activation, since there is little increase in sympathetic tone to other cardiac elements (bradycardia is seen during cerebral ischaemia).

We tested the hypothesis that coronary vasoconstriction is a component of the cerebral ischaemia reflex in a study using anaesthetized cats, producing cerebral ischaemia by occluding the right brachiocephalic and left subclavian arteries for 30 seconds (De Boel and Gutterman, 1993). In this study, cerebral ischaemia reduced cerebral blood flow in all parts of the brain to nearly zero, and induced an increase in arterial pressure and coronary vascular resistance after vagotomy and propranolol (Figure 8.6). After bilateral carotid sinus denervation, the cerebral ischaemia-induced coronary vasoconstriction was attenuated to the same levels seen during mechanical elevations in arterial pressures (Figure 8.6). Thus, a neurogenic reflex coronary vasoconstriction was demonstrated. However, this constriction was the result of baroreceptor unloading, rather than a direct effect of cerebral ischaemia. This study shows that coronary vasoconstriction is not a direct result of cerebral ischaemia but, instead, reflects concurrent *effects on the carotid baroreceptors*.

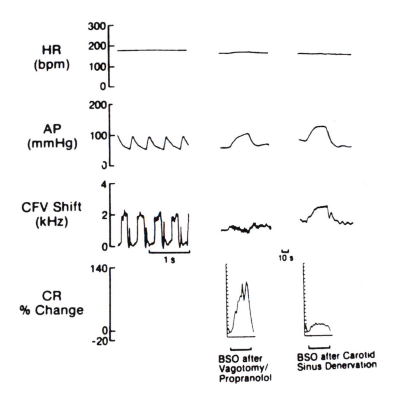

Figure 8.6 Example of the haemodynamic and coronary vascular response to cerebral ischaemia (BSO) in the cat (De Boel and Gutterman, 1993). Phasic tracings are shown in the first panel. In the second panel cerebral ischaemia produced an increase in arterial pressure with modest changes in coronary flow, due to a marked increase in coronary vascular resistance. After bilateral carotid sinus denervation, cerebral ischaemia produced a similar increase in arterial pressure, but this time with a concurrent increase in coronary flow, and no significant increase in coronary vascular resistance, indicating that the coronary constriction during cerebral ischaemia is secondary to concurrent carotid sinus hypotension. HR – heart rate; AP – aortic pressure; CFV shift – coronary flow velocity (kiloHertz shift); CR – coronary vascular resistance. (Reproduced from *Hypertension* (1993) **21** p. 215, Figure 8.2 with permission from the authors and The American Heart Association.)

FUNCTIONAL IMPORTANCE OF NEURAL CONTROL OF THE CORONARY CIRCULATION

It has long been considered curious that the coronary circulation, which regulates a critically vital and highly metabolic active tissue would receive a dense sympathetic vasoconstrictor innervation. Since the sympathetic nervous system does not contribute to resting coronary vasomotor tone, the teleological importance of maintaining a vasoconstrictor mechanism is unclear. Recent studies from several laboratories have shed light on this "paradox".

In the resting state, myocardial perfusion is transmurally homogeneous. However, in situations where vasodilator reserve is reduced (coronary stenosis, exercise, pharmacological vasodilatation) the ratio of flow in the endocardium:epicardium (endo/epi flow ratio) can decrease substantially (Marcus, 1983; Laxson *et al.*, 1989). This transmural heterogeneity in perfusion may have adverse consequences in conditions such as exercise, where the metabolic needs of the relatively underperfused subendocardium are greater than those of the subepicardial tissue.

Recent evidence suggests that neural control of myocardial perfusion optimizes the distribution of flow during such situations. The first evidence for a difference in the transmural effects of sympathetic activation was from Johannsen, Mark and Marcus (1982). These investigators showed that during maximum coronary vasodilatation with adenosine, sympathetic stimulation constricted subepicardial more than subendocardial vessels. This would tend to redistribute flow from the relatively overperfused subepicardial layers. Specificity was demonstrated, since infusion of other vasoconstrictor substances did not redistribute flow in this manner. More recently Baumgart *et al.* (1993) confirmed that sympathetic activation but not humoral activation produces a favorable transmural distribution of myocardial flow. This effect occurred only when vasodilator reserve was depressed.

Observations by Chilian and Ackell (1988) and Huang and Feigl (1988), confirmed greater sympathetic constriction in the subepicardium, using conscious exercising dogs to more closely mimic physiological conditions. Both investigators showed that, in exercising dogs, sympathetic noradrenergic constriction was greater in the subepicardium than in the subendocardium. This would tend to optimize myocardial perfusion during exercise, a condition where subendocardial flow should be maximized. *These observations demonstrate a physiologically important feature of the sympathetic coronary innervation, namely, that during times of stress and increased myocardial demand the sympathetic nervous system fine tunes myocardial perfusion by optimizing transmural flow in the heart.*

Miyashiro and Feigl (1993), have recently put forth another theory to explain the physiological importance of the sympathetic coronary innervation, integrating the effects of simultaneous activation of α- and β-adrenoceptors on the coronary arteries. These investigators demonstrated that intracoronary administration of noradrenaline produced a metabolic coronary vasodilatation by activation of β_1-adrenoceptors on the cardiac myocytes, and by a direct β_1- and β_2-adrenoceptor-mediated coronary vasodilatation. They hypothesize that the direct, or "feed forward" activation of β-adrenoceptors prepares the heart for the increase in metabolic demand associated with simultaneous activation of β_1-adrenoceptors on the myocytes. This was demonstrated by observing excellent match between flow and metabolic demand (little change in coronary venous pO_2) in animals where intracoronary noradrenaline was given following α-adrenoceptor blockade (Miyashiro and Feigl, 1993). In these animals, "feed forward" β-adrenoceptor-mediated mechanisms nicely compensated for the increase in metabolic demand associated with myocardial noradrenoceptor-mediated activation. These authors postulate that microvascular coronary β-adrenoceptors facilitate flow adjustments for changes in myocardial oxygen demand, while simultaneous activation of conduit coronary α-adrenoceptors adjusts for the phasic oscillations in coronary flow to preserve flow to the inner layers of the left ventricle. Thus, β-noradrenoceptor-mediated mechanisms appear to operate more distally, while α-adrenoceptor-mediated mechanisms act proximally in the coronary tree, providing a synergistic effect to maintain subendocardial perfusion, while at the same time optimizing coronary flow adjustments for metabolic needs. Whether this intriguing hypothesis holds true for neural activation, either direct or reflex, remains to be tested.

CENTRAL CONTROL OF THE CORONARY CIRCULATION

Most prior studies of neural control of the coronary circulation examined the effects of applied neurotransmitters or direct stimulation of efferent cardiac nerves. The central nervous system pathways responsible for initiating all physiological sympathetic coronary vascular responses were largely unknown. Over the past several years our laboratory has utilized a feline model to define the central neural circuitry which innervates the coronary vasculature.

Through a series of studies outlined below, we have characterized a descending polysynaptic central pathway, traversing hypothalamic, midbrain, medullary and spinal regions, along which electrical or chemical stimulation produces sympathetic coronary vasoconstriction as part of a more generalized sympathoexcitation. This section will discuss the elements of the coronary vasomotor pathway including brain and spinal components. The potential functional role of this pathway in physiological responses, including the baroreflex and behavioral stresses such as the defence reaction, will also be addressed. Finally, clinical observations regarding central control of the coronary circulation will be described.

BRAIN SITES REGULATING SYMPATHETIC CORONARY VASOCONSTRICTION

These studies were performed in chloralose-anaesthetized adult cats, instrumented for continuous recordings of heart rate and arterial pressure. A specialized, suction-attached, piezoelectric crystal, mounted in a cupped Silastic housing, was placed onto the epicardium over the anterior descending artery (Wangler et al., 1981). Right femoral blood flow velocity was measured with a circumferentially-housed piezoelectric crystal for comparison. In all experiments reported, atenolol was administered and vagotomy performed to minimize the direct and secondary confounding influences of vagal and β-adrenergic activation. Cats were prepared for stereotoxically guided brain stimulation and microinjection.

Effect of electrical stimulation in CNS

Three sites were chosen for initial studies because of their known involvement in autonomic responses, namely lateral hypothalamus, ventral posterolateral thalamus, and medullary lateral reticular formation. Electrical stimulation in each of these areas produced an intensity-dependent increase in arterial pressure and reduction in hindquarter flow velocity. In a discrete subregion of lateral hypothalamus (Bonham et al., 1987) (Figure 8.7) and medullary lateral reticular formation (Figure 8.8) (Gutterman et al., 1989), electrical stimulation also reduced coronary flow velocity. The reduction in coronary flow was similar in both duration and magnitude to that seen with direct stimulation of the stellate ganglia (Bonham et al., 1987). Although the coronary constriction was similar in both regions, the magnitude of the pressor response was greater with medullary stimulation.

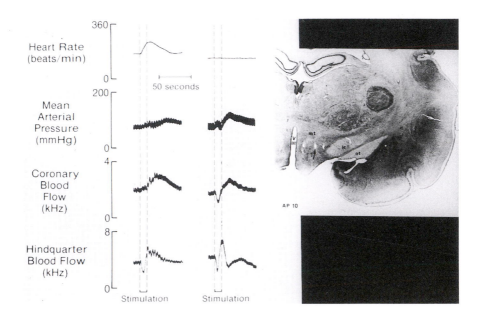

Figure 8.7   Example of the haemodynamic and coronary vascular response to electrical stimulation in lateral hypothalamus (Bonham *et al.*, 1987). Electrical stimulation was performed in three separate sites (inset). Stimulation in the central electrode site (arrow), but not in the adjacent medial or lateral sites, produced a frank decrease in coronary blood flow with a concurrent increase in coronary resistance following β-adrenoceptor blockade (right set of panels). In the absence of β-adrenoceptor blockade (left panel) no decrease in coronary flow was observed primarily because of the concurrent increase in heart rate and myocardial contractility, producing an overriding myocardial metabolic response. ot – optic tract; VIII – third ventricle; mt – mamillothalamic tract; ic$_2$ – internal capsule. (Reproduced from *Am J Physiol* (1987) **252** p. H477, Figure 8.1 with permission from The American Physiological Society.)

The hindquarter response also differed in that only constriction was seen to medullary stimulation, while constriction with a superimposed dilatation was seen during stimulation in lateral hypothalamus.

To determine whether cell bodies or fibres of passage were responsible for the decrease in coronary flow velocity, L-glutamate was injected into the same site where electrical stimulation produced coronary constriction. Microinjection of L-glutamate produced no haemodynamic response in either lateral hypothalamus or medullary lateral reticular formation, indicating that fibres passing through these areas were primarily responsible for the observed coronary constriction.

MECHANISM OF CENTRALLY-INDUCED CORONARY VASOCONSTRICTION

Since arterial pressure increased during central stimulation, we tested whether coronary autoregulation may have contributed to the early increase in coronary vascular resistance.

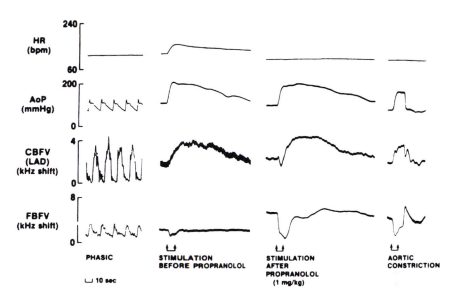

Figure 8.8 Example of the haemodynamic response to electrical stimulation in lateral medullary reticular formation in cat (Gutterman *et al.*, 1989). Phasic tracings of heart rate (HR), aortic pressure (AoP), coronary blood flow velocity (CBFV), and femoral blood flow velocity (FBFV) are shown in the first panel. Electrical stimulation in a discrete region of lateral reticular formation produced an increase in heart rate, arterial pressure, coronary flow and femoral resistance (second panel). Following β-adrenoceptor blockade (propranolol) the tachycardia and myocardial inotropic responses were attenuated, and a frank transient reduction in coronary flow velocity was seen (third tracing) at a time when arterial pressure was rising. This marked increase in coronary resistance was not observed during mechanical elevation in arterial pressure (aortic snare, fourth panel) demonstrating that extracardiac compressive forces and autoregulation do not contribute significantly. (Reproduced from *Am J Physiol* (1989) **256** p. H1221, Figure 8.1 with permission from The American Physiological Society.)

Mechanically-induced increases in arterial pressure (aortic snare) mimicked the pressor response to central stimulation effectively (Figures 8.8, 8.9). However no frank reduction in coronary flow velocity was seen during aortic constriction. Instead, an increase in coronary flow, following the increase in pressure, was always observed. Thus, autoregulatory or myocardial compressive changes in coronary resistance could not explain the early transient reduction in coronary flow velocity.

The receptor mechanism and peripheral neural pathways responsible for hypothalamic and medullary-induced coronary constriction were examined in separate experiments. Ablation of the contralateral stellate ganglion did not alter the centrally-induced coronary constriction (Figure 8.10). However, transection of the ipsilateral stellate ganglion abolished coronary constriction to stimulation in either central site (Bonham *et al.*, 1987; Gutterman *et al.*, 1989). When the ipsilateral sympathetic fibres were transected first the constriction was also prevented. These data demonstrate that the centrally induced coronary constriction is neurally, as opposed to humorally, mediated, involving activation of ipsilateral sympathetic fibres.

In other studies, the selective α_1-adrenoceptor blocking agent, prazosin, was administered. Figure 8.11 demonstrates that electrical stimulation in lateral reticular formation

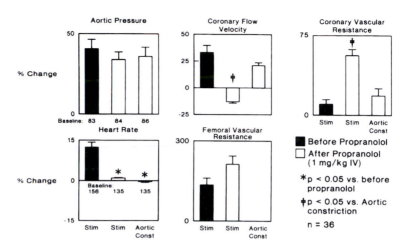

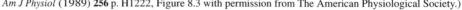

Figure 8.9 Summary of the effects of β-adrenoceptor blockade on the coronary response to electrical stimulation in the lateral reticular formations (Gutterman *et al.*, 1989). Electrical stimulation before and after propranolol and mechanical compression of the aorta produced similar increases in arterial pressure (upper left panel). Electrical stimulation after propranolol resulted in a frank decrease in coronary flow velocity with a corresponding increase in coronary vascular resistance which was significantly greater than the autoregulatory increase in resistance seen during constriction of the aorta following β-adrenoceptor blockade (upper right panel). (Reproduced from *Am J Physiol* (1989) **256** p. H1222, Figure 8.3 with permission from The American Physiological Society.)

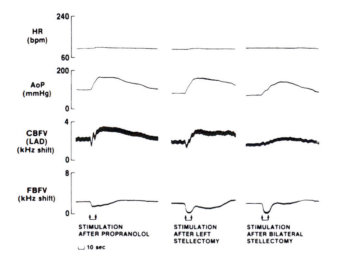

Figure 8.10 Example of the effect of stellate ganglionectomy on coronary constriction to electrical stimulation in lateral reticular formation (Gutterman *et al.*, 1989). In the first panel, electrical stimulation in the right lateral reticular formation produced a characteristic transient decrease in coronary flow in this cat treated with propranolol. In the second panel a similar coronary constriction was observed following contralateral stellate ganglionectomy. However, after bilateral stellate ganglionectomy (third panel) a similar pressor response was seen, but without frank decrease in coronary flow. When ipsilateral stellate ganglionectomy was performed first, abolition of the constriction was also seen (data not shown). CBFV – coronary blood flow velocity; FBFV – femoral blood flow velocity. (Reproduced from *Am J Physiol* (1989) **256** p. H1223, Figure 8.5 with permission from The American Physiological Society.)

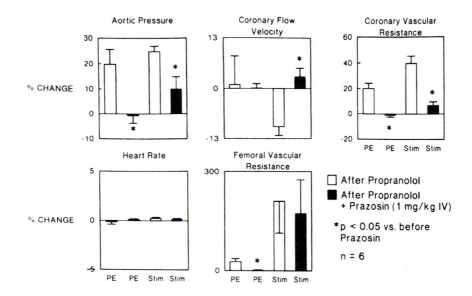

Figure 8.11   Effect of α-adrenoceptor blockade on coronary response to central stimulation and infusion of phenylephrine (PE). The left two bars in each panel represent the response to phenylephrine while the right two bars represent the response to electrical stimulation in lateral reticular formation. A dose of prazosin (1 mg/kg IV), which abolished the pressor and hindquarter flow response to phenylephrine, also abolished the increase in coronary vascular resistance and attenuated the pressor response to central stimulation. Hindquarter vasoconstriction was not altered by prazosin. In other studies, yohimbine, in a dose that selectively antagonised α_2- but not α_1 adrenoceptor agonists did not attenuate the increase in coronary resistance to central stimulation (Bonham *et al.*, 1987). (Reproduced with permission.)

produced coronary constriction, which was abolished following the administration of prazosin (0.1 mg/kg). This dose also attenuated the pressor response to phenylephrine (Gutterman *et al.*, 1989). In a dose selective for α_2-adrenoceptors, yohimbine did not affect the pressor response to phenylephrine or the coronary constriction to central stimulation (Bonham *et al.*, 1987). Only with a higher dose of yohimbine (0.2–0.3 mg/kg) were the pressor response to phenylephrine and the coronary constriction to central stimulation attenuated (Bonham *et al.*, 1987). These data show that central stimulation activates ipsilateral sympathetic fibres coursing through the stellate ganglion which produce an α_1-adrenoceptor-mediated coronary vasoconstriction in cat.

With histological analysis, the central sites were identified from which electrical stimulation produced coronary constriction. The medullary site was located in the lateral reticular formation just ventral to the facial nerve nucleus and lateral to the gigantocellular region (Figure 8.12). Effective sites in lateral hypothalamus were confined to the perifornical region.

Electrical stimulation in the third site selected, the ventral posterolateral nucleus of the thalamus, produced increases in arterial pressure and hindquarter vasoconstriction but no reduction in coronary flow velocity.

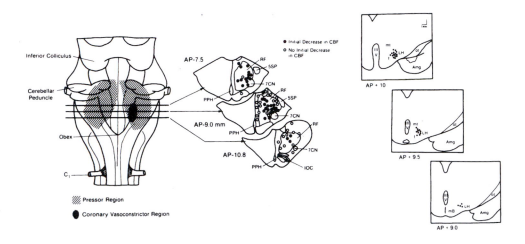

Figure 8.12 Composite of brainstem sites in lateral reticular formation (left panels) and lateral hypothalamus (right panels) in which electrical stimulation produced coronary vasoconstriction (Gutterman *et al.*, 1989). Three coronal sections through the brainstem and hypothalamus at different rostrocaudal levels are shown. On the far left a dorsal view of the brainstem is seen after removal of the cerebellum. The hatched area represents the classic pressor region of the medulla while the filled oval shaped region is a site from which coronary vasoconstriction was elicited. Filled circles in both sets of panels represent discrete sites within one animal in which electrical stimulation produced frank decreases in coronary flow. Stimulation outside these areas (open circles, medulla; not shown for hypothalamus) produced similar increases in arterial pressure and hindquarter vasoconstriction but without an initial decrease in coronary flow velocity. (Reproduced from *Am J Physiol* (1989) **256** p. H1224, Figure 8.6 from The American Physiological Society.)

Projections of central coronary vasomotor regions

To determine the location of cell bodies which project through the coronary vasomotor region of the lateral hypothalamus, the retrograde tracer, Fast Blue, was microinjected into the lateral hypothalamus. This agent is taken up by nerve terminals and damaged fibres, and transported retrogradely to the neuronal soma. Several days later the animal was killed and fluorescent cell bodies were noted in the paraventricular nucleus of the hypothalamus. Horseradish peroxidase conjugated to wheat-germ agglutinin, was microinjected into lateral hypothalamus to trace efferent fibres. Nerve terminals were identified in the ventrolateral periaqueductal gray (Gutterman *et al.*, 1990). Interestingly, electrical stimulation in the hypothalamic paraventricular nucleus failed to elicit the expected coronary vasoconstriction. Instead, coronary vasoconstriction could be elicited just lateral to the paraventricular nucleus in a dense fibre tract region of the anterior hypothalamus (Arthur *et al.*, 1991). Microinjections of L-glutamate into this area did not produce either a pressor response or coronary constriction, however, the effects of electrical stimulation mimic those seen during stimulation in the lateral hypothalamus. Additional preliminary studies suggest that the cell bodies of origin may reside in the amygdala, adjacent to the optic tract (Arthur *et al.*, 1990).

Microinjection of Fast Blue into the vasoconstrictor region of the lateral reticular formation traced the origin of the medullary fibres to cell bodies in two regions:

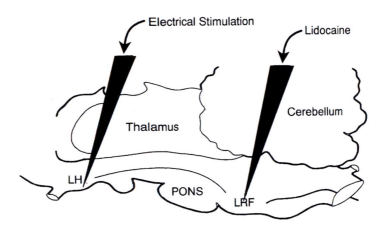

Figure 8.13 Method for evaluating functional connections between hypothalamic and medullary coronary vasomotor regions. This schematic shows a sagittal section of the brainstem. Electrical stimulation in the lateral hypothalamus (LH) and in the lateral reticular formation (LRF) produces coronary vasoconstriction. To determine whether these sites are functionally connected as part of the same pathway, electrical stimulation was performed in the lateral hypothalamus (LH) before and after microinjection of the neural inhibitory agent lidocaine in the lateral reticular formation (LRF).

(1) ventrolateral periaqueductal gray and (2) ventromedial parabrachial nucleus. Coupled with the studies described above using horseradish peroxidase, this result provides a strong rationale for the hypothesis that the lateral hypothalamus and medullary lateral reticular formation are part of the common descending pathway mediating coronary vasoconstriction, as well as other sympathoexcitatory responses. To test this hypothesis, we performed functional studies in which electrical stimulations were performed in the lateral hypothalamus before and after microinjecting lidocaine, an inhibitor of neural transmission, in the ipsilateral lateral reticular formation (Figure 8.13). An example of the response is shown in Figure 8.14. Four important observations are seen. First, ipsilateral injection of lidocaine produced no significant effect on baseline haemodynamics. Second, lidocaine prevented the neurogenic coronary constriction to stimulation in the lateral hypothalamus. Third, this inhibition was reversible in that 45 minutes after injection of lidocaine, repeat stimulation in the hypothalamus produced coronary constriction. Fourth, the hindquarter vasodilatation associated with hypothalamic stimulation was also prevented by lidocaine although the superimposed constriction was not affected. These data demonstrate that the lateral reticular formation is an integral portion of the pathway traversing the lateral hypothalamus along which coronary vasoconstrictor information travels.

We have identified other discrete central sites in which electrical stimulation produces coronary vasoconstriction. These are located in the ventromedial parabrachial nucleus (Miller *et al.*, 1991), which projects through the lateral reticular formation (see above), rostroventrolateral medulla (i.e., RVLM) (Paul *et al.*, 1989), and rostrodorsomedial medulla (Paul *et al.*, 1989). A similar experiment to that described above using lidocaine was

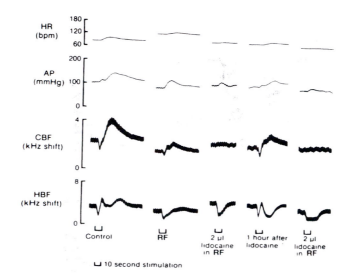

Figure 8.14   Example of the effect of lidocaine in the lateral reticular formation (RF) on the coronary response to electrical stimulation in the interior hypothalamus (Gutterman *et al.*, 1990). All stimulations were performed after β-adrenoceptor blockade. In the first panel, electrical stimulation in the anterior hypothalamus produces a decrease in coronary blood flow (CBF) and hindquarter blood flow (HBF) with small increases in heart rate (HR) and aortic pressure (AP). Stimulation in the lateral reticular formation (second panel) elicits a similar transient decrease in coronary flow. After removing the electrical stimulator in the reticular formation and replacing it with a similarly located microinjection cannula, 2 μl of lidocaine were injected into the site. Subsequent electrical stimulation in the anterior hypothalamus (third panel) failed to elicit coronary constriction. One hour later (panel 4) after the effect of lidocaine had abated, hypothalamic stimulation again produced a decrease in coronary flow velocity. This could subsequently be abolished by a second injection of lidocaine (panel 5). (Reproduced from *Am J Physiol* (1990) **259** p. H919, Figure 8.1 with permission from The American Physiological Society.)

performed with electrical stimulation in the most rostral identified central site (anterior hypothalamus) with microinjection of lidocaine into the most caudal site (RVLM) (Goodson, LaMaster and Gutterman, 1993). Similar inhibition of coronary vasoconstriction was observed after ipsilateral injection of lidocaine, again providing functional demonstration of connections between the coronary vasomotor regions of these brain sites. More importantly, microinjection of the inhibitory neurotransmitter, γ-aminobutyric acid, into RVLM, also blocked the coronary constrictor response to stimulation in the anterior hypothalamus (Figure 8.15). This suggests that cell bodies in RVLM are a necessary component of the central coronary vasoconstrictor pathway. Direct chemical stimulation in RVLM and the parabrachial nucleus also produced a neurogenic coronary vasoconstriction, confirming the importance of cell bodies in mediating the coronary vasomotor response to stimulation in these regions. Cell bodies are also involved in the coronary response elicited from the parabrachial nucleus, since chemical activation in this region produced coronary vasoconstriction. A summary of the central coronary pathway is illustrated in Figure 8.16.

Brain sites which mediate coronary constriction were further characterized by systematically stimulating different anatomical subregions of those sites (Jones, Gutterman

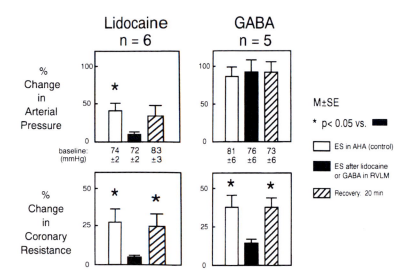

Figure 8.15 Summary of the effects of GABA in the rostroventrolateral medulla (RVLM) on the coronary response to electrical stimulation in the anterior hypothalamus (AHA) (Goodson, LaMaster and Gutterman, 1993). Inhibiting synaptic transmission in the RVLM (GABA) prevented coronary constriction to electrical stimulation in the anterior hypothalamus. This suggests that the descending coronary vasomotor pathway from the hypothalamus projecting through the RVLM synapses in the RVLM. (Reproduced with permission.)

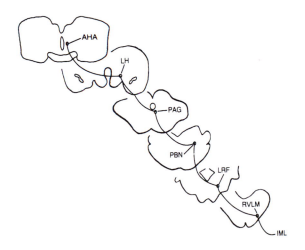

Figure 8.16 Summary of central sites in which electrical or chemical activation produces coronary vasoconstriction as part of a more generalized haemodynamic response. Sites in which electrical stimulation alone produce coronary vasoconstriction include the anterior hypothalamus (AHA), lateral hypothalamus (LH) and lateral reticular formation (LRF). Discrete sites in parabrachial nucleus (PBN), rostroventrolateral medulla (RVLM), and the intermediolateral column of the spinal cord at the T2 level (IML) may be activated with chemical agents as well as electrical stimulation to produce coronary vasoconstriction. In these latter sites cell bodies appear to mediate, in part, the coronary constrictor response to activation. All sites appear to be connected as part of a common descending vasomotor pathway which also has a synapse in periaqueductal gray (PAG), although the diffuseness of the projections in this region prevent direct elicitation of coronary vasoconstriction.

and Brody, 1992). Changes in BP, HR and coronary, femoral, renal and mesenteric flow were examined. Different patterns of regional vascular response were produced during electrical stimulation of discrete areas of the anterior hypothalamus, parabrachial nucleus and rostroventrolateral medulla. Stimulation in the coronary vasoconstrictor region of these brain sites produced a patterned regional vascular response indicative of the defense reaction. This included an atropine-sensitive decrease in hindquarter resistance, increases in renal and mesenteric vascular resistances, and a pressor response. Electrical stimulation in sites outside the coronary vasoconstrictor area did not produce the same regional vascular response. Thus, some organization of coronary and other vasomotor responses exists within RVLM, the anterior hypothalamus, and the region of parabrachial nucleus. These data also suggest that coronary vasoconstriction is a component of the defense reaction (Jones, Gutterman and Brody, 1992).

SPINAL CORD SITES MODULATING CORONARY BLOOD FLOW

The intermediolateral cell column from T1–T6 is the source of virtually all sympathetic preganglionic neurons which innervate the stellate ganglion and heart. The most dense concentration of these cell bodies is located at the T2 level (Coote, 1988). We have performed systematic electrical stimulation in the spinal cord in regions of the intermediolateral cell column as well as in the dorsolateral funiculus where descending fibres from RVLM travel (Paul et al., 1990; Paul, Gutterman and Brody, 1990). Stimulations were made along a long rostral-caudal region from T1 to T4. Despite increases in arterial pressure throughout this region to stimulation in the dorsolateral funiculus, a frank reduction in coronary flow was seen only at the level of T2. In the intermediolateral cell column, electrical stimulation produced only a decrease in coronary flow without changes in arterial pressure or hindquarter flow velocity. Similar reductions in coronary flow were elicited by microinjections of L-glutamate into the same intermediolateral region (Paul et al., 1990). Electrical stimulation, but not L-glutamate, in the dorsolateral funiculus at the T2 level elicited a pressor response with coronary vasoconstriction. All coronary constrictions from the spinal stimulation were abolished by ipsilateral stellate ganglionectomy or administration of prazosin.

Preliminary data suggest that coronary vasoconstriction can only be elicited in the cat by a stimulation in the right IML (Paul, Gutterman and Brody, 1990). Multiple attempts at stimulation in the left IML did not produce a reduction in coronary flow velocity. Interestingly, however, stimulation in either right *or left* RVLM produced coronary vasoconstriction which was abolished by ipsilateral stellate ganglionectomy. The interpretation of these findings is unclear, but they suggest that lateral heterogeneity exists in the spinal cord with respect to coronary vasoconstriction. This is similar to the well-known heterogeneity of spinally-elicited effects on heart rate and contractility (Barman and Wurster, 1975; Taylor and Weaver, 1992).

FUNCTIONAL IMPORTANCE OF CENTRAL CORONARY
VASOCONSTRICTOR PATHWAY

The identification of a brain pathway along which electrical or chemical stimulation produces coronary vasoconstriction as part of a more general sympathoexcitation is of interest in terms of identifying central neural projections. However, the presence of such a pathway does not confer physiological relevance. Therefore, we sought to determine whether this coronary vasoconstrictor pathway is activated during physiological forms of coronary constriction.

One well-described physiological mechanism of coronary vasoconstriction is baroreceptor unloading. Following bilateral carotid occlusion, arterial pressure and systemic vascular resistance increases; neurogenic coronary vasoconstriction is a component of this response. Since the reflex arc includes the brain, with primary afferents entering at the nucleus of the tractus solitarius (NTS), we undertook experiments to determine whether sites along the central coronary vasoconstrictor pathway were involved in baroreflex coronary vasoconstriction.

The carotid sinus nerves terminate in the nucleus of the tractus solitarius. Secondary and tertiary projections are less well-characterized, but regions of the parabrachial nucleus and lateral reticular formation (Miura and Reis, 1969) appear to receive input from the nucleus of the tractus solitarius. Since the lateral reticular formation is also a component of the coronary constrictor pathway, our examination of baroreflex-mediated coronary vasoconstriction was initiated in this medullary site.

Baroreflex-mediated, coronary vasoconstriction was elicited by bilateral carotid artery occlusion (Gutterman et al., 1991). This produced increases in arterial pressure, with less prominent increases in coronary flow and a net increase in coronary resistance (Figure 8.17). A smaller increase in coronary resistance was observed when the aorta was snared to mimic the pressor response to carotid artery occlusion. The difference between the autoregulatory increase in coronary resistance and the increase in resistance during carotid occlusion represented the neurogenic reflex component. This difference could be abolished by stellate ganglionectomy. To assess the role of medullary lateral reticular formation in the baroreflex-mediated coronary constriction, bilateral microinjections of lidocaine were made into the medullary region (Gutterman et al., 1991). Immediately after injection, the coronary constriction to carotid occlusion was attenuated. Forty-five minutes to one hour later, the magnitude of the reflex coronary constriction returned to control levels, demonstrating reversibility of the effects of lidocaine. Interestingly, the pressor response to carotid occlusion was also attenuated, suggesting that many of the fibres mediating the pressor response also traverse the lateral reticular formation. However, bilateral microinjections of lidocaine into the medullary lateral reticular formation did not change baseline arterial pressure. Thus, the lateral reticular formation is a critical component of the central baroreflex arc mediating coronary vasoconstriction, but is not necessary for maintaining basal sympathetic tone.

In separate studies we have demonstrated that the parabrachial nucleus is also a component of the baroreflex coronary constrictor arc, and that cell bodies within this region are involved in the reflex coronary constriction (Gutterman, Marcus and Brody, in press). These data provide the first functional evidence for a physiological role of portions of the coronary vasomotor pathway described above. Specifically, medullary and pontine portions of this pathway are involved in baroreflex-mediated coronary vasoconstriction.

The components of the pathway along which coronary vasoconstriction may be activated (Figure 8.16) are strikingly similar to the previously described "defense reaction" pathway (Ainsworth et al., 1977; Hilton and Smith, 1984; Yardley and Hilton, 1986). This, together

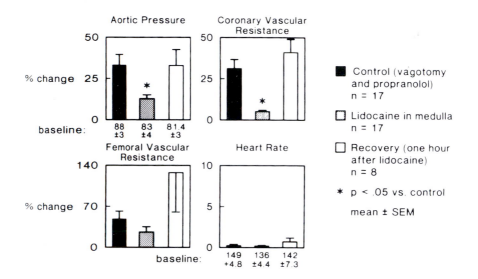

Figure 8.17   Summary of the effects of bilateral carotid occlusion on the coronary vascular response before and after microinjection of lidocaine into the lateral reticular formation (Gutterman *et al.*, 1991). After vagotomy and propranolol bilateral carotid occlusion produce increases in arterial pressure, coronary vascular resistance and hindquarter vascular resistance. The coronary vasoconstriction was abolished following bilateral microinjections of lidocaine into lateral reticular formation. Reversibility and recovery of lidocaine-induced neural inhibition was observed one hour later (third bar of each panel). These data demonstrate the important role of fibres passing through lateral reticular formation in mediating the coronary vasoconstriction to baroreceptor hypotension. (Reproduced from *Brain Research* (1991) **551** p. 204, Figure 8.2 from the authors and Elsevier Science Publishers BV.)

with the similar functional response to stimulation in coronary constrictor areas and defense reaction regions, led us to postulate that coronary vasoconstriction may be a component of behavioral responses such as the defense reaction.

To test this hypothesis, mongrel cats were instrumented for continuous recordings of coronary flow velocity, arterial pressure and heart rate, and for electrical stimulation in the anterior hypothalamus. Cats were trained to rest comfortably in a cage with three opaque walls and one made of Plexiglas. To elicit the defense reaction a dog was brought into the room for visual contact with a cat. Haemodynamics and coronary flow were monitored before and during the cat's behavioral response to the dog. In cats which exhibited piloerection, pupillary dilatation, arching of the back and hissing, frank coronary vasoconstriction was also observed usually late during the one minute exposure period and often lasting several minutes into the recovery period after removal of the dog. This stress-induced reduction in coronary flow was abolished with the α-noradrenoceptor antagonist, prazosin, suggesting that coronary vasoconstriction is a component of the defense reaction. The purpose of this coronary vasomotor response may relate to the improvement in transmural distribution of coronary flow described above.

Other investigators have demonstrated behaviorally-induced coronary vasoconstriction. Carpeggiani and Skinner (1991), showed evidence for coronary vasoconstriction during psychological stress in pigs. Billman and Randall (1981), demonstrated behaviorally-induced increases in coronary vascular resistance during stress in dogs; the observed constriction in their study was transient, similar to that described in our experiments. The neurogenic coronary constriction was most prominent after β-adrenoceptor blockade (Billman and Randall, 1981; Billman and Bickerstaff, 1986) and was not generally seen in the absence of β-adrenoceptor blockade (Marchetti, Merlo and Noseda, 1968; Billman and Bickerstaff, 1986). In a more recent study, Verrier, Hagestad and Lown (1987), described coronary vasoconstriction following provocation of anger in dogs. The anger paradigm involved placing a fasting experimental dog's food dish just out of reach. Then another dog was brought into the room to eat from the bowl. This provoked "anger-like" behavior in the experimental dog. When a coronary stenosis was present in the experimental dogs, a three-fold increase in coronary vascular resistance was observed following, but not during, the period of stress-induced anger. Neurally-invoked changes in vascular tone contributed to this behaviorally-induced coronary vasoconstriction.

In humans with coronary artery disease, vasoconstriction of conduit and resistance coronary vessels is observed in response to stress. Mudge and colleagues (1976), described decreases in coronary flow during a cold-pressor test, and Brown et al. (1984) demonstrated reductions in diameters of coronary conduit vessels, with resultant left ventricular dysfunction in response to a similar stress. Both responses were felt to be neurogenic in origin. These data provide direct clinical evidence that neurogenic coronary vasoconstriction may have adverse effects on cardiac function in humans. It remains to be determined if sites within the central coronary constrictor pathway are involved.

CLINICAL IMPLICATIONS OF CENTRALLY-MEDIATED CORONARY CONSTRICTION

A vast amount of clinical evidence supports a prominent role for the brain in the mechanism of cardiac disease. Clinical evaluation of patients with stroke, brain trauma and intracranial tumors demonstrate marked and sustained changes in the electrocardiogram, consistent with myocardial ischaemia. These changes include ST segment depressions, development of frank Q waves, nonspecific T wave abnormalities, and QT prolongation (Melville et al., 1963; Hersch, 1964; Greenhoot and Reichenbach, 1969; Hammermeister and Reichenbach, 1969). Similar electrocardiographic abnormalities have been demonstrated in animals following brain trauma. Transection of the spinal cord at the cervical level can abolish the ECG abnormalities, demonstrating a neurogenic aetiology (Greenhoot and Reichenbach, 1969). Cases have even been reported of patients presenting with classical symptoms of myocardial infarction, including diagnostic electrocardiographic changes, who were found, to have normal coronary arteries, and subarachnoid haemorrhage as the aetiology (Beard, Robertson and Robertson, 1959). Tumors and intracranial bleeds in autonomic brainstem centers are primarily responsible for these cardiac changes, supporting a specific role for autonomic sites in these pathophysiological cardiac responses.

These observations led numerous investigators to conclude that activation of specific central regions may produce a profound and sustained reduction in coronary flow, often with myocardial infarction. Only recently has the question been tested directly, with the advent of methods for measuring coronary blood flow in humans. Recent clinical studies performed in patients with coronary artery disease clearly demonstrate a pathophysiological role of the brain in coronary vasomotor regulation. As described above, psychological stress has been shown to reduce coronary conductance in patients with coronary disease (Carpeggiani and Skinner, 1991). The cold-pressor test can also evoke a reflex coronary vasoconstriction (Mudge et al., 1976), with induction of cardiac pain. The mechanism of the centrally-induced coronary vasoconstriction is multifactorial. Reflex stimuli such as the cold-pressor test can produce vasoconstriction within the narrowed orifice of a stenosed epicardial coronary artery (Brown et al., 1984). Reductions in flow that occur are likely mediated by downstream arteriolar vasoconstriction (Mudge et al., 1976). Mental arithmetic in patients with coronary artery disease produces myocardial ischaemia by vasoconstriction of the arteriolar, but not large, epicardial segments (L'Abbate et al., 1991). Mental arithmetic is a form of psychological stress that was applied to patients with coronary disease and ischaemia. Forty-four percent of patients developed ischaemic ECG changes similar to those seen during exercise provocation, but at lower rate-pressure products, suggesting a primary reduction in flow. Epicardial diameter either in or adjacent to the stenotic segment was not affected by mental stress, indicating that the constriction occurred in the microcirculation.

Myocardial ischaemia secondary to mental stress (decreased supply of blood) is mechanistically different from ischaemia during exercise (increased metabolic demand); the clinical presentation of the two may also differ. Stress-induced reductions in coronary blood flow may be of similar, or greater, magnitude than the exercise-induced impairments in flow, but generally occur with fewer symptoms (Rozanski et al., 1988; Giubbini et al., 1991). This is consistent with the observation that silent myocardial ischaemia is more prominent during sedentary activities than during exercise (Cecchi et al., 1983). Thus, it may be advantageous to tailor treatment of myocardial ischaemia to eliminate reductions in supply (centrally evoked vasoconstriction) since these episodes have a higher propensity for going unrecognized by the patient. Future investigations into central control of the coronary circulation should strive to identify specific inhibitors of neurotransmitters which selectively prevent the increase in coronary vasomotor tone during behavioral or reflex activation.

NEURAL CONTROL OF THE CORONARY CIRCULATION IN DISEASE

DIABETES MELLITUS

Prominent vascular alterations characterize the diabetic and hyperglycaemic states (Ruderman, Williamson and Brownlee, 1992). The most characteristically observed changes include enhanced production of vasoconstrictor prostanoids (Tesfamariam, Jakubowski and Cohen, 1989; Mayhan, Simmons and Sharpe, 1991) from endothelium, and possibly underlying smooth muscle, enhanced (Gebremedhin et al., 1988; Martin, Knuepfer and Westfall, 1991) or decreased (Gerritsen, 1987; Hattori et al., 1991) production of vasodilator prostanoids, and impairment of endothelium-dependent vasodilatation (Gebremedhin *et al.*, 1988). Enhanced production of thromboxane A_2 and PGH_2 are prominent effects of chronic hyperglycaemia (Tesfamariam, Jakubowski and Cohen, 1989; Mayhan, Simmons and Sharpe, 1991). These changes are observed in both conduit and resistance vessels. In addition, conduit vessels suffer accelerated atherosclerosis.

Evidence for altered neural control of the coronary circulation in diabetes is derived from animal and human studies. Although neurogenic coronary constriction appears to be enhanced in diabetes, it is difficult to draw specific conclusions with regard to these studies because of the variable results reported. For example, Koltai *et al.*, 1988, observed that α-adrenoceptor activation increased prostacyclin production in diabetic, but not control, animals. However, in other studies, phenylephrine was shown to enhance prostacyclin production in normal, but not diabetic dogs (Koltai, Rosen and Pogatsa, 1989).

Koltai *et al.* (1984), examined the effects of electrical stimulation of the sympathetic nerves to the heart in dogs made diabetic three months earlier with an injection of alloxan. In the diabetic animals sympathetic stimulation increased left ventricular dP/dt and increased coronary vascular resistance. In metabolically normal animals, electrical stimulation produced similar elevations in dP/dt but decreased coronary vascular resistance (Koltai *et al.*, 1984). This would suggest enhanced coronary constrictor responses to neural stimuli in diabetes.

In an *in vitro* study, rat coronary arteries constricted similarly to noradrenaline when isolated from either metabolically normal or diabetic animals. Interestingly, the constriction to prostaglandin $F_{2\alpha}$ and to KCl were diminished in the diabetic animals. This would argue that noradrenergic responses are normal, but that constriction to other agents may be reduced in the diabetic state. Downing and colleagues (1983), observed enhanced sensitivity of the diabetic heart to α-adrenoceptor stimulation in the newborn lamb. Thus, diabetic lambs exhibited an increase in left ventricular dP/dt compared to control lambs in response to methoxamine. Coronary blood flow was also measured in these studies and no change was observed.

In preliminary studies, we have examined the effect of stellate nerve stimulation on coronary vasomotor responses in non-diabetic dogs and in dogs made diabetic for one week. Stellate stimulation produced a dose-dependent decrease in coronary flow and increase in coronary vascular resistance which was similar in both diabetic and metabolically normal animals. Intracoronary noradrenaline, however, produced dose-dependent coronary constriction in control dogs which was much greater than the constriction produced in diabetic dogs (Gutterman, Morgan and Dellsperger, 1992). These data would seem to suggest that marked differences exist in release of noradrenaline during nerve stimulation or that other substances released with noradrenaline (e.g., neuropeptide Y) more potently constrict the coronary vasculature of diabetics than normal animals.

In summary, diabetes and hyperglycaemia produce complex metabolic changes in the heart and coronary vasculature. Many of these alterations may be species-dependent or dependent on the method of experimentation (*in vivo* versus *in vitro*). Responses to noradrenaline may be different than those to sympathetic nerve stimulation. A general trend exists toward enhancement of vasoconstrictor stimuli and impairment of vasodilator stimuli in the coronary circulation of diabetic animals.

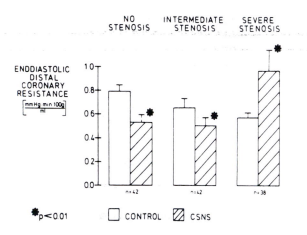

Figure 8.18 Effect of increasing stenosis severity on the coronary vascular response to stellate stimulation in anaesthetized dogs (Heusch and Deussen, 1983). Sympathetic stimulation in the presence of small or no stenosis produced a decrease in coronary vascular resistance while stimulation in the presence of a severe stenosis significantly increased end diastolic distal coronary resistance in these animals. Thus, presence of a coronary stenosis may amplify the magnitude of neurogenic coronary vasoconstriction. CSNS – cardiac sympathetic nerve stimulation. (Reproduced from *Circulation Research* (1983) **53** p. 9, Figure 8.1 with permission from the authors and The American Heart Association.)

CORONARY STENOSIS AND NEUROGENIC VASOCONSTRICTION

As described previously, in anaesthetized dogs cardiac sympathetic activation produces coronary vasodilatation due to stimulation of the myocardium and subsequent release of metabolic factors. However, when coronary vasodilator reserve is exhausted, as in the presence of a severe coronary stenosis, α-adrenoceptor-mediated constriction can overwhelm metabolic dilator stimuli and frank reductions in coronary flow ensue. Heusch and Deussen (1983), studied this phenomenon in an anaesthetized dog model. Bilateral stellate stimulation increased coronary flow and decreased coronary vascular resistance in the control state. In the presence of a mild or moderate coronary stenosis a similar dilatation was observed. However, in the presence of a severe coronary stenosis sympathetic stimulation decreased coronary flow, increasing coronary vascular resistance with resultant lactate production (Figure 8.18). This constriction could be abolished by α_2- but not by α_1-adrenoceptor blockade, suggesting that postjunctional α_2-adrenoceptors activated during sympathetic stimulation competed effectively with the metabolic vasodilatation, reducing coronary flow with subsequent myocardial ischaemia.

This important observation has also been reported by others. Residual α-adrenoceptor-mediated coronary tone has been demonstrated in dogs during exercise in the presence of a stenosis (Laxson, *et al.*, 1989). Buffington and Feigl (1981), examined the range of oxygen consumptions over which α-adrenoceptor-mediated constriction could compete with metabolic vasodilatation. Even at high metabolic rates a persistent and significant α-adrenoceptor-mediated constriction was observed (Figure 8.19). As described above

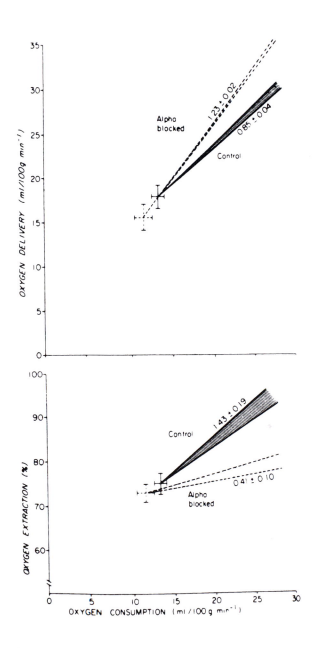

Figure 8.19 Effect of α-adrenoceptor blockade on myocardial responses to noradrenaline and carotid sinus reflex sympathetic activation (Mohrman and Feigl, 1978). For the same degree of oxygen consumption, greater oxygen delivery and less oxygen extraction was noted in animals treated with α-adrenoceptor antagonist. This suggests that, over a wide range of myocardial metabolism, α-noradrenoceptor-mediated influences act to constrict the coronary vasculature. (Reproduced from *Circulation Research* (1978) **42**(1) p. 84, Figure 8.7 with permission from the authors and The American Heart Association.)

(cardiocoronary reflex), myocardial ischaemia distal to a coronary stenosis can reflexly activate sympathetic nerves to further reduce flow in the ischaemic bed (Heusch, Deussen and Thamer, 1985). This observation clearly suggests that neurogenic coronary vasoconstriction, which may be of small magnitude in normal circumstances, can evoke profound detrimental effects when flow reserve is exhausted (Heusch, Deussen and Thamer, 1985). The clinical importance of this neurogenic coronary constriction has been demonstrated in studies by Mudge *et al.* (1979), in which the cold-pressor test increased coronary vascular resistance in patients with coronary disease, but not in controls. This reflex response was associated with angina pectoris in several of the patients.

In summary, neurogenic coronary vasoconstriction may be enhanced in the presence of a coronary stenosis where vasodilator reserve is exhausted. This, neurogenic constriction can evoke lactate production, decrease myocardial function (Seitelberger *et al.*, 1988), and provoke angina pectoris in patients with coronary disease.

ISCHAEMIA AND NEURAL CARDIAC FUNCTION

Peripheral nerves are characteristically refractory to prolonged episodes of ischaemia. Sustained nerve recordings with normal conduction velocities have been reported for 1–2 hours following cessation of tissue perfusion. However, in the heart, evidence for neural dysfunction can be seen as early as several minutes after coronary occlusion (Inoue, Skale and Zipes, 1988).

Martins *et al.* (1980), examined the effects of acute myocardial infarction on cardiac innervation. Because of the differential course of vagal and sympathetic cardiac fibres (Figure 8.1) subendocardial myocardial infarction produces more widespread dysfunction of parasympathetic than sympathetic fibres. Thus, overlying regions of the myocardium and coronary vasculature are affected only by sympathetic fibres.

We have examined the effects of brief periods of myocardial ischaemia followed by reperfusion on the coronary innervation (Gutterman, Morgan and Miller, 1992). Coronary constriction to sympathetic stimulation is inhibited following 15 minutes of coronary artery occlusion and thirty minutes of reperfusion. Responses to intracoronary noradrenaline are maintained suggesting that end-organ function is intact and that the abnormality occurs prejunctionally (Figure 8.20). Tyramine and bretylium are equally effective at producing coronary constriction before and after brief ischaemia suggesting that mechanisms involved in cytosolic and vesicular release of noradrenaline are intact in the postischaemic state (Gutterman, Morgan and Miller, 1992). Taken together with data from Barber *et al.* (1985), Inoue, Skale and Zipes (1988), demonstrating that cardiac afferent fibres are also inhibited following ischaemia, we conclude that myocardial ischaemia likely releases cardiac metabolic products which then act upon the nerve fibres to inhibit neurotransmission. This inhibition appears to be temporary, with recovery occurring variably from 2–4 hours into reperfusion.

From the work of Heusch and Deussen (1983), one may speculate on functional importance of ischaemic inhibition of sympathetic coronary vasoconstriction. Since, in the presence of severe stenosis, neurogenic coronary constriction can further reduce flow, early ischaemic inhibition of nerve conduction would have a protective effect on the distal coronary vasculature.

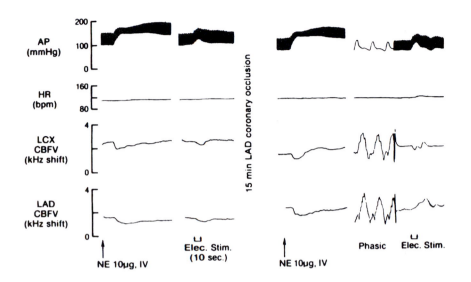

Figure 8.20 Example of the effect of a brief period of myocardial ischaemia on the coronary response to intravenous noradrenaline and electrical stimulation of the stellate ganglia (Gutterman, Morgan and Miller, 1992). On the left panel noradrenaline given after β-adrenoceptor blockade produced increases in arterial pressure and decreases in circumflex and LAD (left anterior descending) blood flow velocities (LCx CBFV (left circumflex coronary blood flow velocity), LAD CBFV respectively). After 15 minutes of LAD occlusion and 30 minutes of reperfusion, noradrenaline similarly constricted LAD and LCx beds and electrical stimulation also produced a characteristic transient decrease in circumflex blood flow. However, the constrictor response initially seen in the postischaemic LAD bed was abolished during reperfusion. These data demonstrate "neural stunning" of the coronary efferent sympathetic innervation. (Reproduced from *Circulation Research* (1992) **71** p. 963, Figure 8.1 from the authors and The American Heart Association.)

The mechanism of this "neural stunning" is unknown. Presumptive evidence exists that adenosine, potassium ions, or hydrogen ions are involved (Miyazaki and Zipes, 1990). Superfusion of the epicardium or subselective coronary injection of these substances alone or together produces a functional denervation in the distal tissue (Miyazaki and Zipes, 1990). Studies from our laboratory suggests that adenosine plays a prominent role in the mechanism of neural coronary stunning (Pettersen, Morgan and Gutterman, 1994). In these studies, adenosine deaminase administered during the coronary occlusion prevented the reduction in sympathetic coronary vasoconstriction. Conversely, intracoronary administration of adenosine for fifteen minutes inhibited subsequent coronary vasoconstriction to sympathetic activation, while intracoronary infusions of papaverine did not alter the neurogenic coronary response (Pettersen, Morgan and Gutterman, 1994).

In summary, although nerves are refractory to ischaemia, in a highly metabolic tissue such as the heart nerves exist in a milieu where ischaemic metabolites may impair neurotransmission, producing a functional denervation in the ischaemic region.

SUMMARY

The coronary arteries receive a dense, sympathetic innervation. Direct stimulation and numerous reflex stimuli can evoke a sympathetic coronary vasoconstriction mediated by α_1- and/or α_2-adrenoceptors. Under normal circumstances, this constriction is overwhelmed by a concurrent metabolic vasodilatation but under conditions where vasodilator reserve is reduced (exercise, coronary stenosis), sympathetic activation may produce frank coronary vasoconstriction, often with haemodynamic and metabolic decompensation. The vagal innervation also participates in coronary vasomotor regulation through muscarinic release of EDRF from the coronary vascular endothelium with resultant vasodilatation.

Neurogenic coronary responses may be altered in diseased states such as hypertension, diabetes, and myocardial ischaemia. However, the exact mechanisms and extent of these alterations remain to be determined.

ACKNOWLEDGEMENT

The expert secretarial assistance provided by Marlene Blakley is greatly appreciated.

REFERENCES

Ainsworth, A., Dostrovsky, J.O., Merrill, E.G. and Millar, J. (1977). An improved method for insulating tungsten micro-electrodes with glass. *J Physiol*, **269**, 4P–5P.

Arthur, J.M. (1990). Studies on the participation of the coronary circulation in the defense reaction. Iowa City: University of Iowa Press.

Arthur, J.M., Bonham, A.C., Gutterman, D.D., Gebhart, G.F., Marcus, M.L. and Brody, M.J. (1991). Coronary vasoconstriction during stimulation in hypothalamic defense region. *Am J Physiol*, **260**, R335–R345.

Aung-Din, R., Mitchell, J.H. and Longhurst, J.C. (1981). Reflex α-adrenergic coronary vasoconstriction during hindlimb static exercise in dogs. *Circ Res*, **48**, 502–509.

Barber, M.J., Mueller, T.M., Davies, B.G., Gill, R.M. and Zipes, D.P. (1985). Interruption of sympathetic and vagal-mediated afferent responses by transmural myocardial infarction. *Circulation*, **72**, 623–631.

Barman, S.M. and Wurster, R.D. (1975). Viseromotor organization within descending spinal sympathetic pathways in the dog. *Circ Res*, **37**, 209–214.

Baumgart, D., Ehring, T., Kowallik, P., Guth, B.D., Krajcar, M. and Heusch, G. (1993). Impact of α-adrenergic coronary vasoconstriction on the transmural myocardial blood flow distribution during humoral and neuronal adrenergic activation. *Circ Res*, **73**, 869–886.

Beard, E.F., Robertson, J.W. and Robertson, R.C.L. (1959). Spontaneous subarachnoid haemorrhage simulating acute myocardial infarction. *Am Heart J*, **58**, 755–759.

Billman, G.E. and Bickerstaff, L.V. (1986). Regulation of the right coronary circulation during a controlled behavioral stress in the conscious dog. *J Auton Nerv Syst*, **17**, 45–61.

Billman, G.E. and Randall, D.C. (1981). Mechanisms mediating the coronary vascular response to behaviorial stress in the dog. *Circ Res*, **48**, 214–223.

Bonham, A.C., Gutterman, D.D., Arthur, J.M., Marcus, M.L., Gebhart, G.F. and Brody, M.J. (1987). Electrical stimulation in perifornical lateral hypothalamus decreases coronary blood flow in cats. *Am J Physiol*, **252**, H4740–H4784.

Boucek, R.J., Takshita, R. and Fojaco, R. (1963). Relation between microanatomy and functional properties of the coronary arteries (dog). *Anat Rec*, **147**, 199–207.

Broten, T.P., Miyashiro, J.K., Moncada, S. and Feigl, E.O. (1992). Role of endothelium-derived relaxing factor in parasympathetic coronary vasodilatation. *AFP*, **262**, H1579–H1584.

Brown, A.M. and Malliani, A. (1971). Spinal sympathetic reflexes initiated by coronary receptors. *J Physiol*, **212**, 685–705.

Brown, B.G., Lee, A.B., Bolson, E.L. and Dodge, H.T. (1984). Reflex constriction of significant coronary stenosis as a mechanism contributing to ischemic left ventricular dysfunction during isometric exercise. *Circulation*, **70**, 18–24.

Buffington, C.W. and Feigl, E.O. (1981). Adrenergic coronary vasoconstriction in the presence of coronary stenosis in the dog. *Circ Res*, **48**, 416–423.

Carpeggiani, C. and Skinner, J.E. (1991). Coronary flow and mental stress. *Circulation*, **83**, II-90–II-93.

Cecchi, A.C., Dovellini, E.V., Marchi, F., Pucci, P., Santoro, G. and Fazini, P.F. (1983). Silent myocardial ischemia during ambulatory electrocardiographic monitoring in patients with effort angina. *J Am Coll Cardiol*, **1**, 934–939.

Chen, D.G., Dai, X.Z., Zimmerman, B.G. and Bache, R.J. (1988). Postsynaptic α_1- and α_2-adrenergic mechanisms in coronary vasoconstriction. *J Cardiovasc Pharmacol*, **11**, 61–67.

Chilian, W.M. and Ackell, P.H. (1988). Transmural differences in sympathetic coronary constriction during exercise in the presence of coronary stenosis. *Circ Res*, **62**, 216–225.

Chilian, W.M., Boatwright, R.B., Shoji, T. and Griggs, D.M., Jr. (1981). Evidence against significant resting sympathetic vasoconstrictor tone in the conscious dog. *Circ Res*, **49**, 866–878.

Chilian, W.M., Layne, S.M., Eastham, C.L. and Marcus, M.L. (1989). Heterogeneous microvascular coronary α-adrenergic vasoconstriction. *Circ Res*, **64**, 376–388.

Cohen, R.A., Shepherd, J.T. and Vanhoutte, P.M. (1984). Effects of the adrenergic transmitter on epicardial coronary arteries. *Fed Proc*, **43**, 2862–2866.

Cohen, R.A., Zitnay, K.M. and Wiesbrod, R.M. (1987). Accumulation of 5-hydroxytryptamine leads to dysfunction of adrenergic nerves in canine coronary artery following intimal damage *in vivo*. *Circ Res*, **61**, 829–833.

Coote, J.H. (1988). The organisation of cardiovascular neurons in the spinal cord. *Rev Physiol Biochem Pharmacol*, **110**, 148–285.

Cox, D.A., Hintze, T.H. and Vatner, S.F. (1983). Effects of acetylcholine on large and small coronary arteries in conscious dogs. *J Pharmacol Exp Ther*, **225**, 764–769.

Dahlstrom, A., Fuxe, K., Mya-Tu, M. and Zetterstrom, B.E.M. (1965). Observation on adrenergic innervation of dog heart. *Am J Physiol*, **209**, 689–692.

Dai, X.Z., Sublett, E., Lindstrom, P., Schwartz, J.S., Homans, D.C. and Bache, R.J. (1989). Coronary flow during exercise after selective α_1- and α_2-adrenergic blockade. *Am J Physiol*, **256**, H1148–H1155.

De Boel, S.L. and Gutterman, D.D. (1993). Coronary vascular response to the cerebral ischemia reflex. *Hypertension*, **21**, 216–221.

Denn, M.J. and Stone, H.L. (1976). Autonomic innervation of dog coronary arteries. *J Appl Physiol*, **41**, 30–35.

Deussen, A., Heusch, G. and Thamer, V. (1985). α_2-adrenoceptor-mediated coronary vasoconstriction persists after exhaustion of coronary dilator reserve. *Eur J Pharmacol*, **115**, 147–153.

DiSalvo, J., Parker, P.E., Scott, J.B. and Haddy, F.J. (1971). Carotid baroreceptor influence on coronary vascular resistance in the anaesthetized dog. *Am J Physiol*, **221**, 156–159.

Downing, S.E., Lee, J.C. and Fripp, R.R. (1983). Enhanced sensitivity of diabetic hearts to α-adrenoceptor stimulation. *Am J Physiol*, **245**, H808–H813.

Downing, S.E., Mitchell, J.H. and Wallace, A.G. (1963). Cardiovascular responses to ischemia, hypoxia, and hypercapnia of the central nervous system. *Am J Physiol*, **204**, 881–887.

Ely, S.W., Sawyer, D.C., Anderson, D.L. and Scott, J.B. (1981). Carotid sinus reflex vasoconstriction in right coronary circulation of dog and pig. *Am J Physiol*, **241**, H149–H154.

Feigl, E.O. (1968). Carotid sinus reflex control of coronary blood flow. *Circ Res*, **23**, 223–237.

Feigl, E.O. (1975). Reflex parasympathetic coronary vasodilatation elicited from cardiac receptors in the dog. *Circ Res*, **37**, 175–182.

Feigl, E.O. (1975). Control of myocardial oxygen tension by sympathetic coronary vasoconstriction in the dog. *Circ Res*, **37**, 88–95.

Feigl, E.O. (1983). Coronary physiology. *Physiol Rev*, **63**, 1–205.

Feigl, E.O. (1987). The paradox of adrenergic coronary vasoconstriction. *Circulation*, **76**, 737–745.

Felder, R.B. and Thames, M.D. (1981). The cardiocardiac sympathetic reflex response during coronary occlusion in anaesthetized dogs. *Circ Res*, **48**, 685–692.

Feldman, R.L., Whittle, J.L., Marx, J.D., Pepine, C.J. and Conti, C.R. (1982). Regional coronary haemodynamic responses to cold stimulation in patients without variant angina. *Am J Cardiol*, **49**, 665–673.

Feldman, R.L., Whittle, J.L., Pepine, C.J. and Conti, C.R. (1981). Regional coronary angiographic observations during cold stimulation in patients with exertional chest pain: comparison of diameter responses in normal and fixed stenotic vessels. *Am Heart J*, **102**, 822–830.

Furchgott, R.F., Zawadzki, J.V. and Cherry, P.D. (1981). Role of endothelium in the vasodilator response to acetylcholine. In *Vasodilatation*, edited by P.M. Vanhoutte and I. Leusen, pp. 49–66. New York: Raven Press.

Gebremedhin, D., Koltai, M.Z., Pogatsa, G., Magyar, K. and Hadhazy, P. (1988). Influence of experimental diabetes on the mechanical responses of canine coronary arteries: role of endothelium. *Cardiovasc Res*, **22**, 537–544.

Gerritsen, M.E. (1987). Eicosanoid production by the coronary microvascular endothelium. *Fed Proc*, **46**, 47–53.

Gilbert, N.C., Fenn, G.K. and LeRoy, G.V. (1940). The effect of distention of abdominal viscera. *JAMA*, **115**, 1962–1967.

Ginsburg, R., Bristow, M.R. and Davis, K.B. (1984). Receptor mechanisms in the human epicardial coronary artery. *Circ Res*, **55**, 416–421.

Giubbini, R., Galli, M., Campini, R., Bosimini, E., Beneivelli, W. and Tavazzi, L. (1991). Effects of mental stress on myocardial perfusion in patients with ischemic heart disease. *Circulation*, **83**, II-100–II-107.

Giudicelli, J.F., Berdeaux, A., Tato, F. and Garnier, M. (1980). Left stellate stimulation-regional myocardial flows and ischemic injury in dogs. *Am J Physiol*, **239**, H359–H364.

Goodson, A.R., LaMaster, T.S. and Gutterman, D.D. (1993). Coronary constrictor pathway from anterior hypothalamus includes neurons in rostroventrolateral medulla. *Am J Physiol*, **265**, R1311–R1317.

Gorman, M.W. and Sparks, H.V., Jr. (1982). Progressive coronary vasoconstriction during relative ischemia in canine myocardium. *Circ Res*, **51**, 411–420.

Greenhoot, J.H. and Reichenbach, D.D. (1969). Cardiac injury and subarachnoid haemorrhage: a clinical, pathological, and physiological correlation. *J Neurosurg*, **30**, 521–531.

Gutterman, D.D., Bonham, A.C., Arthur, J.M., Gebhart, G.F., Marcus, M.L. and Brody, M.J. (1989). Characterization of coronary vasoconstrictor site in medullary reticular formation. *Am J Physiol*, **256**, H1218–H1227.

Gutterman, D.D., Bonham, A.C., Gebhart, G.F., Marcus, M.L. and Brody, M.J. (1990). Connections between hypothalamus and medullary reticular formation mediate coronary vasoconstriction. *Am J Physiol*, **259**, H917–H924.

Gutterman, D.D., Gebhart, G.F., Arthur, J.M., Clothier, J.L., Pardubsky, P., Marcus, M.L., *et al.* (1991). Baroreflex-mediated coronary vasoconstriction involves relays through medullary lateral reticular formation. *Brain Res*, **557**, 202–209.

Gutterman, D.D., Marcus, M.L. and Brody, M.J. (1996). Participation of parabrachial nuclear region in baroreflex coronary vasoconstriction. *Am J Physiol*, in press.

Gutterman, D.D., Morgan, D.A. and Dellsperger, K.C. (1992). Differential coronary response to norepinephrine and sympathetic stimulation in diabetic dogs. *Circulation*, **84**, II-558 (Abstract).

Gutterman, D.D., Morgan, D.A. and Miller, F.J. (1992). Effect of brief myocardial ischemia on sympathetic coronary vasoconstriction. *Circ Res*, **71**(4), 960–969.

Guyton, A.C. (1948). Acute hypertension in dogs with cerebral ischemia. *Am J Physiol*, **154**, 45–54.

Hackett, J.G., Abboud, F.M., Mark, A.L., Schmid, P.G. and Heistad, D.D. (1972). Coronary vascular responses to stimulation of chemoreceptors and baroreceptors. *Circ Res*, **31**, 8–17.

Hamilton, F.N. and Feigl, E.O. (1976). Coronary vascular sympathetic β-receptor innervation. *Am J Physiol*, **230**, 1569–1576.

Hammermeister, K.E. and Reichenbach, D.D. (1969). QRS changes, pulmonary edema, and myocardial necrosis associated with subarachnoid haemorrhage. *Am Heart J*, **78**, 94–100.

Hattori, Y., Kawasaki, H., Abe, K. and Kanno, M. (1991). Superoxide dismutase recovers altered endothelium-dependent relaxation in diabetic rat aorta. *Am J Physiol*, **261**, H1086–H1094.

Hayashi, M., Aizawa, Y., Satoh, M., Suzuki, K. and Shibata, A. (1986). Effect of nifedipine on neuropeptide Y-induced coronary vasoconstriction in anaesthetized dogs. *Jpn Heart J*, **27**, 251–257.

Hersch, C. (1964). Electrocardiographic changes in subarachnoid haemorrhage, meningitis, and intracranial space-occupying lesions. *Br Heart J*, **26**, 785–793.

Heusch, G. and Deussen, A. (1983). The effects of cardiac sympathetic nerve stimulation on perfusion of stenotic coronary arteries in the dog. *Circ Res*, **53**, 8–15.

Heusch, G., Deussen, A., Schipke, J. and Thamer, V. (1984). α_1- and α_2-adrenoceptor-mediated vasoconstriction of large and small canine coronary arteries *in vivo*. *J Cardiovasc Pharmacol*, **6**, 961–968.

Heusch, G., Deussen, A. and Thamer, V. (1985). Cardiac sympathetic nerve activity and progressive vasoconstriction distal to coronary stenoses: feed-back aggravation of myocardial ischemia. *J Auton Nerv Syst*, **13**, 311–326.

Hilton, S.M. and Smith, P.R. (1984). Ventral medullary neurones excited from the hypothalamic and mid-brain defence areas. *J Auton Nerv Syst*, **11**, 35–42.

Hirsch, E.F. and Borghard-Erdle, A.M. (1961). The innervation of the human heart. I The coronary arteries and the myocardium. *Arch Path*, **71**, 384–407.

Hodgson, J.M. and Marshall, J.J. (1989). Direct vasoconstriction and endothelium-dependent vasodilatation. Mechanisms of acetylcholine effects on coronary flow and arterial diameter in patients with nonstenotic coronary arteries. *Circulation*, **79**(5), 1043–1051.

Horio, Y., Yasue, H., Rokutanda, M., Nakamura, N., Ogawa, H., Takaoka, K., *et al.* (1986). Effects of intracoronary injection of acetylcholine on coronary arterial diameter. *Am J Cardiol*, **57**, 984–989.

Huang, A.H. and Feigl, E.O. (1988). Adrenergic coronary vasoconstriction helps maintain uniform transmural blood flow distribution during exercise. *Circ Res*, **62**, 286–298.

Inoue, H., Skale, B.T. and Zipes, D.P. (1988). Effects of ischemia on cardiac afferent sympathetic and vagal reflexes in dog. *Am J Physiol*, **255**, H26–H35.

Ito, B.R. and Feigl, E.O. (1985). Carotid baroreceptor reflex coronary vasodilatation in the dog. *Circ Res*, **56**, 486–495.

Ito, Y., Kitamura, K. and Kuriyama, H. (1979). Effects of acetylcholine and catecholamines on the smooth muscle cell of the porcine coronary artery. *J Physiol (Lond)*, **294**, 595–611.

Johannsen, U.J., Mark, A.L. and Marcus, M.L. (1982). Responsiveness to cardiac sympathetic nerve stimulation during maximal coronary dilation produced by adenosine. *Circ Res*, **50**, 510–517.

Jones, L.F., Gutterman, D.D. and Brody, M.J. (1992). Patterns of haemodynamic responses associated with central activation of coronary vasoconstriction. *Am J Physiol*, **262**, R276–R283.

Joyce, E.E. and Gregg, D.E. (1967). Coronary artery occlusion in the intact unanaesthetized dog: Intercoronary reflexes. *Am J Physiol*, **213**, 64–70.

Kelley, K.O. and Feigl, E.O. (1978). Segmental α-receptor-mediated vasoconstriction in the canine coronary circulation. *Circ Res*, **43**, 908–917.

Knight, D.R., Shen, Y.T., Young, M.A. and Vatner, S.F. (1987). Cholinergic coronary vasoconstriction in conscious calves. *Fed Proc*, **46**, 1240 (Abstract).

Koltai, M.Z., Jermendy, G., Kiss, V., Wagner, M. and Pogatsa, G. (1984). The effects of sympathetic stimulation and adenosine on coronary circulation and heart function in diabetes mellitus. *Acta Physiol Hung*, **63**, 119–125.

Koltai, M.Z., Rosen, P., Hadhazy, P., Ballagi-Pordany, G., Koszeghy, A. and Pogatsa, G. (1988). Relationship between vascular adrenergic receptors and prostaglandin biosynthesis in canine diabetic coronary arteries. *Diabetologia*, **31**, 681–686.

Koltai, M.Z., Rosen, P. and Pogatsa, G. (1989) Diminished vasodilatation; imbalance of synthesized cyclooxygenase products by adrenergic mediation in diabetic coronaries of the dog. In *Prostaglandins in Clinical Research: Cardiovascular System*, Anonymous, pp. 449–453. Alan R. Liss, Inc.

Krokhina, E.M. (1969). The adrenergic component of the effector heart innervation. *Acta Anat*, **74**, 214–227.

L'Abbate, A., Simonetti, I., Carpeggiani. C. and Michelassi, C. (1991). Coronary dynamics and mental arithmetic stress in humans. *Circulation*, **83**, II-94–II-99.

Laxson, D.D., Dai, X.Z., Homans, D.C. and Bache, R.J. (1989). The role of α_1- and α_2-adrenergic receptors in mediation of coronary vasoconstriction in hypoperfused ischemic myocardium during exercise. *Circ Res*, **65**, 1688–1697.

Levy, M.N., Ng, M.L. and Zieske, H. (1968). Cardiac response to cephalic ischemia. *Am J Physiol*, **215**, 169–175.

Lundberg, J.M., Pernow, J. and Lacroix, J.S. (1989). Neuropeptide Y: sympathetic cotransmitter and modulator. *NIPS*, **4**, 13–17.

Malliani, A., Schwartz, P.J. and Zanchetti, A. (1969). A sympathetic reflex elicited by experimental coronary occlusion. *Am J Physiol*, **217**, 703–709.

Manning, G.W., McEachem, C.G. and Hall, G.E. (1939). Reflex coronary artery spasm following sudden occlusion of other coronary branches. *Arch Int Med*, **64**, 661–674.

Marchetti, G., Merlo, L. and Noseda, V. (1968). Response of coronary blood flow to some natural stresses of excitement in the conscious dog. *Pflügers Arch*, **298**, 200–212.

Marcus, M.L. (1983). The coronary circulation in health and disease. New York: McGraw Hill.

Martin, J.R., Kneupfer, M.M. and Westfall, T.C. (1991). Haemodynamic effects of posterior hypothalamic injection of neuropeptide Y in awake rats. *Am J Physiol*, **261**, H814–H824.

Martins, J.B., Kerber, R.E., Marcus, M.L., Laughlin, D.E. and Levy, D.M. (1980). Inhibition of adrenergic neurotransmission in ischaemic regions of the canine left ventricle. *Cardiovasc Res*, **14**, 116–124.

Martins, J.B., Lewis, R.M., Lund, D.D. and Schmid, P.G. (1987). A thin subendocardial infarction produces cholinergic denervation overlying normal epicardium. *J Am Coll Cardiol*, **9**, 94A (Abstract).

Martins, J.B. and Zipes, D.P. (1980). Epicardial phenol interrupts refractory period responses to sympathetic but not vagal stimulation in canine left ventricular epicardium and endocardium. *Circ Res*, **47**, 33–40.

Matsumoto, T., Kinoshita, M. and Toda, N. (1993). Mechanisms of endothelium-dependent responses to vasoactive agents in isolated porcine coronary arteries. *J Card Pharmacol*, **22**, 228–234.

Maturi, M.F., Greene, R., Speir, E., Burrus, C., Dorsey, L.M.A., Markle, D.R., *et al.* (1989). Neuropeptide Y. *J Clin Invest*, **83**, 1217–1224.

Mayhan, W.G., Simmons, L.K. and Sharpe, G.M. (1991). Mechanism of impaired responses of cerebral arterioles during diabetes mellitus. *Am J Physiol*, **260**, H319–H326.

McKibben, J.S. and Getty, R. (1968). A comparative morphologic study of the cardiac innervation in domestic animals. ii. The feline. *Am J Anat*, **122**(3), 545–553.

McRaven, D.R., Mark, A.L., Abboud, F.M. and Mayer, H.E. (1971). Responses of coronary vessels to adrenergic stimuli. *J Clin Invest*, **50**, 773–778.

Melville, K.I., Blum, B., Shister, H.E. and Silver, M.D. (1963). Cardiac ischemic changes and arrhythmias induced by hypothalamic stimulation. *Am J Cardiol*, **12**, 781–791.

Miller, F.J., Marcus, M.L., Brody, M.J. and Gutterman, D.D. (1991). Activation in the region of parabrachial nucleus elicits neurogenically mediated coronary vasoconstriction. *Am J Physiol*, **261**, H1585–H1596.

Miura, M. and Reis, D.J. (1969). Termination and secondary projections of carotid sinus nerve in the cat brainstem. *Am J Physiol*, **217**, 142–153.

Miyashiro, J.K. and Feigl, E.O. (1993). Feedforward control of coronary blood flow via coronary β-receptor stimulation. *Circ Res*, **73**, 252–263.

Miyazaki, T. and Zipes, D.P. (1990). Presynaptic modulation of efferent sympathetic and vagal neurotransmission in the canine heart by hypoxia, high K^+, low pH, and adenosine. *Circ Res*, **66**, 289–301.

Mohrman, D.E. and Feigl, E.O. (1978). Competition between sympathetic vasoconstriction and metabolic vasodilatation in the canine coronary circulation. *Circ Res*, **42**(1), 79–86.

Moore, G.E. and Parratt, J.R. (1977). The effects of distension of the small intestine on myocardial blood flow in anaesthetised cats: possible relevance to coronary vasospasm. *Basic Res Cardiol*, **72**(5), 437–443.

Mudge, G.H., Jr., Grossman, W., Mills, R.M., Jr., Lesch, M. and Braunwald, E.B. (1976). Reflex increase in coronary vascular resistance in patients with ischemic heart disease. *NEJM*, **295**, 1333–1337.

Murray, P.A., Lavallee, M. and Vatner, S.F. (1984). α adrenergic-mediated reduction in coronary blood flow secondary to carotid chemoreceptor reflex activation in conscious dogs. *Circ Res*, **54**, 96–106.

Murray, P.A. and Vatner, S.F. (1981). Carotid sinus baroreceptor control of right coronary circulation in normal, hypertrophied, and failing right ventricles of conscious dogs. *Circ Res*, **49**, 1339–1349.

Nagata, M., Pichet, R. and Lavallee, M. (1988). Coronary dilation with carotid chemoreceptor stimulation in cardiac-denervated dogs. *Am J Physiol*, **255**, H1330–H1335.

Neely, B.H. and Hageman, G.R. (1990). Differential cardiac sympathetic activity during acute myocardial ischemia. *Am J Physiol*, **258**, H1534–H1541.

Ordway, G.A. and Pitetti, K.H. (1986). Stimulation of pulmonary C fibres decreases coronary arterial resistance in dogs. *J Physiol*, **371**, 277–288.

Paul, R.K., Gutterman, D.D. and Brody, M.J. (1990). Induction of neurogenic coronary vasoconstriction from spinal cord is asymmetrical. *Circulation*, **82**, III-636 (Abstract).

Paul, R.K., Gutterman, D.D., Marcus, M.L. and Brody, M.J. (1989). Medullary sites projecting to spinal preganglionic neurons mediate coronary constriction in cat. *Circulation*, **80**, II-311 (Abstract).

Paul, R.K., Gutterman, D.D., Marcus, M.L. and Brody, M.J. (1990). Coronary vasoconstriction results from site-specific activation of thoracic spinal cord. *Faseb J*, **4**, A402 (Abstract).

Peronnet, F., Nadeau, R., Boudreau, G., Cardinal, R., Lamontagne, D., Yamaguchi, N., *et al.* (1988). Epinephrine release from the heart during left stellate ganglion stimulation in dogs. *Am J Physiol*, **254**, R659–R662.

Pettersen, M.D., Morgan, D.A. and Gutterman, D.D. (1995). Role of adenosine in postischemic dysfunction of coronary innervation. *Circ Res*, **76**, 95–101.

Reid, J.V.O., Ito, B.R., Huang, A.H., Buffington, C.W. and Feigl, E.O. (1985). Parasympathetic control of transmural coronary blood flow in dogs. *Am J Physiol*, **249**, H337–H343.

Reimer, K.A., Lowe, J.E., Rasmussen, M.M. and Jennings, R.B. (1977). The wavefront phenomenon of ischemic cell death. I Myocardial infarct size vs duration of coronary occlusion in dogs. *Circulation*, **56**, 786–794.

Rodger, J.C., Railton, R., Parekh, P. and Newman, P.P. (1984). Effect of cold stimulation on myocardial perfusion. An investigation using thallium-201 scintigraphy. *Br Heart J*, **52**, 57–62.

Ross, G. (1976). Adrenergic responses of the coronary vessels. *Circ Res*, **39**, 461–465.

Rozanski, A., Bariey, C.N., Krantz, D.S., Friedman, J., Resser K.J., Morrell, M., *et al.* (1988). Mental stress and the induction of silent myocardial ischemia in patients with coronary artery disease. *NEJM*, **318**, 1105–1012.

Ruderman, N., Williamson, J. and Brownlee. M. (1992). Hyperglycemia, diabetes, and vascular disease. New York: Oxford University Press.

Seitelberger, R., Guth, B.D., Heusch, G., Lee, J.D., Katayama, K. and Ross, J.M., Jr. (1988). Intracoronary α_2-adrenergic receptor blockade attenuates ischemia in conscious dogs during exercise. *Circ Res*, **62**, 436–442.

Shaffer, R.A., Davisson, R.L., Murphy, S.P., Boutelle, S.L.P. and Lewis, S.J. (1993). Immunohistochemical evidence that post-ganglionic sympathetic neurons innervating hindlimb vasculature in rat contain nitric oxide synthase. *Circulation*, **88**, I-425 (Abstract).

Shepherd, J.T. and Vanhoutte, P.M. (1984). Why nerves to coronary vessels. *Fed Proc*, **43**, 2855–2856.

Taira, N., Satoh, K., Maruyama, M. and Yamashita, S. (1983). Sustained coronary constriction and its antagonism by calcium-blocking agents in monkeys and baboons. *Circ Res*, **52**, I40–I46.

Taylor, R.B. and Weaver, L.C. (1992). Spinal stimulation to locate preganglionic neurons controlling the kidney, spleen, or intestine. *Am J Physiol*, **263**, H1026–H1033.

Tesfamariam, B., Jakubowski, J.A. and Cohen, R.A. (1989). Contraction of diabetic rabbit aorta caused by endothelium-derived pgh2-txa2. *Am J Physiol*, **257**, H1327–H1333.

Thomas, J.X., Jr., Jones, C.E. and Randall, W.C. (1988). Neural modulation of coronary blood flow. In *Anonymous*, pp. 178–198.

Tiedt, N. and Religa, A. (1979). Vagal control of coronary blood flow in dogs. *Basic Res Cardiol*, **74**, 267–276.

Toda, N. and Okamura, T. (1989). Endothelium-dependent and independent responses to vasoactive substances of isolated human coronary arteries. *Am J Physiol*, **257**, H988–H995.

Trimarco, B., Vigorito, C., Cuocolo, A., Ricciardelli, B., De Luca, N., Volpe, M., *et al.* (1988). Reflex control of coronary vascular tone by cardiopulmonary receptors in humans. *J Am Coll Cardiol*, **11**, 944–952.

Van Winkle, D.M. and Feigl, E.O. (1989). Acetylcholine causes coronary vasodilatation in dogs and baboons. *Circ Res*, **65**, 1580–1593.

Vatner, S.F., Franklin, D., Van Citters, R.L. and Braunwald, E.B. (1970). Effects of carotid sinus nerve stimulation on the coronary circulation of the conscious dog. *Circ Res*, **27**, 11–21.

Vatner, S.F. and McRitchie, R.J. (1975). Interaction of the chemoreflex and the pulmonary inflation reflex in the regulation of coronary circulation in conscious dogs. *Circ Res*, **37**, 664–673.

Verrier, R.L., Hagestad, E.L. and Lown, B. (1987). Delayed myocardial ischemia induced by anger. *Circulation*, **75**(1), 249–254.

Volpe, M., Trimarco, B., Cuocolo, A., Vigorito, C., Cicala, M., Ricciardelli, B., *et al.* (1985). Carotid sinus reflex control of coronary blood flow in human subjects. *J Am Coll Cardiol*, **5**(6), 1312–1318.

Wangler, R.D., Peters, K.G., Laughlin, D.E., Tomanek, R.J. and Marcus, M.L. (1981). A method for continuously assessing coronary blood flow velocity in the rat. *Am J Physiol*, **241**, H816–H820.

Wilson, R.F., Marcus, M.L., Laughlin, D.E., Hartley, C.J. and White, C.W. (1984). The pulmonary inflation reflex: its physiological significance in conscious humans. *Fed Proc*, **43**, 1003 (Abstract).

Yardley, C.P. and Hilton, S.M. (1986). The hypothalamic and brainstem areas from which the cardiovascular and behavioural components of the defence reaction are elicited in the rat. *J Auton Nerv Syst*, **15**, 227–244.

Yasue, H., Matsuyama, K., Okumura, K., Morikami, Y. and Ogawa, H. (1990). Responses of angiographically normal human coronary arteries to intracoronary injection of acetylcholine by age and segment. *Circulation*, **81**, 482–490.

Yonekura, S., Watanabe, N. and Downey, H.F. (1988). Transmural variation in autoregulation of right ventricular blood flow. *Circ Res*, **62**, 776–781.

9 Skeletal Muscle Circulation

Paul Hjemdahl[1] and Thomas Kahan[2]

[1]*Department of Clinical Pharmacology, Karolinska Hospital,*
  S-171 76 Stockholm, Sweden
[2]*Division of Internal Medicine, Karolinska Institute, Danderyd Hospital,*
  S-182 88 Danderyd, Sweden

Electrical or reflex activation of sympathetic nerves evokes intensity-dependent, and marked vasoconstriction in skeletal muscle. Precapillary resistance increases considerably more than postcapillary resistance. Venous responses may, at least in part, be related to changes in flow. The effects are mediated mainly by the principal transmitter noradrenaline (NA), but non-adrenergic vasoconstriction contributes. NA and adrenaline (ADR) are non-selective α-adrenoceptor agonists, but the transmitter NA is β_1-adrenoceptor selective, and the circulating hormone, ADR, is β_2-adrenoceptor selective. Neuronal NA seems to preferentially stimulate α_1-adrenoceptors, and circulating catecholamines α_2-adrenoceptors. Circulating ADR is a potent vasodilator in skeletal muscle (through β_2-adrenoceptor stimulation), but variations of neurogenic influences are usually more important for blood flow regulation. Microcirculatory responses related to β_2-adrenoceptor stimulation, which promote fluid mobilization during haemorrhage, seem to be caused by NA. Prejunctional α_2-adrenoceptor-mediated inhibition of NA release is pronounced, whereas the evidence for important prejunctional β_2-adrenoceptor-mediated facilitation of NA release is weak. Circulating angiotensin (Ang) II may enhance sympathetic neurotransmission postjunctionally, but does not influence NA overflow from canine skeletal muscle. Locally generated Ang II may enhance NA release slightly. The effects of angiotensin-converting enzyme inhibition are complex and also involve bradykinin accumulation and prostaglandin formation (which enhance and reduce NA release, respectively). Skeletal muscle sympathetic nerve activity is tonically regulated by cardiopulmonary receptors and phasically by high-pressure receptors. Sympathetic nerve activity to skeletal muscle increases with a wide variety of stimuli, including mental stress, although the latter elicits vasodilatation. ADR explains only part of this stress-induced vasodilatation. Cholinergic vasodilator fibres may be involved in neurogenic skeletal muscle vasodilatation in several species, and seem to exist also in man. Peptidergic vasodilator nerves exist, but their physiological importance is unknown. Local metabolic and myogenic mechanisms also influence skeletal muscle blood flow. Activation of the sympathetic nervous system may result in markedly differentiated changes in nerve activity, with differences even between arm and leg muscle. Studies of sympathetic mechanisms should therefore focus specifically on a well-defined region and extrapolation to other regions is hazardous.

KEY WORDS: sympathetic neurotransmission; renin-angiotensin system; adrenoceptors; non-adrenergic neuro-transmission; cholinergic vasodilatation; physiological provocations.

GENERAL

Skeletal muscle comprises a large part of the body and contributes importantly to the regulation of the total peripheral resistance. Sympathetic postganglionic noradrenergic nerves supply smooth muscle cells of arteries and arterioles in skeletal muscle (Falck, 1962; Fuxe and Sedvall, 1965; Marshall, 1982). Sympathetic nerve stimulation increases vascular resistance in skeletal muscle in a frequency-dependent manner (Mellander and Johansson, 1968; Shepherd, 1984). The finding that sympathetic nerve stimulation reduced the tissue volume of the hindquarters of the cat, blood perfused at constant pressure, suggested that the veins in skeletal muscle are also under sympathetic neurogenic control (Mellander, 1960). However, the changes are relatively small, and may also be related to constriction of arterial resistance vessels and flow-dependent reductions of venous distending pressures (Öberg, 1964). The latter explanation is supported by observations in, e.g., the rat spinotrapezius muscle (Marshall, 1982), and in the canine isolated hindleg (Hainsworth et al., 1983). Thus, evidence favouring an important neurogenic control of venous tone in skeletal muscle seems to be weak (Hainsworth, 1986), even if opinions do differ in this respect (Mellander and Johansson, 1968). Whichever mechanism predominates, it is clear that sympathetic stimulation does mobilize blood from the tissue by decreasing the venous volume.

Sympathetic nerve function is important in the regulation of skeletal muscle resistance and microcirculatory function, including solute exchange and fluid balance (Renkin, 1984). Consistent with histochemical findings, the whole arterial vascular tree seems to be constricted upon sympathetic nerve stimulation (Marshall, 1982; Dodd and Johnson, 1991). The increase in proximal arterial resistance, which appears to be a major determinant for the elevation of the total skeletal muscle vascular resistance during sympathetic nerve stimulation, develops gradually and is well maintained (Figure 9.1). The rapid and pronounced increase in microvessel resistance, on the other hand, gradually wanes and returns to basal levels, even though nerve stimulation is sustained (Folkow, Sonnenschein and Wright, 1971; Lundvall and Järhult, 1976; Marshall, 1982; Dodd and Johnson, 1991).

Precapillary resistance increases more markedly than postcapillary resistance during sympathetic nerve stimulation in skeletal muscle. This lowers the capillary pressure and promotes the mobilization of interstitial fluid into the blood stream (Öberg, 1964). The exchange of fluid and solutes between tissue and blood depends on hydrostatic forces, the perfused capillary area and the permeability of the capillaries, in addition to the colloid osmotic pressure. Sympathetic nerve stimulation reduces the exchange of diffusible solutes between blood and tissue in skeletal muscle, mainly due to a reduction of the perfused capillary area, as the filtration coefficient decreases only transiently (Renkin, 1984). Autoregulation of blood flow in skeletal muscle is both myogenic and metabolic (Mellander and Johansson, 1968; Renkin, 1984; Shepherd, 1984). These powerful autoregulatory mechanisms rapidly counteract the effects of vasoconstriction on capillary permeability. Exercise hyperaemia increases capillary perfusion, diffusion capacity and solute exchange in the muscle. Many factors contribute to the hyperaemia in connection with muscular exercise, which can be quite pronounced (Shepherd, 1984; Saltin, 1988).

Previous more extensive reviews on blood flow to skeletal muscle and the mechanisms controlling it (e.g., Mellander and Johansson, 1968; Renkin, 1984: Shepherd, 1984) contain more complete references to the vast literature in the field than those given by us.

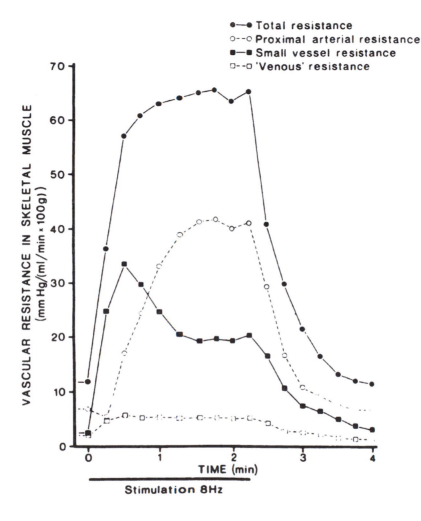

Figure 9.1   Time courses for the development of vascular resistances of various segments of the vascular tree in skeletal muscle during and after high-frequency (8 Hz) nerve stimulation. (From Lundvall and Järhult (1976), with permission.)

SYMPATHO-ADRENAL MECHANISMS

Sympathetic nerves to the skeletal muscle vascular bed display activity, even at rest (Delius *et al.*, 1972a, 1972b; Wallin and Fagius, 1988). Nerve stimulation at constant frequencies of 0.5–2 Hz produces vasoconstriction comparable to the resting tone in skeletal muscle (Folkow, 1952; Renkin, 1984). The average discharge rate in sympathetic vasomotor fibres to skeletal muscle rarely exceeds 8–10 Hz under physiological conditions, and 85% of the maximal vasoconstrictor response is attained at about 6–8 Hz (Folkow, 1952; Mellander and Johansson, 1968). However, individual bursts of impulses in such nerves may display very high frequencies even at a low average firing rate (Wallin and Fagius, 1988). It seems reasonable to assume that the average impulse frequencies in sympathetic nerves to skeletal muscle are approximately 0.5–6 Hz under most conditions, even if higher frequencies occur intermittently. Sympathetic nerve stimulation releases noradrenaline (NA), the principal transmitter in sympathetic nerves. There is also a small amount of dopamine in skeletal muscle (Kahan, Hjemdahl and Dahlöf, 1984); this probably represents precursor dopamine used for the synthesis of NA and no importance has yet been attributed to neurogenic dopamine in skeletal muscle. There are also both pre- and postjunctional dopaminergic receptors in skeletal muscle, but they are mainly targets for pharmacological manipulation and we will, therefore, not dwell on them. Adrenaline (ADR) acts as a circulating hormone released from the adrenal medullae. In canine skeletal muscle we have found that ADR levels are only about 2% of those of NA (Kahan, Hjemdahl and Dahlöf, 1984) and that only 1% of the catecholamines released from skeletal muscle upon nerve stimulation represents ADR (Kahan, Hjemdahl and Dahlöf, 1987). We are unaware of studies showing preferential or substantial release of ADR from sympathetic nerves under physiological conditions, which is of importance when discussing the possible role of ADR as a cotransmitter (*see below*).

METHODS USED TO ASSESS SYMPATHETIC ACTIVITY

Axonal muscle sympathetic nerve activity (MSA) can be evaluated electrophysiologically. The technically demanding, but very valuable, microneurographic recording technique of Wallin and coworkers (Delius *et al.*, 1972a, 1972b) has gained considerable popularity in the past few years, and has provided us with important information on the neurogenic regulation of the vasculature of human skeletal muscle. MSA occurs in pulse-synchronous bursts, which appear to serve an important role to buffer blood pressure variability. The strength of individual bursts may be integrated in order to obtain better information concerning the changes in nerve impulse activity than that obtained in earlier studies, which only quantitated burst frequency. However, single unit recordings are rare, and the actual impulse frequency can, therefore, seldom be determined (recruitment of more nerve fibres cannot be distinguished from increased firing of individual nerve fibres in these recordings). For a recent account of methodological considerations and comparisons with activity in sympathetic nerves supplying skin, the other region that can be evaluated in man, see Wallin and Fagius (1988).

Sympathetic activity is often evaluated in terms of catecholamine levels in plasma. In support of this, several studies have shown frequency-related overflows of NA from individual organs to plasma upon sympathetic nerve stimulation; we have shown this for skeletal muscle (Kahan, Hjemdahl and Dahlöf, 1984). "Plasma NA" is usually used as an ill-defined measure of sympathetic activity in the literature. It is often said that plasma NA is a poor marker for sympathetic activity when results are disappointing, and the authors have not appreciated the complexity of this variable. Another confounding factor is, of course, poor assay precision (Hjemdahl, 1984), which may represent a considerable problem and explain many "negative" findings in the literature.

Sympathetic nerve activity is highly differentiated and may differ between organs and regions of the body, which means that a measurement of NA in plasma derived from an undefined source cannot be used to measure the discrete changes in various regions of the body which occur during physiological activation (Folkow et al., 1983; Hjemdahl, 1993). Actually, the term "sympathetic tone" should be abandoned, as it implies that sympathetic activity occurs in a synchronized fashion.

Plasma NA can be quite a good marker for sympathetic activity if its physiological determinants are understood. Arterial plasma NA concentrations usually reflect whole-body sympathetic nerve activity, but variations in NA clearance from plasma may necessitate measurements of NA "spillover" to plasma (Esler et al., 1988) in some situations. NA turnover in plasma is studied by radiotracer infusion techniques (^{3}H-NA), which might be influenced by back-diffusion of tracer taken up in the tissues to plasma (Henriksen and Christensen, 1989). The latter methodological objection has, however, been refuted (Eisenhofer et al., 1991).

When using plasma NA as a marker for sympathetic activity, it is important to understand the determinants of the NA actually measured in the sample. Due to the high extraction of NA in the human forearm ($\approx 50\%$ during one passage of blood) half of conventionally sampled antecubital venous plasma NA is derived from the arm, and half from the rest of the body (Hjemdahl et al., 1984; Hjemdahl, 1987). Thus, clinical and experimental studies using antecubital venous plasma NA levels as an index of sympathetic activity overemphasize local sympathetic activity in the arm, i.e. mainly forearm muscle sympathetic activity (skin and adipose tissue seem to contribute less). Indeed, venous plasma NA concentrations correlate quite well with MSA in humans (Wallin and Fagius, 1988).

The best approach for biochemical assessments of sympathetic nerve activity is to measure the local overflow of NA (veno-arterial concentration difference x plasma flow) from an individual organ of physiological or pathophysiological interest, i.e. from a defined region of the body. The extraction of NA from arterial plasma should then be evaluated, preferably by use of radiotracer techniques (Esler et al., 1988), in order to separate the arterial contribution to venous NA levels and locally derived NA. If that is not possible, ADR may be used as a marker for NA removal by the tissue (Brown et al., 1981; Hjemdahl, 1993: Lindqvist et al., 1993). The importance of evaluating the arterial contribution to NA overflow from the tissue is underscored by findings that the extraction of NA may vary with the blood flow (Chang et al., 1986; Goldstein et al., 1987; Hjemdahl et al., 1989). When comparing NA overflow from the leg and MSA in the same region, we found reasonably good correlations between the two parameters in humans, even though the biochemical one is based on several variables, each one with its experimental error (Hjemdahl et al., 1989).

Microneurographic recordings of MSA give valuable information on relative levels of (and changes in) axonal impulse activity. However, only a small fraction of all impulses that invade a sympathetic nerve varicosity actually releases the transmitter and evokes a postjunctional response (Brock and Cunnane, 1987; Stjärne, 1989). Thus, regulatory mechanisms at the prejunctional level may also be quite important for the end effect. Furthermore, MSA may display differentiated activity, with different responses to stressors in the arm and leg (Anderson, Wallin and Mark, 1987), even though MSA is highly correlated in the two regions at rest (Wallin and Fagius, 1988). Thus, as for catecholamines, conclusions regarding MSA should be restricted to the area actually studied.

Evaluation of sympathetic mechanisms in skeletal muscle (as in other organs) is thus complex and should preferably involve assessments of nerve activity and prejunctional events possibly modulating transmitter release, as well as the postjunctional sensitivity to the neurotransmitters involved and to circulating catecholamines. No single method gives complete and undebatable evidence. In addition, the large mass of skeletal muscle may be heterogenously regulated.

ADRENOCEPTOR CLASSIFICATION

NA and ADR will stimulate receptors, which initially were categorized into α- and β-adrenoceptors (Ahlquist, 1948). The β-adrenoceptors were later subdivided into β_1- and β_2-adrenoceptors (Lands et $al.$, 1967). α-Adrenoceptors have been subdivided into α_1- and α_2-adrenoceptors, initially based on post- and prejunctional anatomical localizations, respectively (Langer, 1974), but later based on their relative affinities for agonists and antagonists (Berthelsen and Pettinger, 1977). The latter classification has been generally accepted (Langer, 1981; Starke, 1981). A further subclassification of α_1- and α_2-adrenoceptors has been proposed more recently (Bylund, 1988: Minneman, 1988). Developments in molecular biology and pharmacology have led to a further subclassification of α-adrenoceptors into α_{1A-D} and α_{2A-D} (Flavahan and Vanhoutte, 1986; Lomasney et $al.$, 1991; Michel, Philipp and Brodde, 1992). The possible roles of all these new receptor subtypes in physiological responses have not yet been determined (Lomasney et $al.$, 1991; Wilson, Brown and McGrath, 1991). There are also atypical β-adrenoceptors, which have been classified as β_3, and seem to mediate sympathetic influences on metabolic processes in adipose tissue, the digestive tract and skeletal muscle (Emorine et $al.$, 1989; Zaagsma and Nahorski, 1990). In skeletal muscle, the atypical β_3-adrenoceptors may contribute to glycogenolysis, a response previously considered to be mediated by β_2-adrenoceptors (Emorine et $al.$, 1989).

   NA and ADR stimulate α-adrenoceptors non-selectively (Berthelsen and Pettinger, 1977; Starke, 1981), although ADR may display some selectivity for α_2-adrenoceptors in some systems (Hjemdahl, 1991). With regard to β-adrenoceptors, NA is clearly β_1-adrenoceptor selective (Lands et $al.$, 1967), whereas the selectivity of ADR is debated. In various biochemical and in $vitro$ based assay systems, where all receptors may be easily accessed, ADR seems to be non-selective (Lefkowitz, Caron and Stiles, 1984). However, when ADR reaches tissues via the blood stream it seems to be quite β_2-adrenoceptor selective from a functional point of view (Ariëns and Simonis, 1983; Hjemdahl and Schwieler, 1991), and even radioligand binding studies have shown β_2-adrenoceptor selectivity for ADR (Stiles, Caron and Lefkowitz, 1984). Thus, both the inherent properties of the agonist and the neuroanatomical localization of the receptors (in relation to the site of neurotransmitter release or blood, respectively) are of importance for the mechanisms studied.

POSTJUNCTIONAL ADRENERGIC MECHANISMS

α-Adrenoceptors

Nerve stimulation-evoked vasoconstriction in skeletal muscle is mediated via activation of both α_1- and α_2-adrenoceptors (Timmermans and van Zwieten, 1981; McGrath, 1982), but a non-adrenergic component can also be revealed (*see below*). Studies of vascular responses to sympathetic nerve stimulation and exogenous NA in the presence of various selective antagonists have suggested that postjunctional α_1-adrenoceptors are mainly activated by neuronally released NA, whereas postjunctional α_2-adrenoceptors play a dominant role in responses to circulating catecholamines (Langer, Massingham and Shepperson, 1980; Yamaguchi and Kopin, 1980; Wilffert, Timmermans and van Zwieten, 1982; Kahan, Hjemdahl and Dahlöf, 1987). This may be taken as support for a mainly extrajunctional localization of the α_2-adrenoceptors (Langer, Massingham and Shepperson, 1980; Wilffert, Timmermans and van Zwieten, 1982). However, postjunctional α_2-adrenoceptors also seem to participate in the nervous control of vascular tone in skeletal muscle (Gardiner and Peters, 1982; Elsner *et al.*, 1984; Kahan, Hjemdahl and Dahlöf, 1987). This may reflect moderate diffusion distances from the neuroeffector junction to more distantly located receptors. Indeed, nerve stimulation may evoke quite marked elevations of NA, even in the venous effluent from skeletal muscle.

Whereas both α-adrenoceptor subtypes seem to participate in the adrenergic regulation of large arteries and larger arterioles and venules, adrenergic vasoconstriction in precapillary arterioles may depend mainly on α_2-adrenoceptors; the latter may also predominate in large veins (Faber, 1988).

Circulating NA acts mainly as an α-adrenoceptor agonist reducing blood flow to skeletal muscle. Non-selective β-adrenoceptor blockade does not enhance vasoconstrictor responses to exogenous NA in denervated canine skeletal muscle (Hjemdahl and Fredholm, 1976), in agreement with the β_1-adrenoceptor selectivity of NA and the predominance of vascular β_2-adrenoceptors (see below).

In humans, locally infused NA reduces forearm blood flow (Barcroft *et al.*, 1954). After non-selective β-blockade, NA and ADR evoke similar, dose-dependent reductions of forearm blood flow (Jie *et al.*, 1986). Systemically infused NA also reduces blood flow in denervated or nerve-blocked forearms (Barcroft *et al.*, 1954), whereas flow may actually increase when the nerves are intact (Barcroft *et al.*, 1954; Chang *et al.*, 1988); the latter presumably relates to the elevation of the blood pressure and the baroreceptor-mediated withdrawal of vasoconstrictor nerve activity, as seen with other pressor substances (discussed below). In human calf skeletal muscle, however, circulating NA elicits a vasoconstrictor response which is similar to that seen in adipose tissue (Hjemdahl and Linde, 1983).

α-Adrenoceptors controlling muscle blood flow in man are of both subtypes, as intraarterial infusions of α_1- and α_2-adrenoceptor-selective antagonists both elicit forearm vasoconstriction (Jie *et al.*, 1984, 1986; Taddei, Salvetti and Pedrinelli, 1988). Vasoconstriction in the forearm evoked by NA or ADR after β-adrenoceptor blockade is mediated by both α-adrenoceptor subtypes, the dominating component being α_2-adrenoceptor-mediated (Jie *et al.*, 1987) in agreement with a preferential localization of these receptors extrajunctionally (see above). ADR evokes marked and dose-dependent α_2-adrenoceptor-mediated vasoconstriction in the forearm after β- and α_1-adrenoceptor blockade (Bolli *et al.*, 1988). Selective α_1-adrenoceptor blockade, by locally infused prazosin (Bühler *et al.*, 1983) or doxazosin (Jie *et al.*, 1987) attenuates neurogenic vasoconstriction in the forearm, whereas α_2-adrenoceptors are much less important for neurogenic forearm vasoconstriction in humans (Jie *et al.*, 1987).

β-Adrenoceptors

There seems to be a predominance of β_2-adrenoceptors in the skeletal muscle vasculature (Russel and Moran, 1980). Some authors have suggested that there may also be a subset of postjunctional β_1-adrenoceptors in the canine skeletal muscle vasculature (Vatner, Knight and Hintze, 1985; Dahlöf, Kahan and Åblad, 1987). Other studies point towards a pure population of vascular β_2-adrenoceptors in cat skeletal muscle (e.g. Hillman, 1983). Radioligand binding studies in biopsies of human skeletal muscle (which contain both vascular smooth muscle and other cells) have revealed a uniform population of β_2-adrenoceptors (Liggett, Shah and Crier, 1988). ADR would be expected to be the natural agonist for these receptors.

Non-selective (Kahan et al., 1988) or β_2-selective (Kahan and Hjemdahl, 1987b) β-adrenoceptor blockade elevates basal vascular tone in the denervated canine skeletal muscle, suggesting a physiological role for circulating ADR in the control of basal vascular tone in the tissue. Arterial ADR levels were only 0.2–0.3 nM in these experiments. However, locally infused propranolol does not influence blood flow to the human forearm (Brick et al., 1966), suggesting no β_2-adrenoceptor-mediated vasodilator activity (i.e., no ADR effect) at rest. Systemic β-adrenoceptor blockade, on the other hand, elevates basal vascular tone in innervated human skeletal muscle (Linde et al., 1989). β_1-Adrenoceptor-selective blockade had approximately half the effect of non-selective blockade in this respect, suggesting that reflexogenically increased vasoconstrictor nerve activity contributes to the flow reduction in order to compensate for the reduction of cardiac output following systemic β-adrenoceptor blockade (Linde et al., 1989).

There are marked vasodilator responses to circulating ADR in skeletal muscle in animals (Russel and Moran, 1980; Shepherd, 1984; Kahan, Hjemdahl and Dahlöf, 1987) and in humans (Allen, Barcroft and Edholm, 1946; Brick et al., 1966; Johnsson, 1975; Freyschuss et al., 1986), suggesting that the postjunctional vascular β_2-adrenoceptors are exquisitely sensitive to the mixed α- and β-adrenoceptor agonist, ADR. Experiments with i.v. or i.a. infusions of relatively high doses of ADR in humans have shown transient, marked, vasodilator responses to ADR in both the arm and leg, followed by only modestly increased flow (in some instances even vasoconstriction) during continued infusion (Allen, Barcroft and Edholm, 1946). This pattern persists in the forearm after nerve block or cervical sympathectomy (Whelan, 1952). Vasodilator responses to ADR are enhanced by the α-adrenoceptor antagonist, dibenamine (Nickerson, Henry and Nomaguchi, 1953), or by chlorpromazine (de la Lande and Whelan, 1959), suggesting that there is indeed a mixed influence of β-adrenocepor-mediated vasodilator and α-adrenoceptor-mediated vasoconstrictor components in muscle blood flow responses to ADR. There may also be a delayed and sustained increase in blood flow, which may be related to metabolic activation in the muscle (Barcroft and Cobbold, 1956).

Further analyses of the receptors mediating the vascular responses to ADR in humans were performed when more specific antagonists were developed. Following non-selective β-adrenoceptor blockade, potent vasoconstriction is revealed in the forearm during ADR infusions (Brick et al., 1966; Johnsson, 1975). Metoprolol attenuates this vasodilator response to ADR (Johnsson, 1975; van Heerwarden et al., 1977). This may be due to lack of β_1-adrenoceptor selectivity of metoprolol at the doses used, as we have found that a more β_1-adrenoceptor-selective antagonist (pafenolol) did not antagonize vasodilator responses to ADR (unpublished results). Thus, in humans, as in most animals, ADR-induced vasodilatation is β_2-adrenoceptor-mediated.

Postjunctional vascular β_2-adrenoceptors in skeletal muscle do not seem to be under neurogenic control (Russel and Moran, 1980; Wilffert, Timmermans and van Zwieten, 1982; Kahan and Hjemdahl, 1987b), although there are some conflicting results. These findings are compatible with an extrajunctional localization of the postjunctional β_2-adrenoceptors, which would be stimulated by circulating ADR (Russel and Moran, 1980; Wilffert, Timmermans and van Zwieten, 1982; Ariëns and Simonis, 1983). However, NA may also stimulate vascular β_2-adrenoceptors in skeletal muscle (Viveros, Garlick and Renkin, 1968; Hillman, 1983) and in other tissues (Hyman, Lipton and Kadowitz, 1990) under some conditions.

When hypotensive agents are given to rats in order to elicit marked reductions of blood pressure, the vasodilatation in skeletal muscle is attenuated by adrenal demedullation or by β_2-adrenoceptor antagonism, indicating a role for reflexogenically released ADR in this response (Gardiner and Bennett, 1988; Gardiner et al., 1992).

Vascular β_2-adrenoceptors may also be involved in the control of vascular volume. β-Adrenoceptor blockade by propranolol reduces nerve stimulation-induced increases in transcapillary fluid absorption (Lundvall and Järhult, 1976). Activation of β_2-adrenoceptors increases the capillary surface area available for fluid exchange and decreases the capillary hydrostatic pressure (Hillman, 1983; Gustafsson and Lundvall, 1984; Maspers and Björnberg, 1991), even though precapillary dilatation might be expected to increase the latter. This leads to transfer of extracellular fluid into the circulation, and thereby an increased intravascular volume (Hillman, Gustafsson and Lundvall, 1982; Hillman, 1983; Gustafsson and Lundvall, 1984). The effects may be elicited by circulating ADR, but neurogenically-released NA may contribute to the β_2-adrenoceptor-mediated increase in the functional capillary area and fluid transport in skeletal muscle; β_1-adrenoceptors do not seem to participate in these responses (Hillman, 1983). These mechanisms may contribute importantly to the intravascular volume restitution following haemorrhagic hypotension (Hillman, 1983; Gustafsson and Lundvall, 1984).

γ-Receptors

It has also been proposed that neuronally released NA may cause an α-adrenoceptor-independent vasoconstrictor response, via activation of adrenoceptors distinct from the classical receptors (i.e. γ-receptors; Hirst and Neild, 1980). However, the non-adrenergic component of sympathetic vasoconstriction can be elicited *in vivo* and *in vitro* following pretreatment with reserpine, which produces extensive loss of NA in the nerves (Kirkpatrick and Burnstock, 1987; Pernow, Kahan and Lundberg, 1988). These findings do not favour a role for γ-receptor stimulation by NA in the α-adrenoceptor-independent vasoconstrictor response to sympathetic nerve stimulation. In a later review, Hirst is more undecided as to whether fast excitatory junction potentials are related to non-typical NA receptors (i.e. γ-receptors) or to ATP (Hirst and Edwards, 1989). Possible non-adrenergic mechanisms are discussed below.

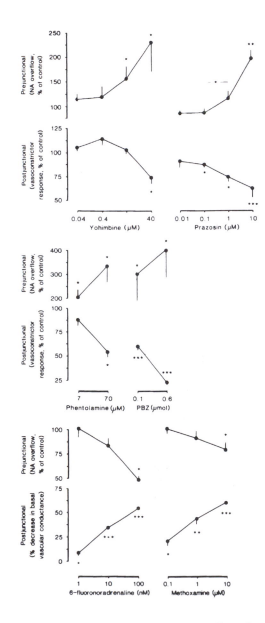

Figure 9.2   Pre- (NA overflow) and postjunctional (vasoconstriction) effects of α_1- and α_2-adrenoceptor-selective agonists and antagonists in canine skeletal muscle *in situ*. Neuronal uptake was inhibited by desipramine and possible muscarinic effects by atropine. The gracilis muscle used was acutely denervated and isolated from all surrounding tissues. Vasoconstriction was measured in terms of increases in perfusion pressure during constant flow perfusion. Both α_1- (methoxamine) and α_2-adrenoceptor-stimulation (6-fluoro-NA) had pre- and postjunctional effects, the former being predominantly (but not exclusively) α_2-adrenoceptor-mediated. Data with α_1-adrenoceptor-selective (prazosin), α_2-adrenoceptor-selective (yohimbine) or non-selective [phentolamine and phenoxybenzamine (PBZ) at the locally infused dose given] antagonists support this view. Significant changes are shown: *$P < 0.05$, **$P < 0.01$, ***$P < 0.001$. (From Kahan (1987), with permission.)

PREJUNCTIONAL ADRENERGIC MECHANISMS

The release of NA from sympathetic nerves in skeletal muscle is modulated by several local mechanisms. Activation of prejunctional α_2-adrenoceptors inhibits NA release (Langer, 1981; Starke, 1981, 1987). Data from canine skeletal muscle *in vivo* are shown in Figure 9.2. Some findings *in vitro* and *in vivo* suggest that there may be a subset of prejunctional α_1-adrenoceptors as well (Cavero *et al.*, 1979; Kobinger and Pichler, 1980; Docherty, 1984; Story, Standford-Starr and Rand, 1985; Hicks *et al.*, 1986). As shown in Figure 9.2, selective α_1-adrenoceptor blockade by prazosin enhanced, and selective α_1-adrenoceptor stimulation by methoxamine reduced sympathetic nerve stimulation-evoked NA overflow in canine skeletal muscle *in situ*, which would be compatible with this idea (Kahan, Dahlöf and Hjemdahl, 1987; Kahan and Hjemdahl, 1987a). However, lack of selectivity of the agents used and/or altered diffusion of NA from the neuroeffector junction to the blood stream may have contributed to the findings. Furthermore, prazosin possesses a relatively high affinity for the α_{2B}-adrenoceptor binding site (Turner, Pierce and Bylund, 1984; Nahorski, Barnett and Cheung, 1985), which may influence transmitter release. α_2-Adrenoceptor blockade by various agents causes pronounced increases in NA overflow from canine skeletal muscle (Kahan, Dahlöf and Hjemdahl, 1987) (Figure 9.2). Taken together, the findings indicate that skeletal muscle is richly endowed with inhibitory prejunctional α-adrenoceptors, which are mainly of the α_2-adrenoceptor subtype.

Studies *in vitro* provide considerable experimental evidence for prejunctional β_2-adrenoceptor-mediated facilitation of NA release (Dahlöf, 1981; Langer, 1981). In the cat hindleg, non-selective β-adrenoceptor blockade by propranolol reduces the vasoconstrictor response to sympathetic nerve stimulation slightly, indicating a prejunctional, β-adrenoceptor-mediated component in the response (Dahlöf, 1981). NA overflow studies in canine skeletal muscle *in situ* confirm the existence of this mechanism (Kahan and Hjemdahl, 1987b). Pharmacological β_2-adrenoceptor stimulation by isoprenaline or rimiterol produces increases in NA overflow at doses producing considerable vasodilatation (Figure 9.3). However, the effect of β_2-adrenoceptor stimulation on NA overflow is small, and α-adrenoceptor-mediated inhibition of NA release seems to be considerably more important (Kahan, Dahlöf and Hjemdahl, 1987; Kahan and Hjemdahl, 1987a) than β-adrenoceptor-mediated enhancement (Kahan and Hjemdahl, 1987b; Kahan, Hjemdahl and Dahlöf, 1987; Kahan *et al.*, 1988) in canine skeletal muscle.

Although β_2-adrenoceptor-mediated facilitation of NA release can be activated pharmacologically, and β-adrenoceptor blockade can reduce NA overflow (usually under conditions with very pronounced NA overflow, and in the presence of α-adrenoceptor blockade), we believe that the role for β-adrenoceptor-mediated prejunctional facilitation of NA release is weak compared to other regulatory mechanisms, and that its physiological importance remains to be demonstrated. The case for an important negative feedback mediated by prejunctional α_2-adrenoceptors is much stronger.

DOES ADRENALINE MODULATE SYMPATHETIC NEUROTRANSMISSION?

Low concentrations of ADR can enhance NA release from isolated tissues *in vitro*; thus circulating ADR may be the naturally occurring agonist for the prejunctional

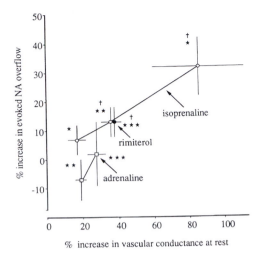

Figure 9.3 β-adrenoceptor-mediated alterations of NA overflow in relation to vasodilator responses (increases in vascular conductance) in canine skeletal muscle *in situ*. Experimental procedures as in Figure 9.2. Local infusions of isoprenaline (non-selective; 3, 15 and 42 nM in plasma) and rimiterol (β_2-selective; 50 nM in plasma) enhanced NA overflow at doses causing substantial vasodilatation. It should be noted that isoprenaline in humans causes considerable haemodynamic responses at ≈ 1 nM in plasma (cf. Hjemdahl, 1991). Intravenous infusions of the mixed α- and β_2-adrenoceptor-agonist, ADR, elicited vasodilatation, but did not influence NA overflow at arterial plasma concentrations of 1.7–6.3 nM. Not shown are findings with the β_2-adrenoceptor-selective antagonist ICI 118,551 that the responses to isoprenaline were indeed β_2-adrenoceptor-mediated (Kahan and Hjemdahl, 1987b). Significant changes are shown for vasodilator responses (*P < 0.05, **P < 0.01, ***P < 0.001) and for the enhancement of NA overflow (†P < 0.05). (Adapted from Kahan and Hjemdahl (1987b) and Kahan, Hjemdahl and Dahlöf (1987), with permission.)

β_2-adrenoceptor (Stjärne and Brundin, 1975). However, the nerves are more easily accessible in *in vitro* systems than they are from the blood stream (see Section on angiotensin, below). In our canine model, with blood-perfused skeletal muscle *in situ*, circulating ADR failed to enhance sympathetic nerve stimulation-induced NA overflow at arterial concentrations up to 6–10 nM (i.v. infusion rates of 0.4 nmol or 75 ng/kg/min), i.e., at concentrations that are seen only under extreme conditions (see Figure 9.3) (Kahan, Hjemdahl and Dahlöf, 1987; Schwieler *et al.*, 1992). These results might have been anticipated. First, relatively high concentrations of β_2-adrenoceptor agonists (based on postjunctional responses) were required to obtain fairly modest effects on NA overflow (Figure 9.3); the corresponding plasma concentration of ADR would most likely have been far above the physiological concentration range. Second, ADR would simultaneously activate prejunctional inhibitory α-adrenoceptors, which would counteract any β-adrenoceptor-mediated facilitation of NA release. We have recently tested the latter hypothesis and found that ADR also fails to enhance NA overflow in the presence of irreversible α-adrenoceptor blockade (Schwieler *et al.*, 1992). Thus, circulating ADR is a potent postjunctional β-adrenoceptor agonist in skeletal muscle, but mechanisms involving β_2-adrenoceptors may be questioned.

It is possible that NA may be the natural agonist for prejunctional β_2-adrenoceptors after all, since NA may cause postjunctional β_2-adrenoceptor-stimulation (see below). In agreement with this idea, propranolol causes a slight reduction of the stimulation-evoked overflow of NA from the canine gracilis muscle (Kahan et al., 1988; Schwieler et al., 1992), even though no responses to ADR could be demonstrated.

Elevations of plasma NA in an intact organism during infusions of ADR can not be taken as evidence for a prejunctional facilitatory action on NA release (Hjemdahl, 1991), as the pronounced vasodilator response to ADR elicits the expected reflexogenic activation of the sympathetic vasoconstrictor nerves (Persson et al., 1989) and knowledge of nerve impulse activity is mandatory when evaluating prejunctional mechanisms. The increase in NA overflow was somewhat larger than the increase in muscle sympathetic nerve activity, which might favour prejunctional facilitation of NA release. However, enhanced diffusibility from the neuroeffector junction to the blood stream cannot be ruled out.

Circulating ADR can be taken up into sympathetic nerves and re-released as a cotransmitter with NA (Guimaraes, Brandao and Paiva, 1978; Rand et al., 1979; Majewski, Rand and Tung, 1981; Floras, 1992); this would provide close access to prejunctional β_2-adrenoceptors. The ADR cotransmitter hypothesis has recently been reviewed and the interpretation was that cotransmitter ADR may be physiologically important, even if several data in the literature are incompatible with the theory (Floras, 1992).

When interpreting results obtained with ADR infusions as evidence for a cotransmitter role for ADR, it must be excluded that phenomena seen during or after an infusion of ADR are caused by postjunctional alterations, or changes in sympathetic axonal nerve impulse activity. For example, we (Persson et al., 1989) have observed a marked and long-lasting increase in muscle sympathetic nerve activity *after* the termination of ADR infusion in humans; this response was most likely caused by a sustained reduction of central venous pressure. Nerve impulse activity also increased during infusion, as mentioned above. Long-lasting reductions of plasma magnesium and calcium after ADR infusions (Joborn et al., 1990) might well be paralleled by intracellular events of importance for various after-effects following ADR infusion, which have been interpreted as evidence for cotransmitter actions of ADR. Thus, after-effects with enhanced responsiveness to physiological provocations and persisting increases in heart rate following ADR infusion (cf. Floras, 1992) may well be related to postjunctional changes in responsiveness or alterations of transmitter release, unrelated to prejunctional β_2-adrenoceptor stimulation by cotransmitter ADR.

If cotransmitter ADR were to facilitate sympathetic neurotransmission it would have to display selectivity for the prejunctional β_2-adrenoceptors after its release. Otherwise, it would also activate inhibitory α-adrenoceptors, which would offset the β-adrenoceptor-mediated enhancing effect. Preferential actions on prejunctional β_2-adrenoceptors would seem to require that they were localized closer to the site of transmitter release than the prejunctional α-adrenoceptors. We are unaware of such neuroanatomical findings.

As mentioned above, the overflow of ADR from skeletal muscle upon sympathetic nerve stimulation is quite small (Kahan, Hjemdahl and Dahlöf, 1987). This is not surprising, as the low circulating levels of ADR have to compete with higher circulating levels of NA and much higher junctional (i.e., neuronally-derived) concentrations of NA for the neuronal uptake mechanism. In addition, the affinity of ADR for neuronal uptake is lower than that of NA (Iversen, 1975), which works against the hypothesis. Thus, there is no preferential accumulation of ADR in sympathetic nerves, and it is not likely to be a cotransmitter of importance, unless ADR levels in plasma are very high during long periods of time; this is probably uncommon.

Taken together, these findings and arguments make us question the role of ADR as a prejunctional facilitator of sympathetic neurotransmission (whether acting from the circulation or released as a cotransmitter), at least in skeletal muscle.

INFLUENCE OF THE NERVE DISCHARGE PATTERN ON NORADRENALINE RELEASE AND VASCULAR RESPONSES

Sympathetic mechanisms have almost invariably been examined experimentally by means of continuous nerve activation at constant impulse frequencies. There is, however, a frequency-dependent increase in the amount of NA released per nerve impulse (Stjärne, 1975); this is also seen in skeletal muscle (Kahan, Hjemdahl and Dahlöf, 1984). The amount of transmitter released per nerve impulse may also be enhanced by an increase in pulse train length (Hughes and Roth, 1974; Stjärne, 1978). Direct recordings of sympathetic nerve impulse traffic show that the normal pattern of firing in sympathetic nerves to skeletal muscle is highly irregular (Wallin and Fagius, 1988). However, the integrated overflows of NA per nerve impulse were similar when sympathetic nerve stimulation was triggered by authentic recordings of the normal irregular discharge or delivered either at constant frequency or as intermittent bursts in our model (Kahan et al., 1988). Thus, the release of NA is fairly constant at a given average frequency, also with physiological variations in the sympathetic discharge pattern.

Variations in nerve impulse activity are closely paralleled by rapid changes in vascular tone. When integrated over time, however, vasoconstrictor responses to irregular, continuous and regular burst activites are similar in magnitude (Andersson, 1983; Kahan et al., 1988). Thus, data obtained with constant frequency stimulation may well be physiologically relevant with regard to both pre- and postjunctional events.

α-Adrenoceptor blockade also enhanced NA overflow when elicited by the authentic irregular sympathetic nerve discharge pattern (Kahan et al., 1988). Interestingly, this effect was less pronounced than during continuous nerve stimulation, which suggests that the degree of α-adrenoceptor-mediated feedback inhibition of NA release may be related to the nerve impulse pattern (Kahan et al., 1988). β-Adrenoceptor blockade reduced NA overflow evoked by stimulation similarly, whether elicited by the authentic irregular nerve impulse pattern, or by continuous or burst stimuli (Kahan et al., 1988).

SYMPATHETIC NON-ADRENERGIC VASOCONSTRICTOR MECHANISMS

Sympathetic nerve stimulation elicits a vasoconstrictor response partially resistant to non-competitive α-adrenoceptor blockade in skeletal muscle (Figure 9.4; Folkow and Uvnäs, 1948; Pernow et al., 1988) The non-adrenergic vasoconstriction is characterized by its delayed onset and prolonged action (Figure 9.5), which is also characteristic of

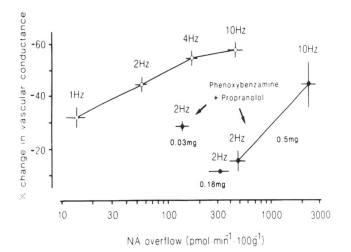

Figure 9.4 Relationships between NA overflow and decreases in vascular conductance during sympathetic nerve stimulation at 1–10 Hz in canine skeletal muscle (experimental procedures as in Figure 9.2) before and after β-adrenoceptor-blockade by propranolol and irreversible α-adrenoceptor-blockade by increasing doses of phenoxybenzamine (0.03–0.5 mg infused locally to the tissue). There is frequency-dependent vasoconstriction which is shifted considerably to the right, but still quite pronounced after combined adrenoceptor blockade. Responses to exogenous NA were markedly reduced (> 90%), but not entirely abolished by adrenoceptor blockade.
(From Pernow et al., 1988, with permission)

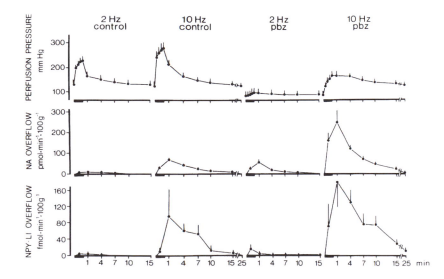

Figure 9.5 Time courses of vasoconstrictor responses and the overflows of NA and NPY-LI from canine skeletal muscle (experimental procedures as in Figure 9.2) during and after sympathetic stimulation at 2 and 10 Hz before (control) and after combined adrenoceptor blockade by propranolol and phenoxybenzamine (pbz). Adrenoceptor blockade enhances the overflows of both NA and NPY-LI, and results in a more slowly developing and waning vasoconstrictor response. (Data from Pernow et al., 1988, with permission)

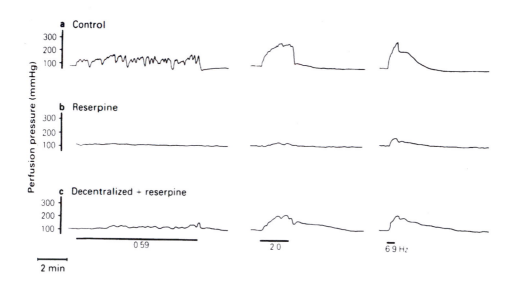

Figure 9.6 Vasoconstrictor responses to sympathetic nerve stimulation with irregular impulse frequencies governed by a recording of MSA from a healthy human volunteer. The average frequencies delivered were 0.59, 2.0 and 6.9 Hz. The same number of pulses were delivered at each frequency. *Control*: an animal studied according to standard procedures (see Figure 9.2); *reserpine*: an animal pretreated with reserpine to deplete NA and NPY from the nerves; *decentralized + reserpine*: reserpine pretreatment after cutting of the preganglionic nerves in order to preserve NPY when NA is depleted (NPY is otherwise depleted from the nerve terminals due to the sympathetic activation caused by reserpine). It can be seen that reserpine alone almost abolished the irregular vasoconstrictor response, but that decentralization lead to the reestablishment of a vasoconstrictor response which was more "sluggish" than without pretreatment. NPY-LI is released under the conditions of panel c. (From Pernow, Kahan and Lundberg, 1988, with permission).

the response to exogenous neuropeptide Y (NPY). This potent vasoconstrictor peptide (Tatemoto, Carlquist and Mutt, 1982; Edvinsson *et al.*, 1987; Potter, 1988; Lundberg *et al.*, 1990) is stored together with NA in sympathetic neurons in several tissues, including skeletal muscle (Pernow *et al.*, 1987). NPY has more pronounced effects on resistance vessels than on capacitance vessels in skeletal muscle (Pernow, Lundberg and Kaijser, 1987; Pernow *et al.*, 1987), and may be involved in the regulation of skeletal muscle microcirculation (Öhlén *et al.*, 1988, 1990). High-frequency sympathetic nerve stimulation is accompanied by a measurable overflow of NPY-like immunoreactivity (NPY-LI) from skeletal muscle *in situ* (Pernow *et al.*, 1988, 1989). Thus, non-adrenergic vasoconstriction may be related to the release of NPY.

Additional evidence that NPY may be involved in the non-adrenergic sympathetic vascular control in skeletal muscle was obtained in dogs, in which the tissue was selectively depleted of its neuronal content of NA by pretreatment with reserpine (to markedly reduce neuronal NA) together with preganglionic denervation (to preserve neuronal NPY). Under these conditions sympathetic nerve stimulation evoked frequency-dependent vasoconstriction (Figure 9.6), which was closely associated with the overflow of NPY-LI (Pernow, Kahan and Lundberg, 1988). The release of NPY-LI from skeletal muscle may be inhibited by activation of prejunctional α_2-adrenoceptors (Figure 9.5; Pernow *et al.*, 1988). NPY can also inhibit NA release prejunctionally (Pernow *et al.*, 1988), but high concentrations of NPY are required and this may not be a physiologically important mechanism, at least not in the skeletal muscle vascular bed.

Studies *in vitro* suggest that low concentrations of NPY may potentiate the vasoconstrictor responses to other pressor stimuli (Edvinsson *et al.*, 1987; Potter, 1988). Findings *in vivo* are less consistent (Dahlöf, Dahlöf and Lundberg, 1985; Potter, 1988; Revington and McCloskey, 1988). In man, exogenous NPY failed to influence the actions of neurogenic activation or locally infused NA in the forearm (Clarke *et al.*, 1991). Several vasoconstrictor agents can "potentiate" each other under *in vitro* conditions. This may simply reflect non-specific summation related to subthreshold elevations of smooth muscle tone in the otherwise atonic *in vitro* preparation.

There are NPY receptor subtypes. Presently a terminology has been proposed, whereby Y1 receptors are those activated by intact NPY, and Y2 receptors are those activated by C-terminal fragments of NPY (Wahlestedt *et al.*, 1990). Y1 receptors were initially thought to be postjunctionally located (e.g. on vascular smooth muscle), with Y2 receptors being prejunctional NPY receptors; however, as for adrenoceptors, this classification is too simplistic (Michel *et al.*, 1990: Wahlestedt *et al.*, 1990). Development of good NPY receptor antagonists is needed to enhance our understanding of possible NPY-related mechanisms.

Adenosine triphosphate (ATP) is another possible sympathetic cotransmitter which may participate in non-adrenergic vasoconstriction (Burnstock and Kennedy, 1986; Pelleg and Burnstock, 1990). It may play an important role in the sympathetic vascular control of several tissues (Sneddon and Burnstock, 1984; Burnstock and Kennedy, 1986; Burnstock and Warland, 1987; Ramme *et al.*, 1987), but there are species differences, organ differences and state-dependent variation (Stjärne, 1989).

In the skeletal muscle vascular bed a high concentration (10 μM) of the stable purinergic receptor agonist α, β-methylene-ATP (which is used to desensitize the receptors) failed to attenuate non-adrenergic vasoconstrictor responses to sympathetic nerve stimulation (Pernow *et al.*, 1988; Pernow, Kahan and Lundberg, 1988). Furthermore, the purinergic vasoconstrictor component is rapid, and seems to be relatively more important at low-stimulation frequencies, and when stimulation is of short duration (Kennedy, Saville and Burnstock, 1986: Burnstock and Warland, 1987). The non-adrenergic vasoconstrictor component in canine skeletal muscle is slow in onset, of prolonged duration and more important with stimulation at high frequencies of long duration (Figures 9.5 and 9.6). Definite conclusions concerning a purinergic component in the non-adrenergic vasoconstrictor response to sympathetic stimulation in canine skeletal muscle cannot be reached without studies using a selective receptor antagonist.

In humans, sympathetic reflex activation by lower body negative pressure elicits a vasoconstrictor response, even in the presence of adrenoceptor blockade (Taddei, Salvetti and Pedrinelli, 1989). This, presumably non-adrenergic, vasoconstrictor response is sympathetically mediated, as bretylium abolishes it (Taddei, Salvetti and Pedrinelli, 1989). Following adrenoceptor blockade, the vasoconstrictor response to nerve activation was associated with an overflow of NPY-LI from the forearm (following α-adrenoceptor blockade), which suggests an involvement of NPY in a non-adrenergic component of the sympathetic control of the skeletal muscle vasculature in man also (Kahan *et al.*, 1992). With regard to the putative purinergic component in this response, Taddei and coworkers have shown effects of the adenosine receptor antagonist theophylline which they interpreted as evidence of neurogenic ATP release (ATP is rapidly metabolized to the vasodilator substance adenosine) in man also (Taddei, Pedrinelli and Salvetti, 1990). However, the evidence is circumstantial and it cannot be ruled out that the adenosine apparently formed was derived from sources other than nerves (Pelleg and Burnstock, 1990).

The mechanistic evidence presented above is largely circumstantial, and the roles of ATP and NPY in sympathetic neurotransmission and non-adrenergic vasoconstriction will be more clearly delineated when efficient and specific receptor antagonists become available.

SYMPATHETIC CHOLINERGIC MECHANISMS

A cholinergic vasodilator pathway originating in the motor cortex and descending via the hypothalamus, has been demonstrated in some species. Activation of these fibres, either by stimulation of specific regions in the brain, which in unanaesthetized animals will elicit a defence reaction, or by stimulation of peripheral sympathetic nerves to skeletal muscle will cause transient vasodilatation mediated by acetylcholine (Uvnäs, 1960; Renkin, 1984; Shepherd, 1984). The sympathetic cholinergic innervation is directed to small arteries and arterioles. Sympathetic cholinergic vasodilatation has been convincingly demonstrated in several species, including the cat and dog, but not in rodents. Its existence in humans has been debated, but it may participate in vasodilator responses in forearm muscles to stress and isometric exercise (see below). The sympathetic cholinergic fibres to skeletal muscle are ordinarily quiescent, but they may play a role in skeletal muscle vasodilatation in anticipation of muscular exercise, or in the defence reaction (Brod, 1963; Shepherd, 1984).

Acetylcholine may reduce NA release via activation of prejunctional, inhibitory muscarinic receptors (Muscholl, 1980; Vanhoutte and Levy, 1980); this has also been shown in skeletal muscle (Kahan, Dahlöf and Hjemdahl, 1985), and may contribute to the vasodilator responses associated with stimulation of sympathetic cholinergic fibres. In skeletal muscle it is also conceivable that acetylcholine from motor nerves may influence NA release from sympathetic nerves, if they are in close proximity. This might be relevant during exercise, but such a mechanism does not seem to have been tested experimentally.

OTHER VASODILATOR MECHANISMS

There is also non-cholinergic neurogenic vasodilatation in skeletal muscle (Hilton, Spyer and Timms, 1979; Öhlén et al., 1990). Obvious candidates in this respect are peptides, like substance P and calcitonin gene-related peptide (Öhlén et al., 1987, 1990). Both peptides produce vasodilatation in skeletal muscle when administered intravenously (Gardiner, Compton and Bennett, 1989; Gardiner et al., 1990b; Bachelard et al., 1992), but their roles in the local neurogenic regulation of skeletal muscle blood flow need to be further delineated by studies of the effects of specific antagonists.

Histamine is present in sympathetic nerves and in blood vessels, and sympathetic nerve stimulation elicits an overflow of radiotracer in skeletal muscle labelled with ^{14}C-histamine

(Tuttle, 1967). Whether this histamine is released from sympathetic nerves or from extraneuronal stores has not been established (Heitz, Schafer and Brody, 1975). Nerve stimulation-evoked dilatation of resistance vessels in skeletal muscle is antagonized by antihistamines (Shepherd, 1984; Bevan and Brayden, 1987). However, little is known about the possible physiological role of sympathetic histaminergic vasodilatation (Shepherd, 1984; Bevan and Brayden, 1987).

A large number of agents, including acetylcholine, ATP, bradykinin, histamine, NA and serotonin, can produce smooth muscle relaxation and vasodilatation mediated by the release of endothelial-derived relaxing factors (Furchgott and Zawadzki, 1980), of which nitric oxide (Palmer, Ferrigo and Moncada, 1987) seems to account for the main part of the biological actions (Furchgott and Vanhoutte, 1989). Continuous endothelial formation of nitric oxide seems to counteract the intrinsic vascular tone in skeletal muscle (Ekelund and Mellander, 1990; Gardiner *et al.*, 1990a). This may play an important role in the physiological control of basal vascular tone; less is known about its importance of a modulator of neurogenic influences on vascular tone *in vivo*. Nitric oxide seems to influence mainly the larger arterial resistance vessels.

THE RENIN-ANGIOTENSIN SYSTEM

Angiotensin (Ang) II is a potent vasoconstrictor, which also has plasma concentration-dependent vasoconstrictor effects in skeletal muscle (e.g., Schwieler *et al.*, 1991a). In addition, there are several ways in which the renin–angiotensin system may reinforce the effects of sympathetic nerve stimulation (Starke, 1977; Westfall, 1977; Zimmerman, 1981). It has been suggested that Ang II might inhibit the neuronal uptake of NA (Starke, 1977; Westfall, 1977), but this seems less likely to occur physiologically (Hjemdahl and Schwieler, 1991; Schwieler *et al.*, 1992). The hypothesis that Ang II might enhance NA synthesis has not gained much support (Westfall, 1977). Circulating Ang II may release ADR from the adrenal medullae (Reit, 1972), but this seems to occur only at pharmacological levels of Ang II in plasma (Schwieler *et al.*, 1992). More interestingly, however, circulating Ang II may elicit central effects, and an increase in efferent vasoconstrictor nerve activity has been demonstrated in man when Ang II was infused at subpressor doses (see Hjemdahl and Schwieler, 1991).

Considerable interest has focused on the effects of Ang II at the peripheral sympathetic neuroeffector junction, and it is often stated that one of the important effects of Ang II is to enhance sympathetic neurotransmission. We have, however, examined this in canine skeletal muscle *in situ*, and found that the effects are not of the magnitude commonly believed.

INTERACTIONS WITH SYMPATHETIC NEUROTRANSMISSION AT THE POSTJUNCTIONAL LEVEL

Ang II may enhance α-adrenoceptor-mediated vasoconstrictor responses at the postjunctional level, as indicated by studies performed *in vitro* (Starke, 1977: Westfall, 1977) and *in vivo* in the pithed rat (Grant and McGrath, 1988a; Wong, Reilly and Timmermans, 1989), i.e. in models with low vascular tone. Both α_1- and α_2-adrenoceptor-mediated pressor responses to exogenous agonists may be enhanced by Ang II. However, this may represent non-specific enhancement related to subthreshold elevations of vascular tone, as discussed above. The physiological importance of Ang II-mediated potentiation of vasoconstrictor effects elicited by exogenous α_2-adrenoceptor agonists, or by neuronally released NA in pithed animals, has indeed been questioned, and attributed to the low vascular tone of the model (de Jonge et al., 1982; Grant and McGrath 1988b).

Data from pithed animal models should be interpreted with caution, in part because of the low vascular tone, and in part due to the markedly stimulated renin-angiotensin system in this model (de Jonge et al., 1982; Grant and McGrath, 1988b). In canine skeletal muscle in situ, Ang II does not seem to influence vasopressor responses to exogenous NA, whereas responses to neuronally released NA may be enhanced (Schwieler et al., 1992, 1993). This may be taken to suggest that Ang II might interact differently with postjunctional α_1- and α_2-adrenoceptors, which seem to be activated mainly by neuronally released NA and circulating catecholamines, respectively.

INTERACTIONS WITH SYMPATHETIC NEUROTRANSMISSION AT THE PREJUNCTIONAL LEVEL

Activation of prejunctional Ang II-receptors may facilitate NA release. This concept is based mainly on findings in vitro and, to some extent, in isolated, saline-perfused tissues. In blood-perfused skeletal muscle in situ, specific Ang (AT_1) receptor antagonism by losartan or inhibition of angiotensin-converting enzyme (ACE) can reduce the sympathetic nerve stimulation-evoked overflow of NA (Schwieler et al., 1993). These findings suggest that endogenous Ang II is likely to participate in the prejunctional modulation of NA release under physiological conditions. However, the effects are modest (10–25% reductions of NA overflow) in comparison to the powerful α-adrenoceptor-mediated modulation of sympathetic neurotransmission. In fact, ACE inhibition only decreases NA overflow in the presence of α-adrenoceptor blockade in this in vivo model (Schwieler et al., 1991a, 1992, 1993).

Based on results obtained in vitro (Nakamaru, Jackson and Inagami, 1986; Ziogas and Story, 1991) and in the pithed rat (Schlicker, Erkens and Göthert, 1988) it has been hypothetized that β_2-adrenoceptor-mediated facilitation of NA release may involve enhanced local generation of Ang II, which in turn would act on facilitatory Ang II-receptors. However, findings by others in vitro (Musgrave and Majewski, 1987; Kuwahara, Kubo and Misu, 1989), and in vivo (Schwieler et al., 1992), do not support this hypothesis.

CIRCULATING VS LOCALLY GENERATED ANGIOTENSIN II

Following ACE inhibition, circulating Ang II failed to facilitate sympathetic nerve stimulation-evoked NA overflow from skeletal muscle in situ in the dog at plasma levels both within and far above the physiological concentration range (Schwieler et al., 1991a, 1992), thus confirming earlier observations in this tissue without measurements of the plasma levels of Ang II actually studied (Zimmerman and Whitmore, 1967). It is likely that Ang II in the circulation has limited access to the neuroeffector junction in vivo, due to the diffusion

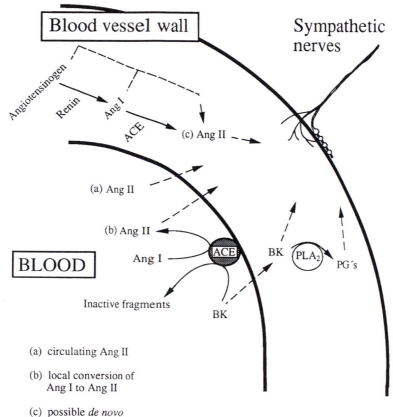

Blood vessel wall

Sympathetic nerves

Angiotensinogen

Renin

Ang I

ACE

(c) Ang II

(a) Ang II

(b) Ang II

Ang I

ACE

BK

PLA₂

PG's

BLOOD

Inactive fragments

BK

(a) circulating Ang II

(b) local conversion of
    Ang I to Ang II

(c) possible *de novo*
    synthesis of Ang II

Figure 9.7 A schematic representation of the perivascular sympathetic nerves and mechanisms possibly relating to the renin–angiotensin system. ACE is predominantly located on the endothelium. Non-ACE-related formation of Ang II may also occur in the vessel wall (dashed lines). Bradykinin (BK) accumulates as the result of ACE inhibition. This may have direct effects and/or stimulate prostaglandin (PG) synthesis via activation of phospholipase A$_2$ (PLA$_2$). Effects of ACE-inhibition on sympathetic neurotransmission may be related to all of these phenomena (which is borne out by our recent findings; Schwieler *et al.*, 1993 and 1994b). It is also interesting to note the diffusion distances from the blood to the perivascular nerves (the role of the vasa vasorum in this context is unclear), which may explain why circulating Ang II and ADR are inefficient with respect to actions on NA release. (From Schwieler and Hjemdahl, 1992, with permission)

barrier offered by the blood vessel wall (Figure 9.7; Hjemdahl and Schwieler, 1991). It is, however, also possible that enhanced formation of inhibitory prostaglandins masks a facilitatory effect of Ang II (Schwieler and Hjemdahl, 1992; Schwieler *et al.*, 1993).

A local renin–angiotensin system has been invoked, and it has been suggested that Ang II generated in the vessel wall may influence vascular tone and structure (Dzau, 1989). For example, local formation and release of Ang II can take place in the isolated rat hindleg (Mizuno *et al.*, 1988; Hilgers *et al.*, 1989). We have found a positive veno-arterial concentration difference for Ang II over the canine gracilis muscle *in situ* (Schwieler *et al.*, 1991b). Whether the Ang II was formed by conversion of circulating Ang I to Ang II (via endothelial ACE) or by *de novo* synthesis in the tissue could not be established. Data from a carefully conducted follow-up study, however, indicate that the endothelial ACE-related mechanism is responsible for Ang II formation in the skeletal muscle (Schwieler *et al.*, 1994a). Whatever mechanism is responsible, locally generated Ang II may be involved in the modulation of sympathetic neurotransmission in skeletal muscle, as we saw no effects of circulating Ang II.

ANGIOTENSION-CONVERTING ENZYME INHIBITION AND SYMPATHETIC NEUROTRANSMISSION

ACE is an important enzyme for the formation of Ang II from Ang I, but other enzymes may also participate in the formation of Ang II (Okamura *et al.*, 1990; Urata *et al.*, 1990; Hjemdahl and Schwieler, 1991; Husain, 1993). ACE also catalyzes the degradation and inactivation of other peptides, including bradykinin, substance P and other tachykinins, and enkephalins (Unger *et al.*, 1989; Husain, 1993). In addition, ACE inhibition may enhance prostaglandin production, possibly via bradykinin accumulation (cf. Schwieler and Hjemdahl, 1992). Thus, the mechanisms by which ACE inhibition may interact with sympathetic neurotransmission are complex. Reduced Ang II formation and enhanced prostaglandin formation might reduce NA release, whereas enhanced bradykinin accumulation might facilitate NA release (Schwieler and Hjemdahl, 1992) (Figure 9.7). There is experimental evidence, from our canine skeletal muscle model, which suggests that all three mechanisms contribute to the prejunctional modulation of sympathetic vascular control by ACE inhibition (Schwieler *et al.*, 1993). The relative contributions of these modulating mechanisms may vary with the experimental conditions.

MUSCLE SYMPATHETIC NERVE ACTIVITY AND BLOOD FLOW IN HUMANS

There is an immense literature on skeletal muscle blood flow in various species under different physiological conditions. The reader is referred to previous excellent overviews on this subject for detailed information (e.g., Ross, 1971; Abboud *et al.*, 1976; Rowell, 1984; Shepherd, 1984; Saltin, 1988). We will concentrate on sympatho-adrenal aspects, and thereby emphasize more recent studies evaluating MSA by microneurography during commonly used stimuli in humans.

Central venous pressure and cardiopulmonary receptors are important in the regulation of muscle sympathetic activity and blood flow. It seems as if there is rather pronounced and tonic regulation of MSA (Wallin and Fagius, 1988) and muscle blood flow by these factors. Various physiological stimuli influence MSA and blood flow in a synchronized and logical fashion, but mental stress seems to enhance muscle blood flow in parallel with increased MSA and/or NA overflow. Some examples will be given to illustrate the sympathetic regulation of muscle blood flow in humans, as well as some discrepancies.

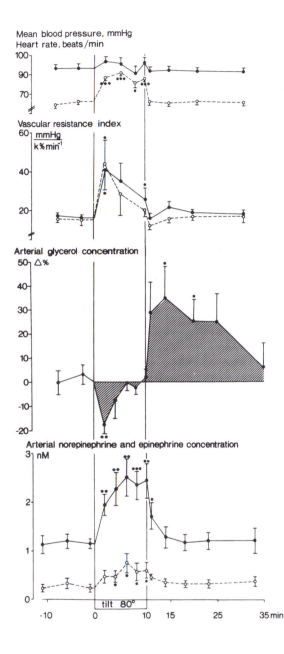

Figure 9.8 Arterial blood pressure, arterial plasma catecholamine and glycerol concentrations, and vascular resistances in skeletal muscle and adipose tissue (measured by the local clearances of radiolabelled pertechnetate; $^{99m}TcO_4^-$) during tilting to 80° for 10 min in eight healthy volunteers. Rapid and equally pronounced vasoconstriction is seen in skeletal muscle and adipose tissue. The plasma glycerol response resembles the glycerol outflow (lipolytic) response in isolated canine subcutaneous adipose tissue in connection with sympathetic nerve stimulation. (From Linde and Hjemdahl, 1982, with permission)

REDUCTIONS OF CENTRAL VENOUS PRESSURE

Orthostatic stress produces rapid vasoconstriction in skeletal muscle (e.g. Linde and Hjemdahl, 1982; Shepherd, 1984); similarly rapid and pronounced responses are seen in adipose tissue (Figure 9.8; Linde and Hjemdahl, 1982). These responses are, most likely, elicited mainly by unloading of volume receptors (arterial baroreceptors may, however, contribute). Local veno-arterial reflexes may also be involved, especially in adipose tissue (Henriksen et al., 1983). These vasoconstrictor responses are paralleled by immediate and sustained increases in MSA (Delius et al., 1972b; Burke, Sundlöf and Wallin, 1977), which are linearly related to the degree of stimulation, i.e. to the angle of tilting (Iwase, Mano and Saito, 1987).

Lower body negative pressure (LBNP) is an elegant manoeuvre that permits studies of various vascular beds during graded reductions of venous return (Wolthuis, Bergman and Nicogossian, 1974). The forearm responds with vasoconstriction during LBNP (e.g. Beiser et al., 1970; Zoller et al., 1972), even at levels low enough not to influence heart rate or blood pressure (Zoller et al., 1972). There is vasoconstriction in the skin and skeletal muscle of the forearm (Beiser et al., 1970; Rowell, Wyss and Brengelmann, 1973; Tripathi and Nadel, 1986). A separate analysis of adipose tissue blood flow has not been performed, but the techniques used to elucidate skin blood flow may have included subcutaneous adipose tissue flow. There may be a slight enhancement of venous tone in the forearm which, together with the decrease in flow, results in a reduced forearm venous volume during LBNP (Tripathi, Mack and Nadel, 1989). However, results have previously not been conclusive in this respect (Wolthius, Bergman and Nicogossian, 1974).

It has been believed that LBNP-induced vasoconstriction in the forearm is moderate. However, using short-lasting bouts of LBNP at increasing intensities (up to −85 mm Hg), Lundvall and Edfeldt (1993) recently showed quite pronounced reflexogenic vasoconstriction in this region (Figure 9.9). Their study also suggested that arterial baroreceptors may be more important for responses to LBNP than previously believed. Others have also questioned whether only cardiopulmonary receptors are involved in the responses to LBNP (Bennett, 1987).

MSA in the peroneal nerve is stimulation-dependently increased by LBNP (Victor and Leimbach, 1987; Fløistrup Vissing, Scherrer and Victor, 1989). With regard to the representativeness of forearm blood flow, for skeletal muscle blood flow responses elsewhere, to reductions in venous return, it has been claimed that the calf responds less markedly than the forearm (Essandoh et al., 1986; Essandoh, Duprez and Shepherd, 1987). However, radial and peroneal MSA seem to respond similarly (Rea and Wallin, 1989), and other authors have seen clear-cut effects of LBNP on calf blood flow, with even larger effects in the calf than in the forearm (Figure 9.10; Fløistrup Vissing, Scherrer and Victor, 1989). The reasons behind these discrepancies have, to our knowledge, not been elucidated.

It is interesting to note that biochemical assessments of sympathetic nerve activity can be troublesome during orthostatic testing. Arterial plasma NA concentrations increase rapidly during tilting (see Figure 9.8) and LBNP, but this is to a large extent due to reductions of NA clearance from plasma and not only to increases in NA spillover to plasma (Esler et al., 1988; Baily et al., 1990). However, regional studies still yield dependable information,

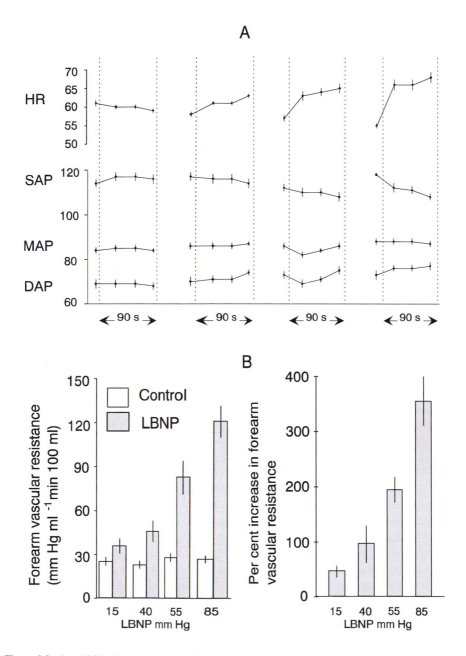

Figure 9.9 Arterial blood pressures [systolic (SAP), mean (MAP) and diastolic (DAP)) and heart rates (HR) (panel A) and vascular resistances — indicated as absolute values and relative changes — in the human forearm (panel B) in connection with 1.5 min bouts of LBNP at −15, −40, −55 and −85 mmHg in 10 healthy volunteers. Note the pronounced vasoconstrictor responses during intense stimulation for brief periods, which are in agreement with pronounced vasoconstrictor responses to sympathetic nerve stimulation in skeletal muscle in animal experiments. (From Lundvall and Edfeldt, 1993, with permission)

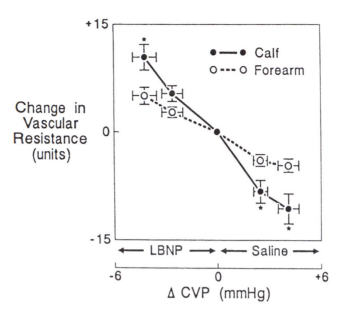

Figure 9.10 Changes in vascular resistance in the calf and forearm during graded changes in central venous pressure (Δ CVP) by LBNP and saline infusion, respectively, in healthy volunteers. In this study the calf demonstrates more marked responses than the forearm. MSA in the peroneal nerve changed in a corresponding fashion. (From Fløistrup Vissing, Scherrer and Victor, 1989, with permission)

as there is an increased net NA overflow from the forearm during LBNP (Hjemdahl, Eklund and Kaijser, 1982). The apparent "spillover" of NA, unfortunately not taking flow into account, has also been found to increase (Baily et al., 1990). Non-adrenergic sympathetic vasoconstrictor mechanisms may participate, and an overflow of NPY-LI from the forearm to plasma can also be demonstrated during LBNP after α-adrenoceptor blockade (Kahan et al., 1992).

INCREASES IN CENTRAL VENOUS PRESSURE

Central volume expansion, by e.g., elevating the lower limbs, leads to increases in forearm blood flow that are not influenced by atropine, and so are presumably mediated by reduced vasoconstrictor nerve activity (Roddie, Shepherd and Whelan, 1957). In agreement with this, leg raising (Delius et al., 1972b), or volume expansion by infusions of blood (Agewall et al., 1990), or saline (Fløistrup Vissing, Scherrer and Victor, 1989), lead to graded reductions of peroneal MSA. Concomitantly, vascular tone is reduced in both the forearm and calf (Figure 9.10). Thus increased central venous pressure reduces nerve activity and vascular tone in skeletal muscle.

Following the release of LBNP, vasodilatation in the forearm may also be observed; this has been attributed to β_2-adrenoceptor activation in the blood vessels (Rahman and

Bennett, 1990), on the basis of results obtained after systemic β-adrenoceptor blockade. However, β_1-selective adrenoceptor blockade by atenolol elicited almost the same degree of inhibition as did non-selective blockade by propranolol (Rahman and Bennett, 1990); ADR levels in plasma were not reported. Systemic β-adrenoceptor blockade may also influence sympathetic nerve activity, via reflexogenic mechanisms elicited by the reduction of cardiac output (Freyschuss et al., 1988). The post-LBNP dilator response in skeletal muscle may well be related to a rapid increase in venous return and a reflexogenic reduction of nerve activity, in analogy with the volume loading situation; systemic β-adrenoceptor blockade might also influence such mechanisms.

INFLUENCE OF ARTERIAL BARORECEPTORS

MSA is not tonically influenced by the input from high-pressure receptors, i.e. receptors regulated by the blood pressure and carotid artery dimensions, as variations in arterial baroreceptor activity cause rather short-lasting responses (Wallin and Fagius, 1988). There is pulse-synchronous burst activity of MSA, which is triggered during diastole and rapidly fades when systolic blood pressure builds up (Wallin and Fagius, 1988). This probably serves as an important beat-to-beat blood pressure-buffering mechanism. However, there is no relationship between the average blood pressure level and MSA (Wallin and Fagius, 1988).

Elevation of blood pressure by infusion of the α-adrenoceptor-agonist, phenylephrine, or lowering of blood pressure by the vasodilator, sodium nitroprusside, elicit dose-dependent decreases and increases, respectively, in peroneal MSA (Eckberg et al., 1988). However, these drugs also influence venous tone and cardiopulmonary receptors. Rea and Hamdan (1990) therefore counteracted drug-induced changes in central venous pressure (by simultaneous application of LBNP or saline infusion, respectively) to achieve selective arterial baroreceptor influences of phenylephrine and sodium nitroprusside on MSA. They found marked effects of elevating or lowering blood pressure also in this experimental setting. Thus, arterial baroreceptors seem to influence MSA in the immediate (beat-to-beat) and short (unclear how long) term, but not chronically.

With regard to biochemical measures of sympathetic nerve activity it has been shown that sodium nitroprusside causes a rapid, and not fully sustained increase of peroneal MSA, whereas simultaneously measured antecubital venous plasma NA concentrations increase much more sluggishly, but to almost the same extent (Rea et al., 1990). This is in line with observations in connection with other stimuli. Eckberg and coworkers (1988) also found changes in forearm venous plasma NA and NPY-LI levels which agreed with their MSA data during pharmacological alterations of blood pressure.

ISOMETRIC EXERCISE

Isometric exercise is a much-studied stimulus, which causes initial vasodilatation followed by vasoconstriction in the non-exercising forearm (Eklund, 1974; Shepherd et al., 1981). The calf, on the other hand, only responds with somewhat delayed vasoconstriction during handgrip exercise (Rusch et al., 1981). With leg exercise, however, the vasoconstrictor response of the resting calf may be preceded by transient vasodilatation (Gaffney, Sjøgaard and Saltin, 1990), and peroneal MSA seems to decrease (Ray *et al.*, 1992). When contractions are sustained to fatigue, however, leg exercise also elicits increases in MSA to the resting leg (Ray and Mark, 1993). Interestingly, the coherence between MSA to the two legs is good at rest and during apnoea, but reduced by single-leg exercise (Wallin, Burke and Gandevia, 1992), indicating that active and passive muscle may be differentially influenced by MSA. Thus, vascular responses to isometric exercise are complex and probably depend on which muscles are contracted, which region is studied, and the intensity of the contraction.

The initial vasodilator response of the forearm during contralateral handgrip exercise is partly blocked by local infusions of propranolol, indicating a β-adrenoceptor-mediated component, and the late vasoconstrictor component is antagonized by local α-adrenoceptor-blockade by phentolamine (Eklund and Kaijser, 1976). There is also a cholinergic component, as combined local infusion of propranolol and atropine abolishes this vasodilator response (L. Kaijser, personal communication). Circulating ADR is probably not involved, as isometric exercise of moderate intensity causes only minor increases of ADR in arterial plasma (Eklund *et al.*, 1983), and the response is so rapid that a neurogenic basis is more likely.

The gradually developing vasoconstrictor response in the resting calf during handgrip is paralleled by a gradually developing, intensity-dependent increase in MSA in the peroneal nerve (Seals, Chase and Taylor, 1988; Seals, 1989; Saito, Mano and Iwase, 1990), whereas skin sympathetic activity follows an entirely different time course with a rapid and maintained increase (Figure 9.11; Saito, Naito and Mano, 1990). Chemoreceptor stimulation by arterial occlusion of the exercising arm after handgrip exercise results in maintained elevations of MSA, calf vascular resistance and blood pressure (Figure 9.11; Mark *et al.*, 1985; Seals, 1989; Saito, Naito and Mano, 1990), but not skin sympathetic activity or heart rate (Saito, Naito and Mano, 1990).

Conversely, isometric leg muscle contractions may increase MSA in the arm (Delius *et al.*, 1972b). Ray *et al.* (1992) have, however, recently shown that leg exercise is a much poorer stimulus for enhanced MSA than handgrip exercise; in fact, MSA appears to decrease in the arm and resting leg during isometric leg exercise of moderate intensity.

Handgrip exercise also increases NA concentrations in venous plasma from the contralateral forearm, with a time lag of about 1 min compared to the MSA response of the leg (Wallin, Mörlin and Hjemdahl, 1987); the peak response of NA in plasma occurred 1–2 min after the end of a 2 min handgrip exercise bout. There is an increased net overflow of NA from the resting forearm during contralateral handgrip of different intensities and duration (Hjemdahl, Eklund and Kaijser, 1982; Kaijser, Eklund and Hjemdahl, unpublished). Again there seems to be a good temporal relationship between the development of vasoconstriction and the overflow of NA, with a lag period of 1–2 min for the transmitter to appear in the venous effluent. Isometric exercise has not been strong enough a stimulus to enhance the overflow of NPY-LI in our experience (Pernow *et al.*, 1986).

DYNAMIC EXERCISE

Vasodilatation occurs in anticipation of muscular exercise; this may be mediated by sympathetic cholinergic vasodilator fibres (Brod, 1963; Shepherd, 1984). During exercise there are intensity-dependent, and potentially very large, increases in sympathetic nerve

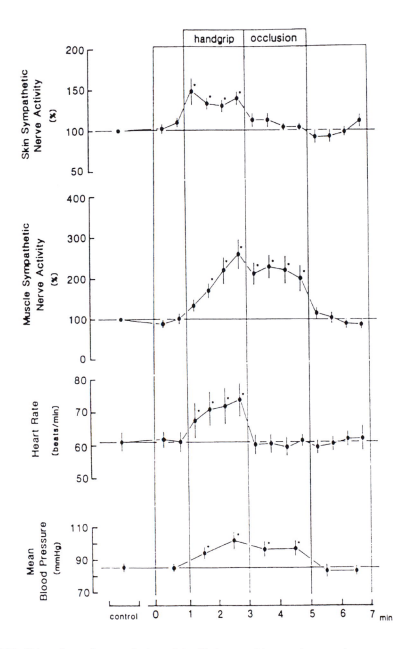

Figure 9.11 Skin and muscle sympathetic activity (% changes of integrated mean voltage neurograms), and heart rate and mean arterial pressure, during and after 2 min of handgrip at 30% of maximal voluntary force in eight healthy volunteers. Cessation of handgrip was in this experiment followed by 2 min of occlusion to cause chemoreceptor stimulation in the exercising forearm. Note the different time courses for the muscle and skin sympathetic nerve activity responses and the persistence of MSA and blood pressure elevations, despite normalization of the heart rate in the ischemic post-contraction period. (From Saito, Naito and Mano, 1990, with permission)

activity to skeletal muscle (Saltin, 1988). This results in vasoconstriction in non-exercising muscle, whereas local metabolic factors override this neurogenic influence, and allow flow to increase markedly in the exercising muscle. This increase in blood flow is important to maintain local homeostasis.

Several factors have been suggested to mediate the exercise-induced, functional hyperaemia. There is no simple solution to this problem and multifactorial metabolic control mechanisms are in all likelihood involved (Renkin, 1984; Shepherd, 1984). The initial vasodilatation during exercise may be related to K^+ release and hyperosmolarity, whereas adenosine seems to be more important during more prolonged (10–15 min) exercise. The persistence of hyperaemia following cessation of exercise may depend on adenosine and prostaglandins; histamine may also contribute. Additional factors may participate as well, but experimental evidence is less supportive (Renkin, 1984; Shepherd, 1984). Local β-adrenoceptor blockade does not influence muscle blood flow during exercise in humans (Juhlin-Dannfelt and Åström, 1979), suggesting that local factors and not ADR are responsible for the hyperaemia.

During exercise involving large muscles the decrease in total peripheral resistance, which is related to the reduction of vascular resistance in working muscle, is counteracted by a reflexogenic increase in sympathetic nerve activity, which also occurs in the exercising muscle and buffers the vasodilatory response (O'Leary, Rowell and Scher, 1991). The sympathetically evoked vasoconstrictor response in resting skeletal muscle seems to develop progressively during sustained exercise (Rowlands and Donald, 1968). The degrees of vasoconstriction in e.g. skeletal muscle (O'Leary, Rowell and Scher, 1991) and the kidney (Tidgren et al., 1991) are positively related to the level of exertion, and such vasoconstriction may be an important factor in the control of arterial blood pressure, i.e., perfusion pressure, during exercise (O'Leary, Rowell and Scher, 1991).

Animal studies have shown that local metabolic changes may depress transmitter release and/or reduce responsiveness at the postjunctional level in exercising muscle (Burcher and Garlick, 1973, 1975; Shepherd, 1984). In humans, sympathetic activation in exercising skeletal muscle has been assessed in terms of local NA overflow. There is an intensity-dependent overflow of NA which is larger from the exercising leg than from the resting leg (Savard et al., 1987, 1989). The enhancement of NA overflow may be as large as 25-fold in the resting leg and 35-fold in the exercising leg in humans (Savard et al., 1989). It is perhaps of interest to note that similarly large increases in NA overflow occur in other organs without confounding factors such as the local hyperaemia, as, e.g., in the human kidney (Tidgren et al., 1991). It is, unfortunately, not possible to establish if the difference in NA overflow between resting and active muscle is due to differences in impulse activity (neurographic studies require stable recording conditions) or prejunctional control mechanisms, or if it is merely a result of enhanced wash-out of NA from the neuroeffector junction to blood. In animals, there is a marked enhancement of NA wash-out from skeletal muscle during simultaneous sympathetic and motor stimulation, and the difference in NA overflow from active and resting muscle is almost abolished by neuronal uptake inhibition, suggesting that wash-out during hyperaemia influences neuronal NA uptake (Folkow, Häggendal and Lisander, 1967).

NPY-LI in plasma increases markedly during exercise (Lundberg et al., 1985; Pernow et al., 1986; Tidgren et al., 1991), but an increment over the forearm could not be demonstrated for NPY-LI, as it could for NA (Pernow *et al.*, 1986). Thus muscle sympathetic nerves in this region do not seem to attain very high levels of activity during moderate exercise.

CONTROL OF MUSCLE BLOOD FLOW DURING MENTAL STRESS

The centrally elicited haemodynamic responses to mental stress seem to be mainly neurogenically mediated, with ADR contributing only marginally to most responses (cf. Hjemdahl, 1991, 1993). Responses seem to be qualitatively similar in different studies, but they may vary quantitatively, depending on the stress test used and how it is administered (as well as on how relaxed the subjects were during resting measurements — the basal measurement is perhaps the most important one in physiologically oriented stress research). The pattern is that of cardiac stimulation, renal and splanchnic vasoconstriction, and an elevation of blood pressure, despite a reduction of total peripheral vascular resistance.

Limb blood flow increases during stress, as demonstrated both in the forearm (Blair *et al.*, 1959; Brod *et al.*, 1959; Barcroft *et al.*, 1960; Brod, 1963; Rusch *et al.*, 1981; Goldstein *et al.*, 1987) and in the leg (Rusch *et al.*, 1981). When directly compared, a reduction of vascular resistance was only seen in the forearm during mental arithmetic or an echo stress test (Rusch *et al.*, 1981). The modified Stroop colour word conflict test used in our laboratory usually elicits more marked stress responses, and also elicits vasodilatation in the leg (Hjemdahl *et al.*, 1989; Linde *et al.*, 1989). Recently, we have also found marked vasodilatation with this stress test in the forearm (Lindqvist *et al.*, 1993). With regard to the different tissues involved, Brod and coworkers have shown vasoconstriction in the skin and vasodilatation in skeletal muscle (cf. Brod, 1963) and we have found vasodilatation in skeletal muscle and adipose tissue (Linde *et al.*, 1989). Skeletal muscle is, most likely, the main contributor to limb blood flow responses to stress. It is of interest to note that even anticipation of various strenuous or unpleasant experiences, such as exercise or cold (Brod, 1963), or stress testing or a loss of blood (Blair *et al.*, 1959), elicits forearm vasodilatation. Forearm veins, on the other hand, seem to constrict during mental stress, as evidenced by a reduced venous volume and distensibility during mental arithmetic (Brod *et al.*, 1976; Robinson *et al.*, 1989).

Which mechanisms can, then, explain limb blood flow responses to mental stress? ADR is a potent vasodilator of skeletal muscle and adipose tissue (Hjemdahl and Linde, 1983; Freyschuss *et al.*, 1986), but constricts skin vessels. However, the arterial plasma ADR response is too small to explain more than a fraction of the vasodilator responses seen (Linde *et al.*, 1989; Hjemdahl, 1993; Lindqvist *et al.*, 1993). The poor or non-existent, antecubital venous plasma NA response to stress (Eliasson, Hjemdahl and Kahan, 1983, and several other studies in our and other groups) suggested to us that vasoconstrictor nerve activity might be unchanged or even reduced in skeletal muscle during our mental stress testing (cf. Hjemdahl, 1991). In the leg, however, we found increased MSA and NA overflow during the colour word conflict test (Hjemdahl *et al.*, 1989). Interestingly, MSA recordings have shown unchanged nerve activity in the arm (Delius *et al.*, 1972b; Anderson, Wallin and Mark, 1987), but increased activity in the leg (Anderson, Wallin and Mark, 1987) during mental arithmetic (Figure 9.12). This pattern is in good agreement with plasma NA concentration data obtained during stress. Plasma NA may, however, increase

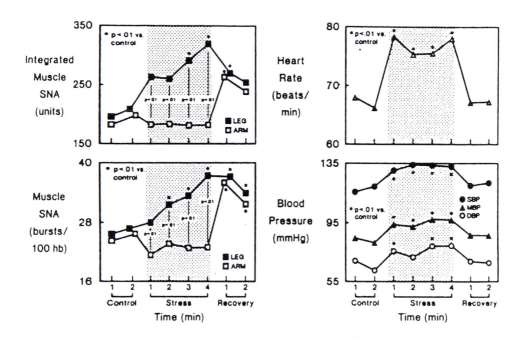

Figure 9.12 MSA (muscle SNA) in the arm and leg (left panel; data presented in absolute terms and in relation to heart rate, i.e. bursts per 100 heart beats) and heart rate and blood pressures (right panel) during mental arithmetic stress. Note the increase in leg MSA during, and in arm MSA after, the stress test. This corresponds to plasma NA concentration responses in the two regions, but not to NA overflow from the forearm during another stress test (see text). (From Anderson, Wallin and Mark, 1987, with permission)

in antecubital venous plasma *after* stress, even if there is no increase during stress (Eliasson, Hjemdahl and Kahan, 1983). Surprisingly, we recently found an increased NA overflow from the forearm during the colour word conflict test as well (Lindqvist, *et al.*, 1993); a similar tendency was found during stress evoked by a video game (Goldstein *et al.*, 1987). The flow response thus dilutes the NA released from the arm during stress. Enhanced nerve activity and NA release therefore seem to (paradoxically) accompany vasodilatation in the forearm and calf during mental stress.

Forearm vasodilator responses to mental stress and arousal are attenuated by i.a. infusions of atropine (Blair *et al.*, 1959; Barcroft *et al.*, 1960), suggesting that stress activates cholinergic vasodilator nerves in this region. Whether this is also true for the leg, thereby explaining our findings, is not known. Peptidergic and other vasodilator nerves may, of course, also be involved. Thus, vasodilator responses to mental stress are not due to withdrawal of sympathetic vasoconstrictor nerve activity, but seem to be related to neurogenic cholinergic and, possibly, peptidergic mechanisms; ADR may contribute to some extent.

PERSPECTIVES

As is evident from the present overview, there is rather detailed knowledge concerning sympatho-adrenal control of the skeletal muscle circulation and the mechanisms involved in animals and in humans. The microneurographic technique is extremely valuable and has provided us with a large data base on sympathetic axonal nerve activity to skeletal muscle in man during various provocations. However, the accumulating data on MSA, plasma NA and vascular resistance have also reinforced the danger of extrapolating from one region to another with regard to sympathetic activity. We believe that sympathetic nerve activity occurs in highly differentiated patterns — in fact, even MSA in the arm and leg seems to differ. Thus, it is quite clear that studies should concern individual organs, if possible, and that conclusions should be restricted to the organ/area actually studied.

With regard to skeletal muscle it is, therefore, questionable if data pertaining to the forearm or calf regions in man are always representative of skeletal muscle as a whole. The present knowledge concerning skeletal muscle derives mainly from the forearm for circulatory variables and from the peroneal nerve for nerve recordings. Methodological developments are needed to establish how representative they are of skeletal muscle in regions of the body other than the limbs. In addition, the possibly confounding fact that limbs also contain skin and adipose tissue needs to be addressed in somewhat greater detail.

It has been pointed out that neurotransmission encompasses more than axonal nerve activity, as there is prejunctional modulation of transmitter release, and postjunctional sensitivity to the transmitter(s) released may vary. The biochemical approach to the assessment of sympathetic neurotransmission currently provides us with valuable data, especially if studies are focused on the local overflows of these transmitters, but better information on the actual relationships between transmitter concentrations in the neuroeffector junction and blood, respectively, would be valuable. Measurements of extracellular tissue concentrations of the neurotransmitters, especially NA, using microdialysis techniques can be foreseen in the near future. This may bring us one step closer to the neuroeffector junction. Also, techniques for assessments of neuropeptide-related mechanisms (especially the development of selective and potent receptor antagonists) are needed to understand the importance of peptidergic neurotransmission — today, evidence in this field is mainly circumstantial.

The physiological roles of the various new adrenoceptor subtypes that have recently been characterized need to be established. This probably requires the development of even more selective adrenoceptor antagonists than those available today. Finally, the importance of the endothelium in the regulation of skeletal muscle blood flow in relation to sympatho-adrenal mechanisms needs to be adressed in detail. Thus, even though we know a great deal about the regulation of skeletal muscle blood flow, we can look forward to stimulating further developments in the field.

REFERENCES

Abboud, F.M., Heistad, D.D., Mark, A.L. and Schmid, P.G. (1976). Reflex control of the peripheral circulation. *Progress in Cardiovascular Diseases*, **18**, 371–403.

Agewall, S., Rhea, B., Persson, B., Karlberg, B., Wallin, G. and Andersson, O.K. (1990). Reflexogenic neuronal and humoral responses to selective stimulation of low-pressure cardiopulmonary receptors in man. *Journal of Internal Medicine*, **228**, 151–158.

Ahlquist, R.P. (1948). A study of the adrenotropic receptors. *American Journal of Physiology*, **153**, 586–600.

Allen, W.J., Barcroft, H. and Edholm, O.G. (1946). On the action of adrenaline on the blood vessels in human skeletal muscle. *Journal of Physiology (London)*, **105**, 255–267.

Anderson, E.A., Wallin, B.G. and Mark, A.L. (1987). Dissociation of sympathetic nerve activity in arm and leg muscle during mental stress. *Hypertension*, **9**(Suppl. 3), 114–119.

Andersson, P.O. (1983). Comparative vascular effects of stimulation continuously and in bursts of the sympathetic nerves to cat skeletal muscle. *Acta Physiologica Scandinavica*, **118**, 343–348.

Ariëns, E.J. and Simonis, A.M. (1983). Physiological and pharmacological aspects of adrenergic receptor classification. *Biochemical Pharmacology*, **32**, 1539–1545.

Bachelard, H., Gardiner, S.M., Kemp, P.A. and Bennett, T. (1992). Involvement of capsaicin-sensitive neurons in the haemodynamic effects of exogenous vasoactive peptides: studies in conscious, adult Long Evans rats treated neonatally with capsaicin. *British Journal of Pharmacology*, **105**, 202–210.

Baily, R.G., Prophet, S.A., Shenberger, J.S., Zelis, R. and Sinoway, L.I. (1990). Direct neurohumoral evidence for isolated sympathetic nervous system activation to skeletal muscle in response to cardiopulmonary baroreceptor unloading. *Circulation Research*, **66**, 1720–1728.

Barcroft, H. and Cobbold, A.F. (1956). The action of adrenaline on muscle blood flow and blood lactate in man. *Journal of Physiology (London)*, **132**, 372–378.

Barcroft, H., Gaskell, P., Shepherd, J.T. and Whelan, R.F. (1954). The effect of noradrenaline infusions on the blood flow through the human forearm. *Journal of Physiology (London)*, **123**, 443–450.

Barcroft, H., Brod, J., Hejl, Z., Hirsjärvi, E.A. and Kitchin, A.H. (1960). The mechanism of the vasodilatation in the forearm during stress (mental arithmetic). *Clinical Science*, **19**, 577–586.

Beiser, G.D., Zelis, R., Epstein, S.E., Mason, D.T. and Braunwald, E. (1970). The role of skin and muscle resistance vessels in reflexes mediated by the baroreceptor system. *Journal of Clinical Investigation*, **49**, 225–231.

Bennett, T. (1987). Cardiovascular responses to central hypovoaemia in man: physiology and pathophysiology. *The Physiologist*, **30**, S-143–S-146.

Berthelsen, S. and Pettinger, W.A. (1977). A functional basis for classification of α-adrenergic receptors. *Life Sciences*, **21**, 595–606.

Bevan, J.A. and Brayden, J.E. (1987). Nonadrenergic neural vasodilator mechanisms. *Circulation Research*, **60**, 309–326.

Blair, D.A., Glover, W.E., Greefield, A.D.M. and Roddie, I.C. (1959). Excitation of cholinergic vasodilator nerves to human skeletal muscles during emotional stress. *Journal of Physiology (London)*, **148**, 633–647.

Bolli, P., Kiowski, W., Amann, F.W. and Bühler, F.R. (1988). Adrenaline and enhanced vasoconstriction in patients with essential hypertension. *Pharmacology and Toxicology*, (Suppl. 1), 41–44.

Brick, I., Glover, W.E., Hutchison, K.J. and Roddie, I.C. (1966). Effects of propranolol on peripheral vessels in man. *American Journal of Cardiology*, **18**, 329–332.

Brock, J.A. and Cunnane, T.C. (1987). Relationship between the nerve action potential and transmitter release from sympathetic postganglionic nerve terminals. *Nature*, **326**, 605–607.

Brod, J. (1963). Haemodynamic basis of acute pressor reactions and hypertension. *British Heart Journal*, **25**, 227–245.

Brod, J., Fencl, V., Hejl, Z. and Jirka, J. (1959). Circulatory changes underlying blood pressure elevation during acute emotional stress (mental arithmetic) in normotensive and hypertensive subjects. *Clinical Science*, **18**, 269–279.

Brod, J., Cachovan, M., Bahlman, J., Bauer, G.E., Celsen, B., Sippel, R., *et al.* (1976). Haemodynamic response to an emotional stress (mental arithemetic) with special reference to the venous side. *Australian and New Zealand Journal of Medicine*, **6**(Suppl. 2), 19–25.

Brown, M.J., Jenner, D.A., Allison, D.J. and Dollery, C.T. (1981). Variations in individual organ release of noradrenaline measured by an improved radioenzymatic technique; limitations of peripheral venous measurements in the assessment of sympathetic nerve activity. *Clinical Science*, **61**, 585–590.

Burcher, E. and Garlick, D. (1973). Antagonism of vasoconstrictor responses by exercise in the gracilis muscle of the dog. *Journal of Pharmacology and Experimental Therapeutics*, **187**, 78–85.

Burcher, E. and Garlick, D. (1975). Effects of exercise metabolites on adrenergic vasoconstriction in the gracilis muscle of the dog. *Journal of Pharmacology and Experimental Therapeutics*, **192**, 149–156.

Burke, D., Sundlöf, G. and Wallin, B.G. (1977). Postural effects on muscle sympathetic nerve activity in man. *Journal of Physiology (London)*, **272**, 399–414.

Burnstock, G. and Kennedy, C. (1986). A dual function for adenosine 5′-triphosphate in the regulation of vascular tone. *Circulation Research*, **58**, 319–330.

Burnstock, G. and Warland, J.J.I. (1987). A pharmacological study of the rabbit saphenous artery *in vitro*: a vessel with large purinergic contractile response to sympathetic nerve stimulation. *British Journal of Pharmacology*, **90**, 111–120.

Bühler, F.R., Bolli, P., Hulthén, U.L., Amann, F.W. and Kiowski, W. (1983). α-adrenoceptors, adrenaline, and exaggerated vasoconstrictor response to stress in essential hypertension. *Chest*, **83**, 304–306.

Bylund, D. (1988). Subtypes of α_2-adrenoceptors: pharmacological and molecular biological evidence converge. *Trends in Pharmacological Sciences*, **9**, 356–361.

Cavero, I., Dennis, T., Lefèvre-Borg, D.T., Perrot, P., Roach, A.G. and Scatton, B. (1979). Effects of clonidine, prazosin and phentolamine on heart rate and coronary sinus catecholamine concentration during cardio-accelerator nerve stimulation in spinal dogs. *British Journal of Pharmacology*, **67**, 283–292.

Chang, P.C., van der Krogt, J.A., Vermeij, P. and van Brummelen, P. (1986). Norepinephrine removal and release in the forearm of healthy subjects. *Hypertension*, **8**, 801–809.

Chang, P.C., Kriek, E., van der Krogt, J.A., Blauw, G.-J. and van Brummelen, P. (1988). Haemodynamic effects of physiological concentrations of circulating noradrenaline in man. *Clinical Science*, **75**, 469–475.

Clarke, J., Benjamin, N., Larkin, S., Webb, D., Maseri, A. and Davies, G. (1991). Interaction of neuropeptide Y and the sympathetic system in vascular control in man. *Circulation*, **83**, 774–777.

Dahlöf, C. (1981). Studies on β-adrenoceptor-mediated facilitation of sympathetic neurotransmission. *Acta Physiologica Scandinavica*, (Suppl. 500), 1–147.

Dahlöf, C., Dahlöf, P. and Lundberg, J.M. (1985). Neuropeptide Y (NPY): enhancement of blood pressure increase upon α-adrenoceptor activation and direct pressor effects in pithed rats. *European Journal of Pharmacology*, **109**, 289–292.

Dahlöf, C., Kahan, T. and Åblad, B. (1987). Prejunctional β_2-adrenoceptor blockade reduces nerve stimulation evoked release of endogenous noradrenaline in skeletal muscle *in situ. Acta Physiologica Scandinavica*, **129**, 499–503.

de Jonge, A., Knape, J.T.A., van Meel, J.C.A., Kalkman, H.O., Wilffert, B., Thoolen, M.J.M., *et al.* (1982). Effect of converting enzyme inhibition and angiotensin receptor blockade on the vasoconstriction mediated by α_1- and β_2-adrenoceptor stimulation in pithed normotensive rats. *Naunyn-Schmiedeberg's Archives of Pharmacology*, **321**, 309–313.

de la Lande, I.S. and Whelan, R.F. (1959). The effect of antagonists on the response of the forearm vessels to adrenaline. *Journal of Physiology (London)*, **148**, 548–553.

Delius, W., Hagbarth, K.-E., Hongell, A. and Wallin, B.G. (1972a). General characteristics of sympathetic activity in human muscle nerves. *Acta Physiologica Scandinavica*, **84**, 65–81.

Delius, W., Hagbarth, K.-E., Hongell, A. and Wallin, B.G. (1972b). Manoeuvres affecting sympathetic outflow in human muscle nerves. *Acta Physiologica Scandinavica*, **84**, 82–94.

Docherty, J. R. (1984). An investigation of presynaptic α-adrenoceptor subtypes in the pithed rat heart and in the rat isolated vas deferens. *British Journal of Pharmacology*, **82**, 15–23.

Dodd, L. R. and Johnson, P.C. (1991). Diameter changes in arteriolar networks of contracting skeletal muscle. *American Journal of Physiology*, **260**, H662–H670.

Dzau, V. J. (1989). Short- and long-term determinants of cardiovascular function and therapy: contributions of circulating and tissue renin-angiotensin systems. *Journal of Cardiovascular Pharmacology*, **14**(Suppl. 4), S1–S5.

Eckberg, D. L., Rea, R.F., Andersson, O.K., Hedner, T., Pernow, J., Lundberg, J.M., *et al.* (1988). Baroreflex modulation of sympathetic activity and sympathetic neurotransmitters in humans. *Acta Physiologica Scandinavica*, **133**, 221–231.

Edvinsson, L., Håkanson, R., Wahlstedt, C. and Uddman, R. (1987). Effects of neuropeptide Y on the cardiovascular system. *Trends in Pharmacological Sciences*, **8**, 231–235.

Eisenhofer, G., Esler, M.D., Goldstein, D.S. and Kopin, I.J. (1991). Neuronal uptake, metabolism, and release of tritium-labeled norepinephrine during assessment of its plasma kinetics. *American Journal of Physiology*, **261**, E505-E515.

Ekelund, U. and Mellander, S. (1990). Role of endothelium-derived nitric oxide in the regulation of tonus in large-bore arterial resistance vessels, arterioles and veins in cat skeletal muscle. *Acta Physiologica Scandinavica*, **140**, 301–309.

Eklund, B. (1974). Influence of work duration on the regulation of muscle blood flow. *Acta Physiologica Scandinavica*, (Suppl. 411), 1–64.

Eklund, B. and Kaijser, L. (1976). Effect of regional α- and β-adrenergic blockade on blood flow in the resting forearm during contralateral isometric handgrip. *Journal of Physiology (London)*, **262**, 39–50.

Eklund, B., Hjemdahl, P., Seideman, P. and Atterhög, J.-H. (1983). Effects of prazosin on haemodynamics and sympatho-adrenal activity in hypertensive patients. *Journal of Cardiovascular Pharmacology*, **5**, 384–391.

Eliasson, K., Hjemdahl, P. and Kahan, T. (1983). Circulatory and sympatho-adrenal responses to stress in borderline and established hypertension. *Journal of Hypertension*, **1**, 131–139.

Elsner, D., Saeed, M., Sommer, O., Holtz, J. and Bassenge, E. (1984). Sympathetic vasoconstriction sensitive to α_2-adrenergic receptor blockade. No evidence for preferential innervation of α_1-adrenergic receptors in the canine femoral bed. *Hypertension*, **6**, 915–925.

Emorine, L.J., Marullo, S., Briend-Sutren, M.-M., Patey, G., Tate, K., Delavier-Klutchko, C., et al. (1989). Molecular characterization of the human β_3-adrenergic receptor. *Science*, **245**, 1118–1121.

Esler, M., Jennings, G., Korner, P., Willett, I., Dudley, F., Hasking, G., et al. (1988). Assessment of human sympathetic nervous system activity from measurements of noradrenaline turnover. *Hypertension*, **11**, 3–20.

Essandoh, L. K., Houston, D. S., Vanhoutte, P. M. and Shepherd, J.T. (1986). Differential effects of lower body negative pressure on forearm and calf blood flow. *Journal of Applied Physiology*, **61**, 994–998.

Essandoh, L. K., Duprez, D.A. and Shepherd, J.T. (1987). Postural cardiovascular reflexes: comparison of responses of forearm and calf resistance vessels. *Journal of Applied Physiology*, **63**, 1801–1805.

Faber, J.E. (1988). *In situ* analysis of α-adrenoceptors on arteriolar and venular smooth muscle in rat skeletal muscle microcirculation. *Circulation Research*, **62**, 37–50.

Falck, B. (1962). Observations on the possibilities of the cellular localization of monoamines by a fluorescent method. *Acta Physiologica Scandinavica*, (Suppl. 197), 1–25.

Flavahan, N.A. and Vanhoutte, P.M. (1986). α_1-Adrenoceptor subclassification in vascular smooth muscle. *Trends in Pharmacological Sciences*, **7**, 347–349.

Floras, J.S. 1992. Epinephrine and the genesis of hypertension. *Hypertension*, **19**, 1–18.

Fløistrup Vissing, S., Scherrer, U. and Victor, R.G. (1989). Relation between sympathetic outflow and vascular resistance in the calf during perturbations in central venous pressure; evidence for cardiopulmonary afferent regulation of calf vascular resistance in humans. *Circulation Research*, **65**, 1710–1717.

Folkow, B. (1952). Impulse frequency in sympathetic vasomotor fibres correlated to the release and elimination of the transmitter. *Acta Physiologica Scandinavica*, **25**, 49–76.

Folkow, B. and Uvnäs, B. (1948). The chemical transmission of vasoconstrictor impulses to the hind limbs and the splanchnic region of the cat. *Acta Physiologica Scandinavica*, **15**, 365–388.

Folkow, B., Häggendal, J. and Lisander, B. (1967). Extent of release and elimination of noradrenaline at peripheral adrenergic nerve terminals. *Acta Physiologica Scandinavica*, (Suppl. 307), 1–38.

Folkow, B., Sonnenschein, R.R. and Wright, D.L. (1971). Loci of neurogenic and metabolic effects on precapillary vessels of skeletal muscle. *Acta Physiologica Scandinavica*, **81**, 459–471.

Folkow, B., DiBona, G.F., Hjemdahl, P., Thorén, P. and Wallin, B.G. (1983). Measurements of plasma norepinephrine concentrations in human primary hypertension — a word of caution on their applicability for assessing neurogenic contributions. *Hypertension*, **5**, 399–403.

Freyschuss, U., Hjemdahl, P., Juhlin-Dannfelt, A. and Linde, B. (1986). Cardiovascular and metabolic responses to low dose adrenaline infusion: an invasive study in humans. *Clinical Science*, **70**, 199–206.

Furchgott, R.F. and Vanhoutte, P.M. (1989). Endothelium-derived relaxing and contracting factors. *FASEB Journal*, **3**, 2007–2018.

Furchgott, R.F. and Zawadzki, J.V. (1980). The obligatory role of endothelial cells in the relaxation of arterial smooth muscle by acetylcholine. *Nature*, **288**, 373–376.

Fuxe, K. and Sedvall, G. (1965). The distribution of adrenergic nerve fibres to the blood vessels in skeletal muscle. *Acta Physiologica Scandinavica*, **64**, 75–86.

Gaffney, F.A., Sjøgaard, G. and Saltin, B. (1990). Cardiovascular and metabolic responses to static contraction in man. *Acta Physiologica Scandinavica*, **138**, 249–258.

Gardiner, J.C. and Peters, C.J. (1982). Postsynaptic α_1- and α_2-adrenoceptor involvement in the vascular responses to neuronally released and exogenous noradrenaline in the hindlimb of the dog and cat. *European Journal of Pharmacology*, **84**, 189–198.

Gardiner, S.M., and Bennett, T. (1988). Regional haemodynamic responses to adrenoceptor antagonism in conscious rats. *American Journal of Physiology*, **255**, H813–H824.

Gardiner, S.M., Compton, A.M. and Bennett, T. (1989). Regional haemodynamic effects of calcitonin gene-related peptide. *American Journal of Physiology*, **256**, R332–R338.

Gardiner, S.M., Compton, A.M., Bennett, T., Palmer, R.M.J. and Moncada, S. (1990a). Control of regional blood flow by endothelium-derived nitric oxide. *Hypertension*, **15**, 486–492.

Gardiner, S.M., Compton, A.M., Kemp, P.A., Bennett, T., Bose, C., Foulkes, R., et al. (1990b). Antagonistic effect of human α-CGRP [8–37] on the *in vivo* regional haemodynamic actions of human α-CGRP. *Biochemical and Biophysical Research Communications*, **171**, 938–943.

Gardiner, S.M., Kemp, P.A., Bennett, T., Bose, C., Foulkes, R. and Hughes, B. (1992). Involvement of β_2-adrenoceptors in the regional haemodynamic responses to bradykinin in conscious rats. *British Journal of Pharmacology*, **105**, 839–848.

Goldstein, D.S., Eisenhofer, G., Sax, F.L., Keiser, H.R. and Kopin, I.J. (1987). Plasma norepinephrine pharmacokinetics during mental challenge. *Psychosomatic Medicine*, **49**, 591–605.

Grant, T.L. and McGrath, J.C. (1988a). Interactions between angiotensin II and α-adrenoceptor agonists mediating pressor responses in the pithed rat. *British Journal of Pharmacology*, **95**, 1229–1240.

Grant, T.L. and McGrath, J.C. (1988b). Interactions between angiotensin II, sympathetic nerve-mediated pressor response and cyclo-oxygenase products in the pithed rat. *British Journal of Pharmacology*, **95**, 1220–1228.

Guimaraes, S., Brandao, F. and Paiva, M.Q. (1978). A study of the adrenoceptor-mediated feedback mechanisms by using adrenaline as a false transmitter. *Naunyn-Schmiedebergs's Archives of Pharmacology*, **305**, 185–188.

Gustafsson, D. and Lundvall, J. (1984). β_2-adrenergic vascular control in haemorrhage and its influence on cardiac performance. *American Journal of Physiology*, **246**, H351–H359.

Hainsworth, R. (1986). Vascular capacitance: its control and importance. *Reviews in Physiology, Biochemistry and Pharmacology*, **105**, 102–171.

Hainsworth, R., Karim, F., McGregor, K.H. and Wood, L.M. (1983). Hind-limb vascular capacitance responses in anaesthetized dogs. *Journal of Physiology (London)*, **337**, 417–428.

Heitz, D.C., Schafer, R.A. and Brody, M.J. (1975). Possible mechanism of histamine release during active vasodilatation. *American Journal of Physiology*, **238**, 1351–1357.

Henriksen, J.H. and Christensen, N.J. (1989). Plasma norepinephrine in humans: limitations in assessment of whole body norepinephrine kinetics and plasma clearance. *American Journal of Physiology*, **257**, E743–E750.

Henriksen, O., Skagen, K., Haxholdt, O. and Dyrberg, V. (1983). Contribution of local blood flow regulation mechanisms to the maintenance of arterial pressure in upright position during epidural blockade. *Acta Physiologica Scandinavica*, **118**, 271–280.

Hicks, P.E., Najar, M., Vidal, M. and Langer, S.Z. (1986). Possible involvement of presynaptic α_1 adrenoceptors in the effects of idazoxan and prazosin on ^{3}H-noradrenline release from tail arteries of SHR. *Naunyn-Schmiedeberg's Archives of Pharmacology*, **333**, 354–361.

Hilgers, K.F., Kuczera, M., Wilhelm, M.J., Wiecek, A., Ritz, E., Ganten, D., et al. (1989). Angiotensin formation in the isolated rat hindlimb. *Journal of Hypertension*, **7**, 789–798.

Hillman, J. (1983). β_2-adrenergic control of transcapillary fluid absorption and plasma volume in haemorrhage. *Acta Physiologica Scandinavica*, (Suppl. 516), 1–62.

Hillman, J., Gustafsson, D. and Lundvall, J. (1982). β_2-adrenergic control of plasma volume in haemorrhage. *Acta Physiologica Scandinavica*, **116**, 175–180.

Hilton, S.M., Spyer, K.M. and Timms, R.J. (1979). The origin of the hind limb vasodilatation evoked by stimulation of the motor cortex in the cat. *Journal of Physiology (London)*, **287**, 545–557.

Hirst, G.D.S. and Edwards, F.R. (1989). Sympathetic neuroeffector transmission in arteries and arterioles. *Physiological Reviews*, **69**, 546–604.

Hirst, G.D.S. and Neild, T.O. (1980). Evidence for two populations of excitatory receptors for noradrenaline on arteriolar smooth muscle. *Nature*, **283**, 767–768.

Hjemdahl, P. (1984). Inter-laboratory comparison of plasma catecholamine determinations using several different assays. *Acta Physiologica Scandinavica*, (Suppl. 527), 43–54.

Hjemdahl, P. (1987). Physiological aspects on catecholamine sampling. *Life Sciences*, **41**, 841–844.

Hjemdahl, P. (1991). Physiology of the autonomic nervous system as related to cardiovascular function: implications for stress research. In *Anxiety and the Heart*. edited by D.G. Byrne and R.H. Rosenman, pp. 95–158. New York: Hemisphere Publishing Corporation.

Hjemdahl, P. (1993). Plasma catecholamines — analytical challenges and physiological limitations. *Baillière's Clinical Endocrinology and Metabolism*, **7**, 307–353.

Hjemdahl, P. and Fredholm, B.B. (1976). Influence of acidosis on noradrenaline-induced vasoconstriction in adipose tissue and skeletal muscle. *Acta Physiologica Scandinavica*, **97**, 319–324.

Hjemdahl, P. and Linde, B. (1983). Influence of circulating NE and Epi on adipose tissue vascular resistance and lipolysis in humans. *American Journal of Physiology*, **245**, H447–H452.

Hjemdahl, P. and Schwieler, J.H. (1991). Modulation of sympatho-adrenal function by the renin-angiotensin system. In *Current Advances in ACE Inhibition 2*, edited by G.A. MacGregor and P.S. Sever, pp. 98–105. Edinburgh: Churchill Livingstone.

Hjemdahl, P., Eklund, B. and Kaijser, L. (1982). Catecholamine handling by the human forearm at rest and during isometric exercise and lower body negative pressure. *British Journal of Pharmacology*, **77**, 324p.

Hjemdahl, P., Freyschuss, U., Juhlin-Dannfelt, A. and Linde, B. (1984). Differentiated sympathetic activation during mental stress evoked by the Strrop test. *Acta Physiologica Scandinavica*, (Suppl. 527), 25–29.

Hjemdahl, P., Fagius, J., Freyschuss, U., Wallin, B.G., Daleskog, M., Bohlin, G., et al. (1989). Muscle sympathetic nerve activity and norepinephrine release during mental challenge in humans. *American Journal of Physiology*, **257**, E654–E664.

Hughes, J. and Roth, R.H. (1974). Variation in noradrenaline output with changes in stimulus frequency and train length: role of different noradrenaline pools. *British Journal of Pharmacology*, **51**, 373–381.

Husain, A. (1993). The chymase-angiotensin system in humans. *Journal of Hypertension*, **11**, 1155–1159.

Hyman, A.L., Lipton, H.L. and Kadowitz, P.J. (1990). Analysis of pulmonary vascular responses in cats to sympathetic nerve stimulation under elevated tone conditions: evidence that neuronally released norepinephrine acts on α_1-, α_2- and β_2-adrenoceptors. *Circulation Research*, **67**, 862–870.

Iversen, L.L. (1975). Uptake processes for biogenic amines. In *Handbook of Psychopharmacology, Vol. 3*, edited by L.L. Iversen, S.D. Iversen and S.H. Snyder, pp. 381–442. New York: Plenum Press.

Iwase, S., Mano, T. and Saito, M. (1987). Effects of graded head-up tilting on muscle sympathetic activities in man. *The Physiologist*, **30**, S62-S63.

Jie, K., van Brummelen, P., Vermeij, P., Timmermans, P.B.M.W.M. and van Zwieten, P.A. (1984). Identification of vascular postsynaptic α_1- and α_2-adrenoceptors in man. *Circulation Research*, **54**, 447–452.

Jie, K., van Brummelen, P., Vermeij, P., Timmermans, P.B.M.W.M. and van Zwieten, P.A. (1986). α_1- and α_2-adrenoceptor-mediated vasoconstriction in the forearm of normotensive and hypertensive subjects. *Journal of Cardiovascular Pharmacology*, **8**, 190–196.

Jie, K., van Brummelen, P., Vermeij, P., Timmermans, P.B.M.W.M. and van Zwieten, P.A. (1987). Postsynaptic α_1- and α_2-adrenoceptors in human blood vessels: interactions with exogenous and endogenous catecholamines. *European Journal of Clinical Investigation*, **17**, 174–181.

Joborn, H., Hjemdahl, P., Larsson, P.T., Olsson, G., Wide, L., Bergström, R., *et al.* (1990). Effects of prolonged adrenaline infusion and mental stress on plasma minerals and parathyroid hormone. *Clinical Physiology*, **10**, 37–53.

Johnsson, G. (1975). Influence of metoprolol and propranolol on hemodynamic effects induced by adrenaline and physical work. *Acta Pharmacologica et Toxicologica*, **36**(Suppl. 5), 59–68.

Juhlin-Dannfelt, A. and Åström, H. (1979). Influence of β-adrenoceptor blockade on leg blood flow and lactate release in man. *Scandinavian Journal of Clinical and Laboratory Investigation*, **39**, 179–183.

Kahan, T. (1987). Prejunctional adrenergic receptors and sympathetic neurotransmission: studies in canine skeletal muscle *in situ*. *Acta Physiologica Scandinavica*, (Suppl. 560), 1–38.

Kahan, T. and Hjemdahl, P. (1987a). Pre- and postjunctional α-adrenoceptor-mediated effects of prazosin, methoxamine and 6-fluoronoradrenaline in blood-perfused canine skeletal muscle *in situ*. *European Journal of Pharmacology*, **133**, 9–20.

Kahan, T. and Hjemdahl, P. (1987b). Prejunctional β_2-adrenoceptor-mediated enhancement of noradrenaline release in skeletal muscle vasculature *in situ*. *Journal of Cardiovascular Pharmacology*, **10**, 433–438.

Kahan, T., Hjemdahl, P. and Dahlöf, C. (1984). Relationship between the overflow of endogenous and radiolabelled noradrenaline from canine blood perfused gracilis muscle. *Acta Physiologica Scandinavica*, **122**, 571–582.

Kahan, T., Dahlöf, C. and Hjemdahl, P. (1985). Influence of acetylcholine, peptides and other vasodilators on endogenous noradrenaline overflow in canine blood perfused gracilis muscle. *Acta Physiologica Scandinavica*, **124**, 457–465.

Kahan, T., Dahlöf, C. and Hjemdahl, P. (1987). Prejunctional α-adrenoceptor-mediated inhibition of norepinephrine release in blood-perfused skeletal muscle *in situ*. *Journal of Cardiovascular Pharmacology*, **9**, 555–562.

Kahan, T., Hjemdahl, P. and Dahlöf, C. (1987). Facilitation of nerve stimulation evoked noradrenaline overflow by isoprenaline but not by circulating adrenaline in the dog *in vivo*. *Life Sciences*, **40**, 1811–1818.

Kahan, T., Pernow, J., Schwieler, J., Wallin, B.G., Hjemdahl, P. and Lundberg, J.M. (1988). Noradrenaline release evoked by the physiological irregular sympathetic nerve discharge is modulated by prejunctional α- and β-adrenoceptors *in vivo*. *British Journal of Pharmacology*, **95**, 1101–1108.

Kahan, T., Taddei, S., Pedrinelli, R., Hjemdahl, P. and Salvetti, A. (1992). Nonadrenergic sympathetic vascular control of the human forearm in hypertension: possible involvement of neuropeptide Y. *Journal of Cardiovascular Pharmacology*, **19**, 587–592.

Kennedy, C., Saville, V.L. and Burnstock, G. (1986). The contributions of noradrenaline and ATP to the responses of the rabbit central ear artery to sympathetic stimulation depend on the parameters of stimulation. *European Journal of Pharmacology*, **122**, 291–300.

Kirkpatrick, K. and Burnstock, G. (1987). Sympathetic nerve-mediated release of ATP from the guinea-pig vas deferens is unaffected by reserpine. *European Journal of Pharmacology*, **138**, 207–214.

Kobinger, W. and Pichler, L. (1980). Investigation into different types of post- and presynaptic α-adrenoceptors at cardiovascular sites in rats. *European Journal of Pharmacology*, **65**, 393–402.

Kuwahara, M., Kubo, T. and Misu, Y. (1989). Isoproterenol induced facilitation of norepinephrine release does not primarily involve a local angiotensin II mechanism in guinea pig pulmonary arteries. *Japanese Journal of Pharmacology*, **51**, 302–305.

Lands, A.M., Arnold, A., Mc Auliff, J.P., Luduena, F.P. and Brown, T.G. (1967). Differentiation of receptor systems activated by sympathomimetic amines. *Nature*, **214**, 597–598.

Langer, S.Z. (1974). Presynaptic regulation of catecholamine release. *Biochemical Pharmacology*, **23**, 1793–1800.

Langer, S.Z. (1981). Presynaptic regulation of the release of catecholamines. *Pharmacological Reviews*, **32**, 337–362.

Langer, S.Z., Massingham, R. and Shepperson, N.B. (1980). Presence of postsynaptic α_2-adrenoceptors of predominantly extrasynaptic location in the vascular smooth muscle of the dog hind limb. *Clinical Science*, **59**, 225s–228s.

Lefkowitz, R.J., Caron, M.G. and Stiles, G.L. (1984). Mechanisms of membrane-receptor regulation — biochemical, physiological, and clinical insights from studies of the adrenergic receptors. *New England Journal of Medicine*, **310**, 1570–1579.

Liggett, S.B., Shah, S.D. and Cryer, P.E. (1988). Characterization of β-adrenoceptors of human skeletal muscle obtained by needle biopsy. *American Journal of Physiology*, **254**, E795–E798.

Linde, B. and Hjemdahl, P. (1982). Effect of tilting on adipose tissue vascular resistance and sympathetic activity in humans. *American Journal of Physiology*, **242**, H161–H167.

Linde, B., Hjemdahl, P., Freyschuss, U. and Juhlin-Dannfelt, A. (1989). Adipose tissue and skeletal muscle blood flow during mental stress. *American Journal of Physiology*, **256**, E12–E18.

Lindqvist, M., Kahan, T., Melcher, A. and Hjemdahl, P. (1993). Cardiovascular and sympatho-adrenal responses to mental stress in primary hypertension. *Clinical Science*, **85**, 401–409.

Lomasney, J.W., Cotecchia, S., Lefkowitz, R.J. and Caron, M.G. (1991). Molecular biology of α-adrenergic receptors: implications for receptor classification and structure-function relationships. *Biochimica et Biophysica Acta*, **1095**, 127–139.

Lundberg, J.M., Franco-Cereceda, A., Lacroix, J.-S. and Pernow, J. (1990). Neuropeptide Y and sympathetic neurotransmission. *Annals of the New York Academy of Science*, **611**, 166–174.

Lundberg, J.M., Martinsson, A., Hemsén, A., Theodorsson-Norheim, E., Svedenhag, J., Ekblom, B., *et al.* (1985). Co-release of neuropeptide Y and catecholamines during physical exercise in man. *Biochemical Biophysical Research Communications*, **133**, 30–36.

Lundvall, J. and Edfeldt, H. (1993). Much more potent sympathetic control of vascular resistance in the forearm in man than previously believed. *Acta Physiologica Scandinavica*, **147**, 185–193.

Lundvall, J. and Järhult, J. (1976). Changes of the pressure drop curve and of resistance along the vascular bed of skeletal muscles evoked by sympathetic stimulation. *Microvascular Research*, **12**, 43–54.

Majewski, H., Rand, M.J. and Tung, L.H. (1981). Activation of prejunctional β-adrenoceptors in rat atria by adrenaline applied exogenously or released as a co-transmitter. *British Journal of Pharmacology*, **73**, 669–679.

Mark, A.L., Victor, R.G., Nerhed, C. and Wallin, B.G. (1985). Microneurographic studies of the mechanisms of sympathetic nerve responses to static exercise in humans. *Circulation Research*, **57**, 461–469.

Marshall, J.M. (1982). The influence of the sympathetic nervous system on individual vessels of the microcirculation of skeletal muscle of the rat. *Journal of Physiology (London)*, **322**, 169–186.

Maspers, M. and Björnberg, J. (1991). β_2-adrenergic attenuation of capillary pressure autoregulation during haemorrhagic hypotension, a mechanism promoting transcapillary fluid absorption in skeletal muscle. *Acta Physiologica Scandinavica*, **142**, 11–20.

McGrath, J.C. (1982). Evidence for more than one type of postjunctional α-adenoceptor. *Biochemical Pharmacology*, **31**, 467–484.

Mellander, S. (1960). Comparative studies on the adrenergic neurohumoral control of resistance and capacitance blood vessels in the cat. *Acta Physiologica Scandinavica*, (Suppl. 176), 1–86.

Mellander, S. and Johansson, B. (1968). Control of resistance, exchange, and capacitance functions in the peripheral circulation. *Pharmacological Reviews*, **20**, 117–196.

Michel, M.C. (1991). Receptors for neuropeptide Y: multiple subtypes and multiple second messengers. *Trends in Pharmacological Sciences*, **12**, 389–394.

Michel, M.C., Philipp, T. and Brodde, O.-E. (1992). α- and β-Adrenoceptors in hypertension: molecular biology and pharmacological studies. *Pharmacology & Toxicology*, **70**(Suppl. 2), s1–s10.

Minneman, K. (1988). α_1-adrenergic receptor subtypes, inositol phosphates, and sources of cell Ca^{2+}. *Pharmacological Reviews*, **40**, 87–119.

Mizuno, K., Nakamaru, M., Higashimori, K. and Inagami, T. (1988). Local generation and release of angiotensin II in peripheral vascular tissue. *Hypertension*, **11**, 223–229.

Muscholl, E. (1980). Peripheral muscarinic control of norepinephrine release in the cardiovascular system. *American Journal of Physiology*, **239**, H713–H720.

Musgrave, I. and Majewski, H. (1987). Facilitation of noradrenaline release by isoprenaline in mouse atria does not involve angiotensin II. *Blood Vessels*, **24**, 217.

Nahorski, S.R., Barnett, D.B. and Cheung, Y.-D. (1985). α-Adrenoceptor-effector coupling: afinity states or heterogeneity of the α_2 adrenoceptor? *Clinical Science*, **68**(Suppl. 10), 39s–42s.

Nakamaru, M., Jackson, E. and Inagami, T. (1986). Role of vascular angiotensin II released by β-adrenergic stimulation in rats. *Journal of Cardiovascular Pharmacology*, **8**(Suppl. 10), S1–S5.

Nickerson, M., Henry, J.W. and Nomaguchi, G.M. (1953). Blockade of responses to epinephrine and nore-pinephrine congeners. *Journal of Pharmacology*, **107**, 300–309.

Öberg, B. (1964). Effects of cardiovascular relexes on net capillary fluid transfer. *Acta Physiologica Scandinavica*, (Suppl. 229), 1–98.

Öhlén, A., Lindbom, L., Staines, W., Hökfelt, T., Hedqvist, P., Fischer, J.A., *et al.* (1987). Substance P and calcitonin gene-related peptide: immunohistochemical localization and microvascular effects in rabbit skeletal muscle. *Naunyn-Schmiedberg's Archives of Pharmacology*, **336**, 87–93.

Öhlén, A., Thureson-Klein, Å., Lindbom, L., Hökfelt, T. and Hedqvist, P. (1988). Substance P and NPY innervation of microvessels in the rabbit tenuissimus muscle. *Microvascular Research*, **36**, 117–129.

Öhlén, A., Persson, M.G., Lindbom, L., Gustafsson, L.E. and Hedqvist, P. (1990). Nerve-induced nonadrenergic vasoconstriction and vasodilatation in skeletal muscle. *American Journal of Physiology*, **258**, H1334–H1338.

Okamura, T., Okunishi, H., Ayajiki, K. and Toda, N. (1990). Conversion of angiotensin I to angiotensin II in dog isolated renal artery: role of two different angiotensin II-generating enzymes. *Journal of Cardiovascular Pharmacology*, **15**, 353–359.

O'Leary, D.S., Rowell, L.B. and Scher, A.M. (1991). Baroreflex-induced vasoconstriction in active skeletal muscle of conscious dogs. *American Journal of Physiology*, **260**, H37–H41.

Palmer, R.M.J., Ferrigo, A.G. and Moncada, S. (1987). Nitric oxide release accounts for the biological activity of endothelium-derived relaxing factor. *Nature*, **327**, 524–525.

Pelleg, A. and Burnstock, G. (1990). Physiological importance of ATP released from nerve terminals and its degradation to adenosine in humans. *Circulation*, **82**, 2269–2272.

Pernow, J., Lundberg, J., Kaijser, L., Hjemdahl, P., Theodorsson-Norheim, E., Martinsson, A., *et al.* (1986). Plasma neuropeptide Y-like immunoreactivity and catecholamines during various degrees of sympathetic activation in man. *Clinical Physiology*, **6**, 561–578.

Pernow, J., Lundberg, J.M. and Kaijser, L. (1987). Vasoconstrictor effects *in vivo* and plasma disappearance rate of neuropeptide Y in man. *Life Sciences*, **40**, 47–54.

Pernow, J., Öhlén, A., Hökfelt, T., Nilsson, O. and Lundberg, J.M. (1987). Neuropeptide Y: presence in perivascular noradrenergic neurons and vasoconstrictor effects on skeletal muscle blood vessels in experimental animals and man. *Regulatory Peptides*, **19**, 313–324.

Pernow, J., Kahan, T., Hjemdahl, P. and Lundberg, J.M. (1988). Possible involvement of neuropeptide Y in sympathetic vascular control in canine skeletal muscle. *Acta Physiologica Scandinavica*, **132**, 43–50.

Pernow, J., Kahan, T. and Lundberg, J. (1988). Neuropeptide Y and reserpine-resistant vasoconstriction evoked by sympathetic nerve stimulation in dog skeletal muscle. *British Journal of Pharmacology*, **94**, 952–960.

Pernow, J., Schwieler, J., Kahan, T., Hjemdahl, P., Oberle, J., Wallin, B.G., *et al.* (1989). Influence of sympathetic discharge pattern on norepinephrine and neuropeptide Y release and vasoconstriction *in vivo*. *American Journal of Physiology*, **257**, H866–H872.

Persson, B., Andersson, O.K., Hjemdahl, P., Wysocki, M., Agerwall, S. and Wallin, G. (1989). Adrenaline infusion in man increases muscle sympathetic activity and noradrenaline overflow to plasma. *Journal of Hypertension*, **7**, 747–756.

Potter, E.K. (1988). Neuropeptide Y as an autonomic neurotransmitter. *Pharmacology and Therapeutics*, **37**, 251–273.

Rahman, M.A. and Bennett, T. (1990). The effects of propranolol and atenolol on the cardiovascular responses to central hypovolaemia in Europeans and Bengalees. *British Journal of Clinical Pharmacology*, **29**, 69–77.

Ramme, D., Regenold, J.T., Starke, K., Busse, R. and Illes, P. (1987). Identification of the neuroeffector transmitter in jejunal branches of the rabbit mesenteric artery. *Naunyn-Schmiedeberg's Archives of Pharmacology*, **336**, 267–273.

Rand, M.J., Majewski, H., McCulloch, M.W. and Story, D.F. (1979). An adrenaline mediated positive feedback loop in sympathetic transmission and its possible role in hypertension. In *Advances in the Biosciences*, Vol. 18: Presynaptic receptors, pp. 263–269. Oxford: Pergamon Press.

Ray, C.A. and Mark, A.L. (1993). Augmentation of muscle sympathetic nerve activity during fatiguing isometric leg exercise. *Journal of Applied Physiology*, **75**, 228–232.

Ray, C.A., Rea, R.F., Clary, M.P. and Mark, A.L. (1992). Muscle sympathetic nerve responses to static leg exercise. *Journal of Applied Physiology*, **73**, 1523–1529.

Rea, R.F. and Hamdan, M. (1990). Baroreflex control of muscle sympathetic nerve activity in borderline hypertension. *Circulation*, **82**, 856–862.

Rea, R.F. and Wallin, B.G. (1989). Sympathetic nerve activity in arm and leg muscles during lower body negative pressure in humans. *Journal of Applied Physiology*, **66**, 2778–2781.

Rea, R.F., Eckberg, D.L., Fritsch, J.M. and Goldstein, D.S. (1990). Relation of plasma norepinephrine and sympathetic traffic during hypotension in humans. *American Journal of Physiology*, **258**, R982–R986.

Reit, E. (1972). Actions of angiotensin on the adrenal medulla and the autonomic ganglia. *Federation Proceedings*, **31**, 1338–1343.

Renkin, E.M. (1984). Control of microcirculation and blood-tissue exchange. In *Handbook of Physiology, Section 2, vol IV, Part 1: The Cardiovascular System*, edited by E.M. Renkin and C.C. Michel, pp. 627–687. Bethesda, Maryland: American Physiological Society.

Revington, M. and McCloskey, D.I. (1988). Neuropeptide Y and control of vascular resistance in skeletal muscle. *Regulatory Peptides*, **23**, 331–342.

Robinson, V.J.B., Manyari, D.E., Tyberg, J.V., Fick, G.H. and Smith, E.R. (1989). Volume-pressure analysis of reflex changes in forearm venous function; a method by mental arithmetic stress and radionuclide plethysmography. *Circulation*, **80**, 99–105.

Roddie, I.C., Shepherd, J.T. and Whelan, R.F. (1957). Reflex changes in vasoconstrictor tone in human skeletal muscle in response to stimulation of receptors in a low-pressure area of the intrathoracic vascular bed. *Journal of Physiology (London)*, **139**, 369–376.

Ross, G. (1971). The regional circulation. *Annual Review of Physiology*, **33**, 445–478.

Rowell, L.B. (1984). Reflex control of regional circulations in humans. *Journal of the Autonomic Nervous System*, **11**, 101–114.

Rowell, L.B., Wyss, C.R. and Brengelmann, G.L. (1973). Sustained human skin and muscle vasoconstriction with reduced baroreceptor activity. *Journal of Applied Physiology*, **34**, 639–643.

Rowlands, D.J. and Donald, D.E. (1968). Sympathetic vasoconstriction during exercise- or drug-induced vasodilatation. *Circulation Research*, **23**, 45–60.

Rusch, N.J., Shepherd, J.T., Webb, R.C. and Vanhoutte, P.M. (1981). Different behaviour of the resistance vessels of the human calf and forearm during contralateral isometric exercise, mental stress, and abnormal respiratory movements. *Circulation Research*, **48**, I-118–I-130.

Russel, M.P. and Moran, N.C. (1980). Evidence for lack of innervation of β_2-adrenoceptors in the blood vessels of the gracilis muscle of the dog. *Circulation Research*, **46**, 344–352.

Saito, M., Mano, T. and Iwase, S. (1990). Changes in muscle sympathetic nerve activity and calf blood flow during static handgrip exercise. *European Journal of Applied Physiology*, **60**, 277–281.

Saito, M., Naito, M. and Mano, T. (1990). Different responses in skin and muscle sympathetic nerve activity to static muscle contraction. *Journal of Applied Physiology*, **69**, 2085–2090.

Saltin, B. (1988). Capacity of blood flow delivery to exercising skeletal muscle in humans. *American Journal of Cardiology*, **62**, 30E–35E.

Savard, G., Strange, S., Kiens, B., Richter, E.A., Christensen, N.J. and Saltin, B. (1987). Noradrenaline spillover during exercise in active versus resting skeletal muscle. *Acta Physiologica Scandinavica*, **131**, 507–515.

Savard, G.K., Richter, E.A., Strange, S., Kiens, B., Christensen, N.J. and Saltin, B. (1989). Norepinephrine spillover from skeletal muscle during exercise in humans: role of muscle mass. *American Journal of Physiology*, **257**, H1812–H1818.

Schlicker, E., Erkens, K. and Göthert, M. (1988). Probable involvement of vascular angiotensin II formation in the β_2 adrenoceptor-mediated facilitation of the neurogenic vasopressor response in the pithed rat. *Naunyn-Schmiedeberg's Archives of Pharmacology*, **338**, 536–542.

Schwieler, J.H. and Hjemdahl, P. (1992). Influence of angiotensin converting enzyme inhibition on sympathetic neurotransmission: possible roles of bradykinin and prostaglandins. *Journal of Cardiovascular Pharmacology*, **20**(Suppl. 9), S39–S46.

Schwieler, J.H., Kahan, T., Nussberger, J. and Hjemdahl, P. (1991a). Influence of the renin-angiotensin system on sympathetic neurotransmission in canine skeletal muscle *in vivo*. *Naunyn-Schmiedeberg's Archives of Pharmacology*, **343**, 166–172.

Schwieler, J.H., Nussberger, J., Kahan, T. and Hjemdahl, P. (1991b). Release of angiotensin II in canine skeletal muscle *in vivo*. *Journal of Hypertension*, **9**, 487–490.

Schwieler, J.H., Kahan, T., Nussberger, J., Johansson, M.-C. and Hjemdahl, P. (1992). Influence of angiotensin II, α- and β-adrenoceptors on peripheral noradrenergic neutrotransmission in canine gracilis muscle *in vivo*. *Acta Physiologica Scandinavica*, **145**, 333–343.

Schwieler, J.H., Kahan, T., Nussberger, J. and Hjemdahl, P. (1993). Coverting enzyme inhibition modulates sympathetic neurotransmission via multiple mechanisms. *American Journal of Physiology*, **264**, E631–E637.

Schwieler, J.H., Nussberger, J., Kahan, T. and Hjemdahl, P. (1994a). Angiotensin II overflow from canine skeletal muscle *in vivo*: importance of plasma angiotensin I. *American Journal of Physiology*, **266**, R1664–R1669.

Schwieler, J.H., Kahan, T., Nussberger, J. and Hjemdahl, P. (1994b) Participation of prostaglandins and bradykinin in the effects of angiotensin II and angiotensin converting enzyme-inhibition on sympathetic neurotransmission *in vivo*. *Acta Physiol Scand*, **152**, 83–92.

Seals, D.R. (1989). Sympathetic neural discharge and vascular resistance during exercise in humans. *Journal of Applied Physiology*, **66**, 2472–2478.

Seals, D.R., Chase, P.B. and Taylor, J.A. (1988). Autonomic mediation of the pressor responses to isometric exercise in humans. *Journal of Applied Physiology*, **64**, 2190–2196.

Shepherd, J.T. (1984). Circulation to skeletal muscle. In *Handbook of Physiology, Section 2, Vol. III, Part 1: The Cardiovascular System*, edited by J.T. Shepherd and F.M. Abboud, pp. 319–370. Bethesda, Maryland: American Physiological Society.

Shepherd, J.T., Blomqvist, C.G., Lind, A.R., Mitchell, J.H. and Saltin, B. (1981). Static (isometric) exercise — retrospection and introspection. *Circulation Research*, **48**, I-179–I-188.

Sneddon, P. and Burnstock, G. (1984). ATP as a cotransmitter in rat tail artery. *European Journal of Pharmacology*, **106**, 149–152.

Starke, K. (1977). Regulation of noradrenaline release by presynaptic receptor systems. *Reviews in Physiology, Biochemistry and Pharmacology*, **77**, 1–124.

Starke, K. (1981). α-Adrenoceptor subclassification. *Reviews in Physiology, Biochemistry and Pharmacology*, **88**, 199–236.

Starke, K. (1987). Presynaptic α-autoreceptors. *Reviews in Physiology, Biochemistry and Pharmacology*, **107**, 73–146.

Stiles, G.L., Caron, M.G. and Lefkowitz, R.J. (1984). β-Adrenergic receptors: biochemical mechanisms of physiological regulation. *Physiological Reviews*, **64**, 661–743.

Stjärne, L. (1975). Basic mechanisms and local feedback control of secretion of adrenergic and cholinergic neurotransmittter. In *Handbook of Psychopharmacology, Vol. 6*, Edited by L.L. Iversen, S.D. Iversen and S.H. Synder, pp. 179–233. New York: Plenum Press.

Stjärne, L. (1978). Inhibitory effects of noradrenaline and prostaglandin E_2 on neurotransmitter secretion evoked by single shocks or by short trains of nerve stimuli. *Acta Physiologica Scandinavica*, **102**, 251–253.

Stjärne, L. (1989). Basic mechanisms and local modulation of nerve impulse-induced secretion of neurotransmitters from individual nerve varicosities. *Reviews in Physiology, Biochemistry and Pharmacology*, **112**, 1–137.

Stjärne, L. and Brundin, J. (1975). Dual adrenoceptor-mediated control of noradrenaline secretion from human vasoconstrictor nerves: facilitation by β-receptors and inhibition by α-receptors. *Acta Physiologica Scandinavica*, **94**, 139–141.

Story, D.F., Standford-Starr, C.A. and Rand, M.J. (1985). Evidence for the involvement of α_1-adrenoceptors in negative feedback regulation of noradrenergic transmitter release in rat atria. *Clinical Science*, **68**(Suppl. 10), 111–115.

Taddei, S., Salvetti, A. and Pedrinelli, R. (1988). Further evidence for α_2-mediated adrenergic vasoconstriction in human vessels. *European Journal of Clinical Investigation*, **34**, 407–410.

Taddei, S., Salvetti, A. and Pedrinelli, R. (1989). Persistence of sympathetic-mediated forearm vasoconstriction after α-blockade in hypertensive patients. *Circulation*, **80**, 485–490.

Taddei, S., Pedrinelli, R. and Salvetti, A. (1990). Sympathetic nervous system-dependent vasoconstriction in humans: evidence for a mechanistic role of endogenous purine compounds. *Circulation*, **82**, 2061–2067.

Tatemoto, K., Carlquist, M. and Mutt, V. (1982). Neuropeptide Y — a novel brain peptide with structural similarities to peptide YY and pancreatic polypeptide. *Nature*, **296**, 659–660.

Tidgren, B., Hjemdahl, P., Theodorsson, E. and Nussberger, J. (1991). Renal responses to dynamic exercise in man. *Journal of Applied Physiology*, **70**, 2279–2286.

Timmermans, P.B.M.W.M. and van Zwieten, P.A. (1981). The postsynaptic α_2-adrenoceptor. *Journal of Autonomic Pharmacology*, **1**, 171–183.

Tripathi, A. and Nadel, E.R. (1986). Forearm skin and muscle vasoconstriction during lower body negative pressure. *Journal of Applied Physiology*, **60**, 1535–1541.

Tripathi, A., Mack, G. and Nadel, E.R. (1989). Peripheral vascular reflexes elicited during lower body negative pressure. *Aviation, Space and Environmental Medicine*, **60**, 1187–1193.

Turner, J.J., Pierce, D.L. and Bylund, D.B. (1984). α_2-Adrenergic regulation of norepinephrine release in the rat submandibular gland as measured by HPLC-EC. *Life Sciences*, **35**, 1385–1394.

Tuttle, R.S. (1967). Physiological release of histamine-^{14}C in the pyramidal cat. *American Journal of Physiology*, **213**, 620–624.

Unger, T., Gohlke, P., Ganten, D. and Land, R. (1989). Converting enzyme inhibitors and their effects on the renin-angiotensin system of the blood vessel wall. *Journal of Cardiovascular Pharmacology*, **13**(Suppl. 3), S8–S16.

Urata, H., Healy, B., Stewart, R.W., Bumpus, M. and Husain, A. (1990). Angiotensin II-forming pathways in normal and failing human hearts. *Circulation Research*, **66**, 883–890.

Uvnäs, B. (1960). Central cardiovascular control. In *Handbook of Physiology, Section 1, Vol II: Neurophysiology*, edited by H.W. Magoun, pp. 1131–1162. Washington DC: American Physiological Society.

van Heerwarden, C.L.A., Fennis, J.F.M., Binkhorst, R.A. and van't Laar, A. (1977). Haemodynamic effects of adrenaline during treatment of hypertensive patients with propranolol and metoprolol. *European Journal of Clinical Pharmacology*, **12**, 397–402.

Vanhoutte, P.M. and Levy, M.N. (1980). Prejunctional cholinergic modulation of adrenergic neurotransmission in the cardiovascular system. *American Journal of Physiology*, **238**, H275–H281.

Vatner, S.F., Knight, D.R. and Hintze, T.H. (1985). Norepinephrine-induced β_1-adrenergic peripheral vasodilatation in conscious dogs. *American Journal of Physiology*, **249**, H49–H56.

Victor, R.G. and Leimbach Jr, W.N. (1987). Effects of lower body negative pressure on sympathetic discharge to leg muscles in humans. *Journal of Applied Physiology*, **63**, 2558–2562.

Viveros, O.H., Garlick, D.G. and Renkin, E.M. (1968). Sympathetic β-adrenergic vasodilatation in skeletal muscle of the dog. *American Journal of Physiology*, **215**, 1218–1225.

Wahlestedt, C., Grundemar, L., Håkanson, R., Heilig, M., Shen, G.H., Zukowska-Grojec, Z., *et al.* (1990). Neuropeptide Y receptor subtypes, Y1 and Y2. *Annals of the New York Academy of Science*, **611**, 7–26.

Wallin, B.G. and Fagius, J. (1988). Peripheral sympathetic neural activity in conscious humans. *Annual Review of Physiology*, **50**, 565–576.

Wallin, B.G., Mörlin, C. and Hjemdahl, P. (1987). Muscle sympathetic nerve activity and venous plasma noradrenaline concentrations during static exercise in normotensive and hypertensive subjects. *Acta Physiologica Scandinavica*, **129**, 489–497.

Wallin, B.G., Burke, D. and Gandevia, S.C. (1992). Coherence between the sympathetic drives to relaxed and contracting muscles of different limbs of human subjects. *Journal of Physiology (London)*, **455**, 219–233.

Westfall, T.C. (1977). Local regulation of adrenergic neurotransmission. *Physiological Reviews*, **57**, 659–728.

Whelan, R.F. (1952). Vasodilatation in human skeletal muscle during adrenaline infusions. *Journal of Physiology (London)*, **118**, 575–587.

Wilffert, B., Timmermans, P.B.M.W.M. and van Zwieten, P.A. (1982). Extrasynaptic location of α_2- and noninnervated β_2-adrenoceptors in the vascular system of the pithed normotensive rat. *Journal of Pharmacology and Experimental Therapeutics*, **221**, 762–768.

Wilson, V.G., Brown, C.M. and McGrath, J.C. (1991). Are there more than two types of α-adrenoceptors involved in physiological responses? *Experimental Physiology*, **76**, 317–346.

Wolthius, R.A., Bergman, S.A. and Nicogossian, A.E. (1974). Physiological effects of locally applied reduced pressure in man. *Physiological Reviews*, **54**, 566–595.

Wong, P.C., Reilly, T.M. and Timmermans, P.B.M.W.M. (1989). Effect of a monoclonal antibody to angiotensin II on haemodynamic responses to noradrenergic stimulation in pithed rats. *Hypertension*, **14**, 488–497.

Yamaguchi, I. and Kopin, I.J. (1980). Differential inhibition of α_1 and α_2 adrenoreceptor-mediated pressor responses in pithed rats. *Journal of Pharmacology and Experimental Therapeutics*, **214**, 275–281.

Zaagsma, J. and Nahorski, S.R. (1990). Is the adipocyte β-adrenoceptor a prototype for the recently cloned atypical 'β_3-adrenoceptor'? *Trends in Pharmacological Sciences*, **11**, 3–7.

Zimmerman, B.G. (1981). Adrenergic facilitation by angiotensin: does it serve a physiological function? *Clinical Science*, **60**, 343–348.

Zimmerman, B.G. and Whitmore, L. (1967). Effect of angiotensin and phenoxybenzamine on release of norepinephrine in vessels during sympathetic nerve stimulation. *International Journal of Neuropharmacology*, **6**, 27–38.

Ziogas, J. and Story, D.F. (1991). Angiotensin II generation in the rat vena cava: Stimulation of local synthesis by β-adrenoceptor activation. *Naunyn-Schmiedeberg's Archives of Pharmacology*, **343**, 31–36.

Zoller, R.P., Mark, A.L., Abboud, F.M., Schmid, P.G. and Heistad, D.D. (1972). The role of low pressure baroreceptors in reflex vasoconstrictor responses in man. *Journal of Clinical Investigation*, **51**, 2967–2972.

10 The Innervation of Skin Vasculature: The Emerging Importance of Neuropeptides

Susan D. Brain

Pharmacology Group, Biomedical Sciences Division, King's College, Manresa Road, London SW3 6LX, UK

The innervation of the skin reflects the multiple roles that the skin has to play as a barrier between the ever-changing external environment and the closely controlled internal environment of the body. A role of cutaneous nerves associated with blood vessels in influencing temperature control has long been recognized. It is generally accepted that the nerves involved are autonomic sympathetic nerves and non-adrenergic, non-cholinergic (NANC) nerves. The NANC nerves include sensory nerves that release peptides peripherally, in addition to transmitting sensory information to the central nervous system. The release of biologically active peptides from sensory nerves, especially unmyelinated C-fibres, has been the subject of much recent research. A large number of peptides (at least 50 have been identified to date) that differ in structure and possess an array of different biological activities are present, and usually colocalized with each other, in sensory nerves. Evidence is presented in this chapter to suggest that neuropeptides contribute physiologically, in providing a nervously mediated vasodilator component, as well as pathologically, as a neurogenic component of inflammation in the skin.

KEY WORDS: skin; innervation; neuropeptides; CGRP.

NORADRENERGIC AND CHOLINERGIC NERVES

Postganglionic sympathetic nerves arise from ganglia in the paravertebral sympathetic chain, from where they travel with sensory nerves to the cutaneous tissue (Abraham, 1989). Their distribution differs substantially from that of sensory nerves.

NORADRENERGIC NERVES

The terminal capillary loops found in the skin form effective heat exchangers and their flow is largely controlled by shunt vessels, the arteriovenous anastomoses (Grant, 1930; Mescon, Hurley and Moretti, 1956). Small arteries and arterioles, as well as the arteriovenous anastomoses, are richly supplied with noradrenergic nerves (Norberg and Hamberger, 1964). Noradrenergic nerves also innervate paravascular mast cells, dermal smooth muscle and sebaceous glands (Weihe and Hartschuh, 1988). The cutaneous beds of the fingers and toes, especially, receive a dense noradrenergic innervation. Noradrenaline, released from the majority of sympathetic nerves that innervate blood vessels, is a potent cutaneous vasoconstrictor, and the continuous intravenous infusion of noradrenaline increases vasomotion (intermittent constriction of arterioles), which can lead to the temporary cessation of flow in the nail bed capillaries (Greishman, 1954).

The exposure of skin to 10–12°C (by immersion in cold water) leads to an initial vasoconstriction, followed after 5–10 min by vasodilatation. This cycle, known as the "hunting reaction" can be repeated and was first described by Lewis in 1930. The mechanism is still not fully understood, but experiments suggest that the responses are dependent on nervous reflexes which result in greater changes when noradrenergic nerves are intact (Shepherd and Thompson, 1953).

Several other activities are known to stimulate vasoconstriction, as a consequence of reflex noradrenergic vasoconstrictor activity (see Wallin and Fagius, 1988). These activities include mental stress and arousal (Abramson and Ferris, 1940). Arterial baroreceptors could have a role in the regulation of the blood flow in the skin, because unloading intrathoracic receptors, which detect volume changes, has been found to decrease the blood flow in the skin (Rowel, 1983). Alternatively, local noradrenergic axon reflexes exist, whereby vasoconstriction is induced in response to venous distension (Henriksen and Sejrsen, 1976). These local reflexes exist in addition to unmyelinated afferent nerve reflexes, which result in vasodilatation following stimulation (see later). Wallin (1990) has recently suggested that if subjects are warm, stimuli such as those described above cause vasoconstriction. However, if the subject is cold, vasodilatation is observed. He suggests that competition between vasodilator and vasoconstrictor components occurs (Wallin, 1990).

The importance of noradrenergic mechanisms in maintaining a constrictor tone is clear when ganglionic blocking agents are used to prevent sympathetic transmission (e.g. hexamethonium). An increase in the cutaneous blood flow is observed, especially in the fingers. A similar response is also observed when α-adrenoceptor antagonists are administered, or agents which interfere with noradrenergic transmission (Abraham, 1989). It is generally assumed that noradrenaline mainly acts via α_1-adrenoceptors on vascular smooth muscle cells in the skin. However, α_1- and α_2-adrenoceptors have been demonstrated in the hand (Coffman and Cohen, 1988), and evidence suggests that vasoconstriction induced by local cooling of vessels in the skin of human fingers is mainly mediated by α_2-adrenoceptors (Ekenvall et al., 1988).

The 36-amino-acid peptide, neuropeptide Y, is found in nerve fibres that contain tyrosine hydroxylase (a major enzyme involved in the synthesis of noradrenaline and used as a marker of noradrenergic nerves) in human skin (Johansson, 1986; Weihe and Hartschuh, 1988). The fibres that contain both neuropeptide Y and noradrenaline innervate arterial blood vessels, strongly suggesting a role for neuropeptide Y as a cotransmitter with noradrenaline in noradrenergic function (Hökfelt et al., 1987).

Neuropeptide Y is also found in noradrenergic sympathetic nerves that innervate para-arterial mast cells (Weihe and Hartschuh, 1988). Neuropeptide Y, like noradrenaline, is an established vasoconstrictor. In addition, it can modify the actions of noradrenaline by acting at both pre- and postjunctional sites (Hökfelt *et al.*, 1987). Neuropeptide Y occurs in high concentrations in fingers and toes (Wallengren, Ekman and Sundler, 1987).

ATP has also been suggested to be colocalized with noradrenaline in sympathetic nerves in skin (see Mione, Ralevic and Burnstock, 1990). It is possible that ATP is involved in the reflex increase in sympathetic tone in cutaneous veins exposed to the cold (Flavahan and Vanhoutte, 1986).

SYMPATHETIC CHOLINERGIC NERVES

There are considerable amounts of acetylcholine in the skin (Scott, 1962) in neuronal as well as extraneuronal sites; the latter have been recently suggested to include endothelial cells (Parnavelas, Kelly and Burnstock, 1985).

The eccrine sweat glands are innervated by sympathetic nerves that release acetylcholine. This was discovered by the classic experiments of Dale and Feldberg (1934). Electrical stimulation of sympathetic nerves was performed whilst the foot pad of the cat was perfused. Electrical stimulation evoked the secretion of sweat and the appearance of acetylcholine in the venous effluent. Megay (1935) showed high concentrations of acetylcholine in the sweat of human skin, and it is now known that acetylcholine acts on muscarinic receptors to stimulate the secretion of sweat (Sato, 1977). Thus, an established function of acetylcholine in the skin is to promote eccrine secretion of sweat. Acetylcholine evokes a more intense sweating response in males compared with females.

The intradermal injection of acetylcholine into the skin stimulates sweating, with accompanying erythema due to an increased blood flow. Higher concentrations of acetylcholine also stimulate an axon-reflex flare which is mediated by the action of acetylcholine on nicotinic receptors (Wada *et al.*, 1952). Receptors for acetylcholine are found in cutaneous blood vessels. However, the cholinergic nerve supply to the skin is sparse (see Zar, 1989). Arteriovenous anastomoses receive a rich noradrenergic supply, but acetylcholinesterase is localized in some nerves, suggestive of some cholinergic involvement (Hurley and Mescon, 1956). In general, the increased cutaneous blood flow is resistant to cholinergic blocking agents and the major vasodilator nervous component in the skin is thought to be mediated by non-adrenergic, non-cholinergic nerves.

The 28-amino-acid peptide, vasoactive intestinal peptide (VIP), is often found colocalized with acetylcholine in parasympathetic nerves and there is evidence for this in the rat lower lip (Kaji *et al.*, 1988).

NON-ADRENERGIC, NON-CHOLINERGIC NERVES

EARLY STUDIES

Discovery of efferent release from sensory nerves

It was suggested in the late 1880s, by the studies of Goltz and Stricker (see Bayliss, 1901), that nerves originating from the dorsal root ganglia release a vasodilator peripherally. The early studies were confirmed by those of Bayliss (1901), who demonstrated that antidromic stimulation of peripheral sensory nerves causes vasodilatation in the skin.

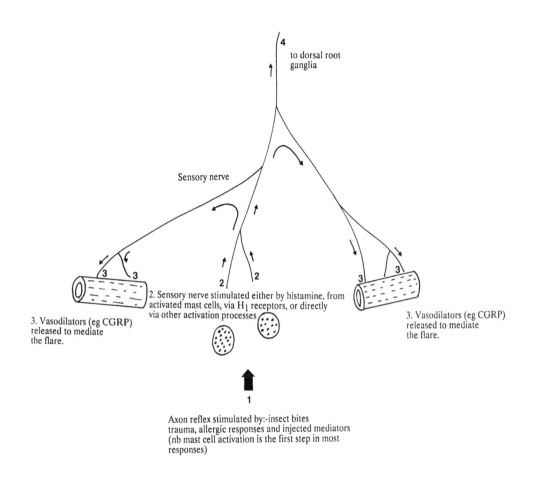

Figure 10.1   The axon-reflex flare in skin.

These results suggest that a sensory nerve, in addition to transmitting sensory information orthodromically, is capable of transmitting motor information antidromically. Furthermore, Bruce (1913) demonstrated that application of mustard oil to the skin stimulates an acute inflammatory response, which does not occur when the sensory nerve supply to the skin has been cut and allowed to degenerate, or when it has degenerated through disease.

The axon-reflex flare

Thomas Lewis (1927) took findings from the studies described above, and together with his own studies suggested a model, involving peripheral axon reflexes, for the inflammatory response to injury to the skin. He suggested that injury to the skin leads to orthodromic stimulation of sensory nerves, resulting in orthodromic transmission of impulses to the spinal cord, as well as antidromic impulses via connecting nerves to adjacent skin (see Figure 10.1).

Antidromic stimulation of these nerve terminals leads to the release of a vasodilator, and thus an increased blood flow in the skin. This increased blood flow is observed as erythema, known as the "axon reflex flare", and can spread for several centimetres around the site of injury in the skin. At an early stage it was realised that the flare is mediated by non-adrenergic, non-cholinergic (NANC) mechanisms. The substance(s) released from the nerve terminals to mediate the increased blood flow observed in the flare area have been the subject of much speculation and is discussed later.

The axon reflex is one component of the "triple response of skin to injury" as defined by Thomas Lewis (1927). The other components are a wheal, due to increased microvascular permeability leading to the formation of oedema, and erythema observed at the site of injection. The triple response is clearly observed in the skin in response to common pin-point injuries (e.g. insect bites) and in response to intradermal injection of mediators (e.g. histamine, as demonstrated by Thomas Lewis).

Capsaicin

The vasodilatation and inflammatory signs that result from antidromic stimulation of sensory nerves have been given the name "neurogenic inflammation". The use of capsaicin (trans-8-methyl-N-vanillyl-6-nonenamide) as a pharmacological tool has allowed us to learn more about these nerves and the contribution of a neurogenic component inflammation (Jancso, Jancso-Gabor and Szolcsanyi, 1967). Capsaicin is the pungent principle extracted from the pepper (capsicum) family. The nerves involved in neurogenic inflammation in the skin appear to be sensitive to capsaicin, although it is possible that not all sensory nerves are affected and this should be remembered when interpreting results. Capsaicin initially stimulates nerves, leading to pain and neurogenic inflammation. This response is not observed in denervated skin (Jancso, Jancso-Gabor and Szolcsanyi, 1967). Subsequent application of capsaicin to innervated skin leads to an attenuation of the response, desensitization of the fibres to stimuli, and, depending on the treatment regime, the degeneration of sensory nerves. For example, the flare component of the triple response in skin is inhibited by prior treatment, over several days, with topical capsaicin (Bernstein *et al.*, 1981; Carpenter and Lynn, 1981; Foreman and Jordan, 1983). Capsaicin acts selectively on sensory nerves; efferent autonomic fibres are not affected, neither by stimulation nor desensitization. Capsaicin has been used extensively in recent research and this is briefly discussed in a later section.

THE AFFERENT ROLE OF SENSORY NERVES

Cutaneous innervation enables the skin to pass sensory information concerning both the external and internal environment to higher nervous centres. This is possible because specialized nerve endings detect changes that can range from innocuous alterations in the temperature or pressure to actual damage that mediates pain. The nerve endings have been studied using electrophysiological techniques and the specialization of different afferent nerve endings in the skin has been extensively reviewed elsewhere (Winkelmann, 1988; Lynn, 1989). The fast-conducting myelinated A-axons (including Aδ-fibres) and the slower conducting unmyelinated C-axons have been studied most. The nerve endings are specialized and can detect changes in pressure and movement (mechanoreceptors), changes in temperature (thermoreceptors) and pain (nociceptors).

Mechanoceptors usually arise from A-fibres and can be further divided into slowly adapting, which respond for several seconds, and rapidly adapting, which respond only initially to stimulation. Thermoreceptors are also divided into two types, those that detect cooling of the skin and those that detect warming of the skin. Cold sensors are associated with $A\delta$-fibres and C-fibres. They are widespread in the skin, especially, in the hands, feet and the face. Warm sensors (C-fibre nerves) are found in distal areas and the face.

Nociceptors are divided into two types: high-threshold mechanoreceptors usually arising from $A\delta$ fibres (Burgess and Perl, 1967), and polymodal nociceptors, associated with 80% of C-fibres. High-threshold mechanoreceptors respond to strong pressure, heat and skin damage (see Lynn, 1989). Polymodal nociceptors are the most common sensory unit in the skin ($10/mm^2$ on the rat paw; Lynn, 1984). They respond to heat, as well as to pressure and irritant chemicals. An important point to note is that polymodal nociceptors, especially, can also be sensitized by the presence of endogenous substances that include acetylcholine, bradykinin, histamine and the prostaglandins. Indeed, the analgesic actions of non-steroidal anti-inflammatory drugs, which inhibit the formation of prostaglandins, is thought to be partly due to the inhibition of the formation of sensitizing prostaglandins (Ferreira, 1972). The exact mechanism by which endogenous substances act varies, depending on the mediator. It is now clear that the mediators act via specific receptor subtypes on afferent nerve terminals and this is the subject of current research for several mediators.

SENSORY-EFFERENT FUNCTION OF NERVES

Sensory afferents primarily transmit information centrally. This is in keeping with experiments where stimulation leads to an enhanced release of neuropeptides at the level of the spinal cord (Duggan et al., 1987). Classically, it has been suggested that the peripheral release of neuropeptides from C-fibre nerves (and $A\delta$ nerves) occurs at a nerve ending which is specialized in releasing the transmitter, separate from the sensory receptor. More recently it has been suggested, from experiments with capsaicin, that sensory nerves can release transmitters from the same terminal that contains sensory receptors (see Holzer, 1988; Maggi and Meli, 1988; Szolcsanyi, 1988). The concept of the sensory-efferent function was suggested as a consequence of experiments carried out with local anaesthetic and the axon conduction blocker, tetrodotoxin. The release of neuropeptides after local anaesthesia and treatment with tetrodotoxin cannot occur as a result of axonal transmission, which is blocked. Thus release can only occur from the stimulated nerve endings. It is obvious from numerous studies of the flare in human skin that the release of neuropeptides occurs as a consequence of axon-reflex stimulation; however, the possibility of a release of neuropeptides from stimulated nerve endings, in the absence of the axon-reflex flare, should also be considered.

EVIDENCE FOR THE EXISTENCE OF SPECIFIC NEUROPEPTIDES IN THE SKIN

Substance P and CGRP

The 11-amino-acid peptide, substance P, was the first neuropeptide to be discovered (von Euler and Gaddam, 1931) and as a result it has been the most extensively studied of all

TABLE 10.1
Structure of the tachykinins and CGRP

Neuropeptide	Amino acid sequence
Substance P	Arg-Pro-Lys-Pro-Gln-Gln-Phe-Phe-Gly-Leu-Met-NH$_2$
Neurokinin A	His-Lys-Thr-Asp-Ser-Phe-Val-Gly-Leu-Met-NH$_2$
Neurokinin B	Asp-Met-His-Asp-Phe-Phe-Val-Gly-Leu-Met-NH$_2$
αCGRP	NH$_2$-Ser-Cys-Asn-Thr-Ala-Thr-Cys-Val-Thr-His-Arg-Leu-Ala-Gly-Leu-Leu-Ser-Arg-Ser-Gly-Gly-Val-Val-Lys-Asp-Asn-Phe-Val-Pro-Thr-Asn-Val-Gly-Ser-Glu-Ala-Phe-amide

the neuropeptides. The structure was elucidated in 1971 (Chang, Leeman and Nrall, 1971; see Table 10.1). It was the first neuropeptide to be demonstrated by immunohistochemical studies to be present in the nerves of skin (Hökfelt *et al.*, 1975). Now it is realised that structurally similar peptides exist, known collectively as the tachykinins or neurokinins. The structures of the principal human neurokinins are shown in Table 10.1. All the neurokinins have identical C-terminal amino acid sequences. Thus, antisera against C-terminal sequences, used in immunohistochemical studies, may also recognize other members of the neurokinin family. Neurokinin A is encoded on the substance P gene (Nawa *et al.*, 1983) and might therefore expected to be colocalized with substance P.

Substance P (and/or neurokinin A) is found in perivascular nerves (Bloom and Polak, 1983) and in free nerve endings in the epidermis and in Meissners corpuscles of digital skin (Bloom and Polak, 1983; Dalsgaard *et al.*, 1983). There is little evidence to date for the existence of nerves that contain neurokinin B in the skin. Substance P and neurokinin A appear to be located in the same nerve fibres, as expected from molecular biological studies (Weihe and Hartschuh, 1988). Some substance P-containing nerves have also been found to innervate sweat glands (Dalsgaard *et al.*, 1983; Tanio, Vaalasti and Rechardt, 1987).

Calcitonin gene-related peptide (CGRP) was discovered through molecular biological studies of the ageing rat (Amara *et al.*, 1982; Rosenfeld, Amara and Evans, 1984). The calcitonin gene encodes for CGRP, but alternative processing of the mRNA of the gene leads to the production of CGRP in nervous tissue and predominantly calcitonin in the thyroid of healthy individuals (Edbrooke *et al.*, 1985). CGRP has been described as one of the most plentiful neuropeptides studied in skin to date (Gibbins, Wattchow and Coventry, 1987). It is found in C- and Aδ-fibres and commonly colocalized with substance P (Gibbins, Wattchow and Coventry, 1987; Wallengren, Eckman and Sundler, 1987). Gibbins and coworkers demonstrated that CGRP is also colocalized with somatostatin in human skin and is found in some nerves alone (e.g. around sweat glands). CGRP is found with substance P in nerves that terminate close to mast cells (Weihe and Hartchuh, 1988) and with VIP in cholinergic sympathetic nerves in the rat (Landis and Fredieu, 1986). There are two forms of human CGRP (α and β) and two forms of rat CGRP. Evidence to date suggests that αCGRP predominates in the periphery (O'Halloran and Bloom, 1991) in organs such as the skin (Mulderry *et al.*, 1988).

VIP

VIP and peptide histidine methionine PHM are found in nerves which are localized at a deeper level in the skin, when compared with substance P and CGRP-containing nerves. The nerves are mainly associated with arteries, arterioles (including arteriovenous anastomoses) and sweat glands (Bloom and Polak, 1983; Hartschuh, Weihe and Reinecke, 1983; O'Shaughnessy et al., 1983; Wallengren, Ekman and Sundler, 1987). A presence in sympathetic cholinergic nerves is common, as discussed above.

Other peptides

Some other neuropeptides have been demonstrated to be present in human skin. These include: somatostatin (Bloom and Polak, 1983; Gibbins, Wattchow and Coventry, 1987; Johansson and Vaalasti, 1987), galanin (Johansson et al., 1988), neurotensin (Hartschuh, Weihe and Reinecke, 1983), bombesin (Bloom and Polak, 1983) and opioids (Weihe and Hartschuh, 1988: Hartschuh, Weihe and Reinecke, 1983). It is generally believed that other neuropeptides remain as yet undiscovered.

THE ACTIVITIES OF NEUROPEPTIDES IN HUMAN SKIN

The actions of the different neuropeptides are complex. Each neuropeptide has its own profile of activity, which can be observed after intradermal injection. The effect of intradermal injection of substance P, CGRP and VIP will be described first, since these neuropeptides have been studied most extensively.

Substance P and the neurokinins

Intradermal injection of substance P into skin induces a response similar to that observed by Thomas Lewis (1927) in response to histamine (see earlier section) Substance P induces the characteristic triple response of wheal, local reddening and axon-reflex flare. The flare component of the response to substance P is inhibited by H_1-receptor antagonists, or by prior depletion of endogenous histamine stores with compound 48/80 (Hagermark, Hökfelt and Pernow, 1978). This suggests that at least part of the response to substance P is a consequence of the release of histamine from mast cells. This is supported by Foreman and colleagues (1983) who investigated the structure-activity relationships of substance P-like peptides in human skin. Only peptides with one or more basic amino acid residues in the N-terminal region were effective in stimulating a flare response. Substance P releases histamine from mast cells isolated from human skin (Benyon, Church and Lowman, 1987). It is possible that activation of mast cells is stimulated via G-proteins (Mousli et al., 1990). The flare in response to substance P is not observed after the injection of local anaesthetic into the skin (Foreman et al., 1983). These combined results suggest that histamine, from substance P-activated mast cells, stimulates the axon-reflex flare, by acting via H_1-receptors situated on afferent nerve terminals. There is little evidence to suggest that substance P directly stimulates nociceptors. However, intradermal injection of substance P is often associated with itch (possibly mediated via histamine). The flare induced by substance P is inhibited when the skin is pretreated with capsaicin at doses that deplete sensory nerves; in contrast, the response to the wheal is unaffected (Carpenter and Lynn, 1981; Foreman *et al.*, 1983).

The ability of peptides to stimulate the formation of a wheal is not dependent on the presence of basic residues. Neurokinin A and B, which possess less basic N-terminals, induce a wheal but do not induce substantial axon-reflex flare in human skin (Devillier *et al.*, 1986; Fuller *et al.*, 1987). Neurokinin A and B have a similar C-terminal structure (see Table 10.1) and have a similar potency to substance P in inducing a wheal in human skin (Devillier *et al.*, 1986; Fuller *et al.*, 1987).

CGRP

The intradermal injection of low doses of CGRP into human skin stimulates a response characteristically different from that induced by substance P. CGRP induces an erythema at the site of intradermal injection, which can be observed for up to 4 h after injection (Brain *et al.*, 1985). "Pseudopodia of erythema" can also often be seen tracking away from the site of injection, which is thought to be due to CGRP that has reached the lymphatics and then acted on perilymphatic blood vessels (Brain *et al.*, 1985). The erythema induced by intradermal CGRP is associated with a prolonged increase in the blood flow, which is considered to occur as a direct consequence of the action of CGRP on microvascular blood vessels (Brain *et al.*, 1986). The cutaneous response to CGRP is similar to that observed after intradermal injection of vasodilator prostanoids prostaglandins E_2 and I_2); but the response to prostaglandin E_2 is considerably shorter lasting (Brain *et al.*, 1986; Brain and Williams, 1988). Higher doses of CGRP can cause a wheal and flare, but these doses are probably not of physiological or pathological, relevance (Brain *et al.*, 1985; Piotrowski and Foreman, 1986).

VIP

VIP produces a response that looks like a combination of the responses to substance P and CGRP. Initially, a wheal and flare response is seen upon injection of VIP in human skin. This response fades within an hour, which is normal, then a local erythema response is observed which fades over the next hour (Anand, Blooms and McGregor, 1983; Brain *et al.*, 1986). The flare response to VIP is inhibited by H_1-receptor antagonists. This suggests that VIP activates mast cells. The local erythema at the site of injection of VIP is due to its ability to directly stimulate the cutaneous blood flow. The local erythema is not inhibited by H_1-receptor antagonists.

Actions of other neuropeptides

There is less well-documented evidence for the action of other neuropeptides in human skin. Neurotensin, which has a structural relationship to substance P (Sydbom, 1982; Foreman and Jordan, 1983), somatostatin (Piotrowski and Foreman, 1986) and opioids (Weihe and Hartschuh, 1988) all stimulate a triple response due to activation of mast cells after intradermal injection into human skin. Evidence is accumulating from experiments, mainly in other tissues, that opioids and some other neuropeptides feed back onto sensory nerves to prevent further release of neuropeptides (see Holzer, 1988; Maggi and Meli, 1988, for reviews).

TABLE 10.2
The effect of some mediators that stimulate the axon-reflex flare

Agent	Response			H_1-receptor antagonists	Reference
Histamine	Flare	Wheal	Local erythema	Inhibition	Foreman and Jordan, 1983
Substance P	"	"	"	"	Hagermark, Hökfelt and Pernow, 1978
VIP	"	"	"	"	Anand, Bloom and McGregor, 1983
CGRP[a]	"	"	"	"	Piotrowski and Foreman, 1986
IgE-mediated	"	"	"	"	Lundblad et al., 1985
PAF	"	"	"	"	Archer et al., 1985
LTC$_4$/D$_4$	"	"	"	—	Camp et al., 1983; Soter et al., 1983
C5a	"	"	"	—	Yancey et al., 1985
Endothelin	"	Constriction	Constriction	"	Crossman, Brain and Fuller, 1991

[a] CGRP induces a wheal and flare at higher doses, but lower doses induce an extremely long-lasting local reddening due to a direct effect of CGRP in increasing blood flow, with no axon reflex (Brain et al., 1985). IgE, immunoglobulin E; PAF, platelet activating factor; LTC$_4$/D$_4$, leukotriene C$_4$/D$_4$.

Thus the pro-inflammatory or vascular actions of these peptides, observed after intradermal injection, might not be their only, or even their most important, cutaneous action (see Barnes, Belvisi and Rogers, 1990).

THE MEDIATION OF THE AXON-REFLEX FLARE

Activation

It is well established that histamine and several neuropeptides stimulate the axon-reflex flare as discussed above. In addition, other endogenous mediators also stimulate a flare as one component of the cutaneous response to intradermal injection, as shown in Table 10.2. The flare component is inhibited by H_1-receptor antagonists in most cases (see Table 10.2). This suggests that activation of cutaneous mast cells and the release of histamine plays a central role in activating sensory axon reflexes in human skin. Thus, there is good evidence that most agents that stimulate an axon-reflex flare in skin do so as a consequence of their ability to stimulate the degranuation of mast cells. Histamine then plays an essential role by acting via H_1-receptors on afferent nerve terminals, as shown in Figure 10.1. The axon-reflex flare induced by some agents (e.g. endothelin) is only partially inhibited by systemic H_1-receptor antagonists (Crossman, Brain and Fuller, 1991). Thus it is possible that endothelin can also act independently of histamine, possibly by stimulating endothelin receptors situated on afferent nerve terminals. Other endogenous substances may also act in this way, but further studies are needed to clarify individual mechanisms. Intradermal capsaicin, which directly activates C-fibre nerves in the skin, stimulates a flare which is independent of histamine (Barnes et al., 1986).

Substances that stimulate an axon-reflex flare in human skin via a histamine-dependent mechanism would be expected to stimulate mast cells isolated from human skin in vitro, but there are some interesting anomalies. Platelet-activating factor does not stimulate mast cells in vitro (Thomas and Church, 1990) and endothelin also lacks this ability (Thomas and Church, unpublished). The reasons for this anomaly are not understood.

In conclusion, in human skin, histamine released from mast cells appears to play a central role in activating sensory nerves. This could be one reason why topical H_1-receptor antagonists play a beneficial role in the treatment of certain skin conditions in man. The role, or even necessity, of an axon-reflex flare is uncertain, but it is generally assumed to be a signalling system which enables adjacent skin sites to be prepared or changes in the immediate environment.

Candidates responsible for mediating the increased blood flow observed in the area of the flare

There is good evidence (as discussed above) that the flare is mediated by the release of vasodilator substances from capsaicin-sensitive nerves in human skin. The nerve endings are situated at sites adjacent to cutaneous microvascular arterioles. Thus, irrespective of how the axon reflex is stimulated, the substance(s) that mediate the flare will always be vasodilators released from the terminal arborizations of sensory nerve terminals. This is often misunderstood and erroneous suggestions made that the substance that stimulates the axon-reflex flare is also responsible for mediating the increased blood flow in the area of the flare.

The identity of the substances that are released from sensory nerve terminals to mediate the flare have been under discussion for many years. The vasodilating substance has been suggested to be; histamine, ATP, substance P, VIP and CGRP, and there was substantial interest in the suggestion that a combination of substance P and histamine could mediate the flare (Lembeck and Gamse, 1982; Foreman and Jordan, 1983). However, substance P is not a potent cutaneous vasodilator in its own right, when injected into skin at doses lower than those required to stimulate the activation of mast cells (Brain and Edwardson, 1989). Furthermore, capsaicin, which activates sensory nerve terminals directly, stimulates pain and an axon-reflex flare. Barnes and co-workers (1986) demonstrated that H_1-receptor antagonists had no effect on the capsaicin-induced flare. This is good evidence that histamine is not the actual vasodilator mediator of the flare response. Thus, substance P and histamine are not ideal candidates and another candidate, VIP, is not commonly localized in capsaicin-sensitive nerves.

CGRP is an extremely potent vasodilator and is found in capsaicin-sensitive nerves. Intradermal injection of low (i.e. femtomole) amounts of CGRP stimulates erythema at the site of injection in the skin for about 20 min, which is the approximate duration of the flare response (Brain et al., 1985; Brain and Edwardson, 1989). Thus, I suggest that low concentrations of CGRP released from peri-arteriolar nerves could mediate the increased blood flow that causes the flare. This hypothesis can be examined more fully when CGRP antagonists which may be used in man are available.

THE CONTRIBUTION OF CAPSAICIN-SENSITIVE NERVES AND THEIR NEUROPEPTIDES TO NEUROGENIC INFLAMMATION: STUDIES IN ANIMALS

The vascular responses of human skin to neuropeptides are similar to the vascular responses in other species. The ability to investigate mechanisms in inflammatory models in animal species has been essential in our quest for determining the importance of changes in the release and activity of neuropeptides in the regulation of cutaneous function.

Vasodilatation and increased microvascular permeability

The tachykinins and CGRP induce similar responses in rat skin to those observed in human skin, although an axon-reflex flare is not as readily demonstrated or measured in animal skin (Lynn and Shakhaneh, 1988). Increases in blood flow and vascular permeability in the skin in response to the release of neuropeptides from capsaicin-sensitive sensory nerves have been been studied most extensively. Capsaicin and antidromic nerve stimulation cause an increased blood flow and the formation of oedema in many animals (Gamse, Holzer and Lembeck, 1980; and see Holzer, 1988; Maggi and Meli, 1988).

Substance P, as in human skin, is a potent mediator of increased microvascular permeability in the rat (Lembeck and Holzer, 1979), although it is inactive in rabbit skin (Brain and Williams, 1985). Oedema (plasma protein extravasation), which results from increased microvascular permeability of the post-capillary venules (Kenins, Hurley and Bell, 1984), can be readily measured in the skin by the extravascular accumulation of either Evans Blue, which binds to plasma proteins (Gamse and Saria, 1985), or the accumulation of radio-labelled albumin (Brain and Williams, 1985). Substance P acts partially via histamine release and partially via substance P receptors on vascular endothelial cells in rat skin (see Foreman and Jordan, 1983; Holzer, 1988; Brain and Williams, 1989). Recently, an inhibitor of the endothelial-derived vasodilator, nitric oxide, has been shown to significantly attenuate substance P-induced oedema in rat skin (Hughes, Williams and Brain 1990). Thus endothelial-derived vasoactive substances modulate neurogenic inflammatory responses.

Neurokinin A and B, as in human skin, are potent mediators of increased microvascular permeability, acting via histamine-independent mechanisms (Gamse and Saria, 1985; Devillier et al., 1986; Brain and Williams, 1989). Receptors for neurokinins have been classified as NK-1, NK-2 and NK-3 on the basis of their affinity for neurokinins (Henry, 1987). Endothelial cells possess NK-1 receptors and there is evidence to suggest that the neurokinins act via NK-1 receptors in rat skin to increase microvascular permeability (Andrews, Thomas and Helme, 1989). Neurokinin B is a more potent mediator of increased microvascular permeability than the other neurokinins, in some models, suggesting an involvement of NK-3 receptors (Couture and Kerouac, 1987). The post-receptor mechanisms have not been extensively studied, but the hydrolysis of inositol phospholipids is involved in post-receptor mechanisms of substance P in rat skin (Thomas et al., 1989).

CGRP, in contrast to the neurokinins, does not mediate increased microvascular permeability in skin (Brain and Williams, 1985). However, as described for human skin, it is an extremely potent vasodilator peptide in the skin of rabbit, rat and other species (Brain et al., 1985; Brain and Williams, 1988; Brain and Williams, 1989). The different forms of CGRP that have been tested to date all have similar actions (Brain, MacIntyre and Williams, 1986).

CGRP, as a consequence of arteriolar vasodilatation, can potentiate the formation of oedema induced by mediators of increased microvascular permeability, such as the neurokinins (Brain and Williams, 1985; Gamse and Saria, 1985). This ability of CGRP to potentiate oedema induced by the neurokinins suggests two things. Firstly, substance P and the neurokinins are not the most potent vasodilators in the skin, contrary to what was originally thought, although their potency as vasodilators when injected intra-arterially or intravenously is well established. Secondly, CGRP can contribute to inflammation as a neurogenically derived component by potentiating the actions of a range of mediators. In this context, CGRP can potentiate oedema induced by direct acting mediators of increased microvascular permeability (e.g. histamine, bradykinin and platelet activating factor) and neutrophil-dependent mediators of increased microvascular permeability (e.g. the complement fragment, C5a, the arachidonate lipoxygenase product, leukotriene B$_4$, and the bacterial peptide, formyl methionyl leucine phenylalanine; Brain and Williams, 1985).

CGRP, although not chemotactic in the rabbit, can potentiate the accumulation of neutrophils induced by chemotactic agents and the cytokine, interleukin-1 (Buckley *et al.*, 1991a, 1991b). Thus, CGRP could contribute indirectly as a damaging neurogenic component to inflammatory responses.

Direct effects on cellular components of inflammation

It has been suggested that substance P is chemotactic for neutrophils, acting via stimulation of the receptor for formyl methionyl leucine phenylalanine (Marasco, Showell and Becker, 1981), but high concentrations are required. More recent studies suggest that substance P is a potent priming agent for neutrophils, making the neutrophils more responsive to subsequent stimulation by chemotactic factors (Perianin, Snyderman and Malfroy, 1989). Human mononuclear leukocytes are chemotactic to substance P (Ruff, Wahl and Pert, 1985) and substance P stimulates the release of interleukin-1 and tumor necrosis factor α from human monocytes (Lotz, Vaughan and Carson 1988).

Substance P and neurokinin A and other neuropeptides have modulatory effects on the function of lymphocytes and of the immune system (Payan, Brewster and Goetzl, 1983; Payan *et al.*, 1987; Scicchitano, Biennenstock and Stanisz, 1988). There is evidence that clearly demonstrates that substance P stimulates arterial smooth muscle cells, human skin fibroblasts (Nilsson, von Euler and Dalsgaard, 1985) and keratinocytes to proliferate (Tanaka *et al.*, 1988).

CGRP, apart from an initial suggestion from preliminary experiments (Piotrowski and Foreman, 1986), is not thought to have potent effects on polymorphonuclear leukocytes. In rabbit skin, CGRP does not directly stimulate the accumulation of neutrophils (Buckley *et al.*, 1991b). Therefore, the most powerful effect of CGRP is thought to be due to an increase in microvascular blood flow, thereby boosting the number of neutrophils arriving at sites where chemotactic agents are present (see the previous section). However, intact rat αCGRP has been shown to be weakly chemotactic for guinea-pig eosinophils *in vitro* (Manley and Haynes, 1989). Perhaps of greater potential importance is the finding that rat αCGRP is broken down by trypsin to fragments that are chemotactic for guinea-pig eosinophils. It is now realised that the eosinophil chemotactic factor of anaphylaxis, previously purified from guinea-pig lung (Goetzl and Austen, 1975), is a tryptic fragment of rat αCGRP (Manley and Haynes, 1989). However, the tryptic digestion of human α- and βCGRP has not been shown to lead to the production of a chemotactic fragment. Thus the importance of the finding of Manley and Haynes (1989) is not yet established.

A depletion of neuropeptides has been detected during wound healing in rat skin (Senapati et al., 1986). The significance of this finding is unknown, but it suggests an involvement of neuropeptides in the process of wound healing.

Use of capsaicin

The activation and subsequent depletion of a large number of sensory neurons by capsaicin has been used extensively to investigate the neurogenic component of inflammation. Capsaicin, given to neonatal rats, causes an irreversible degeneration of a large proportion of sensory nerves (Jancso, Kiraly and Jancso-Gabor, 1977). Capsaicin has been used this way, or given as a pretreatment in adult rats, to determine how the inflammation is altered in models of diseases such as arthritis and delayed hypersensitivity (Colpaert, Donnerer and Lembeck, 1983; Nilsson and Ahlstedt, 1989).

More recently, intensive research has led to an increased knowledge of the mechanisms by which capsaicin activates afferent nerves. It is now realised that capsaicin binds to a membrane ion-channel complex possibly a receptor for an, as yet, unidentified endogenous ligand). Capsaicin stimulates an inward, depolarizing current with inward flow of Ca^{2+} and Na^+ (see Bevan and Szolcsanyi, 1990). The binding and activation of sensory nerves can be inhibited by a cationic dye, ruthenium red. Ruthenium red blocks increased blood flow induced by capsaicin in rabbit skin (Buckley, Brain and Williams, 1990). Research is now being carried out with analogues of capsaicin (e.g. resiniferatoxin and olvanil) in an attempt to learn more about the modulatory effects of capsaicin on sensory nerves (see reviews by Barnes, Belvisi and Rogers, 1990; Bevan and Szolcsanyi, 1990).

IMPORTANCE OF THE SENSORY EFFERENT VASODILATOR RESPONSE FOR THE REGULATION OF CUTANEOUS BLOOD FLOW

Antidromic stimulation of the saphenous nerve leads to an increased blood flow at lower levels of stimulation and the formation of oedema at higher and more sustained levels of stimulation. Antihistamines do not inhibit the cutaneous blood flow produced by antidromic stimulation (Gamse and Saria, 1987). Thus it can be assumed from studies, in the rat at least, that a potent dilator is released in response to a low level of sensory nerve stimulation. In the rabbit, capsaicin stimulates the cutaneous blood flow, which is significantly inhibited by an anti-CGRP antibody and a CGRP antagonist (Buckley et al., 1991c; Hughes and Brain, unpublished), suggesting that CGRP could mediate the vasodilator component in the skin.

Importance of sensory nerves in skin flap survival

Kjartansson and colleagues (1988) demonstrated that transcutaneous electrical nerve stimulation increases the cutaneous blood flow in a musculocutaneous flap in the rat and that the use of capsaicin to selectively deplete sensory nerves led to a decreased flap survival (Kjartansson, Dalsgaard and Jonsson, 1987). Further, local intravenous injection of CGRP increased flap survival, whilst increasing the blood flow (Kjartansson and Dalsgaard, 1987). In an immunocytochemical study of the reinnervation in mouse skin flaps, CGRP and substance P appeared in new nerves in the skin flaps, some days before neuropeptide Y and

VIP (Karanth *et al.*, 1990). These studies suggest that sensory nerves have an important efferent role in releasing vasodilator peptides and protecting against ischaemia.

A role for CGRP in regulating vascular responses to noradrenergic transmission

Studies in the rat perfused mesenteric bed *in vitro* have demonstrated that NANC vasodilator nerves play a role in the regulation of blood flow at the level of the resistance vessel and that the neurogenic vasodilatation is selectively abolished by depleting endogenous CGRP (Kawasaki *et al.*, 1988). The results demonstrate that endogenously released CGRP may play a role as a dilator in controlling peripheral resistance postjunctionally by opposing the pressor response induced by noradrenaline, released from vasomotor nerves (Kawasaki *et al.*, 1990).

Long-term sympathectomy (by pretreatment with guanethidine) leads to marked increases in CGRP-containing nerves in the rat (Aberdeen *et al.*, 1990). A decrease in noradrenaline has been shown to stimulate the production of nerve growth factor (Chun and Patterson, 1977), which in turn stimulates the formation of sensory nerves. Recently, nerve growth factor has been shown to be necessary for the development of myelinated nociceptors *in vivo* (Ritter *et al.*, 1991). Thus, there could be a direct link between the densities of sympathetic and sensory innervations. Few experiments have been carried out in skin to determine whether stimulation of noradrenergic nerves and release of CGRP occur in an actively opposing manner, but this is an interesting area for future research.

Raynaud's disease

Patients with Raynaud's disease exhibit a lack of reflex vasodilatation after exposure to various stresses, in particular, cold. The patients respond normally to CGRP when it is injected into the forearm or digits (Bunker, Foreman and Dowd, 1989; Brain *et al.*, 1990). Intravenous injection of CGRP leads to a flushing of the hands in patients with Raynaud's disease, possibly due to a denervation supersensitivity (Shawket *et al.*, 1989). Evidence suggests that there is a reduction in the number of CGRP-immunoreactive nerves in digital skin in primary Raynaud's phenomenon and in Raynaud's disease associated with systemic sclerosis (Bunker *et al.*, 1990). Thus, the lack of a vasodilator response in patients with Raynaud's disease could be due to a lack of release of vasodilator CGRP. This could be concomitant with increased noradrenergic transmission (sympathectomy is an established treatment for Raynaud's disease; it has led to relief in some cases) or an increase in the release of other vasoconstrictors. The endothelial-derived vasoconstrictor, endothelin, is found in increased levels in the plasma of some Raynaud's sufferers after an attack (Zamora *et al.*, 1990). Endothelin causes constriction at the site of injection when injected intradermally in human skin, although this is accompanied by a surrounding axon-reflex flare in normal individuals (Crossman, Brain and Fuller, 1991).

EVIDENCE FOR THE RELEASE AND ACTION OF NEUROPEPTIDES IN HUMAN SKIN DISEASE

The possibility that neuropeptides play a role in skin disease has been suggested because of the symmetry of the distribution of lesions that can occur (e.g. in psoriasis, Farber *et al.*, 1986). Evidence has been obtained from studies where the innervation and release of neuropeptides have been measured and where capsaicin has been used.

Release of neuropeptides

The amount of neuropeptides that can be measured by radioimmunoassay in skin biopsy extracts is low. However, various, sometimes high, levels of CGRP, somatostatin and neuropeptide Y can be measured in spontaneous blisters in conditions that include bullous pemphigoid and herpes zoster (Wallengren, Ekman and Moller, 1986; Wallengren, Ekman and Sundler, 1987). In a controlled study, substance P, CGRP and VIP were measured in fluid from suction blisters obtained from control and test sites of patients with urticaria, but little difference in levels was seen (Wallengren, Ekman and Sundler, 1987). One problem associated with measuring substances in skin extracts/fluids is that proteases are present which break down the peptides. This is established as a problem associated with neuropeptide research in the lung, where a range of protease inhibitors are used when possible *in vitro* (Sekizawa, *et al.*, 1987). In skin, proteases that include tryptase and chymase from mast cells readily break down peptides. This can be observed under experimental conditions in man. The injection of substance P with CGRP into human skin causes a large initial response due to the combined response to substance P and CGRP. However, the long-lasting erythema normally observed with CGRP is not seen. This is due to the action of tryptase from mast cells activated by substance P in degrading, and thus inactivating, CGRP (Brain and Williams, 1988, 1989). Urticaria is a mast cell-dependent phenomenon where the levels of tryptase released are high (Schwartz, *et al.*, 1987) and, as a consequence, neuropeptides might be expected to be metabolized soon after their release from cutaneous nerves. Therefore, the measurement of neuropeptides in skin samples is probably not a good indicator of either their release or activity.

Capsaicin

Local pretreatment with capsaicin reduces the flare response to intradermal histamine. This is due to the depletion of C-fibre nerves from skin (see earlier sections on capsaicin). This phenomenon has been utilized to enable the involvement of capsaicin-sensitive nerves in some models of human inflammation to be investigated. The flare is inhibited by pretreatment with capsaicin in a model of an immunoglobulin E cutaneous allergic response in man (Lundblad *et al.*, 1985). The local pretreatment with capsaicin attenuates the flare response to intradermal histamine and substance P, but causes an overall enhancement of the erythema responses in ultraviolet irradiation, contact dermatitis and the tuberculin reaction (Wallengren and Moller, 1986). It is possible that this is because modulatory neuropeptides (e.g. opioids and somatostatin) may normally be released from capsaicin-sensitive nerves to modulate responses. Thus, the use of capsaicin to learn about the efferent function of neuropeptides has led to some difficulties in interpretation. However, pretreatment with capsaicin has been used therapeutically to relieve pain in herpes (Bernstein, 1988) and diabetic neuropathy (Ross and Varipapa, 1989).

CONCLUSION

Recent research suggests that the vasoactive neuropeptides play a role in the regulation of cutaneous homeostasis, in wound repair and in the mediation of inflammatory responses. Their precise role is uncertain and research into the role of the neuropeptides is progressing in parallel with research into the actions of vasoactive substances that include the endothelial-derived nitric oxide and endothelin. Interactions occur between these recently discovered vasoactive substances and neuropeptides, which leads to difficulties in interpreting results. However, the role and importance of the various neuropeptides in the functions of skin should be established over the next decade, as improved inhibitors/antagonists are developed.

REFERENCES

Aberdeen, J., Corr, L., Milner, P., Lincoln, J. and Burnstock, G. (1990). Marked increases in calcitonin gene-related peptide-containing nerves in the developing rat following long-term sympathectomy with guanethidine. *Neuroscience*, **35**, 175–184.

Abraham, D.I. (1989). Dermal blood vessels and lymphatics. In *Pharmacology of the Skin I*, edited by M.W. Greaves and S. Shuster, pp. 89–116. Berlin: Springer.

Abramson, D.I. and Ferris, E.B. (1940). Responses of blood vessels in the resting hand and forearm to various stimuli. *American Heart Journal* **19**, 541–553.

Amara, S.G., Jonas, V., Rosenfeld, M.G., Ong, E.S. and Evans, R.M. (1982). Alternative RNA processing in calcitonin gene expression generates mRNAs encoding different polypeptide products. *Nature*, **298**, 240–244.

Anand, A., Bloom, S.R. and McGregor, G.P. (1983). Topical capsaicin pretreatment inhibits axon reflex vasodilatation caused by somatostatin and vasoactive intestinal polypeptide in human skin. *British Journal of Pharmacology*, **78**, 665–669.

Andrews, P.V., Thomas, K.L. and Helme, R.D. (1989). NK-1 receptor mediation of neurogenic plasma extravasation in rat skin. *British Journal of Pharmacology*, **97**, 1232–1238.

Archer, C.B., MacDonald, D.M., Morley, J., Page, C.P., Paul, W. and Sanyar, S. (1985). Effects of serum albumin, indomethacin and histamine H_1-antagonists of Paf-acether-induced inflammatory responses in the skin of experimental animals and man. *British Journal of Pharmacology*, **85**, 109–113.

Barnes, P.J., Belvisi, M.G. and Rogers, D.F. (1990). Modulation of neurogenic inflammation: novel approaches to inflammatory disease. *Trends in Pharmacological Sciences*, **11**, 185–189.

Barnes, P.J., Brown, M.J., Dollery, C.T., Fuller R.W., Heavey, D.J. and Ind, P.W. (1986). Histamine is released from skin by substance P but does not act as the final vasodilator in the axon reflex. *British Journal of Pharmacology*, **88**, 741–745.

Bayliss, W.M. (1901). On the origin from the spinal cord of the vasodilator fibres of the hind limb, and on the nature of these fibres. *Journal of Physiology (London)*, **26**, 173–209.

Benyon, R.C., Church, M.K. and Lowman, M.A. (1987). Histamine release from human dispersed skin mast cells induced by substance P. *British Journal of Pharmacology*, **90**, 102P.

Bernstein, J.E. (1988). Capsaicin in dermatologic disease. *Seminars in Dermatalogy*, **7**, 304–309.

Bernstein, J.E., Swift, R.M., Soltani, K. and Lorincz, A.L. (1981). Inhibition of axon reflex vasodilatation by topically applied capsaicin. *Journal of Investigative Dermatology*, **76**, 394–395.

Bevan, S. and Szolcsanyi, J. (1990). Sensory neuron-specific actions of capsaicin: mechanisms and applications. *Trends in Pharmacology Sciences*, **11**, 330–333.

Bloom, S.R. and Polak, J.M. (1983). Regulatory peptides and the skin. *Clinical and Experimental Dermatology*, **8**, 3–18.

Brain, S.D. and Edwardson, J.A. (1989). Neuropeptides and skin. In *Pharmacology of the Skin I*, edited by M.W. Greaves and S. Shuster, pp. 89–116. Berlin: Springer.

Brain, S.D. and Williams, T.J. (1985). Inflammatory oedema induced by synergism between calcitonin gene-related peptide (CGRP) and mediators of increased vascular permeability. *British Journal of Pharmacology*, **86**, 855–860.

Brain, S.D. and Williams, T.J. (1988). Substance P regulates the vasodilator activity of calcitonin gene-related peptide. *Nature*, **335**, 73–75.

Brain, S.D. and Williams, T.J. (1989). Interactions between the tachykinins and calcitonin gene-related peptide lead to the modulation of oedema formation and blood flow in rat skin. *British Journal of Pharmacology*, **97**, 77–82.

Brain, S.D., Williams, T.J., Tippins, J.R., Morris, H.R. and MacIntyre, I. (1985), Calcitonin gene-related peptide is a potent vasodilator. *Nature*, **313**, 54–56.

Brain, S.D., MacIntyre, I. and Williams, T.J. (1986). A second form of human calcitonin gene-related peptide which is a potent vasodilator. *European Journal of Pharmacology*, **124**, 349–352.

Brain, S.D., Tippins, J.R., Morris, H.R., MacIntyre, I. and Williams, T.J. (1986). Potent vasodilator activity of calcitonin gene-related peptide in human skin. *Journal of Investigative Dermatology*, **87**, 533–536.

Brain, S.D., Petty, R.G., Lewis, J.D. and Williams, T.J. (1990). Cutaneous blood flow responses in the forearms of Raynaud's patients induced by local cooling and intradermal injections of CGRP and histamine. *British Journal of Clinical Pharmacology*, **30**, 853–859.

Bruce, A.N. (1913), Vasodilator axon reflexes. *Quarterly Journal of Experimental Physiology*, **6**, 339–354.

Buckley, T.L., Brain, S.D. and Williams, T.J. (1990). Ruthenium red selectively inhibits oedema formation and increased blood flow induced by capsaicin in rabbit skin. *British Journal of Pharmacology*, **99**, 7–8.

Buckley, T.L., Brain, S.D., Collins, P. and William, T.J. (1991a). Inflammatory oedema induced by interactions between interleukin-1 and the neuropeptide calcitonin gene-related peptide. *Journal of Immunology*, **146**, 3424–3430.

Buckley, T.L., Brain, S.D., Rampart, M. and Williams T.J. (1991b). Time-dependent synergistic interactions between the vasodilator neuropeptide, calcitonin gene-related peptide (CGRP) and mediators of inflammation. *British Journal of Pharmacology*, **103**, 1515–1519.

Buckley, T.L., Jose, P.J., Brain, S.D. and William, T.J. (1991c). The release of calcitonin gene-related peptide (CGRP) by capsaicin in rabbit skin *in vivo*. *British Journal of Pharmacology*, **102**, 76P.

Bunker, C.B., Foreman, J. and Dowd, P.M. (1989). Digital cutaneous vascular responses to histamine, compound 48/80 and neuropeptides in normal subjects and Raynaud's phenomenon. *Journal of Investigative Dermatology*, **92**, 409.

Bunker, C.B., Terenghi, G., Springall, D.R., Polak, J.M. and Dowd, P.M. (1990). Deficiency of calcitonin gene-related peptide in Raynaud's phenomenon. *Lancet*, **2**, 1530–1533.

Burgess, P.R. and Perl, E.R. (1967). Myelinated afferent fibres responding specifically to noxious stimulation of the skin. *Journal of Physiology (London)*, **190**, 541–562.

Camp, R.D.R., Coutts, A.A., Greaves, M.W., Kay, A.B. and Walport, M.J. (1983). Responses of human skin to intradermal injection of leukotrienes C_4, D_4 and B_4. *British Journal of Pharmacology*, **80**, 497–502.

Carpenter, S.E. and Lynn, B. (1981). Vascular and sensory responses of human skin to mild injury after topical treatment with capsaicin. *British Journal of Pharmacology*, **73**, 755–758.

Chang, M.M., Leeman, S.E. and Nrall, H.D. (1971). Amino acid sequence of substance P. *Nature*, **232**, 86–87.

Chun, L.L.Y. and Patterson, P.H. (1977). Role of nerve growth factor in the development of rat sympathetic neurons *in vitro*. Survival, growth and differentiation of catecholamine production. *Journal of Cell Biology*, **75**, 694–704.

Coffman, J.D. and Cohen, R.A. (1988). Role of α-adrenoceptor subtypes mediating sympathetic vasoconstriction in human digits. *European Journal of Clinical Investigation*, **18**, 309–313.

Colpaert, F.C., Donnerer, J. and Lembeck, F. (1983). Effects of capsaicin on inflammation and on the substance P content of nervous tissues; in rats with adjuvant arthritis. *Life Sciences*, **32**, 1827–1834.

Couture, R. and Kerouac, R. (1987). Plasma protein extravasation induced by mammalian tachykinin in rat skin: influence of anaesthetic agents and an acetylcholine antagonist. *British Journal of Pharmacology*, **91**, 265–273.

Crossman, D.C., Brain, S.D. and Fuller, R. (1991). Potent vasoactive effects of endothelin in skin. *American Journal of Physiology*, **70**, 260–266.

Dale, H.H. and Feldberg, W. (1934). The chemical transmission of secretory impulses to the sweat glands of the cat. *Journal of Physiology (London)*, **82**, 121–128.

Dalsgaard, C.J., Johnsson, C.E, Hökfelt, T. and Cuello, A.C. (1983). Localization of substance P-immunoreactive nerve fibers in the human digital skin. *Experientia*, **39**, 1018–1020.

Devillier, P., Regoli, D., Asseraf, A., Descurs, B., Marsac, J. and Renoux, M. (1986). Histamine release and local responses of rat and human skin to substance P and other mammalian tachykinins. *Pharmacology*, **32**, 340–347.

Duggan, A.W., Morton, C.R., Zhao, Z.Q. and Hendry, I.A. (1987). Noxious heating of the skin releases immunoreactive substance P in the substantia gelatinosa of the rat: a study with antibody microprobes. *Brain Research*, **403**, 345–349.

Edbrooke, M.R., Parker, D., McVey, J.H Riley, J.H., Sorenson, G.D., Pettengell, O.S. (1985). Expression of the human calcitonin/CGRP gene in lung and thyroid carcinoma. *EMBO Journal*, **4**, 715–724.

Ekenvall, F., Lindblad, L.E., Norbeck, O. and Etzell, B.-M. (1988). α-adrenoceptors and cold induced vasocon-striction in human finger skin. *American Journal of Physiology*, **255**, H1000–H1003.

Farber, E.M., Nickologg, B.J., Recht, B. and Fraki, J.E. (1986). Stress, symmetry and psoriasis: possible role of neuropeptides. *Journal of American Academy of Dermatology*, **14**, 305–311.

Ferreira, S.H. (1972). Prostaglandins, aspirin-like drugs and analgesia. *Nature*, **240**, 200–203.

Flavahan, N.A. and Vanhoutte, P. (1986). Sympathetic purinergic vasoconstriction and thermosensitivity in a canine cutaneous vein. *Journal of Pharmacology and Experimental Therapeutics*, **239**, 784–789.

Foreman, J.C. and Jordan, C.C. (1983). Histamine release and vascular changes induced by neuropeptides. *Agents and Actions*, **13**, 105–116.

Foreman, J.C., Jordan, C.C., Oehme, P. and Renner, H. (1983). Structure-activity relationships for some substance P-related peptides that cause wheal and flare reactions in human skin. *Journal of Physiology (London)*, **335**, 449–465.

Fuller, R.W., Conradson, T.-B., Dixon, C.M.S., Crossman, D.C. and Barnes, P.J. (1987). Sensory neuropeptide effects in human skin. *British Journal of Pharmacology*, **92**, 781–788.

Gamse, R. and Saria, A. (1985). Potentiation of tachykinin-induced plasma protein extravasation by calcitonin gene-related peptide. *European Journal of Pharmacology*, **114**, 61–66.

Gamse, R. and Saria, A. (1987). Antidronic vasodilation in the rat hindpaw measured by laser Doppler flowmetry: pharmacological modulation. *Journal of Autonomic Nervous System*, **19**, 105–111.

Gamse, R., Holzer, P. and Lembeck, F. (1980). Decrease of substance P in primary afferent neurons and impairment of neurogenic plasma extravasation by capsaicin. *British Journal of Pharmacology*, **68**, 207–213.

Gibbins, I.L., Wattchow, D. and Coventry, G. (1987). Two immuno-histochemically identified populations of calcitonin gene-related peptide (CGRP)-immunoreactive axons in human skin. *Brain Research*, **414**, 143–148.

Goetzl, E.J. and Austen, F. (1975). Purification and synthesis of eosinophilic tetrapeptides of human lung tissue: identification as eosinophil chemotactic factor of anaphylaxis. *Proceedings of the National Academy of Sciences USA*, **72**, 4123–4127.

Grant, R.T. (1930). Observations on direct communications between arteries and veins in the rabbit's ear. *Heart*, **15**, 281–303.

Greishman, S.E. (1954). The reaction of the capillary bed of the nailfold to the continuous intravenous infusion of levo-norepihephrine in patients with normal blood pressure and with essential hypertension. *Journal of Clinical Investigation*, **33**, 975–983.

Hagermark, O., Hökfelt, T. and Pernow, B. (1978). Flare and itch induced by substance P in human skin. *Journal of Investigative Dermatology*, **71**, 233–235.

Hartschuh, W., Weihe, E. and Reinecke, M. (1983). Peptidergic (neurotensin, VIP, substance P) nerve fibres in the skin. Immunohistochemical evidence of an involvement of neuropeptides in nociception, pruritus and inflammation. *British Journal of Dermatology*, **109** (Suppl. 25), 14–17.

Henriksen, O. and Sejrsen, P. (1976). Local reflex in microcirculation in human cutaneous tissue. *Acta Physiologica Scandinavica*, **98**, 227–231.

Henry, J.L. (1987). Discussions of nomenclature for tachykinins and tachykinin receptors. In *Substance P and Neurokinins*, edited by J.L. Henry, R. Couture, A.C. Cuello, G. Pelletier, R. Quirion and D. Regoli. xvii–xviii. New York: Springer.

Hökfelt, T., Kellerth, J.-O., Nilsson, G. and Pernow, B. (1975). Substance P localization in the central nervous system and some primary sensory neurons. *Science*, **190**, 889–890.

Hökfelt, T., Millhorn, D., Seroogy, K., Tsuruo, Y., Ceccatelli, S., Lindh, B., *et al.* (1987). Coexistence of peptides with classical neurotransmitters. *Experientia*, **43**, 768–784.

Hölzer, P. (1988). Local effector functions of capsaicin-sensitive sensory nerve endings: involvement of tachykinins, calcitonin gene-related peptide and other neuropeptides. *Neuroscience*, **24**, 739–768.

Hughes, S.R., Williams, T.J. and Brain, S.D. (1990). Evidence that endogenous nitric oxide modulates oedema formation induced by substance P. *European Journal of Pharmacology*, **191**, 481–484.

Hurley, H.J. and Mescon, H. (1956). Cholinergic innervation of the digital arteriovenous anastomoses of human skin: a histochemical localization of cholinesterase. *Journal of Applied Physiology*, **9**, 82–84.

Jancso, G., Kiraly, E. and Jancso-Gabor, A. (1977). Pharmacologically induced selective degeneration of chemosensitive primary sensory neurons. *Nature*, **270**, 741–743.

Jancso, N., Jancso-Gabor, A. and Szolcsanyi, J. (1967). Direct evidence of neurogenic inflammation and its prevention by denervation and by treatment with capsaicin. *British Journal of Pharmacology*, **31**, 138–151.

Johansson, O. (1986). A detailed account of NPY-immunoreactive nerves and cells of the human skin. Comparison with VIP, substance-P and PHI-containing structures. *Acta Physiologica Scandinavica*, **128**, 147–153.

Johansson, O. and Vaalasti, A. (1987). Immunohistochemical evidence for the presence of somatostatin-containing sensory nerve fibres in the human skin. *Neuroscience Letters*, **73**, 225–230.

Johansson, O., Vaalasti, A., Tainio, H. and Ljungberg, A. (1988). Immunohisto-chemical evidence of galanin in sensory nerves of human digital skin. *Acta Physiologica Scandinavia*, **132**, 261–263.

Kaji, A., Shigematsu, H., Fujita, K., Maeda, T. and Watanabe, S. (1988). Parasympathetic innervation of cutaneous blood vessels by vasoactive intestinal peptide-immunoreactive and acetylcholinesterase-positive nerves: histochemical and experimental study on rat lower lip. *Neuroscience*, **25**, 353–362.

Karanth, S.S., Dhital, S., Springall, D.R. and Polak, J.M. (1990). Reinnervation and neuropeptides in mouse skin flaps. *Journal of Autonomic Nervous System*, **31**, 127–134.

Kawasaki, H., Takasaki, K., Saito, A. and Goto, K. (1988). Calcitonin gene-related peptide acts as a novel vasodilator neurotransmitter in mesenteric resistance vessels of the rat. *Nature*, **335**, 164–167.

Kawasaki, H., Nuki, C., Saito, A. and Takasaki, K. (1990). Role of calcitonin gene-related peptide-containing nerves in vascular adrenergic transmission. *Journal of Pharmacology and Experimental Therapeutics*, **252**, 403–409.

Kenins, P., Hurley, J.V. and Bell, C. (1984). The role of substance P in the axon reflex in the rat. *British Journal of Dermatology*, **111**, 551–559.

Kjartansson, J. and Dalsgaard, C.J. (1987). Calcitonin gene-related peptide increases survival of a musculo cutaneous flap in the rat. *European Journal of Pharmacology*, **142**, 355–358.

Kjartansson, J., Dalsgaard, C.-J. and Jonsson, C.E. (1987). Decreased survival of experimental critical flaps in rats after sensory denervation with capsaicin. *Plastic Reconstuctive Surgery*, **79**, 218–221.

Kjartansson, J., Lindberg, T., Samuelson, V.E., Dalsgaard, C.J. and Heden, P. (1988). Calcitonin gene-related peptide (CGRP) and transcutaneous electrical nerve stimulation (TENS) increase cutaneous blood-flow in a musculo-cutaneous flap in the rat. *Acta Physiologica Scandinavica*, **134**, 89–94.

Landis, S.C. and Fredieu, J.R. (1986). Coexistence of calcitonin gene-related peptide and vasoactive intestinal peptide in cholinergic sympathetic innervation of rat sweat glands. *Brain Research*, **377**, 177–181.

Lembeck, F. and Gamse, R. (1982). Substance P in peripheral sensory processes. In *Substance P in the Nervous System*, Ciba Foundation Symposium, edited by R. Porter and M. O'Connor. pp. 35–49. London: Pitman.

Lembeck, F. and Holzer, P. (1979). Substance P as a mediator of antidromic vasodilatation and neurogenic plasma extravasation. *Naunyn-Schmiedeberg's Archives of Pharmacology*, **310**, 175–183.

Lewis, T. (1927). *The Blood Vessels of the Human Skin and their Responses*. London: Shaw.

Lewis, T. (1930). Observations upon reactions of vessels in human skin to cold. *Heart*, **15**, 177–208.

Lotz, M., Vaughan, J.H. and Carson, D.A. (1988). Effect of substance P and substance K on the growth of cultured keratinocytes. *Journal of Investigative Dermatology*, **241**, 1218–1221.

Lundblad, L., Lundberg, J.M., Anggard, A. and Zetterstom, O. (1985). Capsaicin pretreatment inhibits the flare component of the cutaneous allergic reaction in man. *European Journal of Pharmacology*, **113**, 461–462.

Lynn, B. (1984). The detection of injury and tissue damage. In *Textbook of Pain*, edited by P.D. Wall and R. Melzack. pp. 19–33. Edinburgh: Churchill-Livingstone.

Lynn, B. (1989). Structure, function and control: different nerve endings in the skin. In *Pharmacology of the Skin I*, edited by M.W. Greaves and S. Shuster, pp. 89–116. Berlin: Springer.

Lynn, B. and Shakhanbeh, J. (1988). Neurogenic inflammation in the skin of the rabbit. *Agents and Actions*, **25**, 228–230.

Maggi, C.A. and Meli, A. (1988). The sensory efferent function of capsaicin-sensitive sensory neurons. *General Pharmacology*, **19**, 1–43.

Manley, H.C. and Haynes, L.W. (1989). Eosinophil chemotactic response to rat CGRP-1 is increased after exposure to trypsin or guinea-pig lung particulate fraction. *Neuropeptides*, **13**, 29–34.

Marasco, P.W., Showell, H.J. and Becker, E.L. (1981). Substance P binds to the formylpeptide chemotaxis receptor on the rabbit neutrophil. *Biochemical Biophysical Research Communications*, **99**, 1065–1072.

Megay, K.V. (1935). Versuche an biologischen Testobjekten uber die Natur des im Schweiß vorhanden vagometischen Stoffes. *Pflügers Archives Gestive Physiologica*, **236**, 159–165.

Mescon, H., Hurley, H.J. and Moretti, G. (1956). Anatomy and histochemistry of the arteriovenous anastomes in digital sin. *Journal of Investigative Dermatology*, **27**, 133–145.

Mione, M.C., Ralevic, V. and Burnstock, G. (1990). Peptides and vasomotor mechanisms. *Pharmacology and Therapeutics*, **46**, 429–468.

Mousli, M., Bueb, J.-L., Bronner, C., Rouot, B. and Landry, Y. (1990). G protein activation: a receptor independent mode of action for cationic amphiphilic neuropeptides and venom peptides. *Trends in Pharmacological Sciences*, **11**, 358–362.

Mulderry, R.K., Ghatei, M.A., Spokes, R.A., Jones, P.M., Pierson, A.M., Hamid, Q.A., *et al.* (1988). Differential expression of αCGRP and βCGRP by primary sensory neurons of the rat. *Neuroscience*, **25**, 195–205.

Nawa, H., Hirose, T., Takashima, H., Inayama, S. and Nakamishi, S. (1983). Nucleotide sequences of cloned cDNAs for two types of bovine brain substance P precursor. *Nature*, **306**, 32–36.

Nilsson, G. and Ahlstedt, S. (1989). Increased hypersensitivity reaction in rats neuromanipulated with capsaicin. *International Archives of Applied Immunology*, **90**, 256–260.

Nilsson, J., von Euler, A.M. and Dalsgaard, C.J. (1985). Stimulation of connective tissue cell growth by substance P and substance K. *Nature*, **315**, 61–63.

Norberg, K.-A. and Hamberger, B. (1964). The sympathetic adrenergic neuron: some characteristics revealed by histochemical studies on the intraneuronal distribution of the transmitter. *Acta Physiologica Scandinavica (Supplement)*, **238**, 1–42.

O'Halloran, D. and Bloom, S.R. (1991). Calcitonin gene-related peptide. *British Medical Bulletin*, **302**, 739–740.

O'Shaughnessy, D.J., McGregor, G.P., Ghatei, M.A., Blank, M.A., Springall, D.R., Gu, J., *et al.* (1983). Distribution of bombesin, somatostatin, substance-P and vasoactive intestinal polypeptide in feline and porcine skin. *Life Sciences*, **32**, 2827–2836.

Parnavelas, J.G, Kelly, W. and Burnstock, G. (1985). Ultrastructural localization of choline acetyltransferase in vascular endothelial cells in rat brain. *Nature*, **316**, 724–725.

Payan, D.G., Brewster, D.R. and Goetzl, E.J. (1983). A specific stimulation of human T-lymphocytes by substance P. *Journal of Immunology*, **131**, 1613–1615.

Payan, D.G., McGillis, J.P., Renold, F.K., Mitsuhashi, M. and Goetzl, E.J. (1987). Neuropeptide modulation of leukocyte function. *Annals of the New York Academy of Sciences*, **496**, 182–191.

Perianin, A., Snyderman, R. and Malfroy, B. (1989). Substance P primes human neutrophil activation: mechanism for neurological regulation of inflammation. *Biochemical Biophysical Research Communications*, **161**, 520–524.

Piotrowski, W. and Foreman, J.C. (1986). Some effects of calcitonin gene-related peptide in human skin and on histamine release. *British Journal of Dermatology*, **114**, 37–46.

Ritter, A.M., Lewin, G.R. Kremer, N.E. and Mendell, L.M. (1991). Requirement for nerve growth factor in the development of myelinated nociceptors *in vivo*. *Nature*, **350**, 500–502.

Rosenfeld, M.G., Amara, S.G. and Evans, R.M. (1984). Alternative RNA processing: determining neuronal phenotype. *Science*, **225**, 1315–1320.

Ross, D.R. and Varipapa, R.J. (1989). Treatment of painful diabetic neuropathy with topical capsaicin. *New England Journal of Medicine*, **321**, 474–475.

Rowell, L.B. (1983). Cardiovascular adjustments to thermal stress. In *Handbook of Physiology, Section 2: The Cardiovascular System, Volume III: Peripheral Circulation and Organ Blood Flow*, Part 2, pp. 967–1023. Bethesda, MD: American Physiological Society.

Ruff, M.R., Wahl, S.M. and Pert, C.B. (1985). Substance P- medicated chemotaxis of human monocytes. *Peptides*, **6** (Suppl. 2), 107–111.

Sato, K. (1977). The physiology, pharmacology and biochemistry of the eccrine sweat glands. *Reviews in Physiology, Biochemistry and Pharmacology*, **79**, 51–131.

Schwartz, L.B., Atkins, P.C., Bradford, T.R., Fleekop, P., Shalit, M. and Zweiman, B. (1987). Release of tryptase together with histamine during the immediate cutaneous response to allergen. *Journal of Allergy and Clinical Immunology*, **80**, 850–855.

Scicchitano, R., Biennenstock, J. and Stanisz, A.M. (1988). *In vivo* immunomodulation by the neuropeptide substance P. *Immunology*, **63**, 733–735.

Scott, A. (1962). Acetylcholine in normal and diseased skin. *British Journal of Dermatology*, **7**, 317–322.

Sekizawa, K., Tamaoki, J., Graf, P.D., Basbaum, C.B., Borson, D.B. and Nadel, J.A. (1987). Enkephalinase inhibitor potentiates mammalian tachykinin-induced contraction in ferret trachea. *Journal of Pharmacology and European Therapeutics*, **243**, 1211–1217.

Senapati, A., Anand, P., McGregor, G.P., Ghatei, M.A., Thompson, R.P.H. and Bloom, S.R. (1986). Depletion of neuropeptides during wound healing in rat skin. *Neuroscience Letters*, **71**, 101–105.

Shawket, S., Dickerson, C., Hazleman, B. and Brown, M.J. (1989). Selective suprasensitivity to calcitonin gene-related peptide in the hands in Raynaud's phenomenon. *Lancet*, **ii**, 1354–1357.

Shepherd, J.T. and Thompson, I.D. (1953). The response to cold of the blood vessels of denervated fingers during the regeneration of the nerves. *Irish Journal of Medical Science*, **6**, 208–211.

Soter, N.A., Lewis, R.A., Corey, E.J. and Austen, K.F. (1983). Local effects of synthetic leukotrienes (LTC$_4$, LTD$_4$, LTE$_4$ and LTB$_4$) in human skin. *Journal of Investigative Dermatology*, **80**, 115–119.

Sydbom, A. (1982). Histamine release from isolated rat mast cells by neurotensin and other peptides. *Agents and Actions*, **12**, 91–93.

Szolcsanyi, J. (1988). Antidromic vasodilatation and neurogenic vasodilatation. *Agents and Action*, **23**, 4–11.

Tanaka, T., Danno, K., Ikai, K. and Imamura, S. (1988). Effect of substance P and substance K on the growth of cultured keratinocytes. *Journal of Investigative Dermatology*, **90**, 399–401.

Tanio, H., Vaalasti, A. and Rechardt, L. (1987). The distribution of substance P-, CGRP-, galanin- and ANP-like immunoreactive nerves in human sweat glands. *Histochemical Journal*, **19**, 375–380.

Thomas, G. and Church, M.K. (1990). Platelet activating factor does not release histamine from dispersed cutaneous mast cells. *Clinical and Experimental Allergy*, **20**, 377–382.

Thomas, K.L., Andrews, P.V., Khalil, Z. and Helme, R.D. (1989). Substance P induced hydrolysis of inositol phospholipids in rat skin in an *in vivo* model of inflammation. *Neuropeptides*, **13**, 191–196.

von Euler, V.S. and Gaddum, J.H. (1931). An unidentified depressor substance in certain tissue extracts. *Journal of Physiology (London)*, **72**, 74–87.

Wada, M., Arai, T., Takagaki, T. and Nakagawa, T. (1952). Axon reflex mechanism in sweat responses to nicotine, acetylcholine and sodium chloride. *Journal of Applied Physiology*, **4**, 745–752.

Wallengren, J. and Moller, H. (1986). The effect of capsaicin on some experimental inflammations in human skin. *Acta Dermatologica Venereologica (Stockholm)*, **66**, 375–380.

Wallengren, J., Ekman, R. and Moller, H. (1986). Substance P and vasoactive intestinal peptide in bullous and inflammatory skin diesease. *Acta Dermatologca Venereologica (Stockholm)*, **66**, 23–28.

Wallengren, J., Ekman, R. and Sundler, F. (1987). Occurrence and distribution of neuropeptides in the human skin. *Acta Dermatologica Venereologica (Stockholm)*, **67**, 185–192.

Wallin, B.G. (1990). Neural control of human skin blood flow. *Journal of Autonomic Nervous System*, **30**, S185–S190.

Wallin, B.G. and Fagius, J. (1988). Peripheral sympathetic neural activity in conscious humans. *Annual Review of Physiology*, **50**, 565–576.

Weihe, E. and Hartschuh, W. (1988). Multiple peptides in cutaneous nerves: regulators under physiological conditions and a pathogenetic role in skin disease? *Seminars in Dermatology*, **7**, 284–300.

Winkelmann, R.K. (1988). Cutaneous sensory nerves. *Seminars in Dermatology*, **7**, 236–268.

Yancey, K.B., Hammer, C.H., Hawath, L., Frank, M.M. and Lawley, T.J. (1985). Studies of human C5a as a mediator of inflammation in normal human skin. *Journal of Clinical Investigation*, **75**, 486–495.

Zamora, M.R., O'Brien, R.F., Rutterford, R.B. and Weil, V.Y. (1990). Serum endothelin-1 concentrations and cold provocation in primary Raynaud's phenomenon. *Lancet*, **336**, 1144-1147.

Zar, M.A. (1989). Acetylcholine, atropine and related cholinergic and anticholinergics. In *Pharmacology of the Skin I*, edited by M.W. Greaves and S. Shuster, pp. 331–345. Berlin: Springer.

11 Renal Circulation

Bruce N. Van Vliet[1], John E. Hall[2], Thomas E. Lohmeier[2]
and H. Leland Mizelle[2]

[1] *Faculty of Medicine, Memorial University of Newfoundland,*
  St. John's, Newfoundland, Canada A1B 3V6
[2] *Department of Physiology and Biophysics,*
  University of Mississippi Medical Center,
  2500 North State Street, Jackson, MS 39216–4505, USA

The kidney receives a spinal-afferent and sympathetic-efferent innervation. Renal afferents signal pain, but also provide feedback concerning the renal environment (e.g. the osmolality of the medullary interstitium). Increases in renal sympathetic nerve activity (RSNA) stimulate renin secretion, inhibit sodium and water excretion, and increase renal vascular resistance. Although RSNA is normally not sufficient to restrain renal blood flow or glomerular filtration rate in unstressed animals, both fall during large increases in RSNA associated with the "defence reaction". Renal renin secretion and sodium reabsorption are tonically stimulated by RSNA in unstressed animals. Acute inhibition of RSNA results in up to a threefold increase in renal sodium excretion. However, chronic renal denervation increases renal sodium excretion by only a trivial amount. By mediating short-term adjustments of renal excretory function, the renal sympathetic nerves may help stabilize intravascular volume and accelerate the establishment of renal-body fluid balance.

KEY WORDS: renin angiotensin system; renal sympathetic nerve activity; renal afferents; sodium excretion; fluid balance; renal vasculature; glomerular filtration rate; hypertension; renal nerves.

INTRODUCTION

The sympathetic innervation of the kidney has attracted considerable attention since the responses to denervation and stimulation of the renal nerves were first reported (Bernard, 1859; Bradford, 1889). As the renal nerves are a relatively accessible and homogeneous supply of postganglionic sympathetic vasomotor fibres, they have often been selected for study for practical reasons. Of all of the vasomotor nerves, the activity of the renal nerves appears to have been most frequently recorded in recent years. However, attention to the renal sympathetic innervation has additionally been due to the realization that the renal nerves not only participate in the control of the renal vasculature, but also in regulatory mechanisms with widespread effects on the entire cardiovascular system.

MULTIPLE ROLES OF THE RENAL SYMPATHETIC INNERVATION

The renal sympathetic innervation participates in circulatory control at several levels of cardiovascular organization. At the level of the renal vasculature, the sympathetic innervation of the kidney potentially controls a vascular bed that normally receives approximately one-fifth of the cardiac output. The control of the renal vascular resistance by the renal nerves therefore has the potential to participate in acute adjustments of arterial pressure or cardiac output distribution.

At the organ level, the net influence of activating the renal sympathetic innervation is a biasing of renal function toward the retention of sodium and water. This is achieved not only through the influence of the renal nerves on the renal vasculature, but also through direct effects on renin secretion by the juxtaglomerular apparatus and fluid and electrolyte reabsorption by the renal tubules (Figure 11.1).

Finally, at the level of the entire cardiovascular system, the renal nerves may influence the state of the circulation in two ways. First, the renal nerves have the potential to influence the tone, and hence capacity, of the entire circulation. This effect is achieved through the influence of the renal sympathetic innervation on the renal secretion of renin and the resultant formation of the potent vasoconstrictor, angiotensin II (Figure 11.1). The second way in which renal nerves may affect the state of the circulation is through their influence on the filling of the vascular system. The net effect of activating the renal sympathetic nerves is to bias renal function towards the retention of sodium and water. If such an effect were sustained, this would provide the renal sympathetic nerves with the potential to initiate and maintain an increased filling of the circulation. The significance of such changes is that together, the filling and capacity of the cardiovascular system are determinants of the mean circulatory filling pressure and hence, cardiac preload, cardiac output and the mean arterial pressure (Figure 11.1). As arterial pressure in turn influences the fluid and electrolyte excretion of the kidney (i.e. pressure diuresis and natriuresis, respectively), these processes constitute a feedback loop commonly referred to as the renal–body fluid feedback mechanism (Figure 11.1). The underlying principles of this system and its predominance as a long-term controller of arterial blood pressure were first identified through mathematical modelling (Guyton and Coleman, 1967), and have since been confirmed empirically (Guyton, 1990; Guyton et al., 1990; Hall et al., 1990). It is principally through this connection with the renal–body fluid feedback mechanism that renal nerves have been implicated in pathophysiological states (Janssen and Smits, 1989; Zambraski, 1989; see later section on *Role of the renal-body fluid feedback mechanism*).

SCOPE OF THE REVIEW

The present review provides an overview of the literature on the renal nerves that, except for a brief discussion of renal sensory nerves, focuses on the sympathetic innervation of the kidney. As discussed above, the significance of the renal sympathetic innervation extends well beyond the limits of the renal vasculature or kidney. Therefore, this chapter reviews

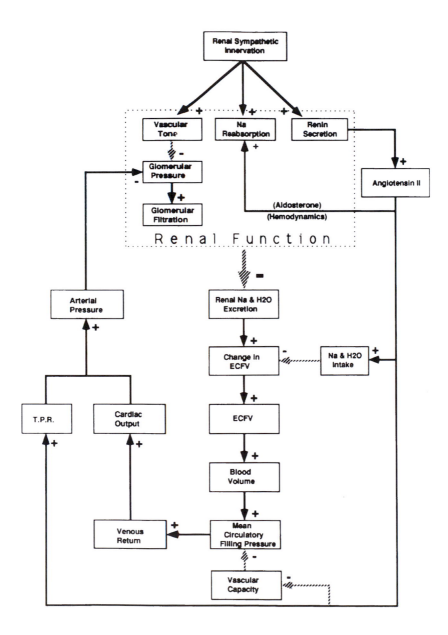

Figure 11.1 Interaction of the renal sympathetic nerves with the renal–body fluid feedback mechanism. Abbreviations: ECFV, extracellular fluid volume; T.P.R., total peripheral resistance.

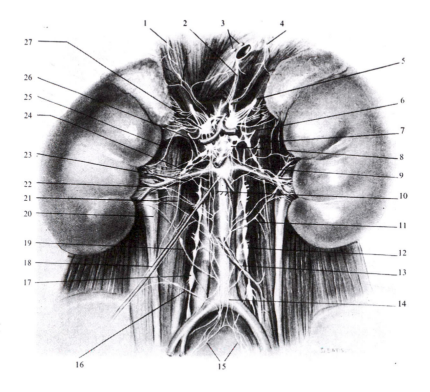

Figure 11.2   The renal plexus in man. Key: 1, right phrenic nerve; 2, coeliac division of posterior vagal trunk; 3, anterior vagal trunks; 4, left phrenic nerve; 5, superior (greater) thoracic splanchnic nerve; 6, middle (lesser) thoracic splanchnic nerve; 7, inferior (least) thoracic splanchnic nerve; 8, superior mesenteric ganglion; 9, posterior renal ganglion; 10, intermesenteric nerves; 11, renal branches from lower ends of intermesenteric nerves; 12, lumbar sympathetic trunk; 13, inferior mesenteric plexus; 14, superior hypogastric plexus; 15, hypogastric nerves; 16, middle ureteric and spermatic nerve; 17, lumbar sympathetic trunk; 18, superior spermatic nerve; 19, renal branch from superior hypogastric plexus; 20, superior ureteric nerve; 21, communication between renal plexus and superior spermatic nerve; 22, small renal ganglion; 23, renal branch from lumbar sympathetic trunk; 24, posterior renal ganglion; 25, communication between renal and suprarenal plexus; 26, aorticorenal ganglion; 27, right coeliac ganglion. (Reproduced with permission from Mitchell, 1950b; see also Mitchell, 1950a.)

the renal innervation in several contexts, including not only the anatomy of its distribution within the kidney and its actions on individual renal tissues, but also its broader influence on the circulation.

INNERVATION OF THE KIDNEY

The extrinsic innervation of the kidney occurs via the nerves of the renal plexus (Figure 11.2), which has been well described in several mammals (cat, Christensen, Lewis and Kuntz, 1951; rat, Drukker *et al.*, 1987; monkey, Marfurt, Echtenkamp and Jones, 1989) including

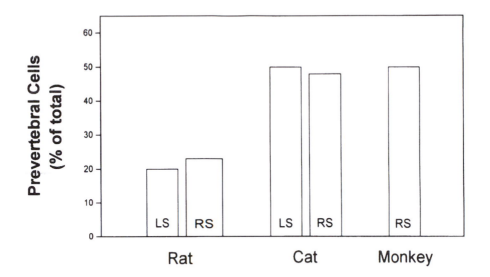

Figure 11.3   Distribution of renal sympathetic postganglionic cell bodies between prevertebral and paravertebral (sympathetic chain) ganglia. The values represent the percentage of all identified renal postganglionic cell bodies that were located in prevertebral ganglia. LS–Left Side, RS–Right Side. References: rat, Sripairojthikoon and Wyss, 1987; cat, Meckler and Weaver, 1984; monkey, Marfurt, Echtenkamp and Jones, 1989.

man (Mitchell, 1950a, 1950b). The renal nerves consist predominantly of pre- and postganglionic renal sympathetic fibres and a smaller number of renal afferent fibres. Ultimately, the nerves of the renal plexus congregate at the renal hilum, where they enter the renal capsule by way of the renal vasculature and proximal ureter.

EFFERENT INNERVATION

Origin of renal postganglionic sympathetic fibres

The postganglionic sympathetic fibres of the renal plexus arise from the paravertebral ganglia of the sympathetic chain directly, by way of the thoracic and lumbar splanchnic nerves, and indirectly, by way of the prevertebral ganglia of the solar plexus. In rats, 70–80% of renal postganglionic cell bodies are found in the sympathetic chain (Figure 11.3; Ferguson, Ryan and Bell, 1986; Sripairojthikoon and Wyss, 1987; Chevendra and Weaver, 1991), whereas an approximately even distribution between pre- and paravertebral ganglia has been described in the cat (Meckler and Weaver, 1984). On average, the cell bodies of postganglionic renal sympathetic neurons in five cynomolgus monkeys (*Macaca fascicularis*) were equally divided between pre- and paravertebral ganglia (49.9% prevertebral, Marfurt, Echtenkamp and Jones, 1989). There is considerable variation between individuals of this species, however. Labelled postganglionic neurons arose entirely from the sympathetic chain in one individual, whereas 94% arose from the prevertebral ganglia in another. Such variation between individuals is much less apparent in rats (Ferguson, Ryan and Bell, 1986;

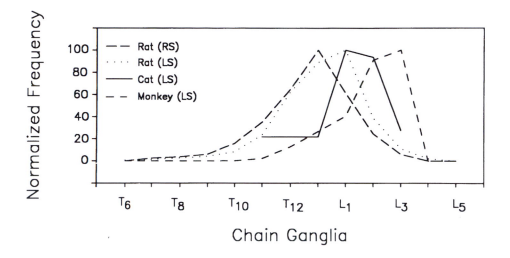

Figure 11.4 Segmental distribution of the cell bodies of renal sympathetic postganglionic neurons within the sympathetic chain ganglia. Individual data values are expressed as a percentage of the highest number of cells/ganglia reported in each study. LS–Left Side, RS–Right Side. References: rat, Sripairojthikoon and Wyss, 1987; cat, Meckler and Weaver, 1984; monkey, Marfurt et al., 1989.

Sripairojthikoon and Wyss, 1987; Chevendra and Weaver, 1991), and may be related to the degree of inbreeding of this species. Considerable variation between individuals may be anticipated in man.

The segmental origin of renal postganglionic sympathetic neurons that arise from the sympathetic chain is species dependent (Figure 11.4). In the rat, the occurrence of retrograde-labelled renal sympathetic neurons within the sympathetic chain is most dense at levels T_{13}–L_1 on the left side, and at level T_{13} on the right side (Ferguson, Ryan and Bell, 1986; Gattone, Marfurt and Dallie, 1986; Sripairojthikoon and Wyss, 1987; Chevendra and Weaver, 1991). The distribution is shifted one to two segments caudally in the cat, in which the peak occurrence of renal postganglionic neurons occurs at levels L_1 and L_2 on both sides (Kuo, de Groat and Nadelhaft, 1982; Meckler and Weaver, 1984), and even more caudally in the cynomolgus monkey, in which peak occurrences were observed at levels L_2 and L_3 on the right side (Marfurt, Echtenkamp and Jones, 1989).

The distribution of renal sympathetic neurons within prevertebral ganglia of the solar plexus is complex. This is a result of variation in the structure of the solar plexus between species, the variable number of ganglia that are recognized by different investigators, and the variable distribution of renal postganglionic neurons within the ganglia of the plexus. Most frequently, renal sympathetic neurons have been described within the superior mesenteric and/or coeliac ganglia, and aorticorenal (splanchnic, suprarenal) and renal ganglia (Mitchell, 1950a, 1950b; Bell and McLachlan, 1982; Kuo, de Groat and Nadelhaft, 1982; Meckler and Weaver, 1984; Ferguson, Ryan and Bell, 1986; Gattone, Marfurt and Dallie, 1986;

Drukker *et al.*, 1987; Sripairojthikoon and Wyss, 1987; Marfurt, Echtenkamp and Jones, 1989; Chevendra and Weaver, 1991). Postganglionic cell bodies are also distributed among numerous small ganglia along the course of the renal nerves or within the kidney itself (Mitchell, 1950a, 1950b; Shvalev, 1966).

Intrinsic sympathetic innervation

The three most conspicuous influences of the sympathetic nervous system on renal function are the modulation of vascular tone, renin secretion and the tubular reabsorption of sodium. Consequently, there has been much interest in the innervation of the renal tissues that mediate each of these functions: renal vascular smooth muscle, granular (renin-secreting) and macula densa (sodium-sensing) cells of the juxtaglomerular apparatus, and the renal tubules. Investigation of the sympathetic innervation of these regions has been facilitated by several characteristics which permit noradrenergic nerves to be distinguished. These characteristics include the presence of noradrenaline, as revealed by induced fluorescence, the presence of noradrenaline uptake, as revealed by autoradiography, the presence of enzymes used in the synthesis of noradrenaline, as distinguished by immunohistochemistry, and the abundance of small dense-core synaptic vesicles, as revealed by electron microscopy. Using such techniques, the sympathetic innervation of the kidney has been described with an exactness and certainty that was not possible in classic studies (reviewed by Mitchell, 1950a, 1950b; Asfoury, 1971) which relied solely on use of the light microscope.

The noradrenergic innervation of the kidney is confined to the cortex and outer medulla, and is most dense in the inner (juxtamedullary) cortex (McKenna and Angelakos, 1968). Sympathetic fibres are distributed to the renal parenchyma by way of periarterial nerve bundles, and form a rich vascular plexus along the entire arterial circulation of the kidney, with the greatest density of innervation occurring at the afferent glomerular arterioles (Barajas and Powers, 1990; Luff *et al.*, 1992). At the glomerulus, neuroeffector junctions are seen to include both granular (renin-containing) and agranular afferent and efferent arterioles and mesangial cells. The renal tubules are sparsely innervated by fine sympathetic fibres arising principally from the nerve supply of neighbouring glomerular arterioles, interstitial capillaries and arteries. With the exception of the earliest segment of the proximal tubule in subcapsular nephrons (Barajas and Powers, 1989), all cortical segments of the tubule appear to be innervated in the rat (Barajas and Powers, 1990). The proximal tubule receives the greatest proportion of the tubule's noradrenergic innervation, followed by the thick ascending loop of Henlé (TALH), distal convoluted tubule and collecting duct, respectively (Barajas, Powers and Wang, 1984). In relative terms, however, the TALH is the most *densely* innervated cortical tubule segment, followed by the distal and proximal tubules, respectively. Overall, TALH segments of juxtamedullary nephrons receive a much heavier and consistent innervation than do mid-cortical or superficial cortical nephrons (Barajas and Powers, 1988). An intriguing feature in mid-cortical and superficial nephrons is the pattern of innervation along the length of the TAHL. In these nephrons, the density of innervation peaks at the level of the macula densa, achieving densities more than five times greater than regions of the TALH leading to the macula densa. The macula region of the TALH in superficial nephrons appears to be the most densely innervated region of the renal tubules in rats.

The presumed site of sympathetic neurotransmission is at varicosities, frequent swellings of the sympathetic axons that characteristically contain mitochondria and synaptic vesicles. In many cases, the basal lamina of the vascular smooth muscle and the axon bundle fuse to form a single layer between the closely (ca. 100 nm) apposed varicosity and the smooth muscle cell membrane. A small proportion (<24%) of such neuromuscular contacts exhibit specialization of the prejunctional membrane (Barajas and Muller, 1973; Luff *et al.*, 1991, 1992). However, not all varicosities conform to this simple arrangement (Barajas, Powers and Wang, 1984; Barajas and Powers, 1990). Some varicosities, for example, fail to form specialized junctions with target cells and are observed to simply overlap or lie adjacent to vascular smooth muscle or tubular cells (Barajas, Powers and Wang, 1984; Barajas and Powers, 1990; Luff *et al.*, 1991, 1992). Furthermore, synaptic vesicles within the varicosities are occasionally found to accumulate adjacent to the membrane facing the interstitium (Barajas and Powers, 1990). These sites may provide for neurotransmission to extrajunctional receptors within the kidney by way of the interstitium. This mode of sympathetic neurotransmission may be highly significant in the kidney, as only a fraction of cells are directly innervated (Barajas and Muller, 1973; Barajas and Powers, 1989), and at least in mouse kidney, electrical coupling between vascular smooth muscle cells is relatively weak (Nobiling *et al.*, 1991).

Recent ultrastructural studies by Luff *et al.* (1991, 1992) have noted an unusual diversity of the size and pattern of varicosities of the sympathetic fibres in the renal vasculature of the rat and rabbit. Two forms of sympathetic axon could be distinguished based on the structure of the varicosities. Type I axons exhibited larger varicosities (0.52 versus 0.36 μm^3) and intravaricosity axon diameters (0.36 versus 0.08 μm), relative to Type II axons. Furthermore, prejunctional membrane specializations were observed more frequently in Type I (24%) than Type II (11%) axons. However, the most prominent distinction was the presence of microtubule clusters in the varicose regions of Type I but not Type II axons. In Type II axons, microtubules were confined to the intervaricose regions, as previously observed for sympathetic vasomotor fibres in other vascular beds. The two axon types also differed in the distribution of their junctions, with afferent arterioles receiving a relatively high density ($14.2 \times 10^3/mm^2$) and preferential distribution of junctions from Type I axons. At present, the functional significance of the two axon types is not known. It has been suggested, however, that the afferent arterioles may receive a particularly effective innervation due to the high proportion of Type I axon junctions in this region, and their tendancy for prejunctional specialization and large varicosities.

The synaptic vesicles identified within the varicosities of the renal sympathetic nerves are of both the granular (dense-core) and agranular (clear) varieties (Barajas, 1978; Luff *et al.*, 1991). The dense-core vesicles contain noradrenaline (Muller and Bell, 1986), which abundant evidence suggests is the principal renal sympathetic neurotransmitter in mammals: it is by far the predominant catecholamine appearing in renal extracts (Holzbauer and Sharman, 1972) or in the renal venous circulation (Bradley, Sollevi and Lagerkranser, 1986). In addition, most actions of the renal nerves on kidney function can be reproduced with adrenergic agonists, including noradrenaline, and the effect of renal nerve activation on renal function can be blocked with adrenergic antagonists (Oswald and Greven, 1981).

Accumulating evidence suggests that noradrenaline may not be the only sympathetic transmitter in the kidney. In the dog, for example, it has been suggested that a subset of renal postganglionic sympathetic neurons may employ dopamine in place of noradrenaline as the transmitter substance (Bell, Lang and Laska, 1978; Dinerstein *et al.*, 1979; Bell, 1987). Furthermore, although the contents of the clear synaptic vesicles that occur in sympathetic varicosities have not been identified in the kidney, studies performed in other organ systems suggest that they may contain neuropeptides that are released during activation of the sympathetic nerves. For example, neuropeptide Y (NPY) is a 36-amino-acid peptide which exerts potent effects on renal function (Persson, Grimpl and Lang, 1991). NPY-immunoreactive nerve fibres are abundant within the kidney of mammals, and are distributed in a pattern parallel to that of renal noradrenergic fibres. NPY immunoreactivity appears to be localized within noradrenergic fibres of the kidney (Knight, Fabre and Beal, 1989), and has been shown to correspond chemically with NPY, which is present in extracts of renal tissue (Ballesta *et al.*, 1984). Although NPY may ultimately prove to function as a renal sympathetic *co*transmitter substance, the physiological importance of neurally released NPY in influencing renal function has not yet been demonstrated.

Renal sympathetic nerve activity

Most studies of reflex alterations of renal sympathetic nerve activity (RSNA) have relied on recordings of multi-unit activity, or the integrated activity of an intact nerve. The use of techniques applied to intact renal nerves has enabled recording of RSNA to be conducted in unanaesthetized, chronically instrumented animals. As shown in Table 11.1, a variety of afferent inputs have been shown to influence RSNA.

The most frequently investigated input has been that of the arterial baroreceptors. The sensitivity of the baroreflex control of RSNA is highest in response to dynamic pressure stimuli. In the dog carotid sinus, for example, the gain of the baroreflex control of RSNA has been shown to peak at stimulus frequencies between 0.1 and 2 Hz. This range of frequencies includes those that compose the normal shape of the arterial pressure pulse (Kedzi and Geller, 1968). Consequently, RSNA is dominated by a conspicuous cardiac rhythm caused by the beat-to-beat inhibition of RSNA. Although the sensitivity of RSNA to slower changes in arterial pressure is lower than it is to dynamic changes, integrated RSNA is nonetheless strongly influenced by sustained changes in mean arterial pressure. Following administration of noradrenaline (1–4 μg/kg) to conscious cats, for example, integrated RSNA is reduced by 1.8% of control levels for each 1 mmHg rise in arterial pressure (Ninomiya, Matsuakawa and Nishiura, 1988).

A potent influence on RSNA also arises from mechanoreceptors in the low-pressure cardiopulmonary regions of the circulation. These receptors are activated by increased filling of the cardiac chambers or vein–atrial junctions, such as may occur following an increase in blood volume or centralization of venous blood (Table 11.1), and their activation reflexively inhibits RSNA. Figure 11.5A illustrates the inhibition of RSNA that accompanies immersion to the mid-cervical level in thermoneutral (37°C) water in conscious dogs. Immersion forces peripheral venous blood centrally, in this case raising central venous pressures by approximately 10 mmHg and inhibiting RSNA by 43–48% throughout the immersion period of 2 h (Figure 11.5A; Miki *et al.*, 1989a). This effect of immersion or volume loading on RSNA is attenuated or abolished following denervation of cardiopulmonary

TABLE 11.1
Reflexes affecting renal sympathetic nerve activity. References cited are single examples,
and are not comprehensive

Input	Stimulus	Renal nerve response	Species	References
Central chemoreceptors	CO_2	↑	Rabbit	Dorward et al., 1987
Arterial chemoreceptors	Hypoxia	↑	Rabbit	Dorward et al., 1987
Arterial baroreceptors	Carotid sinus distension	↓	Dog	Kedzi and Geller, 1968
Cardiopulmonary mechanoreceptors (vagal)	Left atrial baloon inflation	↓	Dog	Karim et al., 1972
	Immersion	↓	Dog	Miki et al., 1989a
	Head-up tilt	↑	Dog	Miki et al., 1989b
Cardiopulmonary chemoreceptors (sympathetic)	Bradykinin	↑	Cat	Reimann and Weaver, 1980
		↓	Monkey	Gorman and Zucker, 1984
		↓	Dog	Felder and Thames, 1982
		↑/↓	Dog	Gorman, Zucker and Gilmore, 1983
Hepatic baroreceptors	Portal vein distension	↑	Dog	Kostreva, Castaner and Kampine, 1980
Hepatic osmoreceptors	↑ osmolarity	↓	Rabbit	Ishiki, Morita and Hosomi, 1991
Renal chemoreceptors	Renal pelvic perfusion with 0.9% NaCl	↑ (C)	Rat	Kopp and Smith, 1987
		— (C)	Dog	Kopp, Olson and DiBona, 1984
Renal mechanoreceptors	Renal pelvic distension	↓ (C)	Rat	Kopp and Smith, 1987
		↑ (C)	Dog	Kopp, Olson and DiBona, 1984
Splenic afferents	Bradykinin	↑	Cat	Stein and Weaver, 1988
Intestinal afferents	Bradykinin	↑	Cat	Stein and Weaver, 1988
Uterine mechanoreceptors	Uterine horn distension	↓	Rat	Robbins and Sato 1991
Bladder mechanoreceptors	Bladder distension	↑	Dog	Drinkhill et al., 1989
Nasopharyngeal receptors	Inhalation of cigarette smoke	↑	Rabbit	Riedel, Kozawa and Iriki, 1982
Cutaneous nociceptors	Squeeze footpad	↑	Rabbit	Dorward et al., 1987
Cutaneous themoceptors	Skin warming	↑	Cat	Ninomiya and Fujita, 1976
Hypothalamic thermoceptors	Hypothalamic warming	↑	Cat	Ninomiya and Fujita, 1976

Abbreviations: C, contralateral kidney.

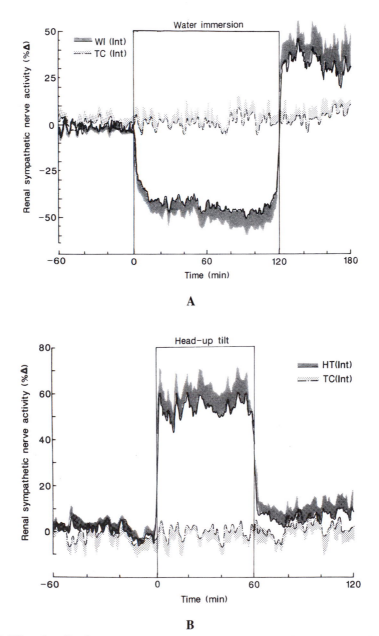

A

B

Figure 11.5   Effect of cardiopulmonary receptors on renal sympathetic nerve activity in chronically instrumented conscious dogs. *A*: Percent change in renal sympathetic nerve activity during immersion to the mid-cervical level in 37°C water (WI) and a time control (TC). Both arterial and central venous pressures rose by 10 mmHg during immersion. Renal responses of renal-denervated and sham-operated groups are shown in Figure 11.12. Data represent the mean and standard error for eight dogs. Reproduced from Miki *et al.* (1989a) with permission. *B*: Per cent change in renal sympathetic nerve activity during a 40° head-up tilt in standing dogs (HT) and a time control (TC). Tilt was accompanied by an 8–19 mmHg increase in renal perfusion pressure and a 7–8 mmHg fall in central venous pressures. (From Miki *et al.*, 1989b, with permission.)

regions, but not following arterial baroreceptor denervation (Thames, Miller and Abboud, 1982; Morita and Vatner, 1985; Hajduczok *et al.*, 1987). Figure 11.5B illustrates an approximately 60% increase in RSNA during a 40° head-up tilt in standing, conscious dogs. A head-up tilt causes venous blood to pool away from the cardiopulmonary regions, resulting in a 7–8 mmHg fall in central venous pressures in this example (Figure 11.5B; Miki *et al.*, 1989b). However, as tilting may also unload the carotid sinus baroreceptors, both arterial baroreceptors and cardiopulmonary receptors may contribute to the stimulation of RSNA during tilting (DiBona, Johns and Osborn, 1981). The importance of arterial and cardiac mechanoreceptors in controlling renal function is discussed in greater detail in subsequent sections (*Physiological importance of the renal nerves in regulating renal vascular resistance*, and *Control of sodium excretion by cardiac reflexes*).

In contrast with the inhibitory influence of cardiovascular mechanoreceptors, with few exceptions, the remaining afferent inputs affecting RSNA are excitatory (Table 11.1). Many of the excitatory inputs listed in Table 11.1, especially stimulation of visceral and somatic nociceptors, may be equated with an alerting or arousal response. Indeed, RSNA has been shown to be greatly influenced by emotional and psychic stress in conscious animals. For example, substantial increases in RSNA have been described during a rat's response to a jet of air (Lundin and Thoren, 1982; Koepke, Jones and DiBona, 1988), a cat's confrontation with a dog (Kirchner, 1974), and a dog's response to the discharging of a gun (Gross and Kirchheim, 1980).

More quantitative descriptions of renal sympathetic nerve activity have been obtained in recordings of the activity of single renal sympathetic fibres in anaesthetized animals. In such preparations, renal sympathetic fibres have been found to discharge at frequencies ranging from one spike every several seconds to several spikes per second under control conditions (Table 11.2). Discharge frequencies as high as 12.6 spikes/s have been recorded during severe hypoxia in rabbits anaesthetized with alphathesin (Dorward *et al.*, 1987). In most preparations, however, the upper range of discharge frequencies is considerably lower (Table 11.2). It is not clear to what extent the renal sympathetic discharge frequencies observed in anaesthetized animals may differ from those in conscious animals, as different anaesthetics have been reported to increase (chloralose, Schad and Seller, 1975; alfathesin, Dorward *et al.*, 1985; pentobarbital, Kirchner, 1974; Morita *et al.*, 1987; see also Berne *et al.*, 1952; Sadowski, Kurkus and Gellert, 1979), decrease (isoflurane, Seagard *et al.*, 1984), or have no effect (halothane, Schad and Seller, 1975; pentobarbital, Morita *et al.*, 1987) on integrated RSNA in chronically instrumented animals. Despite the limitations imposed by the use of anaesthesia, the recording of single unit activity has provided valuable information concerning the absolute level of renal nerve discharge. This has enabled comparisons of RSNA to be made between genetically hypertensive and normotensive rat strains, for example (Table 11.2).

The information provided through single unit recording has also helped to evaluate whether renal sympathetic fibres represent a functionally homogeneous or heterogeneous population of sympathetic fibres. This has been of interest, as discharge characteristics of sympathetic fibres in other organs has been found to be related to the nature of the tissue innervated. For example, fibres destined to innervate cardiovascular structures exhibit certain traits, such as cardiovascular and respiratory modulation, which are absent in those fibres destined for non-cardiovascular (e.g. glandular) targets. This raises the

TABLE 11.2
Measurements of single unit activity in renal nerves under control conditions in anaesthetized animals

Species	Activity (spikes/s)	Anaesthesia	References
Rat (SD)	0.47 (0.06–1.49)	Pentobarbital	Rogenes, 1982
Rat (WKY)	1.7	Chloralose–Urethane	Lundin, Ricksten and Thoren, 1984
Rat (WKY)	1.6 (±0.23)	Chloralose–Urethane	Thoren and Ricksten, 1979
Rat (SHR)	3.8	Chloralose–Urethane	Lundin, Ricksten and Thoren, 1984
Rat (SHR)	3.3 (±0.45)	Chloralose–Urethane	Thoren and Ricksten, 1979
Cat	1.2 (0.03–6.4)	Chloralose	Meckler and Weaver, 1988
Cat	1.3 (0.1–6.4)	Chloralose	Stein and Weaver, 1988
Rabbit	2.0 (0.8–3.4)	Alphathesin	Dorward et al., 1987
Rabbit	2.4 (0.3–6.4)	Chloralose–Urethane	Dorward et al., 1987
Dog	1.27 (0.2–2.58)	Chloralose	Drinkhill et al., 1989
Dog	0.57 (0.24–1.26)	Chloralose	Kidd, Linden and Scott, 1981

SD, Sprague Dawley; SHR, spontaneously hypertensive rats; WKY, Wistar-Kyoto.

possibility that the sympathetic outflow to distinct renal tissues, such as the renal vasculature, juxtaglomerular apparatus and renal tubules, might be independently regulated. Although most studies reveal renal sympathetic fibres to exhibit relatively uniform characteristics, such as cardiac and respiratory modulation, some exceptions have been noted. For example, although renal units are typically inhibited by an increase in arterial pressure (cat, Meckler and Weaver, 1988; Stein and Weaver, 1988; and rabbit, Dorward, et al., 1987), Drinkhill et al. (1989) reported 11 of 37 renal units were unaffected by an increase in the pressure applied to the vascularly isolated carotid sinus. Similarly, four of 40 units failed to respond to noxious stimulation of the footpad in rabbits (Dorward et al., 1987), three of eight units were resistant to inhibition caused by distension of the junction between the pulmonary vein and left atrium in dogs (Kidd, Linden and Scott, 1981), and three of 22 and two of eight units failed to respond to the application of bradykinin to the intestine and spleen, respectively (Meckler and Weaver, 1988: Stein and Weaver, 1988). These exceptions do not provide direct evidence for a heterogeneous population of renal sympathetic neurons, as they can simply be attributed to assorted sensitivities of different units within an otherwise homogeneous population.

Highly heterogeneous behaviour of renal sympathetic fibres was described by Riedel and Peter (1977), who distinguished two types of single unit renal sympathetic activity in rabbits anaesthetized with pentobarbital or alphathesin. Type A activity consisted of relatively small spikes that, if spontaneously active, discharged at approximately 4 spikes/s under control conditions and showed little respiratory modulation. Such units were said to be stimulated by warming and inhibited by cooling of the skin. In addition, type A activity was inhibited during the pressor response to noradrenaline (15 μg), yet was vigorously stimulated (to approximately 20 spikes/s!) by a bolus (3 μg) of angiotensin II (ANGII). In contrast, the larger type B activity discharged at approximately 2 spikes/s under control conditions, was inhibited by the pressor response to both noradrenaline and ANGII, exhibited respiratory modulation of its discharge, and was inhibited by warming and stimulated by cooling the skin of the animal. Despite the marked contrast in the reported characteristics of these subtypes, such heterogeneity has not been confirmed by subsequent studies in this or other species

(Dorward *et al.*, 1987). However, other hints of renal sympathetic heterogeneity were evident in a study of the renal sympathetic response to stimulation of renal R2 chemoreceptors (Rogenes, 1982). In this study, 15 renal units were stimulated, four were inhibited and an additional four showed no change in the response to a reflux of urine into the renal pelvis.

The non-uniform behaviour of renal sympathetic units in these experiments confirms that reflex connections with renal sympathetic fibres may not be entirely homogeneous. However, in comparison with the marked heterogeneity that has been described in the sympathetic supply of other organs in which vasoconstrictor, vasodilator and motility-regulating neurons are readily distinguished and may be even further subclassified (Janig and McLachlan, 1987; Janig, 1988), renal sympathetic fibres behave as a relatively homogeneous population of "vasomotor" fibres. It seems doubtful that the sympathetic nervous system is capable of distinguishing individual target tissues within the kidney.

AFFERENT INNERVATION

The kidney as a sensory organ

Historically, the most conspicuous sensory function of renal afferent neurons has been the mediation of visceral and referred pain of renal origin. In humans, a common cause of renal pain is distension of the renal pelvis due to obstruction of the urinary tract (DeWolf and Fraley, 1975; Elhilali and Winfield, 1989; Ansell and Gee, 1990). Pain of renal origin may also be evoked by a variety of conditions that distort the renal vasculature or compress the kidney. These forms of pain are likely to be mediated by renal mechanoreceptors, which have been shown to be sensitive to mechanical stimulation of the renal vasculature (Pines, 1959; Astrom and Crafoord, 1967, 1968; Beacham and Kunze, 1969; Niijima, 1971; Uchida, Kamisaka and Ueda, 1971; Gilmore and Tomomatsu, 1985) and pelvis (Pines, 1960; Astrom and Crafoord, 1968; Beacham and Kunze, 1969; Gilmore and Tomomatsu, 1985) in several mammalian species. The physiological response to distension of the renal pelvis is species dependent: a reduction of sympathetic tone to the contralateral kidney occurs in rats (Kopp, Olson and DiBona, 1984), whereas sympathetic arousal is observed in dogs and cats (Kopp, Olson and DiBona, 1984; Kopp and Smith, 1987; Ammons, 1988b).

Other stimuli that are known to cause pain of renal origin are ischaemia (e.g. due to an obstructive embolus or thrombus) or inflammation (e.g. due to pyelonephritis). These forms of renal pain may involve the activation or sensitization of renal afferent nerves through the local liberation of chemical mediators. In the rat, rabbit and cat, afferent nerves have been described that discharge in response to severe renal ischaemia (Pines, 1960; Astrom and Crafoord, 1968; Recordatti, Moss and Waselkov, 1978; Ge and Shiu-Yong, 1990b). Their response to ischaemia may be arrested by flushing the renal circulation with saline (Recordatti, Moss and Waselkov, 1978). Endogenous substances that have been implicated in stimulating or sensitizing the renal afferent nerves include purine nucleotides (Miller *et al.*, 1978; Katholi *et al.*, 1983b), prostaglandins (Faber, 1987) and kinins (Smits and Brody, 1984; Faber, 1987).

One subtype of renal chemoreceptor afferent neuron has properties that are clearly inconsistent with an exclusive role in mediating pain: the renal R2 chemoreceptor of rats (Recordati *et al.*, 1980) and rabbits (Ge and Shiu-Yong, 1990b). In addition to responding to severe renal ischaemia, this subtype of renal afferent fibre exhibits a resting discharge and is stimulated by the reflux of urine and artificial hypertonic or potassium-containing solutions into the renal pelvis (Recordatti *et al.*, 1980; Moss, 1989; Ge and Shiu-Yong, 1990b). These characteristics, coupled with the observation that the resting discharge of these receptors can be reduced simply by the induction of a mild water diuresis (Recordatti *et al.*, 1980), suggest that R2 chemoreceptors may function as osmoreceptors situated in close proximity to the renal pelvis and/or interstitium, and may provide feedback concerning physiological alterations in the physicochemical environment of the kidney, even in relatively benign (i.e. pain-free) states. This is consistent with the demonstration that R2 chemoreceptors are activated even during modest reductions in renal perfusion pressure that are well within the autoregulatory range (Barber and Moss, 1990; Rankin, Ashton and Swift, 1992).

Selective stimulation of renal R2 chemoreceptors in rats leads to a contralateral diuresis, natriuresis and reduction in sympathetic tone to the contralateral kidney, with no effect on the mean arterial blood pressure (Kopp, Olson and DiBona, 1984; Kopp and Smith, 1991). In contrast, perfusion of the renal pelvis with hypertonic saline evokes a small pressor response in cats (Kopp and Smith, 1987), a depressor response in rabbits (Ge and Shiu-Yong, 1990a; Rankin, Ashton and Swift, 1992), and is without effect in dogs (Kopp, Olson and DiBona, 1984). In rats, reflex responses to modest reductions in renal perfusion pressure and hypertonic perfusion of the renal pelvis appears to be dependent on the synthesis of prostaglandins (Barber and Moss, 1990; Kopp and Smith, 1991).

Intrinsic afferent innervation

Several approaches have been used to resolve the structure and distribution of afferent nerves within the kidney. A small minority of renal afferent neurons have myelinated axons, and therefore can be readily distinguished from the postganglionic sympathetic innervation of the kidney (Asfoury, 1971; Zimmerman, 1975; Barajas and Wang, 1978). Afferent fibres have also been distinguished by the lack of traits specific to noradrenergic neurons (e.g. Fergusson and Bell, 1985). A widely used approach has been to apply immunohistochemical techniques to distinguish nerves containing neuropeptides such as substance P and calcitonin gene-related peptide (Fergusson and Bell, 1985; Su *et al.*, 1986; Knight *et al.*, 1987; Fergusson and Bell, 1988; Reinecke and Forssmann, 1988; Geppetti *et al.*, 1989; Kurtz *et al.*, 1989), which appear to exist within most anatomically identified renal afferent neurons (Su *et al.*, 1986). Recently, a highly selective technique in which renal afferent fibres are distinguished by the presence of a histochemical label (horseradish peroxidase) transported along afferent axons from an injection site in the dorsal root ganglia has been used with great success in the rat (Marfurt and Echtenkamp, 1991).

The techniques described above have demonstrated that the distribution of renal afferent fibres is strikingly different to that of sympathetic fibres. The most densely innervated region of the kidney is the renal pelvis, which receives its innervation along the interlobar arteries by way of the connective tissue supporting the renal calyces, and directly from the hilus by way of the proximal ureter (Marfurt and Echtenkamp, 1991). The afferent fibres of the pelvis are arranged circumferentially, in contrast to the longitudinal orientation found in the ureter. This arrangement of afferent fibres is likely to include those mechanoreceptors that respond to distension of the renal pelvis (Pines, 1960; Astrom and Crafoord, 1968;

Beacham and Kunze, 1969; Gilmore and Tomomatsu, 1985). The afferent fibres terminate in a plexus in the smooth muscle and subepithelial layers of the pelvic wall. A small number of fibres reach the epithelial lining of the pelvis. Such afferents could potentially include renal chemoreceptors which are presumed to reside near the pelvic epithelium, but have not been specifically localized.

Within the remainder of the kidney, most of the afferent renal innervation is associated with the renal vasculature. Renal veins receive a sparse supply of afferent fibres, except for a plexus on the renal vein proper at the level of the hilus. The renal arterial circulation is more heavily innervated, with the hilar and interlobar arteries receiving the greatest innervation, and decreasing amounts occurring in the arcuate and interlobular arteries. The afferent innervation of the renal parenchyma appears to be sparse. However, presumed afferent fibres have been described in the outer stripe of the renal medulla, in association with the afferent arteriole and juxtaglomerular apparatus, and between the collecting ducts in the papilla (Knight et al., 1987; Reinecke and Forssmann, 1988; Geppetti et al., 1989).

Central projections of renal afferent neurons

The cell bodies of visceral afferent fibres travelling in the renal nerves are primarily distributed among five to six ipsilateral dorsal root ganglia of the lower thoracic and early lumbar segments. Their precise segmental distribution, as revealed by neuronal tract-tracing methods, is highly species dependent (Figure 11.6). In the rat, the greatest incidence of renal afferent cell bodies occurs at levels T_{10} and T_{11} on the right side, and T_{12} and T_{13} on the left side (Ciriello and Calaresu, 1983; Fergusson, Ryan and Bell, 1986). Renal cortical afferents may have a slightly more caudal distribution (Donovan, Wyss and Winternitz, 1983; Gattone, Marfurt and Dallie, 1986). The segmental distribution described for renal afferents in monkey (right side) and cats (left side) are somewhat lower than in rats, peaking at L_1 and L_2, respectively (Kuo et al., 1983; Marfurt, Echtenkamp and Jones, 1989).

The segmental distribution of renal afferents has not been studied using quantitative methods in animals other than the rat, cat and monkey. However, there is indirect evidence that a similar segmental distribution occurs in other animals. In the dog, for example, resection of dorsal roots T_{12} through L_2 has been claimed to satisfactorily alleviate pain arising from the renal pelvis (White, 1942). In man, analysis of the body segments to which pain of renal origin is referred suggests that renal afferents project from T_{11} through L_2 (Head, 1893, as modified by Mackenzie, 1893). According to Ray and Neil (1947), however, painful responses to stimulation of the renal pelvis and pedicle were abolished after interrupting the afferent pathway by resection of the sympathetic chain from T_7 through T_{11}, and cutting the greater and lesser splanchnic nerves. Relief of ureteral pain required the additional resection of T_{12} through L_1.

From the dorsal root ganglia, the central processes of renal afferent neurons pass into the local segments of the spinal cord, where some may be distributed to adjacent spinal segments by way of Lissauer's tract. The central process of most renal afferent neurons terminate on second order afferent neurons in the region of the dorsal grey commissure or in Lamina I and III through VII of the cord. Here, inputs from renal and somatic primary afferent neurons converge on second and higher order neurons that project to the brainstem and thalamus by way of the spinoreticular and spinothalamic pathways,

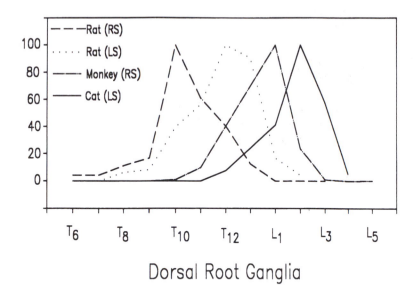

Dorsal Root Ganglia

Figure 11.6 Segmental origin of the renal sensory innervation. The graphs illustrate the segmental distribution of renal afferent cell bodies within the dorsal root ganglia. Individual data values are expressed as a percentage of the highest number of cells/ganglia reported in each study. LS–Left Side, RS–Right Side. References: rat, Ferguson, Ryan and Bell, 1986; cat, Kuo *et al.*, 1983; monkey, Marfurt, Echtenkamp and Jones, 1989.

respectively. Intersection of renal afferents with nociceptive somatic afferent pathways at this level may account for the mechanism by which pain of renal origin is referred to (i.e. interpreted as arising from) the body surface. In addition, the central processes of large myelinated renal mechanoreceptors ascend in the dorsal columns directly to the brainstem (Simon and Schramm, 1984; Wyss and Donovan, 1984; Knuepfer and Schramm, 1985).

Despite the potential for input from renal afferents to be integrated at the spinal level, several lines of evidence suggest that they are integrated predominantly at supraspinal levels, at least in anaesthetized animals; e.g. the numerous supraspinal projections of renal afferents (see below), the long latency of reno-reflexes (Calaresu *et al.*, 1978; Saeki, Terui and Kumada, 1988) and the demonstrated dependence of responses to renal afferent stimulation on the integrity of connections between the spine and brainstem in anaesthetized animals (Kopp, Smith and DiBona, 1985; Webb and Brody, 1987; Saeki, Terui and Kumada, 1988). Projections within the brainstem include the lateral segmental field, the dorsal vagal complex, the paramedian reticular formation, the nucleus tractus solitarius, the nucleus gracilis and fasciculus gracilis, and the ventrolateral medulla (Calaresu and Ciriello, 1981; Simon and Schramm, 1984; Felder, 1986; Ammons, 1988a). Within the hypothalamus, neurons responsive to the activation of renal afferent stimulation are widespread. Responsive cells are largely concentrated in the paraventricular nucleus, and in the lateral hypothalamus and lateral preoptic area. In addition, presumed vasopressin-secreting cells of the supraoptic nucleus in the rat have been shown to be activated by renal afferent neurons sensitive to bradykinin or capsaicin, but not adenosine or severe ischaemia (Day and Ciriello, 1987).

INFLUENCE OF RENAL SYMPATHETIC NERVES ON RENAL HAEMODYNAMICS AND THE RENIN–ANGIOTENSIN SYSTEM

OVERALL EFFECTS OF NORADRENERGIC STIMULATION ON RENAL HAEMODYNAMICS

Noradrenergic stimulation of the kidney, with either intrarenal infusion of catecholamines or electrical stimulation of renal nerves, causes renal vasoconstriction that can be attenuated or abolished by α-adrenoceptor antagonists (Berne *et al.*, 1952; Vander, 1965; Coote *et al.*, 1972; Schrier, 1974; Kopp *et al.*, 1981; DiBona, 1985a, 1989a; Moss *et al.*, 1992). The increase in renal vascular resistance and decrease in renal blood flow is dose dependent, or proportional to the frequency of renal nerve stimulation, with essentially no response occurring at a frequency of 1 Hz, and maximal vasoconstriction occurring at 10 Hz (DiSalvo and Fell, 1971; DiBona, 1982; Moss, Colindres and Gottschalk, 1992). Although the threshold for renal vasoconstrictor effects of sympathetic nerve stimulation occurs at approximately 1–2 Hz, changes in other renal functions, including increases in sodium reabsorption and renin release, can occur at lower frequencies (Table 11.3; DiBona, 1978, 1982, 1989a; Moss, Colindres and Gottschalk, 1992). These changes, in turn, can alter the control of renal haemodynamics indirectly via changes in ANGII formation and tubuloglomerular feedback (TGF), as discussed below. Thus, in considering the overall effects of noradrenergic stimulation on renal haemodynamics, one has to take into account not only the direct effects of the stimulus, but also indirect effects, some of which may be unique for the kidney. Unfortunately, the experimental designs of many studies do not allow a quantitative assessment of the multiple actions of adrenergic stimuli on the control of renal haemodynamics.

The direct vasoconstrictor effects of noradrenergic stimulation are mediated through activation of α-adrenoceptors. Although α_1- and α_2-adrenoceptors are present in the renal vasculature (Gottschalk, 1979; Gottschalk, Moss and Colindres, 1985; DiBona, 1989a; Moss, Colindres and Gottschalk, 1992), multiple studies in isolated vessels, isolated kidneys and anaesthetized animals suggest that vasoconstriction resulting from renal nerve stimulation or the infusion of α-adrenoceptor agonists, such as noradrenaline, is mediated mainly by α_1-adrenoceptors (Drew and Whiting, 1979; Horn *et al.*, 1982; Copper and Malik, 1985; Duval, Hicks and Langer, 1985; DiBona and Sawin, 1987; Wolff, Gesek and Strandhoy, 1987). Recent studies in conscious or areflexic animals, however, suggest that α_2-adrenoceptors could contribute to renal vasoconstriction at very low levels of stimulation (Gellai and Ruffolo, 1987; Richer *et al.*, 1987; Wolff, Colindres and Strandhoy, 1989). In conscious unrestrained rats, intrarenal bolus injections of noradrenaline elicit renal vasoconstriction that is mediated by both α_1 and α_2-adrenoceptors. After administration of the α_2-adrenoceptor antagonist, rauwolscine, the dose of noradrenaline (a mixed agonist) needed to reduce the renal blood flow was markedly increased, indicating that part of the renal vasoconstrictor effect of this agonist was mediated by stimulation of α_2-adrenoceptors (Wolff, Colindres and Strandhoy, 1989). It should be noted, however, that α_2-adrenoceptor antagonists do not oppose the vasoconstrictor response to renal nerve stimulation (Moss, Colindres and Gottschalk, 1992). This suggests that although α_2-adrenoceptors may be activated by circulating noradrenaline, the response to renal nerve stimulation is

TABLE 11.3
Influence of stimulus frequency on response to renal nerve stimulation
(Modified from DiBona, 1989a)

Stimulation frequency (pulses/s)	Renin secretion rate (RSR)	Urinary sodium excretion	Renal blood flow
0.25	↔ Basal RSR	↔	↔
	↑ RSR mediated by non-neural stimuli		
0.5	↑	↔	↔
1	↑	↓	↔
2.5	↑	↓	↓

(↑, increase; ↓, decrease; ↔, no change)

almost entirely mediated by α_1-adrenoceptors. The importance of α_1- and α_2-adrenoceptors in mediating the effects of sustained noradrenergic stimulation, either by circulating catecholamines or renal nerve stimulation, has apparently not been determined.

During prolonged activation of the renal nerves at high frequencies, or infusion of large doses of catecholamines, the renal vasculature begins to "escape" from the adrenoceptor-mediated vasoconstriction (Figure 11.7; Johansson, Sparks and Biber, 1970; McGiff et al., 1972; Van Vliet, Smith and Guyton, 1991). This escape is believed to be caused by an increased release of vasodilators, such as prostaglandins (McGiff et al., 1972), but it seems likely that other factors could also be important. For example, during prolonged nerve stimulation, there is a decrease in the amount of noradrenaline released per impulse (Johansson, Sparks and Biber, 1970), suggesting either a depletion of catecholamine stores or an inhibition of catecholamine release by some additional factor. Also, powerful local regulatory mechanisms, such as TGF, or release of endothelial-derived nitric oxide could play a role in escape from the vasoconstrictor actions of adrenoceptor stimulation.

In most studies where escape has been noted, large doses of catecholamines have been infused or high-frequency nerve stimulation has been used. Therefore, it is not clear whether prolonged renal vasoconstriction can be produced by physiological stimuli. Katholi et al. (1977) and Cowley and Lohmeier (1979) reported that noradrenaline infusion into the renal artery of conscious dogs at a rate of 0.27–0.29 μg/kg/min produced renal vasoconstriction and decreased the renal plasma flow and the glomerular filtration rate (GFR) for as long as the infusion was continued (10–25 days). In addition, the vasoconstrictor effect of noradrenaline also appeared to be related to the daily sodium intake; at high sodium intakes, noradrenaline infusion caused larger increases in renal vascular resistance than at low sodium intakes. However, chronic intrarenal noradrenaline infusion also markedly increased the plasma renin activity (Cowley and Lohmeier, 1979), and it is possible that part of the renal vasoconstriction was mediated by elevated levels of ANGII. Although modest increases in renal vascular resistance have been observed during several hours of renal nerve stimulation (Figure 11.7; Van Vliet, Smith and Guyton, 1991), it is still not clear whether prolonged low levels of renal nerve stimulation can cause sustained increases in

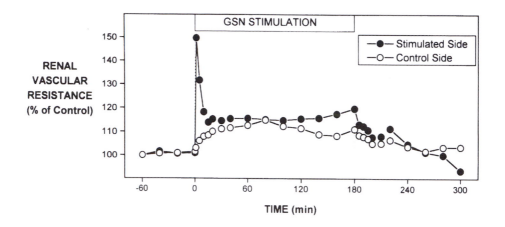

Figure 11.7   Time-dependent changes in renal vascular resistance during activation of renal sympathetic fibres for 3 h in pentobarbital-anaesthetized dogs (n = 9). Renal sympathetic fibres were activated by electrical stimulation of the greater splanchnic nerve (GSN) at 3 Hz after removing the adrenal gland. Note the slow response of the contralateral-denervated kidney (open symbols). Resistance values were calculated from data presented in Van Vliet, Smith and Guyton, 1991.

renal vascular resistance, lasting for days or weeks. Moreover the importance of indirect effects of prolonged sympathetic stimulation, such as increased ANGII formation, compared to direct noradrenergic effects is unknown.

There is some evidence that in certain chronic pathophysiological conditions, such as congestive heart failure, renal vasoconstriction may be mediated to a small extent by enhanced sympathetic nerve activity (Brod, Fejfar and Fejfarova, 1954; Kon, Yared and Ichikawa, 1985). However, other investigators have not found marked differences in renal blood flow in innervated and denervated kidneys during congestive heart failure or other chronic pathophysiological conditions in which sympathetic activity may be increased (Mokotoff and Ross, 1948; Sweet *et al.*, 1985; Mizelle, Hall and Montani, 1989; Lohmeier *et al.*, 1993). Overall, there is little definitive evidence that enhanced sympathetic nerve activity is capable of overriding local regulatory mechanisms to cause long-term changes in renal vascular resistance.

EFFECTS OF NORADRENERGIC STIMULATION ON RENAL SEGMENTAL VASCULAR RESISTANCES

As discussed above (see *Intrinsic sympathetic innervation*), almost all parts of the renal vasculature are innervated, including arteries and veins as well as afferent and efferent arterioles. Most investigators report that mild or moderate adrenoceptor stimulation, due to intrarenal infusion of noradrenaline or renal nerve stimulation, causes greater decreases in renal blood flow than in GFR, suggesting that noradrenergic stimulation may have a greater effect on post- than on preglomerular vessels of the kidney (Schrier, 1974; Johns, Lewis and Singer, 1976). Myers, Deen and Brenner (1975), in a micropuncture study, reported that noradrenaline infusion caused proportional increases in afferent and efferent arteriolar resistances, but that much of the increase in preglomerular resistance was secondary to an autoregulatory response to increased blood pressure. These investigators concluded that the major site of action of exogenous noradrenaline was on the efferent arteriole. However, the response to exogenous noradrenaline may not mimic the responses to physiological stimulation of the renal nerves, particularly when sympathetic tone is already elevated by anaesthesia and surgery. The afferent arterioles seem to be more densely innervated than the efferent arterioles (Selkurt, 1963) and may therefore normally be exposed to higher levels of endogenous noradrenaline, making them less sensitive to exogenous noradrenaline than the efferent arterioles.

Low level stimulation of the renal nerves (2 Hz) apparently elicits proportional increases in afferent and efferent arteriolar resistances, whereas stimulation at higher frequencies (5–10 Hz) causes constriction that is more pronounced in the afferent arterioles (Hermansson et al., 1981). Because afferent arteriolar constriction occurred in the absence of changes in renal artery pressure, these effects were not due to a pressure-dependent autoregulatory mechanism (Hermansson et al., 1981). Thus, sympathetic nerve stimulation or intrarenal noradrenaline infusion constricts both pre- and postglomerular vessels, but the relative changes in the resistance of these segments may depend upon the level of stimulation, the change in arterial pressure that occurs and interactions with local regulatory mechanisms. As discussed below, increases in efferent arteriolar resistance with prolonged stimulation of the renal nerves could be due, in part, to increased levels of ANGII. With low levels of renal nerve stimulation, the constriction of afferent arterioles may be completely offset by efferent arteriolar constriction so that GFR remains relatively constant despite significant reductions in renal blood flow. At higher levels of stimulation, greater constriction of afferent arterioles may lower GFR. Because most micropuncture techniques do not allow discrimination between afferent arteriolar constriction and constriction of other preglomerular vessels, it is possible that part of the preglomerular constrictor response to nerve stimulation may be localized in small arteries, as well as in afferent arterioles.

PHYSIOLOGICAL IMPORTANCE OF RENAL NERVES IN REGULATING RENAL VASCULAR RESISTANCE

It is widely believed that cardiopulmonary and aortic baroreceptor reflexes play an important role in regulating renal vascular resistance. For example, studies in anaesthetized animals suggest that volume expansion reduces RSNA and renal vascular resistance, in part, via reflex mechanisms (Clement, Pelletier and Shepherd, 1972; Mancia, Shepherd and Donald, 1975). Since this response occurred in the absence of input from arterial baroreceptors and was abolished by a vagal deafferentation, low-pressure cardiopulmonary receptors were implicated in mediating the renal vascular responses to volume expansion (Clement, Pelletier and Shepherd, 1972; Karim et al., 1972; Weaver, 1977; Thames and Abboud, 1979). Reflex activation of the sympathetic nervous system by volume depletion is also believed to cause intense renal vasoconstriction via reflex mechanisms. Clement, Pelletier and Shepherd (1972) reported that in rabbits with sinoaortic denervation, haemorrhage of 10% of the blood volume caused a marked increase in the renal vascular resistance that was abolished by vagotomy. With the carotid sinus baroreflex active, the increase in renal vascular resistance was similar to that observed with only the vagi operative, but constriction of hindlimb blood vessels was much greater. These investigators concluded that cardiopulmonary receptors subserved by vagal afferents exert a major influence on the renal and splanchnic circulations during haemorrhage, whereas carotid sinus baroreceptors predominantly affect the hindlimb vessels.

Although these studies suggest that the cardiopulmonary receptors may play an important role in acute regulation of renal haemodynamics under certain experimental conditions, such as reduced blood volume, it is doubtful that these receptors play a major role in regulating renal haemodynamics during increased blood volume or during more physiological conditions in the intact animal. Atrial distension, volume expansion and water immersion decrease RSNA in anaesthetized and conscious animals (Clement, Pelletier and Shepherd, 1972; Thames, Miller and Abboud, 1982; see also Figure 11.5 and the section on *Control of sodium excretion by cardiac reflexes*), but most investigators have found little or no change in GFR or renal vascular resistance during these manoeuvres in conscious animals (Kaczmarczyk *et al.*, 1978, 1981b; Sit, Morita and Vatner, 1984; Morita and Vatner, 1985; Miki *et al.*, 1989a). Gilmore and Zucker (1978b) found, in conscious monkeys, that large increases in left atrial pressure for 40 min caused no significant changes in the effective renal plasma flow, GFR or renal excretion. Also, head-out water immersion does not alter GFR or renal plasma flow in humans or non-human primates (Epstein, 1978; Gilmore and Zucker, 1978a). Morita and Vatner (1985) also found that volume expansion reduced RSNA by approximately 87% in the absence of significant reflex-mediated changes in renal vascular resistance. Thus, there seems to be a non-linearity between cardiopulmonary-mediated changes in RSNA and renal vascular resistance. Most of the available evidence indicates that cardiopulmonary receptors, activated by relatively large increases in atrial pressure, may decrease RSNA and renal vascular resistance in anaesthetized animals, but probably have little effect on renal haemodynamics in conscious, undisturbed animals or humans. Considering that relatively intense levels of renal nerve activation are required to cause a change in renal haemodynamics, the resting RSNA may simply be too low in unstressed conscious subjects to impose a renal vasoconstrictor tone.

The quantitative importance of cardiopulmonary receptors in the long-term regulation of renal haemodynamics has not been widely studied. Although it is clear that cardiopulmonary reflexes may be sustained for several hours (Figure 11.5; Miki *et al.*, 1989a, 1989b), it has not been established whether these receptors, like the arterial baroreceptors, may be reset during long-term changes in cardiopulmonary pressures. Greenberg *et al.* (1973) found that the frequency of atrial receptor discharge in dogs with sustained elevations of central venous pressures caused by chronic cardiac failure was about the same as in normal dogs. Thus, although the cardiopulmonary receptors may be important in the acute regulation of renal haemodynamics under some circumstances, there is currently little evidence that they are of major importance as a long-term regulator of renal vascular resistance.

Likewise, the importance of arterial baroreceptor-mediated activation of the sympathetic nervous system in regulating renal vascular resistance has been questioned. There is general agreement that increased carotid sinus pressure in anaesthetized animals reduces RSNA but has little effect on renal vascular resistance (for review, see Kirchheim, 1976). However, large reductions in carotid artery pressure have been found, in some studies, to increase the renal vascular resistance (Katz and Shear, 1975; Gross, Kirchheim and Ruffman, 1981).

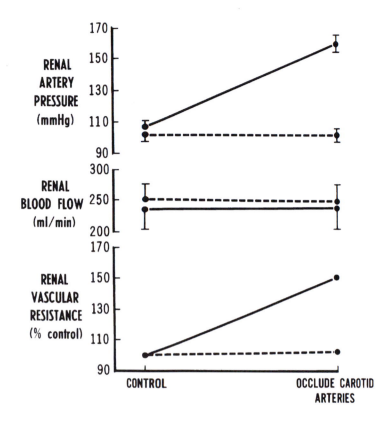

Figure 11.8   Role of arterial pressure in increasing renal resistance when baroreceptors are unloaded. Carotid baroreceptors were unloaded by bilateral carotid occlusion in conscious dogs. Baroreflex unloading produced a rise in both arterial pressure and renal vascular resistance (solid lines). Renal vascular resistance was unchanged when increases in renal perfusion pressure were prevented by controlled constriction of the aorta above the level of the renal arteries (broken lines). The data suggest that the resistance change simply results from a renal autoregulatory response to increased arterial pressure, and not an increase in renal sympathetic nerve activity. (Reproduced from Gross, Kirchheim and Ruffman (1981), with permission.)

Yet, the elevated renal vascular resistance observed during bilateral carotid occlusion may be due primarily to an autoregulatory response elicited by increased blood pressure. For example, Gross, Kirchheim and Ruffman (1981) found that when the renal artery pressure was held constant by a suprarenal aortic constriction, there was no significant change in the renal vascular resistance during bilateral carotid occlusion in conscious dogs (Figure 11.8). These findings suggest that moderate changes in sympathetic nerve activity associated with physiological changes in carotid sinus pressure do not directly cause significant changes in renal blood flow or renal vascular resistance. However, it should be noted that these studies were conducted in dogs maintained on a high sodium diet to suppress possible secondary actions of the nervous system mediated by changes in ANGII formation. It is possible that in animals with an intact renin–angiotensin system, moderate increases in sympathetic nerve activity, comparable to that caused by carotid occlusion, could alter renal haemodynamics indirectly by stimulating renin release. Vatner (1974) also reported that mild or moderate haemorrhage caused intense vasoconstriction in the mesenteric and iliac vasculature beds, but a decrease in the renal vascular resistance that was abolished by inhibition of prostaglandin synthesis. After blockade of prostaglandin synthesis, reflex activation of the renal nerves by mild or moderate haemorrhage did not alter the renal vascular resistance.

Because of the rapid adaptation of arterial baroreceptors to sustained changes in arterial pressure, it is unlikely that they are important in the long-term control of renal haemodynamics, either directly or indirectly. Krieger (1970) found that afferent nerve firing from the arterial baroreceptors increased markedly during acute hypertension, but then decreased back toward control within 24 h. Even more rapid "resetting" of arterial baroreceptors was observed when the blood pressure was reduced (Salgado and Krieger, 1973). Thus, any effect of the arterial baroreceptors on renal haemodynamics (which seems to be mediated mainly through indirect mechanisms such as changes in renin release) is probably limited to the first 24 h after a change in blood pressure.

With extremely large increases in RSNA, elicited by activation of the "defence reaction", there are major changes in the renal vascular resistance. For example, Gross and Kirchheim (1980) found that auditory stimuli, which elicited a 500% increase in RSNA, caused a 40% decrease in renal blood flow. Smith (1939) observed in human subjects exposed to alarming information that renal plasma flow decreased by 50% whereas GFR decreased only slightly and the filtration fraction increased. Furthermore, the renal vasoconstriction was maintained for approximately 1 h until the subject was assured that the alarm was false. In patients with essential hypertension, renal plasma flow decreased by 20% or more, whereas GFR was unchanged when the subject of conversation turned to a traumatic experience (Wolf *et al.*, 1948). Renal vasoconstriction also occurs during pain and emotional responses such as anger (Smith, 1951). Thus, the acute effects of stressful environmental stimulation on renal haemodynamics are well documented. However, it appears that renal vasoconstriction occurs only when RSNA is increased several-fold, in contrast to the changes in the renal sodium excretion and renin release that occur with much lower levels of RSNA.

Thus, some of the most important effects of RSNA in everyday circumstances are probably mediated via indirect mechanisms that involve activation of the renin–angiotensin system or other local control systems. It seems unlikely that basal RSNA has a major direct effect on renal vascular resistance. However, quantitative relationships between sympathetic activity and renal vascular resistance, over a wide range of renal nerve activities, are not available for conscious animals.

HETEROGENEITY OF RENAL VASCULAR RESPONSES TO SYMPATHETIC ACTIVATION

Noradrenergic stimulation has been suggested to elicit a redistribution of intrarenal blood flow from cortical to renal medullary regions (Pomeranz, Birtch and Barger, 1968; Katz *et al.*, 1971). However, others, using microsphere methods, have found no indication of such a redistribution with stimulation of the renal nerves, even when the total renal blood flow was reduced by as much as 50% (Stein *et al.*, 1973). Kaczmarczyk *et al.* (1981b) also found that left atrial distention, which markedly inhibits renal sympathetic activity, had no significant effect on the distribution of the renal blood flow, measured with radioactive microspheres. Aukland (1968), using the hydrogen electrode technique, also concluded that renal nerve stimulation produced parallel reductions in blood flow in all regions of the kidney. Unfortunately, accurate methods for measuring the distribution of the renal blood flow, particularly flow in the renal medulla, are not readily available. Yet, the evidence that is available suggests that changes in RSNA, in the physiological or pathophysiological range, have no major effect on the distribution of the renal blood flow.

INTERACTION BETWEEN THE SYMPATHETIC NERVOUS AND RENIN–ANGIOTENSIN SYSTEMS

Several potential interactions between noradrenergic mechanisms and the renin–angiotensin system have been described that could influence renal circulatory and excretory functions. For example, increased noradrenergic activity stimulates renin secretion and ANGII formation (Davis and Freeman, 1976; Moss, Colindres and Gottschalk, 1992). Since ANGII has potent renal vasoconstrictor and antinatriuretic effects (Hall, 1982; Hall and Brands, 1992), it is not surprising that some of the renal changes associated with noradrenergic stimulation are mediated by ANGII (e.g. Yang and Lohmeier, 1993). Additionally, ANGII has been postulated to stimulate the sympathetic nervous system, either centrally or peripherally (Feldberg and Lewis, 1964; Ferrario, Gildenburg and McCubbin, 1972; Zimmerman, Sybertz and Wong, 1984; Johns, 1989). Obviously, if all of these interactions between the noradrenergic and renin–angiotensin systems were physiologically important, they could provide the basis for a positive feedback whereby activation of the sympathetic nervous system would stimulate ANGII formation which, in turn, would cause further stimulation of the sympathetic nervous system. Thus, a quantitative assessment of the reported interactions between the noradrenergic and renin–angiotensin systems is necessary to understand their physiological relevance.

NORADRENERGIC CONTROL OF RENIN SECRETION

Sympathetic efferent fibres innervate the renal arterioles in the region of the juxtaglomerular cells and there is direct innervation of the epithelioid cells of the juxtaglomerular apparatus (Barajas, 1978). This finding has provided the anatomical basis for the belief that renin release is controlled by the sympathetic nervous system independently of changes in renal haemodynamics or tubular function. However, sympathetic stimulation may also increase renin release through various indirect mechanisms, such as renal vasoconstriction and increased tubular reabsorption, depending upon the intensity of the stimulation (Figure 11.9; DiBona, 1982, 1985b). The exact mechanisms by which sympathetic stimulation increases renin release under different experimental and physiological conditions has been difficult to assess because of the multiple, complex pathways by which renin release is controlled.

Intrarenal baroreceptor control of renin release

At high rates of stimulation, sufficient to cause renal vasoconstriction, the renal nerves could increase renin release via reduced stretch of the intrarenal baroreceptor, believed to reside

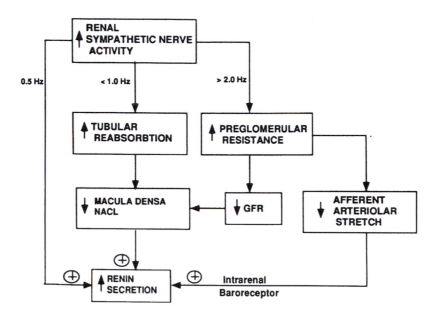

Figure 11.9 Multiple mechanisms by which renal sympathetic nerve activity may increase renal renin secretion. At low (0.5 Hz) intensities of renal nerve stimulation, renin release may be stimulated by a direct effect on the renin-secreting cells of the juxtaglomerular apparatus. At moderate (~1.0 Hz) intensities, increases in the tubular re-absorption of sodium may additionally promote renin secretion. During activation of the renal nerves at high (>2 Hz) intensities, increases in afferent arteriolar tone and resistance may result in further stimulation of renin secretion.

in the afferent arteriole of each nephron and to be associated with the juxtaglomerular cells (Davis and Freeman, 1976; Freeman and Davis, 1983; Kirchheim, Ehmke and Persson, 1988). Changes in renal perfusion pressure, expressed as changes in transmural pressure or wall tension, signal this receptor to alter renin secretion, possibly by changing the transmembrane calcium flux through voltage-dependent channels (Churchill, 1985; Fray, Park and Valentine, 1987). Increased stretch of isolated juxtaglomerular cells depolarizes the cells and inhibits renin secretion, an effect antagonized by calcium-channel blockers (Churchill, 1985). Decreased stretch of the juxtaglomerular cells, mediated by upstream vasoconstriction, would reduce the calcium influx in the juxtaglomerular cells and increase renin secretion.

Although numerous studies have indicated the importance of the intrarenal baroreceptor in acute regulation of renin secretion, its role during sustained changes in pressure is unclear. Some studies suggest that increases in the secretion of renin mediated by intrarenal baroreceptors may be transient following changes in the renal perfusion pressure (Mangelsen and Malvin, 1978). If adaptation of the renal baroreceptor to chronic changes in pressure occur, as has been demonstrated for other mechanoreceptors, then the intrarenal baroreceptor may not play a major role in mediating the renin responses to sustained activation of the renal sympathetic nerves. However, further studies are needed to determine whether the intrarenal baroreceptor adapts and whether it mediates renin responses to chronic activation of the renal sympathetic nerves.

Macula densa control of renin release

Another mechanism by which RSNA may indirectly alter renin secretion is by reducing the delivery of sodium chloride to the macula densa (Vander, 1967; Davis and Freeman, 1976). The macula densa is a specialized portion of the early distal tubule in each nephron that lies near the afferent and efferent arterioles of that same nephron. Together with the associated glomerulus, these structures are collectively referred to as the juxtaglomerular apparatus. Considerable evidence indicates that the macula densa plays a key role in TGF control of glomerular filtration and in the regulation of renin release (Vander, 1967; Davis and Freeman, 1976). For example, afferent arteriolar resistance and renin secretion appear to be inversely related to some function of the delivery of sodium chloride to the macula densa. The exact signal sensed is still unclear, but may be closely related to the transport of sodium chloride across the macula densa cells (Briggs and Schnermann, 1990).

A detailed discussion of TGF is beyond the scope of this chapter and the reader is referred to several excellent reviews for further details (Navar, 1978; Schnermann, Briggs and Weber, 1984; Wright, 1984; Briggs and Schnermann, 1990). Briefly, however, the TGF hypothesis proposes that decreased tubular fluid flow and delivery of sodium chloride to the macula densa cause decreased afferent arteriolar resistance and increased renin secretion (Navar, 1978; Schnermann, Briggs and Weber, 1984; Wright, 1984; Briggs and Schnermann, 1990). The decreased afferent arteriolar resistance raises glomerular hydrostatic pressure and increases GFR, thereby returning distal delivery toward normal. Conversely, increases in distal tubular flow rate raise afferent arteriolar resistance and inhibit renin secretion. Extensive support for TGF control of GFR and renin secretion comes from microperfusion studies in which changes in distal tubular flow rate, and in the delivery of sodium chloride, can be controlled (Navar, 1978; Schnermann, Briggs and Weber, 1984; Wright, 1984; Skott and Briggs, 1987; Briggs and Schnermann, 1990).

Because sympathetic stimulation tends to reduce GFR and enhances reabsorption of sodium chloride in the proximal tubule and the loop of Henlé (DiBona et al., 1977; DiBona and Sawin, 1982; Gottschalk, Moss and Colindres, 1985; DiBona, 1989b; Moss, Colindres and Gottschalk, 1992), it would also tend to reduce the delivery of sodium chloride to the macula densa. This change, in turn, would tend to cause a TGF-mediated decrease in the preglomerular resistance as well as stimulation of renin release. The net effect on renal vascular resistance therefore depends on the relative contribution of each of these adjustments, as well as the direct effects of noradrenergic stimulation. In circumstances associated with attenuation or impairment of TGF, the preglomerular constrictor effects of sympathetic stimulation would be expected to be amplified. For example, because a chronic high sodium intake impairs TGF (Wright, 1984; Briggs and Schnermann, 1990), the renal vasoconstrictor responses to sympathetic stimulation could be amplified because of an attenuated counterbalancing effect of TGF to cause afferent arteriolar vasodilatation in response to a decreased delivery of sodium chloride to the macula densa. In pathophysiological conditions associated with blockage of the tubules (acute renal failure), the TGF mechanism would be severely impaired and the renal vasoconstrictor effects of sympathetic stimulation would be greatly enhanced. Unfortunately, there are very few experimental studies that have quantitated the importance of the interactions between TGF and the sympathetic nervous system in regulating renal haemodynamics under physiological and pathophysiological conditions.

Because the renal sympathetic nerves decrease the delivery of sodium chloride delivery to the macula densa, they could also influence renin release and renal vascular resistance via this indirect mechanism (Figure 11.9). At renal nerve frequencies of approximately 2–3 Hz, renal vasoconstriction and decreased GFR would reduce the delivery of sodium chloride to the macula densa and stimulate renin release. At nerve stimulation frequencies of 1.0 Hz and below, the renal nerves could also stimulate renin release by enhancing reabsorption of sodium chloride in the proximal tubule or loop of Henlé (Gottschalk, 1979; DiBona, 1982; Moss, Colindres and Gottschalk, 1992). These indirect effects appear to be mediated primarily by α_1-adrenoceptors and may be important in contributing to activation of the renin–angiotensin system in acute circumstances such as haemorrhage. The increased renin release and ANGII formation, in turn, would contribute to increased renal vascular resistance, as discussed below.

β-adrenoceptor control of renin secretion

The renal nerves can also directly stimulate renin secretion by activation of β-adrenoceptors, especially β_1-adrenoceptors (Davis and Freeman, 1976; Keeton and Campbell, 1980; Johns, 1989; Moss, Colindres and Gottschalk, 1992). This effect probably enhances renin secretion by reducing intracellular calcium levels secondary to β-adrenoceptor activation of adenylate cyclase and subsequent increases in cyclic adenosine monophosphate, which promotes calcium efflux by stimulation of the sodium-potassium and calcium-ATPases (Freeman and Davis, 1983; Churchill, 1985). Considerable evidence suggests that a direct effect of sympathetic stimulation on renin release, mediated by β-adrenoceptors, occurs at stimulation frequencies as low as 0.5 Hz (DiBona, 1982, 1985b; Moss, Colindres and Gottschalk, 1992); thus, direct stimulation of renin release by the renal sympathetic nerves can occur at frequencies below those needed to directly reduce urinary sodium excretion or cause renal vasoconstriction (Table 11.3; DiBona, 1985b).

Modulation of non-neural stimuli for renin release by renal nerves

In addition to the direct and indirect mechanisms described above by which the renal nerves may enhance renin secretion, renin secretion can also influence the renal nerves less overtly. Renal denervation attenuates the renin secretory response to non-neural stimuli, such as reduced renal perfusion pressure or furosemide administration (Stella, Calaresu and Zanchetti, 1976; Stella and Zanchetti, 1977). In addition, the renin response to these manoeuvres is augmented by background RSNA at a level (0.25 Hz) that does not independently stimulate renin release (Thames and DiBona, 1979). Therefore, although the renal nerves are capable of independently stimulating renin secretion, very low levels of activity also serve to amplify the response to other stimuli.

Several studies have shown that this interaction is dependent upon both the frequency of nerve stimulation as well as the non-neural stimulus imposed (Kopp and DiBona, 1984). For example, at a low renal artery pressure of 50 mmHg, which markedly stimulates the intrarenal baroreceptor and macula densa mechanism, only a very low frequency of renal nerve stimulation is required for augmentation of the renin secretion response (DiBona, 1985b). However, at a higher level of pressure in the renal artery, which stimulates the baroreceptor and macula densa mechanisms to a lesser extent, a higher frequency of renal nerve stimulation is needed to enhance the renin secretory response (DiBona, 1985b). This modulation of renin secretion appears to be dependent on a functional macula densa mechanism, since it is not observed when the kidney is non-filtering (Osborn, Thames and DiBona, 1982). Presumably, with sympathetic nerve stimulation, the effects of non-neural stimuli, such as decreased renal artery pressure, to reduce the delivery of sodium chloride to the macula densa are enhanced, thereby accounting for amplification of the renin secretion response.

In some physiological and pathophysiological disturbances, the various influences of the renal nerves on renin secretion may be additive. For example, with acute haemorrhage, direct sympathetic stimulation of renin release, as well as indirect stimulation via the intrarenal baroreceptor and macula densa mechanisms may all contribute to the marked increases in renin secretion. In other disturbances, such as chronic sodium deprivation, the contribution of the renal nerves to enhanced renin secretion may be more subtle, since measurements of renal noradrenaline overflow in conscious animals suggests that sodium depletion does not increase RSNA (Carroll, Lohmeier and Brown, 1988). Yet, renal denervation markedly attenuates the renin responses to chronic sodium depletion (Mizelle *et al.*, 1987). Therefore, with sodium depletion it seems likely that the primary contribution of the renal nerves may be in modulating the response to other non-neural mechanisms, such as the macula densa and intrarenal baroreceptor mechanisms.

ROLE OF ANGIOTENSIN II IN MEDIATING RENAL EFFECTS OF SYMPATHETIC STIMULATION

Although it is clear that the renal nerves are capable of stimulating renin release, the importance of ANGII in mediating the renal haemodynamic and excretory responses to sympathetic stimulation is less certain, especially during chronic physiological disturbances. There is evidence that the renin–angiotensin system mediates part of the renal haemodynamic responses to acute sympathetic stimulation. For example, the renovascular response to noradrenaline is attenuated when increases in ANGII are prevented (Yang and Lohmeier, 1993). Activation of the renin–angiotensin system during moderate levels of renal nerve stimulation protects against excessive reductions in GFR by causing constriction of efferent arterioles (Figure 11.10; Myers, Deen and Brenner, 1975; Johns, Lewis and Singer, 1976; Johns, 1989). The importance of this interaction is that it allows the renal nerves to elicit renal vasoconstriction and reductions in the excretion of water and electrolytes, while at the same time maintaining relatively normal excretion of waste products, which depend upon glomerular filtration for their removal. This is advantageous in circumstances associated with volume depletion in which reduced excretion of electrolytes and water helps to restore extracellular fluid volume without major changes in the excretion of metabolic waste products.

It is possible that part of the antinatriuretic effect of renal nerve stimulation may be mediated by increased ANGII formation, since ANGII is a powerful antinatriuretic

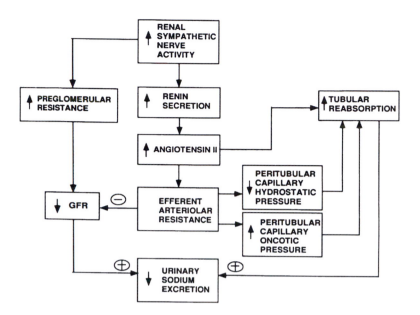

Figure 11.10   Mechanisms by which angiotensin II formation may maintain glomerular filtration while promoting sodium retention. The effect of angiotensin II to constrict efferent arterioles alters downstream peritubular physical factors in favour of increased fluid and sodium reabsorption. At the same time, efferent arteriolar constriction helps maintain glomerular hydrostatic pressure, thereby preserving glomerular filtration in the face of increased preglomerular resistance.

hormone, even at very low concentrations (Hall, 1982; Hall and Brands, 1992). With prolonged (3 h) activation of renal sympathetic fibres, the plasma renin activity is markedly elevated and appears to contribute to a slowly developing renal vasoconstriction and sodium retention (Van Vliet, Smith and Guyton, 1991). Furthermore, sustained hypertension produced by chronic intrarenal arterial infusion of noradrenaline does not occur when plasma ANGII concentrations are prevented from rising above control levels (Reinhart, Lohmeier and Hord, 1993). However, several studies have demonstrated that the acute antinatriuretic response to low level stimulation of the renal nerves is not completely abolished by ANGII blockade (Johns, 1987). These findings indicate that renal nerve stimulation can alter the urinary excretion of water and electrolytes independently of changes in the activity of the renin–angiotensin system. However, under the usual physiological conditions, in which the renal nerves and the renin–angiotensin system are both activated, it seems likely that part of the effects of nerve stimulation on renal electrolyte excretion are mediated by ANGII.

ROLE OF THE RENAL NERVES IN MEDIATING THE RENAL EFFECTS OF ANGII

ANGII has been postulated to stimulate noradrenergic activity through several mechanisms that could alter renal haemodynamics and sodium excretion (Johns, 1989). ANGII may stimulate the release of noradrenaline by the adrenal medulla (Feldberg and Lewis, 1964; Badder *et al.*, 1985) and facilitate noradrenaline release at central and peripheral synapses (Ferrario, Gildenberg and McCubbin, 1972; Zimmerman, Sybertz and Wong, 1984). Moreover, ANGII has been reported to inhibit re-uptake by central and peripheral noradrenergic neurons (Ferrario, Gildenberg and McCubbin, 1972; Zimmerman, Sybertz and Wong, 1984; Badder *et al.*, 1985). ANGII could also sensitize the renal vasculature or tubules to the effects of adrenoceptor stimulation. Thus, there are several potential mechanisms by which ANGII could either stimulate renal sympathetic activity or increase the effects of sympathetic stimulation on renal haemodynamics and electrolyte excretion.

One difficulty in assessing the physiological significance of reported interactions between ANGII and the sympathetic nervous system is that pharmacological, rather than physiological, doses of ANGII have often been used in studies in which ANGII has been found to increase sympathetic activity. Also, in many cases only acute interactions between ANGII and the sympathetic nervous system have been examined. There are very few studies in which the potential role of long-term interactions between ANGII and the sympathetic nervous system in regulating kidney function have been evaluated.

In support of the possibility that ANGII may increase renal sympathetic activity, McGiff and colleagues (McGiff and Fasy, 1965; McGiff, 1980) reported that renal denervation reduced or abolished the renal vasoconstrictor responses to intravenous ANGII injections and that after administration of sympatholytic agents, ANGII caused a natriuretic response instead of reducing sodium excretion. Liu and Cogan (1988), using microperfused proximal tubules of rats, reported that ANGII-mediated increases in sodium chloride and volume reabsorption required intact renal innervation, whereas increases in bicarbonate reabsorption were independent of the renal nerves. These investigators suggested that ANGII modulation of the reabsorption of sodium bicarbonate in the proximal convoluted tubule occurs via epithelial cell receptors, while changes in the reabsorption of sodium chloride occur via presynaptic receptors on renal nerves (Liu and Cogan, 1988).

Other studies, however, indicate that renal denervation or administration of sympatholytic agents does not prevent, or even attenuate, the acute renal responses to ANGII. Pelayo and Blantz (1984) reported that administration of a converting enzyme inhibitor or ANGII antagonist in hydropenic rats increased sodium excretion and reduced absolute as well as fractional proximal sodium reabsorption to a greater extent in acutely renal-denervated rats, compared to rats with intact renal nerves. Also, ANGII increases fluid reabsorption on completely isolated perfused proximal tubules, devoid of sympathetic nerves (Schuster, Kokko and Jacobson, 1984), and stimulates sodium transport in proximal tubules grown in primary culture (Simpson and Goodfriend, 1984). These observations provide clear evidence that the sympathetic nervous system is not essential for ANGII stimulation of sodium reabsorption (for review, see Hall, 1986a, 1986b). However, they do not rule out the possibility that the renal nerves may play at least a partial role in ANGII-mediated increases in sodium reabsorption or that ANGII may have a long-term effect on the sympathetic nervous system that is not revealed in acute studies.

There have only been a few studies in which the long-term interactions between ANGII and the sympathetic nervous system in controlling sodium excretion have been examined. In one study, we found that during chronic infusion of physiological amounts of ANGII (5 ng/kg/min) in dogs, administration of the sympatholytic agent guanethidine for 8 days did

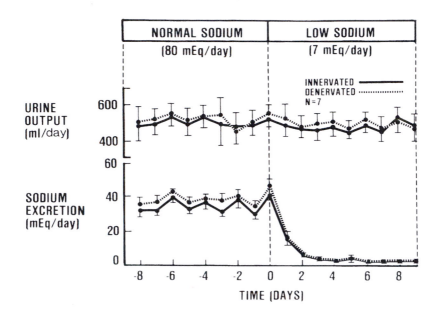

Figure 11.11 Comparison of sodium and water excretion in innervated and denervated kidneys of unilaterally renal-denervated conscious dogs (n = 7) during a reduction in sodium intake from normal (80 mEq/day) to low (7 mEq/day) levels. The dogs were prepared so that the urine produced by each kidney could be collected separately. Innervated and denervated kidneys appeared to be similar in their response to a reduced sodium intake. (Reproduced from Mizelle *et al.* (1987), with permission.)

not attenuate the renal haemodynamic, sodium-retaining, or hypertensive effects of ANGII (Hall and Granger, 1983). In fact, guanethidine reduced the blood pressure considerably more in normal dogs than in ANGII hypertensive dogs, suggesting that chronic infusion of ANGII may have inhibited sympathetic activity. Carroll, Lohmeier and Brown (1984) also found that renal noradrenaline overflow, an index of renal sympathetic activity, was reduced during chronic infusion of ANGII. Although these findings provide no evidence that increased circulating ANGII stimulates RSNA, it is important to note that in these studies infusion of ANGII was associated with increased blood pressure, which could have reflexively inhibited renal sympathetic activity. This effect presumably would not occur with activation of the endogenous renin–angiotensin system as a compensation for low blood pressure or reduced sodium intake.

To quantitate the contribution of the renal nerves in regulating sodium excretion during physiological increases in ANGII formation, Mizelle and colleagues (Mizelle *et al.*, 1987; Mizelle, Hall and Woods, 1988; Mizelle, Hall and Montani, 1989) studied the changes in renal haemodynamics and electrolyte excretion in separate innervated and denervated kidneys when the renin–angiotensin system was activated by chronic sodium depletion (Figure 11.11) or congestive cardiac failure. Comparison of the changes in sodium excretion and renal haemodynamics in innervated and denervated kidneys in the same animals provided a very sensitive means of detecting an effect of ANGII mediated by the renal nerves, since only the innervated kidney could respond to ANGII-induced increases in noradrenergic activity in these studies. Moreover, since both kidneys were exposed to the same blood pressures and circulating hormones in these experiments, any differences in renal function in response to changes in ANGII formation could be attributed to direct or indirect effects of the renal nerves. However, no differences were observed in the renal haemodynamic or sodium excretion response of innervated and denervated kidneys during chronic sodium depletion, after blockade of ANGII formation with converting enzyme inhibitors or subsequent replacement of circulating ANGII, or during chronic congestive cardiac failure (Mizelle *et al.*, 1987; Mizelle, Hall and Woods, 1988; Mizelle, Hall and Montani, 1989). These findings suggest that the renal nerves do not play a significant role in mediating the chronic renal vasoconstrictor or antinatriuretic actions of ANGII.

Although physiological levels of circulating or intrarenal ANGII may not markedly enhance renal sympathetic activity, it is possible that ANGII formed in the central nervous system could in some way enhance the overall sympathetic activity, thereby contributing to renal vasoconstriction and sodium retention. Alternatively, a minimal amount of ANGII may be needed for normal sympathetic nerve function. However, most of the available evidence suggested other actions of ANGII, besides possible interactions with the sympathetic nervous system, play a much more important role in mediating its long-term effects on renal haemodynamics and sodium excretion.

INFLUENCE OF THE RENAL SYMPATHETIC NERVES ON SODIUM EXCRETION

NORADRENERGIC CONTROL OF SODIUM AND WATER EXCRETION

Acute changes in RSNA evoke striking alterations in renal solute and water excretion. The excretion of many solutes are affected, including sodium, calcium, copper, phosphate, bicarbonate, uric acid, p-aminohippurate, and so forth (Szalay, Benscath and Takacs, 1977a, 1977b; Szalay *et al.*, 1977; Cogan, 1986; Johns and Mantius, 1987; Girchev, Toneva and Natcheff, 1989), but most interest has focused on the excretion of sodium and water because of their significance in fluid balance.

Electrical or reflex activation of the renal nerves decreases the renal excretion of sodium and water, and acute interruption of RSNA results in a prompt increase in renal sodium and water excretion. Three major mechanisms may contribute to the antinatriuretic effect of renal nerve activation. As outlined in Figure 11.1, these are: (1) a direct influence of the sympathetic innervation on the renal tubular cells to promote sodium reabsorption; (2) an effect on granular cells of the juxtaglomerular apparatus to facilitate the secretion of renin, thereby indirectly promoting sodium reabsorption through the formation of ANGII and the secretion of aldosterone; (3) vasoconstriction, which not only reduces renal blood flow, but also GFR and peritubular capillary pressures. Each of these mechanisms is recruited at different intensities of acute activation of the renal nerves. Activation of the renal nerves at low frequencies ($\ll 1$ Hz), for example, facilitates renin secretion without causing an immediate effect on sodium excretion (Osborn, DiBona and Thames, 1981; Table 11.3). However, as the secreted renin leads to the formation of two antinatriuretic hormones, ANGII and aldosterone, sustained activation at this level may be expected to reduce sodium excretion in time.

As RSNA is raised, a threshold is reached at which sodium excretion begins to fall. Although the antinatriuretic effect of renal nerve stimulation was once believed to be solely the result of renal haemodynamic effects of the renal nerves, it is now clear that the threshold for antinatriuresis is below the level required to produce measurable changes in GFR or the renal blood flow (Bello-Reuss, Trevino and Gottschalk, 1976; LaGrange, Sloop and Schmid, 1976; DiBona, 1977). This direct influence of the renal nerves on tubular sodium reabsorption has been demonstrated for the proximal tubule, loop of Henlé and distal convoluted tubule, and appears to be mediated virtually exclusively by α-adrenoceptors (Zambraski, DiBona and Kaloyanides, 1976). Specifically, the antinatriuresis appears to be due to the α_1-adrenoceptor subtype, as it is blocked by α_1-adrenoceptor antagonists (e.g. prazosin, Osborn et al., 1983; Hesse and Johns, 1985) but not α_2-adrenoceptor antagonists (e.g. yohimbine, rauwolscine, Osborn et al., 1983; DiBona and Sawin, 1987). The tubular response to exogenous or circulating catecholamines may additionally involve the participation of extrajunctional α_2-adrenoceptors (Pettinger et al., 1987). Unlike α_1-adrenoceptor activation, however, selective activation of α_2-adrenoceptors elicits an increase in sodium and water excretion (Strandhoy, Morris and Buckalew, 1982; Gellai and Ruffolo, 1987). α_2-adrenoceptor activation inhibits adenylate cyclase activity and therefore may interact with other effector systems, such as antidiuretic hormone, which also utilize adenylate cyclase in controlling fluid and electrolyte excretion (Pettinger et al., 1987). Exogenous or circulating catecholamines may also interact with extrajunctional β-adrenoceptors. Like α_1-adrenoceptors, activation of tubular β-adrenoceptors causes a reduction in renal sodium and water excretion. This effect may arise within the loop of Henlé and the distal tubule, where β_2-adrenoceptor agonists have been found to increase sodium, chloride and potassium reabsorption (Morel and Doucet, 1986; Bailly et al., 1990). In the proximal tubule, the effect of β-adrenoceptor agonists remains controversial (Gill and Casper, 1971; Bello-Reuss, 1980; Weinman et al., 1982; Murayama et al., 1985).

Intense activation of the renal nerves causes an abrupt decline in sodium and water excretion, associated with a decline in renal blood flow (Bradford, 1889; Hesse and Johns, 1984; Johns and Mantius, 1987; Echtenkamp and Dandridge, 1989; Van Vliet, Smith and Guyton, 1991). Under these conditions, much of the sodium and water retention may result from a decreased glomerular capillary pressure and filtration rate, due to the dominance of afferent (i.e. preglomerular) arteriolar constriction during intense activation of the renal nerves (Hermansson et al., 1981). Afferent and efferent arteriolar constriction will also reduce peritubular capillary pressures and flows, thereby promoting the contribution of physical factors to fluid and electrolyte reabsorption from the renal tubules. Vasoconstriction will additionally promote renin secretion as a consequence of decreased glomerular filtration, and hence decreased delivery of sodium chloride to the macula densa, and perhaps a direct effect of reduced pressure on the intrarenal baroreceptor control of renin (see section on *Intrarenal baroreceptor control of renin release*).

CONTROL OF SODIUM EXCRETION BY CARDIAC REFLEXES

Cardiovascular mechanoreceptors passing in the vagus and glossopharyngeal nerve are perhaps the most powerful and frequently investigated influence on RSNA. The main function of cardiovascular mechanoreceptors, regardless of their location, is to signal the degree of distension of the vascular segment in which they reside. As a main function of the renal nerves appears to be to influence renal fluid and electrolyte excretion, and therefore the filling of the vasculature, the influence of cardiovascular mechanoreceptors on RSNA represents part of an important feedback loop for controlling the intravascular volume and related variables such as arterial pressure (Figure 11.1). While arterial baroreceptors have a conspicuous beat-to-beat influence on RSNA, and are well established to influence renal function (Kezdi and Geller, 1968; Gross and Kirchheim, 1980; Karim, Mackay and Kappagoda, 1982; Persson *et al.*, 1989), cardiac (cardiopulmonary) receptors appear to be more important in regulating renal sodium excretion in response to physiological changes in body fluid volumes (Clement, Pelletier and Shepherd, 1972; Thames, Miller and Abboud, 1982; Morita and Vatner, 1985).

Atrial reflexes

Classic studies by Gauer and Henry (1963) suggested that cardiac filling may influence plasma volume by atrial reflexes which alter urinary fluid excretion. Their pioneering studies provided the impetus for a large number of studies designed to determine the mechanisms whereby atrial stretch promotes diuresis, and the physiological significance of this reflex. While their studies emphasized the role of reflex suppression of the secretion of arginine vasopressin (AVP) in mediating the diuresis produced by atrial stretch, it is now clear that reflex inhibition of RSNA contributes to the production of renal natriuresis and diuresis when atrial pressure is elevated (Ledsome, 1987; Linden, 1987; Miki *et al.*, 1989a, 1989b; Miki, Hayashida and Shiraki, 1993). The inhibition of RSNA in response to stimulation of atrial receptors may promote the excretion of sodium by both direct renal actions as well as indirect effects which are mediated by the suppression of renin release.

The reflex effects of receptors with myelinated vagal afferents are best characterized and likely account for most of the reflex responses produced by stimulation of atrial receptors in dogs (Ledsome, 1987; Linden, 1987). Unencapsulated receptors with myelinated vagal afferents are present in the subendocardium and are especially prominent in the junctional tissue of the vena cavae and right atrium, and the pulmonary veins and left atrium. The natural stimulus for these receptors is stretch, brought about by increases in atrial volume. The discharge frequency of these receptors correlates well with changes in blood volume and central venous pressure.

Mitral obstruction by either inflation of an atrial balloon or occlusion of the mitral annulus with a purse-string suture has been used to more or less selectively activate left atrial receptors in dogs. Single unit recordings from myelinated nerves in anaesthetized animals show a direct relationship between atrial receptor discharge and atrial pressure (Ledsome, 1987). After initial rapid adaptation, the atrial receptor discharge remains constant for at least 60 min at a rate dependent upon the prevailing atrial pressure. Since mitral obstruction tends to reduce cardiac output and arterial pressure, unloading of the arterial baroreceptors would be expected to stimulate RSNA and thereby attenuate or even override any effect of activation of left atrial receptors. The influence of the arterial baroreflex on RSNA, as well as the direct effects of hypotension on urinary sodium excretion, may account for the inconsistent natriuresis associated with mitral obstruction in anaesthetized animals. In conscious dogs, devoid of the complicating effects of the anaesthesia and surgical trauma on reflex function, arterial pressure and cardiac output are not reduced by degrees of mitral obstruction which increase left atrial pressure up to 6–8 mmHg (Kaczmarczyk *et al.*, 1981a; Fater *et al.*, 1982; Schultz *et al.*, 1982; Miki, Hayashida and Shiraki, 1993). Under these conditions, activation of the left atrial receptors consistently produces natriuresis and diuresis associated with decreased RSNA, renin release and AVP secretion. As would be expected, suppression of RSNA and increments in salt and water excretion in response to increased atrial pressure are abolished by cardiac denervation which removes the afferent limb of this cardiorenal reflex (Kaczmarczyk *et al.*, 1981a; Fater *et al.*, 1982; Miki, Hayashida and Shiraki, 1993). In one of the few studies that have addressed the time-course of change in RSNA during atrial distension, Miki, Hayashida and Shiraki (1993) reported a sustained suppression in RSNA in conscious dogs subjected to a 1 h step increase in left atrial pressure of about 7.5 mmHg. This study demonstrates the non-adaptive nature of this reflex over at least a 1 h period. However, the response to more sustained increases in pressure to which the atria may be exposed in both physiological and pathophysiological circumstances has not been reported.

In addition to reducing RSNA, stimulation of atrial receptors with myelinated vagal afferents causes tachycardia by increasing sympathetic nerve activity to the heart (Karim *et al.*, 1972; Linden, 1987). In a study in conscious dogs subjected to graded distention of the left atrium by balloon inflation, Miki, Hayashida and Shiraki (1991) reported an inverse relationship between changes in RSNA and left atrial pressure (up to 6 mmHg). Increments in heart rate were directly proportional to elevations in left atrial pressure. Other than the heart and kidneys, no effects of stimulation of atrial receptors on sympathetic activity to other vascular beds have been demonstrated (Karim *et al.*, 1972; Ledsome, 1987).

Ventricular reflexes

Mechanoreceptive ventricular vagal afferents respond to manoeuvres which result in ventricular distension, including volume expansion, left ventricular hypertension, asphyxia and ventricular ischaemia (Thoren, 1979; Shepherd and Mancia, 1986; Hainsworth, 1991). Such receptors may also be paradoxically stimulated when ventricular filling is greatly reduced (Thoren, 1979). Some receptors exhibit chemosensitivity, responding to hypoxia as well as exogenous (Veratrum alkaloids, nicotine, capsaicin and phenyldiguanide) and endogenous substances (bradykinin and prostaglandins) (Coleridge and Coleridge, 1977, 1980). The receptor population appears to be heterogeneous, as receptors may exhibit various combinations of mechano- and chemosensitivity.

Because commonly used experimental manoeuvres, such as volume expansion and water immersion also have concomitant effects on atrial and arterial pressures, it has been difficult to assess the specific reflex responses to physiological activation of ventricular receptors. However, from the use of unphysiological yet potent stimuli, such as foreign chemicals (e.g. veratridine, serotonin) or aortic occlusion, it is clear that ventricular receptors are capable of producing profound reflex hypotension and bradycardia (Shepherd and Mancia, 1986;

Zucker, 1986; Hainsworth and McGregor, 1987; Hainsworth, 1991; Minisi and Thames, 1991). Activation of ventricular receptors inhibits sympathetic outflow to the heart, kidneys and skeletal muscle, and causes a decrease in vascular resistance in several areas of the body, including skeletal muscle. However, in the conscious dog with low basal RSNA, stimulation of ventricular receptors by intracoronary injection of veratridine does not decrease renal vascular resistance (Barron and Bishop, 1982; Gorman, Cornish and Zucker, 1984). Studies in dogs subjected to chronic sinoaortic denervation indicate that the lack of renal vasodilatation is not due to the influence of the arterial baroreflex on RSNA in response to the concomitant hypotension during left ventricular stimulation (Gorman, Cornish and Zucker, 1984). Indeed, it is probably simply due to the low level of RSNA and the lack of tonic renal sympathetic vasoconstrictor tone in unstressed conscious dogs (see *Physiological Importance of Renal Nerves in Regulating Renal Vascular Resistance*).

There have been few studies on the reflex effects of ventricular receptor activation on the renal excretion of salt and water. In a recent study in conscious dogs, Chen and Gorman (1990) compared urinary excretory responses during nitroprusside infusion to those that occurred with comparable reductions in arterial pressure during activation of ventricular receptors either by intracoronary infusion of veratrine or by ascending aortic occlusion. In this study, significantly greater reductions in salt and water excretion occurred, in the absence of changes in GFR and renal plasma flow, when hypotension was achieved without activation of ventricular receptors. This was interpreted to indicate that the stimulation of ventricular receptors inhibits neurally induced antinatriuresis and antidiuresis, and is consistent with an earlier observation in conscious dogs that intracoronary administration of veratridine attenuates reflex-induced increments in RSNA associated with nitroprusside-induced hypotension (Zucker, 1986). Other studies in both conscious and anaesthetized dogs have shown that activation of ventricular receptors attenuates reflex-induced increments in RSNA, renin secretion and AVP secretion (Zucker, 1986; Gorman and Chen, 1989; Minisi and Thames, 1991). Taken together, these studies in conscious dogs indicate that although ventricular reflexes have little effect on renal haemodynamics, they increase renal excretory capability by attenuating reflex-induced increments in RSNA, renin release and AVP secretion.

Reflex effects on sodium excretion caused by abrupt changes in cardiac pressures without volume expansion

The renal responses to increases in cardiac pressures throughout the heart have been studied in conscious dogs using thermoneutral (37°C) water immersion (Figures 11.5 and 11.12; Miki *et al.*, 1989a). Head-out water immersion causes central translocation of blood from the periphery, leading to increased cardiac filling pressures and cardiac output. In a study in conscious dogs, water immersion produced an abrupt increase in the central venous pressure of 10 mmHg and a 43% fall in RSNA (Figure 11.5). These changes were sustained throughout the entire 2 h period of water immersion (Miki *et al.*, 1989a). In association with these responses, there was a 10 mmHg rise in mean arterial pressure, and sodium and water excretion increased two- to three-fold in the absence of changes in the GFR (Figure 11.12). When this study was repeated in the same dogs several weeks after bilateral renal denervation, there were similar changes in systemic haemodynamics but salt and

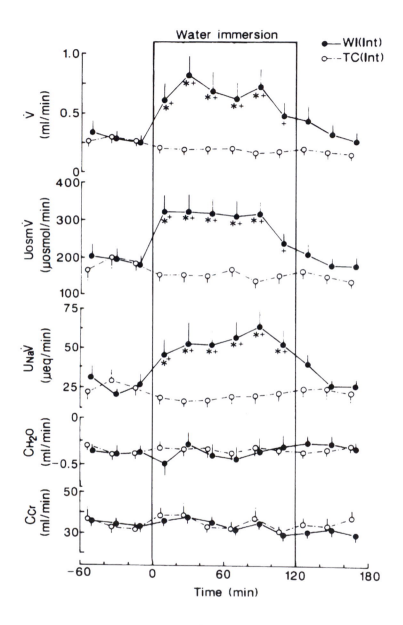

A

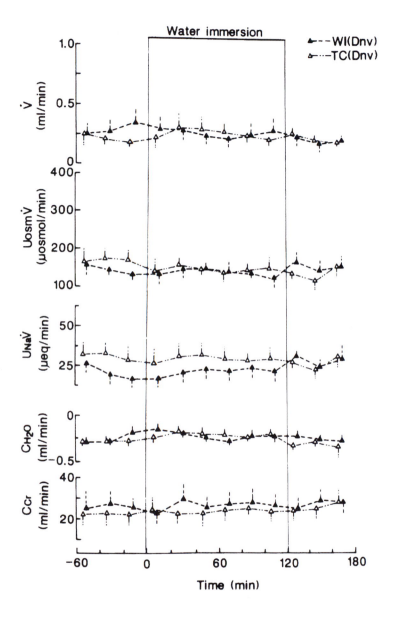

B

Figure 11.12   Comparison of renal excretory response to water immersion in bilaterally renal-denervated (Dnv) and sham-operated (Int, intact) dogs. A: Renal responses to water immersion (WI) and time controls (TC) in sham-operated dogs. Water immersion results in a large increase in urine flow ($\dot{V}$) and total solute ($U_{osm}\dot{V}$) and sodium ($U_{Na}\dot{V}$) excretion, and little change in the clearance of water (C_{H2O}) or creatinine (C_{cr}). B: Renal responses to water immersion are absent following bilateral renal denervation. The effect of immersion on renal sympathetic nerve activity is shown in Figure 11.5A. (Reproduced from Miki et al. (1989a), with permission.)

water excretion failed to increase in response to water immersion (Figure 11.12). Since it was shown in an earlier study that cardiac denervation abolished the natriuretic response to water immersion in conscious dogs (Hajduczok et al., 1987), it appears that cardiac reflexes play a major role in inhibiting RSNA when cardiac filling pressures are elevated by water immersion, and that the attendant natriuresis is greatly dependent upon suppression of RSNA.

The renal responses to abrupt unloading of the cardiac receptors has been studied in conscious dogs by producing head-up tilt, a manoeuvre that translocates blood from the intrathoracic region of the circulation to the lower parts of the body. Miki et al. (1989b) reported that a 40° head-up tilt produced a sharp fall in the central venous pressure of approximately 7 mmHg and an increase in RSNA of 53% (Figure 11.5B). During the 60 min tilting period, these changes were sustained and, in spite of a moderate increase in the mean arterial pressure that would tend to increase sodium excretion, there was a pronounced antinatriuresis and antidiuresis in the absence of changes in GFR. As in their water immersion experiments mentioned above, chronic bilateral denervation abolished the changes in urinary sodium and water excretion induced by cardiac reflexes, indicating their dependence on changes in RSNA.

Reflex effects on sodium excretion in response to acute volume expansion

If cardiorenal reflexes are important in the normal daily regulation of salt and water balance, then they would be expected to participate in the response to the intermittent sodium and volume loads to which animals and humans are exposed following a meal. To mimic the volume-induced increments in cardiac pressures that occur after ingestion of a salty meal (Kaczmarczyk et al., 1979), comparable fluid loads have been imposed by intravenous infusion of isotonic saline. Atrial pressures increase several mmHg and RSNA is inhibited during expansion of the intravenous fluid volume, but both rapidly return to control levels as most of the fluid load is eliminated within 4 h (Kaczmarczyk et al., 1981a; Fater et al., 1982; Morita and Vatner, 1985; Cowley and Skelton, 1991).

Although volume-loading does cause modest increases in arterial pressure, experiments performed in conscious, sinoaortic baroreceptor-denervated dogs demonstrated that the reflex suppression of RSNA and the attendant natriuresis are not mediated by the arterial baroreflex (Sit, Morita and Vatner, 1984; Morita and Vatner, 1985). However, when these same animals were subjected to volume expansion following bilateral cervical vagotomy, the suppression in RSNA, and the natriuretic and diuretic responses were attenuated. Similar findings were reported in conscious primates (Cornish, McCulloch and Gilmore, 1984; Vatner, Manders and Knight, 1986). These results suggest that vagally mediated reflex decreases in RSNA induced by volume-loading exert a significant effect on salt and water excretion. This is consistent with the results of studies in anaesthetized animals, in which decreases in RSNA in response to volume expansion were not affected by sinoaortic denervation but were attenuated by vagotomy alone (Clement, Pelletier and Shepherd, 1972; Thames, Miller and Abboud, 1982). On the other hand, Kaczmarczyk et al. (1981a), and Fater and associates (1982) found no significant difference in the sodium excretory responses to acute isotonic volume expansion when comparing conscious dogs with intact and denervated hearts. It is conceivable that arterial baroreceptors play a

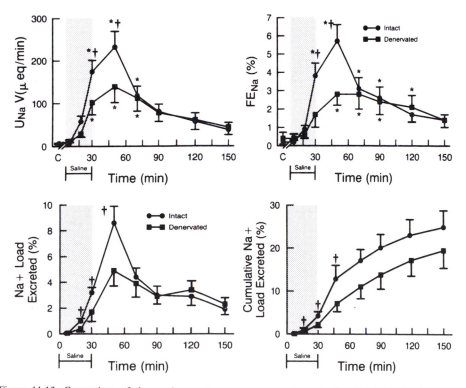

Figure 11.13 Comparison of the renal excretory response to volume loading in chronically instrumented lambs following bilateral renal-denervation or sham surgery. Volume expansion consisted of an infusion of isotonic saline equal to 5% of the animal's body weight over 30 min. (Reproduced from Smith et al. (1989), with permission.) Abbreviations: $U_{Na}V$, sodium excretion; FE_{Na}, fractional excretion of sodium.

more important role in mediating reflex inhibition of RSNA in the chronic absence of cardiac receptors.

A role for reflex withdrawal of RSNA in mediating the natriuretic and diuretic responses to volume expansion is further supported by studies that have employed chronic bilateral renal denervation. Indeed, a number of studies in a wide variety of conscious animals have demonstrated that chronic bilateral denervation blunts the effects of volume expansion on salt and water excretion (Figures 11.13 and 11.14; DiBona and Sawin, 1985; Morita and Vatner, 1985; Peterson, Benjamin and Hurst, 1988; Smith et al., 1989; Peterson et al., 1991). Moreover, Sadowski, Kurkus and Gellert (1979) reported that conscious dogs with one innervated and one denervated kidney had greater increments in sodium excretion from the innervated than the denervated kidney following saline loading. These changes occurred without alterations in GFR and renal plasma flow. Since both the innervated and denervated kidney were exposed to the same systemic haemodynamic and hormonal changes, the greater response of the innervated kidney provides compelling evidence of the contribution of reflex inhibition of RSNA in increasing salt and water excretion in response to a volume load.

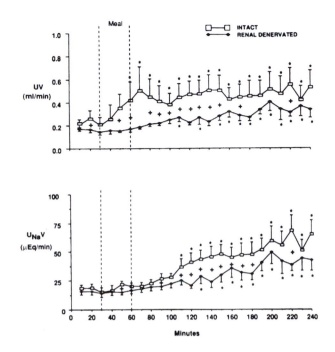

Figure 11.14 Comparison of the effect of a salty meal on the renal salt ($U_{Na}V$) and water (UV) excretion in conscious monkeys before and following bilateral renal-denervation. The meal was administered by nasogastric tube over 30 min, and provided 2.5 mEq Na/kg body weight and approximately 17 ml water/kg body weight. (Reproduced from Peterson *et al.* (1991), with permission.)

Unimportance of reflex effects on sodium excretion during chronic alterations in sodium intake

Although cardiorenal reflexes contribute to the excretion of salt and water during acute volume expansion, these reflexes may normally be relatively unimportant in the chronic regulation of sodium excretion for two reasons. First, as discussed in a subsequent section, the renal–body fluid feedback mechanism for arterial pressure control, working in concert with the renin–angiotensin system, is very efficient in minimizing changes in body fluid volumes during chronic alterations in the sodium intake. Therefore, in spite of the sensitivity of cardiac receptors, such as those located in the atria, to relatively small changes (~ 1 mmHg) in cardiac filling pressures, the small changes in blood volume associated with variations in the sodium intake would not be sufficient to evoke alterations in cardiac receptor activity.

A recent study by Krieger, Liard and Cowley (1990) quantified the small change in body fluid volumes that occurs when the sodium intake is altered. Using elegant techniques for continuous measurement of total body weight (as an index of changes in total body water) and haemodynamics, these investigators reported that a 15-fold increase in the sodium intake over a 7-day period in sodium-depleted dogs produced only approximately a 3%

(250 g) increase in total body water, without significant changes in either blood volume or mean arterial pressure. Cardiac output rose by 10%. As their technique for the measurement of blood volume was capable of detecting small changes in blood volume in the order of 5%, in the absence of a significant increase in blood volume, these investigators concluded that the rise in cardiac output was not related to changes in blood volume, but rather to a fall in total peripheral resistance, due to suppression of the concentration of ANGII in the plasma. Because suppression of the concentration of ANGII in the plasma may also increase vascular capacity, this would attenuate the impact of small increments in blood volume on cardiac filling pressures. As this study indicates that cardiac filling pressures are relatively unaffected in spite of substantial increments in the sodium intake, cardiac receptors are unlikely to be significantly affected by chronic alterations in the sodium intake.

A second factor that limits the importance of cardiac receptors during chronic alterations in the sodium intake is their very ability to respond to a sustained increase in cardiac filling pressure, should this occur. Numerous studies have shown that mechanoreceptors in the large central systemic arteries, the arterial baroreceptors, undergo considerable adaptation or resetting in response to sustained changes in arterial pressure. This resetting phenomenon enables the arterial baroreflex to shift its setpoint and operating range in the direction of the pressure disturbance, thereby allowing the reflex to buffer short-term changes in arterial pressure in spite of changes in the long-term mean arterial pressure that may occur naturally (e.g. as a function of age) or pathologically (e.g. hypertension). Like baroreceptors, cardiac receptors have been shown to elicit effective reflexes for several hours (Ledsome, 1987; Miki et al., 1989a, 1989b; Miki, Hayashida and Shiraki, 1993; Figure 11.5). Although data pertaining to longer periods of time has not been reported, like arterial baroreceptors, cardiac mechanoreceptors may be expected to exhibit resetting in the long term. The more complete the adaptation process, the less important cardiac reflexes would be in the long term control of sodium balance. In the future, establishment of the time course of adaptation of cardiac mechanoreceptors will be important in defining the significance of cardiac reflexes in controlling sodium balance.

Direct evidence that the arterial baroreceptors and cardiac mechanoreceptors are not important in the long term regulation of sodium excretion and arterial pressure comes from studies that have completely abolished their input into the central nervous system. As acute unloading of cardiac receptors increases RSNA, continued unloading of cardiac receptors might be expected to cause sustained increases in RSNA and secretion of AVP, and an impairment of renal sodium and water excretion. If this were to be sustained, this would lead to the development of hypertension through the renal–body fluid feedback mechanism (see next section). However, even the most extreme form of "unloading" of cardiac receptors, cardiac denervation, does not cause chronic hypertension (Persson et al., 1987, 1988). This indicates that even complete elimination of the restraining influences of these areas of the circulation on sympathetic activity does not, in the long term, significantly impair the ability of the kidneys to excrete salt and water. This is also consistent with the results of Mizelle et al. (1987), who found no evidence for a role of the renal nerves in adjusting sodium excretion during chronic reductions in the sodium intake. In this study, the bladder was surgically divided into two hemi-bladders so that sodium excretion could be compared between a denervated kidney and a contralateral innervated control kidney. The advantage of this method is that both kidneys experience the same arterial pressure and plasma composition, and therefore differ only in respect to their innervation. When sodium intake was decreased from normal (80 mEq/day) to 7 mEq/day, sodium excretion fell from 33.6 to 3.5 mEq/day in innervated kidneys, and from 37.6 to 4.0 mEq/day in denervated kidneys. Clearly, the denervated kidney was capable of appropriately adjusting the sodium balance in the absence of the renal nerves.

Because chronic alterations in sodium intake have only minimal effects on body fluid volumes and cardiac filling pressures, and because cardiac receptors may adapt in the long run, it is unlikely that cardiac reflexes play an important role in influencing sodium excretion during long term changes in sodium intake. This conclusion is consistent with the results from chronic studies reviewed above, that indicate that the renal nerves are not important in the chronic regulation of sodium excretion when sodium intake is increased or decreased.

Does impairment of cardiac reflexes lead to sodium and fluid retention in cardiac failure?

There is now considerable evidence from experimental animals and humans that reflexes arising from cardiac mechanoreceptors are impaired in chronic cardiac failure (Greenberg et al., 1973; Zucker, Earle and Gilmore, 1977; Zucker et al., 1985; Dibner-Dunlap and Thames, 1992). Because cardiac reflexes normally exert an important tonic restraining influence on sympathetic activity and on the secretion of renin and AVP, a number of investigators have proposed that the impairment of cardiac reflexes may contribute to, or be responsible for, the fluid retention associated with decompensated cardiac failure (Abboud, 1987; Packer, 1988; Zucker, 1991). This hypothesis assumes that cardiac reflexes would normally respond to the increased central venous pressures caused by the failing heart by inhibiting RSNA and AVP secretion, thereby facilitating renal fluid excretion and the correction of the elevated central venous pressures. Impairment of this mechanism in the later stages of cardiac failure would lead to the loss of the inhibitory influence of cardiac reflexes on sympathetic activity. In turn, this would lead to increases in RSNA, increased secretion of salt and water-retaining hormones such as ANGII and AVP, and pronounced fluid retention. While this is an attractive hypothesis to account for the neurohumoral activation and fluid retention of cardiac failure, there is little direct experimental evidence in its support.

Involvement of the cardiac reflexes in cardiac failure would require that the loss of input from the impaired cardiac mechanoreceptors is capable of causing sustained neurohumoral activation. Although even complete cardiac denervation does not chronically impair renal excretory capability or lead to persistent hypertension, sustained hypertension apparently does occur when denervation of the heart is combined with denervation of sinoaortic baroreceptors (Persson et al., 1987, 1988). Accordingly, a similar mechanism could account for fluid retention in chronic cardiac failure because there is not only dysfunction of cardiac mechanoreceptors, but impairment of the arterial baroreflex as well (Abboud, 1987; Wang, Chen and Zucker, 1990; Minisi and Thames, 1991; Zucker, 1991).

SIGNIFICANCE OF THE RENAL NERVES IN REGULATING RENAL SODIUM EXCRETION: ACUTE VERSUS CHRONIC ROLES

In most anaesthetized animals, acute renal denervation causes a marked increase in renal water and sodium excretion (e.g. Bencsath et al., 1972; Bello-Reuss, Pastoriza-Munoz and Colindres, 1977; Rudd, Grippo and Arendshorst, 1986; Johns and Manitus, 1987). A similar phenomenon can be produced by reflex inhibition of RSNA (e.g. Kaufman and Stelfox, 1987). As the excretion of the innervated kidney is markedly reduced but that of the denervated kidney is relatively unaffected during anaesthesia (Berne, 1952; Sadowski, Kurkus and Gellert, 1979), the pronounced diuresis and natriuresis that accompanies acute renal denervation in anaesthetized animals may, in part, reflect the high levels of RSNA that may occur during anaesthesia (Smith, 1951; Lifshitz, 1978).

The response to acute renal denervation has not been studied in unstressed conscious animals. However, evidence that the renal nerves may normally restrain renal excretory function has been obtained from studies in which the excretory responses of renal denervated and sham-operated animals have been compared during procedures which reflexively inhibit RSNA (Sadowski, Kurkus and Gellert, 1979; Peterson *et al.*, 1988, 1991; Miki *et al.*, 1989a; Smith *et al.*, 1989). As shown in Figure 11.13, for example, the renal excretory response to volume loading is much greater in animals with innervated kidneys than in renal-denervated animals. Consequently, renal excretion of the sodium load is retarded in renal-denervated animals (Figure 11.13). Figure 11.14 illustrates a similar difference in the renal sodium excretion of renal-denervated and sham-operated animals during a more physiological example of volume loading: ingestion of a salty meal. In a variety of circumstances in which RSNA is inhibited, a three-fold difference in sodium excretion between innervated and denervated kidneys is about the upper limit that has been reported (Sadowski, Kurkus and Gellert, 1979; Peterson *et al.*, 1988, 1991; Smith *et al.*, 1989), and can therefore serve as an estimate of the degree to which the renal nerves may acutely influence renal excretory function in chronically instrumented conscious dogs.

To determine to what extent the renal nerves may chronically influence renal excretory function, experiments have been performed in chronically instrumented, unilaterally renal-denervated dogs, prepared such that the urine of the innervated and denervated kidney can be collected separately and compared. The advantage of this preparation is that the innervated and denervated kidneys share a common blood supply, and therefore cannot be influenced by subtle differences in factors such as arterial pressure or hormonal levels. A common finding in such preparations is that the excretory function of innervated and denervated kidneys of conscious, unilaterally renal-denervated dogs is strikingly similar (Gruber, 1933; Mizelle *et al.*, 1987; Mizelle, Hall and Woods, 1988; Peterson, Benjamin and Hurst, 1988; Girchev, Toneva and Natcheff, 1989; Mizelle, Hall and Montani, 1989; Lohmeier *et al.*, 1993). The denervated kidney is consistently reported to excrete from 8 to 35% more sodium and water than the innervated kidney. When comparisons between innervated and denervated kidneys were made over 24 h periods, the average sodium and water excretion of denervated kidneys was reported to be only 12% greater than that of the innervated control kidney (Mizelle *et al.*, 1987; Mizelle, Hall and Woods, 1988; Mizelle, Hall and Montani, 1989).

The influence of the renal nerves on renal sodium and water excretion in the different conditions discussed above is summarized schematically in Figure 11.15. The two- to three-fold increase in sodium and water excretion following acute inhibition of RSNA in innervated kidneys suggests that RSNA does indeed restrain renal excretory function in conscious, chronically instrumented dogs; yet, why do the 24 h sodium excretions of innervated and denervated kidneys differ by only 12%? The lack of a chronic influence of renal denervation on renal sodium excretion cannot be simply due to adaptation of the renal

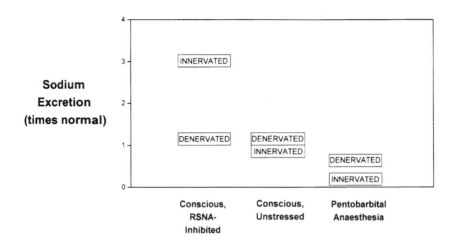

Figure 11.15 Influence of the renal nerves on sodium excretion during reflex inhibition of renal sympathetic nerve activity (left) and anaesthesia (right). Values are approximate. See text for details and references.

response to sympathetic stimulation, as an underlying restraint of renal sodium excretion is revealed following inhibition of RSNA. Although an explanation for this discrepancy has not been established, taken at face value the data suggest that renal excretory function is especially sensitive to acute changes in RSNA, but relatively insensitive to the long-term mean level of RSNA. This form of time-dependent response would facilitate large increases in renal excretion when RSNA is acutely inhibited, such as immediately following a volume load, but minimize the effect of long-term changes in RSNA on renal excretion, body fluid balance or arterial blood pressure. Thus, the main significance of the renal sympathetic nerves in controlling renal sodium excretion may be in mediating short-term adjustments of renal excretory function to help minimize disturbances in intravascular filling, and accelerate the relatively slow process of renal–body fluid balance.

INFLUENCE OF THE RENAL NERVES ON THE LONG-TERM CONTROL OF ARTERIAL BLOOD PRESSURE

ROLE OF THE RENAL–BODY FLUID FEEDBACK MECHANISM

The long-term control of arterial blood pressure is linked to renal excretory function and fluid volume homeostasis by way of the renal–body fluid feedback mechanism (Guyton, 1980; Hall et al., 1990). The basic elements of this mechanism are depicted in Figure 11.1. A main feature of the mechanism is the pressure–natriuresis mechanism, the effect of increased blood pressure to raise renal sodium and water excretion. Normally, disturbances that tend to raise the arterial pressure without altering the renal excretory function cause an increase in sodium and water excretion. Similarly, reductions in the arterial pressure reduce sodium and fluid excretion until the arterial pressure is returned to a normal level. Although the pressure–natriuresis mechanism can be readily demonstrated even in isolated perfused kidneys, the sensitivity of the pressure–natriuresis mechanism is greatly amplified in the intact circulation by the operation of the renin–angiotensin system. During chronic increases in sodium intake, for example, the suppression of ANGII formation helps to increase sodium excretion, thereby ensuring that the sodium balance is maintained with a minimal change in the arterial pressure or vascular volume.

Although the renal–body fluid feedback mechanism is only one of several systems that regulate arterial pressure, a unique feature is that it represents an integral control system (Guyton, 1980). This type of control system is able to completely correct a disturbance, if given sufficient time. For this reason, the kidneys have been considered to be the dominant mechanism in setting the long-term mean arterial blood pressure. A second important characteristic is that integral control systems, and the control of arterial pressure through fluid balance in particular, are inherently slow. Thus, the renal–body fluid feedback mechanism is not effective in the beat-to-beat or hour-to-hour regulation of the arterial blood pressure. Other systems (e.g. arterial baroreflexes) appear to be specialized for the regulation of the arterial pressure over such short time spans. Rather, the body fluid feedback mechanism is thought to be responsible for the consistency of the 24 h mean arterial blood pressure from day-to-day and month-to-month.

A resetting of the pressure–natriuresis mechanism to higher pressures is a consistent feature of all models of hypertension that have been examined (Hall *et al.*, 1990). This is almost self evident, as otherwise the development of hypertension would result in increased fluid and water excretion until the blood pressure was returned to normal. Thus, hypertension produced by any means must include a mechanism that allows the kidney to maintain normal sodium and fluid balance at an elevated arterial pressure.

The significance of the renal nerves in the present context is that the antinatriuretic effect of their activation represents a shift of the acute pressure–natriuresis mechanism to a higher pressure level (Ehmke *et al.*, 1990). This antinatriuresis is sustained for at least 3 h during continued activation of the renal nerves (Van Vliet, Smith and Guyton, 1991). If it were sustained for considerably longer periods of time, sodium and water balance could only be re-established at an elevated level of arterial pressure. Thus, a shift of the pressure–natriuresis mechanism is assumed to be the principle mechanism underlying any influence of the renal nerves on the long-term control of arterial blood pressure.

EFFECT OF RENAL DENERVATION IN VARIOUS RAT MODELS OF EXPERIMENTAL HYPERTENSION

A large number of studies have been performed to investigate the role of the renal nerves in hypertension. Table 11.4 reviews the results of renal denervation studies performed in various rat models of experimental hypertension. Although there is a firm consensus for the impact of renal denervation in some models, such as the Okamoto strain of spontaneously hypertensive rats, the effect of renal denervation is more controversial in most other models that have been studied by several groups of investigators.

A common finding in several models of experimental hypertension is that renal denervation is particularly effective in attenuating the initial development of hypertension.

TABLE 11.4

Impact of renal denervation in various rat models of hypertension. Values are the approximate per cent reduction in hypertension (developing or established hypertension, timing or duration of study, and reference)

Model	Approximate correction of hypertension (%)	
	Complete renal denervation	Selective afferent denervation
SHR (Okamoto strain)	45–55% (DH, 7–12 weeks old)[a] < 40% (EH, 11–14 weeks old)[c] 30–35% (EH, 8–18 weeks old)[e]	0% (DH, 6–12 weeks old)[b] 15% (EH, 18 weeks old)[d]
DAHL	0% (DH, 4–10 weeks old)[f] 0% (DH, 1st 12 days of high salt)[g]	
DOCA–salt	40–50% (DH, 1–4 weeks of treatment)[h] 50–60% (DH, 5–25 days of treatment)[i] 0% (DH and EH, 8 weeks of treatment)[j] < 30% (EH, after 3 weeks of treatment)[k] < 5% (EH, after 10 weeks of treatment)[k]	
ANGII	100% (DH, first 3 days)[l] 10% (EH, from day 9 to 14)[l]	
Aortic denervation (AD)	100% (DH, first 10 days following AD)[m] 100% (EH, after 5 or 19 days of AD)[m]	
Goldblatt 2K1C	60–65% (EH, after 7 weeks of 2K1C)[n]	
Goldblatt 1K1C	70% (EH, after 2 and 9 weeks of 1K1C)[o] 80% (DH, 1st 4 weeks after 1K1C)[q] 0% (EH, after 5 weeks of 1K1C)[q] 0% (DH, 1st 4 weeks of 1K1C)[r] 0% (EH, after 2 and 6–7 weeks of 1K1C)[r]	40–60% (DH, 1–5 weeks after 1K1C)[p]
Renal wrap (RW)		0% (DH, 2 weeks of RW)[s]
New Zealand strain	30–40% (DH, from 7–11 weeks of age)[t]	
Intra–renal noradrenaline		0% (DH and EH, 5 days)[u]

Abbreviations: ANGII, angiotensin-II-treated rats; DH, denervation tested during initial development phase of hypertension; DOCA, desoxy-corticosterone-acetate-treated rats; 1K1C and 2K1C, one- and two-kidney, one-clip Goldblatt models; EH, denervation tested in established hypertension; SHR, spontaneously hypertensive rats.

References: (a): Winternitz, Katholi and Oparil, 1980; (b): Oparil, Sripairojthikoon and Wyss, 1987; (c): Säynävälammi et al., 1982; (d): Janssen et al., 1989a; (e): Norman and Dzielak, 1982; (f): Wyss, Sripairojthikoon and Oparil, 1987; (g): Osborn, Roman and Ewens, 1988; (h): Takahashi et al., 1984; (i): Katholi, Naftilan and Oparil, 1980; (j): Dzielak and Norman, 1985; (k) Katholi et al., 1983a; (l): Vari et al., 1987; (m): Kline et al., 1983; (n): Katholi et al., 1982; (o): Katholi, Winternitz and Oparil, 1981; (p): Wyss, Aboukarsh and Oparil, 1986; (q): Norman et al., 1984; (r): Villarreal et al., 1984; (s): Jing-yun et al., 1985; (t): Diz, Nasjletti and Baer, 1982; (u): Janssen et al., 1989b.

When the time course of the development of hypertension is compared in renal denervated and sham-operated rats, renal denervation often appears to principally delay the onset of hypertension by several weeks. Renal denervation is often much less effective in reducing the arterial blood pressure of rats with established hypertension (Table 11.4). Typically, only a small fraction of the established hypertension can be relieved by renal denervation. In most models of experimental hypertension, therefore, the renal nerves do not appear to be the primary cause of the hypertension. Rather, it may be more appropriate to consider that their presence may exacerbate hypertension caused by other mechanisms.

Several investigators have reported that renal denervation is highly effective in preventing hypertension induced by baroreceptor denervation (Kline *et al.*, 1983; Ryuzaki *et al.*, 1992). Kline *et al.* (1983) demonstrated that renal denervation effectively prevented a 25 mmHg increase in arterial blood pressure following aortic denervation, and that renal denervation 5 or 19 days following aortic denervation was also capable of completely reversing the hypertension. Interpretation of these results is complicated by the nature of the hypertension induced by baroreceptor denervation. Although baroreceptor denervation causes an immediate increase in arterial blood pressure that may be sustained for days or weeks, it has previously been established that the long-term effects of baroreceptor denervation are an increased lability and reactivity of arterial blood pressure, with little or no change in the mean level (Cowley, Laird and Guyton, 1973; Norman, Coleman and Dent, 1980, 1981). Following sinoaortic denervation, for example, the process of assessing blood pressure by the tail-cuff technique in restrained rats causes a marked increase in the mean arterial blood pressure (Norman, Coleman and Dent, 1980, 1981). Despite this increase in blood pressure reactivity and lability, no hypertension is evident when the 24 h mean arterial blood pressure of denervated and control rats are compared (Norman, Coleman and Dent, 1980, 1981). Thus, it is not clear to what extent the results of Kline *et al.* (1983) in aortic denervated rats reflected an effect of renal denervation on the mean arterial blood pressure or its lability.

Effect of selective afferent denervation

Although the consequences of renal denervation are often attributed to renal sympathectomy, the procedure also deprives the kidney of its afferent innervation. Sectioning of the appropriate dorsal roots has been used to achieve permanent denervation of renal afferent fibres (Lappe, Webb and Brody, 1985). Although this technique is selective in that it removes only afferent fibres, it should be noted that this approach removes afferent fibres from all regions of the body wall and viscera innervated by the affected spinal segments.

Renal afferent denervation has been reported to markedly attenuate hypertension in the one-kidney, one-clip Goldblatt model (Wyss, Aboukarsh and Oparil, 1986). The effect appeared to be selective as afferent denervation of the contralateral (i.e. nephrectomized) side was without effect, and afferent denervation had no effect in unclipped rats. A small effect was also observed following afferent denervation in spontaneously hypertensive rats, leading the authors to conclude that the renal afferent nerves did not play an important role in the development of maintenance of hypertension in this model (Janssen *et al.*, 1989a). Negative results were also reported for the renal wrap and intrarenal noradrenaline infusion models (Table 11.4).

IS INCREASED RENAL NERVE ACTIVITY ALONE SUFFICIENT TO CAUSE HYPERTENSION?

Although the results of renal denervation studies suggest that the renal sympathetic nerves contribute to the elevation of the arterial pressure in several models of hypertension, we still do not know whether an increase in the activity of the renal sympathetic nerves is sufficient to produce chronic hypertension.

A study of Kottke, Kubicek and Visscher (1945) has often cited as proof of the importance of the renal nerves in long-term sodium balance and hypertension. The authors of this study described a slowly developing hypertension in response to chronic electrical activation of the renal nerves. Though hypertension was clearly achieved, it was unlikely to have been due to activation of the renal sympathetic fibres. The electrodes used were wrapped around the renal artery and nerve plexus. Hypertension could only be achieved by stimulation with a low-frequency (1.5–5 Hz) alternating current which, in retrospect, was likely to severely damage local tissues because of the tremendous wattage delivered to the tissue. The passage of electrical currents across arteries by this technique may induce thrombosis (Sawyer, Pate and Weldon, 1953). Indeed, such an approach has been adopted as a method of producing coronary thrombi in dogs (Salazar, 1961; Romson, Haack and Lucchesi, 1980). Thus, the hypertension caused by this unusual form of electrical stimulation may have arisen as the result of renal artery thrombosis. This interpretation is consistent with statements that this form of stimulation caused sustained renal vasoconstriction that was not rapidly reversible (Kottke, Kubicek and Visscher, 1945), the hypertension could not be reproduced using conventional stimuli (e.g. rectangular pulse, Kottke, Kubicek and Visscher, 1945) and that sustained responses could not be achieved by applying alternating current to the renal nerves alone (Block, Wakim and Mann, 1952a, 1952b). Thus, it remains to be demonstrated that activation of the renal nerves alone is sufficient to cause hypertension.

CONCLUSION

This chapter has described the afferent and efferent innervation of the kidney, and discussed the role of renal sympathetic nerves in controlling the renal vasculature, renal renin secretion, and renal sodium and water excretion. The main significance of the renal sympathetic nerves is that they are able, by several mechanisms, to influence the overall electrolyte and fluid excretion of the kidney. In this manner, RSNA may impact on the electrolyte and fluid homeostasis of the entire body.

The ability of the renal nerves to facilitate the renal response to sudden changes in vascular filling is well established. The available evidence suggests that the potency of this acute influence is not well sustained with time. Similarly, in most models of experimental hypertension, the most consistent effect of renal denervation is to delay the initial development of hypertension. Like many neural circulatory mechanisms (Guyton, 1980), the renal nerves may be specialized for dealing principally with relatively rapid but short-lived disturbances. That is, their ultimate significance may be in accelerating what are otherwise relatively slow processes of sodium and fluid balance.

REFERENCES

Abboud, F.M. (1987). Role of cardiogenic reflexes in heart failure. In *Cardiogenic reflexes*, edited by R. Hainsworth, P.N. McWilliam and D.A.S.G. Mary, pp. 371–388. Oxford: Oxford University Press.

Ammons, W.S. (1988a). Renal and somatic input to spinal neurons antidromically activated from the ventrolateral medulla. *Journal of Neurophysiology*, **60**, 1967–1981.

Ammons, W.S. (1988b). Spinoreticular cell responses to renal venous and ureteral occlusion. *American Journal of Physiology*, **254**, R268–R276.

Ansell, J.S. and Gee, W.F. (1990). Diseases of the kidney and ureter. In *The management of pain*. Volume II. 2nd edn, edited by J.J. Bonica, pp. 1232–1249. Philadelphia: Lea and Febiger.

Asfoury, Z.M. (1971). *Sympathectomy and the innervation of the kidney*. New York: Appleton-Century-Crofts.

Astrom, A. and Crafoord, J. (1967). Afferent activity recorded in the kidney nerves of rats. *Acta Physiologica Scandinavica*, **70**, 10–15.

Astrom, A. and Crafoord, J. (1968). Afferent and efferent activity in the renal nerve of cats. *Acta Physiologica Scandinavica*, **74**, 69–78.

Aukland, K. (1968). Effects of adrenaline, noradrenaline, angiotensin, and renal nerve stimulation on intrarenal distribution of blood flow in dogs. *Acta Physiologica Scandinavica*, **72**, 498–509.

Badder, E.M., Durate, B., Seaton, J.F., Hamaji, M. and Harrison (1985). Angiotensin II restoration of reflex adrenal medullary secretion to anephric dogs is physiologically dose dependent. *Endocrinology*, **117**, 1920–1929.

Bailly, C., Imbert-Teboul, N., Roinel, N. and Ameil, C. (1990). Isoproterenol increases Ca, Mg, and NaCl reabsorption in mouse thick ascending limb. *American Journal of Physiology*, **258**, F1224–F1231.

Ballesta, J., Polak, J.M., Allen, J.M. and Bloom, S.R. (1984). The nerves of the juxtaglomerular apparatus of man and other mammals contain the potent peptide NPY. *Histochemistry*, **80**, 483–485.

Barajas, L. (1978). Innervation of the renal cortex. *Federation Proceedings*, **37**, 1192–1201.

Barajas, L. and Muller, J. (1973). The innervation of the juxtaglomerular apparatus and surrounding tubules: A quantitative analysis by serial section electron microscopy. *Journal of Ultrastructural Research*, **43**, 107–132.

Barajas, L. and Powers, K. (1988). Innervation of the thick ascending limb of Henlé. *American Journal of Physiology*, **255**, F340–F348.

Barajas, L. and Powers, K. (1989). Innervation of the renal proximal convoluted tubule of the rat. *American Journal of Anatomy*, **186**, 378–388.

Barajas, L. and Powers, K. (1990). Monoaminergic innervation of the rat kidney: a quantitative study. *American Journal of Physiology*, **259**, F503–F511.

Barajas, L. and Wang, P. (1978). Myelinated nerves of the rat kidney. A light and electron microscopic autoradiographic study. *Journal of Ultrastructural Research*, **65**, 148–162.

Barajas, L., Powers, K. and Wang, P. (1984). Innervation of the renal cortical tubules: a quantitative study. *American Journal of Physiology*, **247**, F50–F60.

Barber, J.D. and Moss, N.G. (1990). Reduced renal perfusion pressure causes prostaglandin-dependent excitation of R2 chemoreceptors in rats. *American Journal of Physiology*, **259**, R1243–R1249.

Barron, K.W. and Bishop, V.S. (1982). Reflex cardiovascular changes with veratridine in the conscious dog. *American Journal of Physiology*, **242**, H810–H817.

Beacham, W.S. and Kunze, D.L. (1969). Renal receptors evoking a spinal vasomotor reflex. *Journal of Physiology*, **201**, 73–85.

Bell, C. (1987). Dopamine: precursor or neurotransmitter in sympathetically innervated tissues? *Blood Vessels*, **24**, 234–239.

Bell, C., Lang, W.J. and Laska, F. (1978). Dopamine-containing vasomotor nerves in the dog kidney. *Journal of Neurochemistry*, **31**, 77–83.

Bell, C. and McLachlan, E.M. (1982). Dopaminergic neurons in sympathetic ganglia of the dog. *Proceedings of the Royal Society (London)*, **215**, 175–190.

Bello-Reuss, E. (1980). Effect of catecholamines on fluid reabsorption by the isolated proximal convoluted tubule. *American Journal of Physiology*, **238**, F347–F352.

Bello-Reuss, E., Trevino, D.L. and Gottschalk, C.W. (1976). Effect of renal sympathetic denervation on proximal water and sodium reabsorption. *Journal of Clinical Investigation*, **57**, 1104–1107.

Bello-Reuss, E., Pastoriza-Munoz, E. and Colindres, R.E. (1977). Acute unilateral renal denervation in rats with extracellular volume expansion. *American Journal of Physiology*, **232**, F26–F32.

Bencsath, P., Szalay, L., Debreczeni, L.A., Vajda, L., Takacs, L. and Fischer, A. (1972). Denervation diuresis and renin secretion in the anaesthetized dog. *European Journal of Clinical Investigation*, **2**, 422–425.

Bernard, C. (1859). *Lecons sur les proprietes physiologique et les alterations pathologiques des liquides de l'organisme*. Paris: Balliere.

Berne, R.M. (1952). Haemodynamics and sodium excretion of denervated kidney in anaesthetized and unanaesthetized dog. *American Journal of Physiology*, **171**, 148–158.

Berne, R.M., Hoffman, W.K., Kagan, A. and Levy, M.N. (1952). Response of the normal and denervated kidney to L-adrenaline and L-noradrenaline. *American Journal of Physiology*, **171**, 564–571.

Block, M.A., Wakim, K.G. and Mann, F.C. (1952a). Circulation through the kidney during stimulation of the renal nerves. *American Journal of Physiology*, **169**, 659–669.

Block, M.A., Wakim, K.G. and Mann, F.C. (1952b). Renal function during stimulation of the renal nerves. *American Journal of Physiology*, **169**, 670–677.

Bradford, J.R. (1889). The innervation of the renal blood vessels. *Journal of Physiology (London)*, **10**, 358–407.

Bradley, T., Sollevi, A. and Lagerkranser, M. (1986). Effect of hypotension induced by sodium nitroprusside on catecholamine overflow in the canine kidney. *Acta Physiologica Scandinavica*, **128**, 305–308.

Briggs, J. and Schnermann, J. (1990). The tubuloglomerular feedback mechanism. In *Hypertension: Pathophysiology, Diagnosis, and Management*, edited by J.H. Laragh and B.M. Brenner, pp. 1067–1087. New York: Raven Press.

Brod, J., Fejfar, Z. and Fejfarova, M.H. (1954). The role of neurohumoral factors in the genesis of renal haemodynamic changes in heart failure. *Acta Medica Scandinavica*, **148**, 273–290.

Calaresu, F.R. and Ciriello, J. (1981). Renal afferent nerves affect discharge rate of medullary and hypothalamic single units in the cat. *Journal of the Autonomic Nervous System*, **3**, 311–320.

Calaresu, F.R., Kim, P., Nakamura, H. and Sato, A. (1978). Electrophysiological characteristics of renorenal reflexes in the cat. *Journal of Physiology*, **283**, 141–154.

Carroll, R.G., Lohmeier, T.E. and Brown, A.J. (1984). Chronic angiotensin II infusion decreases renal noradrenaline overflow in conscious dogs. *Hypertension*, **6**, 675–681.

Carroll, R.G., Lohmeier, T.E. and Brown, A.J. (1988). Disparity between renal venous noradrenaline and renin responses to sodium depletion. *American Journal of Physiology*, **254**, F754–F761.

Chen, J.-S. and Gorman, A.J. (1990). Intracoronary veratrine and aortic stenosis modify renal responses to hypotension in conscious dogs. *American Journal of Physiology*, **259**, F18–F25.

Chevendra, V. and Weaver, L.C. (1991). Distribution of splenic, mesenteric and renal neurons in sympathetic ganglia in rats. *Journal of the Autonomic Nervous System*, **33**, 47–54.

Christensen, K., Lewis, E. and Kuntz, A. (1951). Innervation of the renal blood vessels in the cat. *Journal of Comparative Neurology*, **95**, 373–385.

Churchill, P.C. (1985). Second messengers in renin secretion. *American Journal of Physiology*, **249**, F175–F184.

Ciriello, J. and Calaresu, F.R. (1983). Central projections of afferent renal fibers in the rat: an anterograde transport study of horseradish peroxidase. *Journal of the Autonomic Nervous System*, **8**, 273–285.

Clement, D.L., Pelletier, C.L. and Shepherd, J.T. (1972). Role of vagal afferents in the control of renal sympathetic nerve activity in the rabbit. *Circulation Research*, **31**, 824–830.

Cogan, M.G. (1986). Neurogenic regulation of proximal bicarbonate and chloride reabsorption. *American Journal of Physiology*, **250**, F22–F26.

Coleridge, J.C.G. and Coleridge, H.M. (1977). Afferent C–Fibers and cardiorespiratory chemoreflexes. *American Review of Respiratory Disease*, **115**, 251–260.

Coleridge, H.M. and Coleridge, J.C.G. (1980). Cardiovascular afferents involved in regulation of peripheral vessels. *Annual Review of Physiology*, **42**, 413–427.

Coote, J.H., Johns, E.J., MacLeod, V.H. and Singer, B. (1972). Effect of renal nerve stimulation, renal blood flow and noradrenergic blockade on plasma renin activity in the cat. *Journal of Physiology*, **226**, 15–36.

Copper, C.L. and Malik, K.U. (1985). Prostaglandin synthesis and renal vasoconstriction elicited by noradrenergic stimuli are linked to activation of α_1-noradrenergic receptors in the isolated rat kidney. *Journal of Pharmacology and Experimental Therapeutics*, **233**, 24–31.

Cornish, K.G., McCulloch, T. and Gilmore, J.P. (1984). Sinoaortic baroreceptors and the control of blood volume in the nonhuman primate. *American Journal of Physiology*, **247**, F539–F542.

Cowley, A.W. and Lohmeier, T.E. (1979). Changes in renal vascular activity and arterial pressure associated with sodium intake during long-term intrarenal noradrenaline infusion in dogs. *Hypertension*, **1**, 549–558.

Cowley, A.W. Jr. and Skelton, M.M. (1991). Dominance of colloid osmotic pressure in renal excretion after isotonic volume expansion. *American Journal of Physiology*, **261**, H1214–H1225.

Cowley, A.W. Jr., Laird, J.F. and Guyton, A.C. (1973). Role of the baroreceptor reflex in daily control of arterial blood pressure and other variables in dogs. *Circulation Research*, **32**, 564–576.

Davis, J.O. and Freeman, R.H. (1976). Mechanisms regulating renin release. *Physiological Reviews*, **56**, 1–56.

Day, T.A. and Ciriello, J. (1987). Effects of renal receptor activation on neurosecretory vasopressin cells. *American Journal of Physiology*, **253**, R234–R241.

DeWolf, W.C. and Fraley, E.E. (1975). Renal Pain. *Urology*, **6**, 403–408.

Dibner-Dunlap, M.E. and Thames, M.D. (1992). Control of sympathetic nerve activity by vagal mechanoreflexes is blunted in heart failure. *Circulation*, **86**, 1929–1934.

DiBona, G.F. (1977). Neurogenic regulation of renal tubular sodium reabsorption. *American Journal of Physiology*, **233**, F73–F81.

DiBona, G.F. (1978). Neural control of renal tubular sodium reabsorption in the dog. *Federation Proceedings*, **37**, 1214–1217.

DiBona, G.F. (1982). The functions of the renal nerves. *Reviews of Physiology, Biochemistry and Pharmacology*, **94**, 75–181.

DiBona, G.F. (1985a). Neural control of renal function: Role of renal α-adrenoceptors. *Journal of Cardiovascular Pharmacology*, **7**(Suppl. 8), S18–S23.

DiBona, G.F. (1985b). Neural regulation of renal tubular sodium reabsorption and renin secretion. *Federation Proceedings*, **44**, 2816–2822.

DiBona, G.F. (1989a). Sympathetic nervous system influences on the kidney: Role in hypertension. *American Journal of Hypertension*, **2**, 119S–124S.

DiBona, G.F. (1989b). Neural control of renal tubular solute and water transport. *Mineral and Electrolyte Metabolism*, **15**, 44–50.

DiBona, G.F. and Sawin, L.L. (1982). Effect of renal nerve stimulation on NaCl and H_2O transport in Henlé's loop of the rat. *American Journal of Physiology*, **243**, F576–F580.

DiBona, G.F. and Sawin, L.L. (1985). Renal nerve activity in conscious rats during volume expansion and depletion. *American Journal of Physiology*, **248**, F15–F23.

DiBona, G.F. and Sawin, L.L. (1987). Role of renal α_2-adrenergic receptors in spontaneously hypertensive rats. *Hypertension*, **9**, 41–48.

DiBona, G.F., Zambraski, E.J., Aguilera, A.J. and Kaloyanides, G.J. (1977). Neurogenic control of renal tubular sodium reabsorption in the dog. *Circulation Research*, **40**(Suppl. I), I127–I130.

DiBona, G.F., Johns, E.J. and Osborn, J.L. (1981). The effect of vagotomy on sodium reabsorption and renin release in anaesthetized dogs subjected to 60° head-up tilt. *Journal of Physiology (London)*, **320**, 293–302.

Dinerstein, R.J., Vannice, J., Henderson, R.C., Roth, L.J., Goldberg, L.I. and Hoffmann, P.C. (1979). Histofluorescence techniques provide evidence for dopamine-containing neuronal elements in canine kidney. *Science*, **205**, 497–500.

DiSalvo, J. and Fell, C. (1971). Changes in renal blood flow during renal nerve stimulation. *Proceedings of the Society for Experimental Biology and Medicine*, **136**, 150–153.

Diz, D.I., Nasjletti, A. and Baer, P.G. (1982). Renal denervation at weaning retards development of hypertension in New Zealand genetically hypertensive rats. *Hypertension*, **4**, 361–368.

Donovan, M.K., Wyss, J.M. and Winternitz, S.R. (1983). Localization of renal sensory neurons using the fluorescent dye technique. *Brain Research*, **259**, 119–122.

Dorward, P.K., Burke, S.L., Janig, W. and Cassell, J. (1987). Reflex responses to baroreceptor, chemoreceptor and nociceptor inputs in single renal sympathetic neurons in the rabbit and the effects of anaesthesia on them. *Journal of the Autonomic Nervous System*, **18**, 39–54.

Dorward, P.K., Riedel, W., Burke, S.L., Gipps, J. and Korner, P.I. (1985). The renal sympathetic baroreflex in the rabbit: arterial and cardiac baroreflex influences, resetting, and effect of anaesthesia. *Circulation Research*, **57**, 618–633.

Drew, G.M. and Whiting, S.B. (1979). Evidence for two distinct types of postsynaptic α-adrenoceptors in vascular smooth muscle *in vivo*. *British Journal of Pharmacology*, **67**, 207–215.

Drinkhill, M.J., Mary, D.A.S.G., Ramadan, M.R.M. and Vacca, G. (1989). The effect of distension of the urinary bladder on activity in efferent renal fibres in anaesthetized dogs. *Journal of Physiology*, **409**, 357–369.

Drukker, J., Green, G.J., Boekelaar, A.B. and Baljet, B. (1987). The extrinsic innervation of the rat kidney. *Clinical and Experimental Hypertension*, **A9**(Suppl 1), 15–31.

Duval, N., Hicks, P.E. and Langer, S.Z. (1985). Dopamine preferentially stimulates postsynaptic α_2-adrenoceptors in the renal vascular bed of the anaesthetised dog. *European Journal of Pharmacology*, **108**, 265–272.

Dzielak, D.J. and Norman, R.A. Jr. (1985). Renal nerves are not necessary for onset or maintenance of DOC-salt hypertension in rats. *American Journal of Physiology*, **249**, H945–H949.

Echtenkamp, S.F. and Dandridge, P.F. (1989). Influence of renal sympathetic nerve stimulation on renal function in the primate. *American Journal of Physiology*, **257**, F204–F209.

Ehmke, H., Persson, P.B., Seyfarth, M. and Kirchheim, H.R. (1990). Neurogenic control of pressure natriuresis in conscious dogs. *American Journal of Physiology*, **259**, F466–F473.

Elhilali, M.M. and Winfield, H.N. (1989). Genitourinary pain. In *Textbook of pain*, edited by P.D. Wall and R. Melzack, pp. 500–505. New York: Churchill Livingston.

Epstein, M. (1978). Renal effects of head-out water immersion in man: Implications for an understanding of volume homeostasis. *Physiological Reviews*, **58**, 530–558.

Faber, J.E. (1987). Role of prostaglandins and kinins in the renal pressor reflex. *Hypertension*, **10**, 522–532.

Fater, D.C., Schultz, H.D., Sundet, W.D., Mapes, J.S. and Goetz, K.L. (1982). Effects of left atrial stretch in cardiac-denervated and intact conscious dogs. *American Journal of Physiology*, **242**, H1056–H1064.

Feldberg, W. and Lewis, G.P. (1964). The actions of peptides on the adrenal medulla. Release of adrenaline by bradykinin and angiotensin. *Journal of Physiology*, **171**, 98–108.

Felder, R.B. (1986). Excitatory and inhibitory interactions among renal and cardiovascular afferent nerves in dorsomedial medulla. *American Journal of Physiology*, **250**, R580–R588.

Felder, R.B. and Thames, M.D. (1982). Responses to activation of cardiac sympathetic afferents with epicardiac bradykinin. *American Journal of Physiology*, **242**, H148–H153.

Fergusson, M and Bell, C. (1985). Substance P immunoreactive nerves in the rat kidney. *Neuroscience Letters*, **60**, 183–188.

Fergusson, M. and Bell, C. (1988). Ultrastructural localization and characterization of sensory nerves in the rat kidney. *Journal of Comparative Neurology*, **274**, 9–16.

Ferguson, M., Ryan, G.B. and Bell, C. (1986). Localization of sympathetic and sensory neurons innervating the rat kidney. *Journal of the Autonomic Nervous System*, **16**, 279–288.

Ferrario, C.M., Gildenberg, P.L. and McCubbin, J.W. (1972). Cardiovascular effects of angiotensin mediated by the central nervous system. *Circulation Research*, **30**, 257–262.

Fray, J.C.S., Park, C.S. and Valentine, A.N.D. (1987). Calcium and the control of renin secretion. *Endocrine Reviews*, **8**, 53–93.

Freeman, R.H. and Davis, J.O. (1983). Factors controlling renin secretion and metabolism. In *Hypertension*, edited by J. Genest, O. Kuchel, P. Hamet and M. Cantin, pp. 225–250. New York: McGraw-Hill.

Gattone, V.H., Marfurt, C.F. and Dallie, S. (1986). Extrinsic innervation of the rat kidney: a retrograde tracing study. *American Journal of Physiology*, **250**, F189–F196.

Gauer, O.H. and Henry, J.P. (1963). Circulatory basis of fluid volume control. *Physiological Reviews*, **43**, 423–481.

Ge, M. and Shiu-Yong, H. (1990a). Haemodynamic effect of renal interoreceptor and afferent nerve stimulation in rabbit. *Acta Physiologica Sinica*, **42**, 262–268.

Ge, M. and Shiu-Yong, H. (1990b). Observation on the afferent nerve activity induced by stimulation of renal receptors in rabbits. *Acta Physiologica Sinica*, **42**, 269–276.

Gellai, M. and Ruffolo, R.R. Jr. (1987). Renal effects of selective α_1- and α_2-adrenoceptor agonists in conscious, normotensive rats. *Journal of Pharmacology and Experimental Therapeutics*, **240**, 723–728.

Geppetti, P., Baldi, E., Castelucci, A., Del Bianco, E., Santicicoli, P., Maggi, C.A., *et al.* (1989). Calcitonin gene-related peptide in the rat kidney: occurrence, sensitivity to capsaicin, and stimulation of adenylate cyclase. *Neuroscience*, **30**, 503–513.

Gill, J.R. and Casper, A.G.T. (1971). Depression of proximal tubular sodium reabsorption in the dog in response to renal β-adrenergic stimulation by isoproterenol. *Journal of Clinical Investigation*, **50**, 112–118.

Gilmore, J.P. and Tomomatsu, E. (1985). Renal mechanoreceptors in nonhuman primates. *American Journal of Physiology*, **248**, R202–R207.

Gilmore, J.P. and Zucker, I.H. (1978a). Contribution of vagal pathways to the renal responses to head-out immersion in the nonhuman primate. *Circulation Research*, **42**, 263–267.

Gilmore, J.P. and Zucker, I.H. (1978b). Failure of left atrial distension to alter renal function in the nonhuman primate. *Circulation Research*, **42**, 267–270.

Girchev, R., Toneva, Z. and Natcheff, N. (1989). Excretory function after unilateral renal denervation and administration of propranolol to unanaesthetized dogs. *Acta Physiologica Hungarica*, **73**, 53–60.

Gorman, A.J. and Chen, J.-S. (1989). Reflex inhibition of plasma renin activity by increased left ventricular pressure in conscious dogs. *American Journal of Physiology*, **256**, R1299–R1307.

Gorman, A.J. and Zucker, I.H. (1984). Renal nerve and blood pressure responses to stimulation of cardiac receptors in dogs and cats by bradykinin. *Basic Research in Cardiology*, **79**, 142–154.

Gorman, A.J., Zucker, I.H. and Gilmore, J.P. (1983). Renal nerve responses to cardiac receptors stimulation with bradykinin in monkeys. *American Journal of Physiology*, **244**, F659–F665.

Gorman, A.J., Cornish, K. and Zucker, I.H. (1984). Renal and iliac vascular responses to left ventricular receptor stimulation in conscious dogs. *American Journal of Physiology*, **246**, R788–R798.

Gottschalk, C.W. (1979). Renal nerves and sodium excretion. *Annual Review of Physiology*, **41**, 229–240.

Gottschalk, C.W., Moss, N.G. and Colindres, R.E. (1985). Neural control of renal function in health and disease. In *The Kidney: Physiology and Pathophysiology*, edited by D.W. Seldin and G. Giebisch, pp. 581–611. New York: Raven Press.

Greenberg, T.T., Richmond, W.H., Stocking, R.A., Gupta, P.D., Meehan, J.P. and Henry, J.P. (1973). Impaired atrial receptor responses in dogs with heart failure due to tricuspid insufficiency and pulmonary artery stenosis. *Circulation Research*, **32**, 424–433.

Gross, R. and Kirchheim, H. (1980). Effects of bilateral carotid occlusion and auditory stimulation on renal blood flow and sympathetic nerve activity in the conscious dog. *Pflügers Archiv*, **383**, 233–239.

Gross, R., Kirchheim, H. and Ruffman, K. (1981). Effect of carotid occlusion and of perfusion pressure on renal function in conscious dogs. *Circulation Research*, **48**, 777–784.

Gruber, C.M. (1933). The autonomic innervation of the genito-urinary system. *Physiological Reviews*, **13**, 497–609.

Guyton, A.C. (1980). *Arterial pressure and hypertension*. Philadelphia: W.B. Saunders.

Guyton, A.C. (1990). Long-term arterial pressure control: an analysis from animal experiments and computer and graphic models. *American Journal of Physiology*, **259**, R865–R877.

Guyton, A.C. and Coleman, T.G. (1967). Long-term regulation of the circulation; interrelationships with body fluid volumes. In *Physical basis of circulatory transport regulation and exchange*, edited by E.B. Reeve and A.C. Guyton, pp. 179–201. Philadelphia: Saunders Publishing.

Guyton, A.C., Hall, J.E., Coleman, T.G. and Manning, R.D. Jr. (1990). The dominant role of the kidneys in the long-term regulation of arterial pressure in normal and hypertensive states. In *Hypertension: Pathophysiology, diagnosis, and management*, edited by J.H. Laragh and B.M. Brenner. pp. 1029–1052. New York: Raven Press.

Hainsworth, R. (1991). Reflexes from the heart. *Physiological Reviews*, **71**, 617–658.

Hainsworth, R. and McGregor, K.H. (1987). Reflex vascular responses to stimulation of cardiac ventricular receptors. In *Cardiogenic reflexes*, edited by R. Hainsworth, P.N. McWilliam and D.A.S.G. Mary, pp. 45–61. Oxford: Oxford University Press.

Hajduczok, G., Miki, K., Hong, S.K., Claybaugh, J.R. and Krasney, J.A. (1987). Role of cardiac nerves in response to head-out water immersion in conscious dogs. *American Journal of Physiology*, **253**, R242–R253.

Hall, J.E. (1982). Regulation of renal haemodynamics. In *Cardiovascular Physiology IV, International Review of Physiology*, Volume 26, edited by A.C. Guyton and J.E. Hall, pp. 243–321. Baltimore: University Park Press.

Hall, J.E. (1986a). Control of sodium excretion by angiotensin II: Intrarenal mechanisms and blood pressure regulation. *American Journal of Physiology*, **250**, R960–R972.

Hall, J.E. (1986b). Regulation of glomerular filtration rate and sodium excretion by angiotensin II. *Federation Proceedings*, **45**, 1431–1437.

Hall, J.E. and Brands, M.W. (1992). The renin–angiotensin-aldosterone systems. In *The Kidney: Physiology and Pathophysiology*, Second Edition, edited by D.W. Seldin and G. Giebisch, pp. 1455–1504. New York: Raven Press.

Hall, J.E. and Granger, J.P. (1983). Role of peripheral sympathetic nervous system in mediating chronic blood pressure and renal haemodynamic effects of angiotensin II. *Federation Proceedings*, **42**, 589.

Hall, J.E., Mizelle, H.L., Hildebrandt, D.A. and Brands, M.W. (1990). Abnormal pressure natriuresis. A cause or a consequence of hypertension. *Hypertension*, **15**, 547–559.

Head, H. (1893). On disturbances of sensation with especial reference to the pain of visceral disease. *Brain*, **16**, 1–133.

Hermansson, K., Larson, Kallskog, O. and Wolgast, M. (1981). Influence of renal nerve activity on arteriolar resistance, ultrafiltration dynamics and fluid reabsorption. *Pflügers Archives European Journal of Physiology*, **389**, 85–90.

Hesse, I.F. and Johns, E.J. (1984). The effect of graded renal nerve stimulation on renal function in the anaesthetized rabbit. *Comparative Biochemistry and Physiology*, **79A**, 409–414.

Hesse, I.F. and Johns, E.J. (1985). The role of α-adrenoceptors in the regulation of renal tubular sodium reabsorption and renin secretion in the rabbit. *British Journal of Pharmacology*, **84**, 715–724.

Holzbauer, M. and Sharman, D.F. (1972). The distribution of catecholamines in vertebrates. *Handbook of Experimental Pharmacology*, **33**, 110–185.

Horn, P.T., Kohli, J.D., Listinsky, J.J. and Goldberg, L.I. (1982). Regional variations in the α-noradrenergic receptors in the canine resistance vessel. *Naunyn Schmiedeberg's Archives of Pharmacology*, **318**, 166–172.

Ishiki, K., Morita, H. and Hosomi, H. (1991). Reflex control of renal nerve activity originating from the osmoreceptors in the hepato-portal region. *Journal of the Autonomic Nervous System*, **36**, 139–148.

Janig, W. (1988). The function of the autonomic nervous system as interface between body and the environment. Old and new concepts: W.B. Cannon and W.R. Hess revisited. In *Neurobiological approaches to human disease*, edited by D. Helhammer, I. Florin, and H. Weiner, pp. 143–173. Toronto: Han Huber Publishing.

Janig, W. and MacLachlan, E.M. (1987). Organization of lumbar spinal outflow to the distal colon and pelvic organs. *Physiological Reviews*, **67**, 1332–1404.

Janssen, B.J.A. and Smits, J.F.M. (1989). Renal nerves in hypertension. *Mineral and Electrolyte Metabolism*, **15**, 74–82.

Janssen, B.J.A., van Essen, H., Vervoort-Peters, L.H.T.M., Struyker-Boudier, H.A.J. and Smits, J.F.M. (1989a). Role of afferent renal nerves in spontaneous hypertension in rats. *Hypertension*, **13**, 327–333.

Janssen, B.J.A., van Essen, H., Vervoort-Peters, L.H.T.M., Thijssen, H.H.W., Derkx, F.H.M., Struyker-Boudier, H.A.J. and Smits, J.F.M. (1989b). Effects of complete renal denervation and selective afferent renal denervation on the hypertension induced by intrarenal noradrenaline infusion in conscious rats. *Journal of Hypertension*, **7**, 447–455.

Jing-Yun, P., Bishop, V.S., Ball, N.A. and Haywood, J.R. (1985). Inability of dorsal spinal rhizotomy to prevent renal wrap hypertension in rats. *Hypertension*, **7**, 722–728.

Johansson, B., Sparks, H. and Biber, B. (1970). The escape of the renal blood flow response during sympathetic nerve stimulation. *Angiologica*, **7**, 333.

Johns, E.J. (1987). The role of angiotensin II in the antidiuresis and antinatriuresis induced by stimulation of the sympathetic nerves to the rat kidney. *Journal of Autonomic Pharmacology*, **7**, 205–214.

Johns, E.J. (1989). Role of angiotensin II and the sympathetic nervous system in the control of renal function. *Journal of Hypertension*, **7**, 695–701.

Johns, E.J. and Manitius, J. (1987). An investigation into the neural regulation of calcium excretion by the rat kidney. *Journal of Physiology*, **383**, 745–755.

Johns, E.J., Lewis, B.A. and Singer, B. (1976). The sodium-retaining effect of renal nerve activity in the cat: Role of angiotensin formation. *Clinical Science and Molecular Medicine*, **51**, 93–102.

Kaczmarczyk, G., Eigenheer, F., Gatzka, M., Kuhl, U. and Reinhardt, H.W. (1978). No relation between atrial natriuresis and renal blood flow in conscious dogs. *Pflügers Archiv: European Journal of Physiology*, **373**, 49–58.

Kaczmarczyk, G., Schimmrich, B., Mohnhaupt, R. and Reinhardt, H.W. (1979). Atrial pressure and postprandial volume regulation in conscious dogs. *Pflügers Archiv: European Journal of Physiology*, **381**, 143–150.

Kaczmarczyk, G., Drake, A., Eisele, R., Mohnhaupt, R., Noble, M.I.M., Simgen, B., Stubbs, J. and Reinhardt, H.W. (1981a). The role of cardiac nerves in the regulation of sodium excretion in conscious dogs. *Pflügers Archiv: European Journal of Physiology*, **390**, 125–130.

Kaczmarczyk, G., Unger, V., Mohnhaupt, R. and Reinhardt, H.W. (1981b). Left atrial distension and intrarenal blood flow distribution in conscious dogs. *Pfluegers Archives European Journal of Physiology*, **390**, 44–48.

Karim, F., Kidd, C., Malpus, C.M. and Penna, P.E. (1972). The effects of stimulation on the left atrial receptors on sympathetic efferent nerve activity. *Journal of Physiology*, **227**, 243–260.

Karim, F., Mackay, D. and Kappagoda, C.T. (1982). Influence of carotid sinus pressure on atrial receptors and renal blood flow. *American Journal of Physiology*, **242**, H220–H226.

Katholi, R.E., Carey, R.M., Ayers, C.R., Vaughan, E.D. Jr., Yancey, M.R. and Morton, C.L. (1977). Production of sustained hypertension by chronic intrarenal noradrenaline infusion in conscious dogs. *Circulation Research*, **40**(Suppl. II), 118–126.

Katholi, R.E., Naftilan, A.J. and Oparil, S. (1980). Importance of renal sympathetic tone in the development of DOCA-salt hypertension in the rat. *Hypertension*, **2**, 266–273.

Katholi, R.E., Winternitz, S.R. and Oparil, S. (1981). Role of the renal nerves in the pathogenesis of one-kidney renal hypertension in the rat. *Hypertension*, **3**, 404–409.

Katholi, R.E., Whitlow, P.L., Winternitz, S.R. and Oparil, S. (1982). Importance of the renal nerves in established two-kidney, one clip goldblatt hypertension. *Hypertension*, **4**(Suppl. 2), II-166–II-174.

Katholi, R.E., Naftilan, A.J., Bishop, S.P. and Oparil, S. (1983a). Role of the renal nerves in the maintenance of DOCA-salt hypertension in the rat. Influence on the renal vasculature and sodium excretion. *Hypertension*, **5**, 427–435.

Katholi, R.E., Hageman, G.R., Whitlow, P.L. and Woods, W.T. (1983b). Haemodynamic and afferent renal nerve responses to intrarenal adenosine in the dog. *Hypertension*, **5**(Suppl I), 149–154.

Katz, M.A. and Shear, L. (1975). Effects of renal nerves on renal haemodynamics. I. Direct stimulation and carotid occlusion. *Nephron*, **14**, 246–256.

Katz, M.A., Blantz, R.C., Rector, F.C. and Seldin, D.W. (1971). Measurement of intrarenal blood flow: Analysis of microsphere method. *American Journal of Physiology*, **222**, 1903–1913.

Kaufman, S. and Stelfox, J. (1987). Atrial stretch-induced diuresis in Brattleboro rats. *American Journal of Physiology*, **252**, R503–R506.

Keeton, T.K. and Campbell, W.B. (1980). The pharmacologic alteration of renin release. *Pharmacological Reviews*, **32**, 81–277.

Kezdi, P. and Geller, E. (1968). Baroreceptor control and postganglionic sympathetic nerve discharge. *American Journal of Physiology*, **214**, 427–435.

Kidd, C., Linden, R.J. and Scott, E.M. (1981). Reflex responses of single renal sympathetic fibres to stimulation of atrial receptors and carotid baro- and chemoreceptors. *Quarterly Journal of Experimental Physiology*, **66**, 311–320.

Kirchheim, H. (1976). Systemic arterial baroreceptor reflexes. *Physiological Reviews*, **56**, 100–176.

Kirchheim, H., Ehmke, H. and Persson, P. (1988). Physiology of the renal baroreceptor mechanism of renin release and its role in congestive heart failure. *American Journal of Cardiology*, **62**, 68E–71E.

Kirchner, F. (1974). Correlations between changes of activity of the renal sympathetic nerve and behavioural events in unrestrained cats. *Basic Research in Cardiology*, **69**, 343–356.

Kline, R.L., Patel, K.P., Ciriello, J. and Mercer, P.F. (1983). Effect of renal denervation on arterial pressure in rats with aortic nerve transection. *Hypertension*, **5**, 468–475.

Knight, D., Beal, J., Yuon, Z.P. and Fournet, T. (1987). Substance P-immunoreactive nerves in the rat kidney. *Journal of the Autonomic Nervous System*, **21**, 145–155.

Knight, D.S., Fabre, R.D. and Beal, J.A. (1989). Identification of noradrenergic nerve terminals immunoreactive for neuropeptide Y and vasoactive intestinal polypeptide in the rat kidney. *The American Journal of Anatomy*, **184**, 190–204.

Knuepfer, M.M. and Schramm, L.P. (1985). Properties of renobulbar afferent fibers in rats. *American Journal of Physiology*, **248**, R113–R119.

Koepke, J.P., Jones, S. and DiBona, G.F. (1988). Stress increases renal nerve activity and decreases sodium excretion in Dahl rats. *Hypertension*, **11**, 334–338.

Kon, V., Yared, A. and Ichikawa, I. (1985). Role of renal sympathetic nerves in mediating hypoperfusion of renal cortical microcirculation in experimental congestive heart failure and acute extracellular fluid volume depletion. *Journal of Clinical Investigation*, **76**, 1913–1920.

Kopp, U.C. and DiBona, G.F. (1984). Interaction between neural and nonneural mechanism controlling renin secretion rate. *American Journal of Physiology*, **246**, F620–F626.

Kopp, U.C. and Smith, L.A. (1987). Renoreflex responses to renal sensory receptor stimulation in normotension and hypertension. *Clinical and Experimental Hypertension*, **A9**(Suppl 1), 113–125.

Kopp, U.C. and Smith, L.A. (1991). Inhibitory renorenal reflexes: a role for renal prostaglandins in activation of renal sensory receptors. *American Journal of Physiology*, **261**, R1513–R1521.

Kopp, U., Aurell, M., Sjolander, M. and Ablad, B. (1981). The role of prostaglandins in the α and β-adrenoceptor mediated renin release response to graded renal nerve stimulation. *Pflügers Archiv*, **391**, 1–8.

Kopp, U.C., Olson, L.A. and DiBona, G.F. (1984). Renorenal reflex responses to mechano- and chemoreceptor stimulation in the dog and rat. *American Journal of Physiology*, **246**, F67–F77.

Kopp, U.C., Smith, L.A. and DiBona, G.F. (1985). Renorenal reflexes: Neural components of ipsilateral and contralateral renal responses. *American Journal of Physiology*, **249**, F507–F517.

Kostreva, D.R., Castaner, A. and Kampine, J.P. (1980). Reflex effects of hepatic baroreceptors on renal and cardiac sympathetic nerve activity. *American Journal of Physiology*, **238**, R390–R394.

Kottke, F.J., Kubicek, W.G. and Visscher, M.B. (1945). The production of arterial hypertension by chronic renal artery-nerve stimulation. *American Journal of Physiology*, **145**, 38–47.

Krieger, E.M. (1970). Time course of baroreceptor resetting in acute hypertension. *American Journal of Physiology*, **218**, 486–490.

Krieger, J.E., Liard, J.–F. and Cowley, A.W. Jr. (1990). Haemodynamics, fluid volume, and hormonal responses to chronic high-salt intake in dogs. *American Journal of Physiology*, **259**, H1629–H1636.

Kuo, D.C., Groat, W.C. de, and Nadelhaft, I. (1982). Origin of the sympathetic efferent axons in the renal nerves of the cat. *Neuroscience Letters*, **29**, 213–218.

Kuo, D.C., Nadelhaft, I., Hisamitsu, T. and Groat, W.C. de (1983). Segmental distribution and central projections of renal afferent fibers in the cat studied by transganglionic transport of horseradish peroxidase. *Journal of Comparative Anatomy*, **216**, 162–174.

Kurtz, A., Schurek, H., Jelkmann, W., Muff, R., Lipp, H.P., Heckmann, U., *et al.* (1989). Renal mesangium is a target for calcitonin gene related peptide. *Kidney International*, **36**, 222–227.

La Grange, R.G., Sloop, C.H. and Schmid, H.E. (1976). Selective stimulation of renal nerves in the anaesthetized dog. *Clinical Research*, **33**, 704–712.

Lappe, R.W., Webb, R.L. and Brody, M.J. (1985). Selective destruction of renal afferent versus efferent nerves in rats. *American Journal of Physiology*, **249**, R634–R637.

Ledsome, J.R. (1987). Renal responses to stimulation of left atrial receptors in anaesthetized dogs. In *Cardiogenic reflexes*, edited by R. Hainsworth, P.N. McWilliam, and D.A.S.G. Mary, pp. 106–121. Oxford: Oxford University Press.

Lifschitz, M.D. (1978). Lack of a role for the renal nerves in renal sodium reabsorption in conscious dogs. *Clinical Science and Molecular Medicine*, **54**, 567–572.

Linden, R.J. (1987). The function of atrial receptors. In *Cardiogenic reflexes*, edited by R. Hainsworth, P.N. McWilliam, and D.A.S.G. Mary, pp. 18–39. Oxford: Oxford University Press.

Liu, F.-Y. and Cogan, M.G. (1988). Angiotensin II stimulation of hydrogen ion secretion in the rat early proximal tubule. *Journal of Clinical Investigation*, **82**, 601–607.

Lohmeier, T.E., Reinhart, G.A., Mizelle, H.L., Montani, J.-P., Hildebrandt, D.A., Hester, R.L. and Hord, C.E. (1993). Neurohormonal control of sodium excretion during controlled reductions in cardiac output. *FASEB Journal*, **7**, A188.

Luff, S.E., Hengstberger, S.G., McLachlan, E.M. and Anderson, W.P. (1991). Two types of sympathetic axon innervating the juxtaglomerular arterioles of the rabbit and rat kidney differ structurally from those supplying other arteries. *Journal of Neurocytology*, **20**, 781–795.

Luff, S.E., Hengstberger, S.G., McLachlan, E.M. and Anderson, W.P. (1992). Distribution of sympathetic neuroeffector junctions in the juxtaglomerular region of the rabbit kidney. *Journal of the Autonomic Nervous System*, **40**, 239–254.

Lundin, S. and Thoren, P. (1982). Renal function and sympathetic nerve activity during mental stress in normotensive and spontaneously hypertensive rats. *Acta Physiologica Scandinavica*, **115**, 115–124.

Lundin, S., Ricksten, S.E. and Thoren, P. (1984). Renal sympathetic activity in spontaneously hypertensive rats and normotensive controls, as studied by three different methods. *Acta Physiologica Scandinavica*, **120**, 265–272.

Mackenzie, J. (1893). Some points bearing on the association of sensory disorders and visceral disease. *Brain*, **16**, 21.

Mancia, G., Shepherd, J.T. and Donald, D.E. (1975). Role of cardiac, pulmonary and carotid mechanoreceptors in the control of hind-limb and renal circulation in dogs. *Circulation Research*, **37**, 200–208.

Mangelsen, E.L. and Malvin, R.L. (1978). Renin secretion: Transient response to a step reduction in arterial pressure. *Renal Physiology*, **1**, 247–253.

Marfurt, C.F. and Echtenkamp, S.F. (1991). Sensory innervation of the rat kidney and ureter as revealed by the anterograde transport of wheat germ agglutinin–horse radish perioxidase (WGA–HRP) from dorsal root ganglia. *Journal of Comparative Neurology*, **311**, 389–404.

Marfurt, C.F., Echtenkamp, S.F. and Jones, M.A. (1989). Origins of the renal innervation in the primate, *Macaca fascicularis*. *Journal of the Autonomic Nervous System*, **27**, 113–126.

McGiff, J.C. (1980). Interactions of prostaglandins with the kallikrein-kinin and renin–angiotensin systems. *Clinical Science*, **59**, 105s–116s.

McGiff, J.C. and Fasy, T.M. (1965). The relationship of the renal vascular activity of angiotensin II to the autonomic nervous system. *Journal of Clinical Investigation*, **44**, 1911–1923.

McGiff, J.C., Crowshaw, K., Terragno, N.A., Malik, K.U. and Lonigro, A.J. (1972). Differential effect of noradrenaline and renal nerve stimulation on vascular resistance in the dog kidney and the release of a prostaglandin E-like substance. *Clinical Science*, **42**, 223–233.

McKenna, O.C. and Angelakos, E.T. (1968). Adrenergic innervation of the canine kidney. *Circulation Research*, **22**, 345–354.

Meckler, R.L. and Weaver, L. (1984). Comparison of the distributions of renal and splenic neurons in sympathetic ganglia. *Journal of the Autonomic Nervous System*, **11**, 189–200.

Meckler, R.L. and Weaver, L.C. (1988). Characteristics of ongoing and reflex discharge of single splenic and renal sympathetic postganglionic fibres in cats. *Journal of Physiology (London)*, **396**, 139–153.

Miki, K., Hayashida, Y., Sagawa, S. and Shiraki, K. (1989a). Renal sympathetic nerve activity and natriuresis during water immersion in conscious dogs. *American Journal of Physiology*, **256**, R299–R305.

Miki, K., Hayashida, Y., Tajima, F., Iwamoto, J. and Shiraki, K. (1989b). Renal sympathetic nerve activity and renal responses during head-up tilt in conscious dogs. *American Journal of Physiology*, **257**, R337–R343.

Miki, K., Hayashida, Y. and Shiraki, K. (1991). Quantitative and sustained suppression of renal sympathetic nerve activity by left atrial distension in conscious dogs. *Pflügers Archiv: European Journal of Physiology*, **419**, 610–615.

Miki, K., Hayashida, Y. and Shiraki, K. (1993). Cardiac-renal-neural reflex plays a major role in natriuresis induced by left atrial distension in conscious dogs. *American Journal of Physiology*, **264**, R369–R375.

Miller, W.L., Thomas, R.A., Berne, R.M. and Rubio, R. (1978). Adenosine production in the ischaemic kidney. *Circulation Research*, **43**, 390–397.

Minisi, A.J. and Thames, M.D. (1991). Reflexes from ventricular receptors with vagal afferents. In *Reflex control of the circulation*, edited by I.H. Zucker, and J.P. Gilmore, pp. 359–405. Boca Raton: CRC Press.

Mitchell, G.A.G. (1950a). The nerve supply of the kidneys. *Acta Anatomica*, **10**, 1–37.

Mitchell, G.A.G. (1950b). The renal nerves. *British Journal of Urology*, **22**, 269–280.

Mizelle, H.L., Hall, J.E., Woods, L.L., Montani, J-.P., Dzielak, D.J. and Pan, Y.-J. (1987). Role of renal nerves in compensatory adaptation to chronic reductions in sodium intake. *American Journal of Physiology*, **252**, F291–F298.

Mizelle, H.L., Hall, J.E. and Woods, L.L. (1988). Interactions between angiotensin II and renal nerves during chronic sodium deprivation. *American Journal of Physiology*, **255**, F823–F827.

Mizelle, H.L., Hall, J.E. and Montani, J-.P. (1989). Role of renal nerves in control of sodium excretion in chronic congestive heart failure. *American Journal of Physiology*, **256**, F1084–F1093.

Mokotoff, R.G. and Ross, G. (1948). The effect of spinal anaesthesia on renal ischaemia in congestive heart failure. *Journal of Clinical Investigation*, **27**, 335.

Morel, F. and Doucet, A. (1986). Hormonal control of kidney functions at the cell level. *Physiological Reviews*, **66**, 377–468.

Morita, H. and Vatner, S.F. (1985). Effects of volume expansion on renal nerve activity, renal blood flow, and sodium and water excretion in conscious dogs. *American Journal of Physiology*, **249**, F680–F687.

Morita, H., Nishida, Y., Uemura, N. and Hosomi, H. (1987). Effect of pentobarbital anaesthesia on renal sympathetic nerve activity in the rabbit. *Journal of the Autonomic Nervous System*, **20**, 57–64.

Moss, N.G. (1989). Electrophysiological characteristics of renal sensory receptors and afferent renal nerves. *Mineral and Electrolyte Metabolism*, **15**, 59–65.

Moss, N.G., Colindres, R.E. and Gottschalk, C.W. (1992). Neural control of renal function. In *Handbook of Physiology*, section 8, Renal Physiology, edited by E.E. Windhager, pp. 1061–1128. New York: Oxford University Press and the American Physiological Society.

Muller, B.D. and Bell, C. (1986). Vesicular storage of 3,4-dihydroxyphenylethylamine and noradrenaline in terminal sympathetic nerves of dog spleen and kidney. *Journal of Neurochemistry*, **47**, 1370–1375.

Murayama, N., Ruggles, B.T., Gapstur, S.M., Werness, J.L. and Dousa, T.P. (1985). Evidence for β-adrenoceptors in proximal tubules: isoproterenol-sensitive adenylate cyclase in pars recta of canine nephron. *Journal of Clinical Investigation*, **76**, 474–481.

Myers, B.D., Deen, W.M. and Brenner, B.M. (1975). Effects of noradrenaline and angiotensin II on the determinants of glomerular ultrafiltration and proximal tubule fluid reabsorption in the rat. *Circulation Research*, **37**, 101–110.

Navar, L.G. (1978). Renal autoregulation: Perspectives from whole kidney and single nephron studies. *American Journal of Physiology*, **234**, F357–F370.

Niijima, A. (1971). Afferent discharges from arterial mechanoreceptors in the kidney of the rabbit. *Journal of Physiology*, **219**, 477–485.

Ninomiya, I. and Fujita, S. (1976). Reflex effects of thermal stimulation on sympathetic nerve activity to skin and kidney. *American Journal of Physiology*, **230**, 271–278.

Ninomiya, I., Matsuakawa, K. and Nishiura, N. (1988). Central and baroreflex control of sympathetic nerve activity to the heart and kidney in the daily life of the cat. *Clinical and Experimental Hypertension*, **A10**(Suppl 1), 19–31.

Nobiling, R., Gabel, M., Persson, P.B., Dietrich, M.S. and Buhrle, C.P. (1991). Differential effect of neuropeptide-Y on membrane potential of cells in renal arterioles of the hydronephrotic mouse. *Journal of Physiology*, **444**, 317–327.

Norman, R.A. Jr. and Dzielak, D.J. (1982). Role of renal nerves in onset and maintenance of spontaneous hypertension. *American Journal of Physiology*, **243**, H284–H288.

Norman, R.A. Jr., Coleman, T.G. and Dent, A.C. (1980). Pseudohypertension in sinoaortic-denervated rats. *Clinical Science*, **59**, 303–306.

Norman, R.A. Jr., Coleman, T.G. and Dent, A.C. (1981). Continuous monitoring of arterial pressure indicates sinoaortic denervated rats are not hypertensive. *Hypertension*, **3**, 119–125.

Norman, R.A. Jr., Murphy, W.R., Dzielak, D.J., Khraibi, A.A. and Carroll, R.G. (1984). Role of the renal nerves in one-kidney, one clip hypertension in rats. *Hypertension*, **6**, 622–626.

Oparil, S., Sripairojthikoon, W. and Wyss, J.M. (1987). The renal afferent nerves in the pathogenesis of hypertension. *Canadian Journal of Physiology and Pharmacology*, **65**, 1548–1558.

Osborn, J.L., DiBona, G.F. and Thames, M.D. (1981). β_1 receptor mediation of renin secretion elicited by low frequency renal nerve stimulation. *Journal of Pharmacology and Experimental Therapeutics*, **216**, 265–269.

Osborn, J.L., Thames, M.D. and DiBona, G.F. (1982). Role of macula densa in renal nerve modulation of renin secretion. *American Journal of Physiology*, **242**, R367–R371.

Osborn, J.L., Holdaas, H., Thames, M.D. and DiBona, G.F. (1983). Renal adrenoceptor mediation of antinatriuretic and renin secretion responses to low frequency renal nerve stimulation in the dog. *Circulation Research*, **53**, 298–305.

Osborn, J.L., Roman, R.J. and Ewens, J.D. (1988). Renal nerves and the development of Dahl salt-sensitive hypertension. *Hypertension*, **11**, 523–528.

Oswald, H. and Greven, J. (1981). Effects of adrenergic activators and inhibitors on renal function. *Handbook of Experimental Pharmacology*, **54**, 243–288.

Packer, M. (1988). Neurohormonal interactions and adaptations in congestive heart failure. *Circulation*, **77**, 721–730.

Pelayo, J.C. and Blantz, R.C. (1984). Analysis of renal denervation in the hydropenic rat: Interactions with angiotensin II. *American Journal of Physiology*, **246**, F87–F95.

Persson, P.B., Ehmke, H., Kirchheim, H. and Seller, H. (1987). The influence of cardiopulmonary receptors on long-term blood pressure control and plasma renin activity in conscious dogs. *Acta Physiologica Scandinavica*, **130**, 553–561.

Persson, P.B., Ehmke, H., Kirchheim, H. and Seller, H. (1988). Effect of sino-aortic denervation in comparison to cardiopulmonary deafferentiation on long-term blood pressure in conscious dogs. *Pflügers Archiv: European Journal of Physiology*, **411**, 160–166.

Persson, P.B., Ehmke, H., Koegler, U. and Kirchheim, H. (1989). Modulation of natriuresis by sympathetic nerves and angiotensin II in conscious dogs. *American Journal of Physiology*, **256**, F485–F489.

Persson, P.B., Gimpl, G. and Lang, R.E. (1991). Importance of neuropeptide Y in regulation of kidney function. *Annals of the New York Academy of Sciences*, **611**, 156–165.

Peterson, T.V., Benjamin, B.A. and Hurst, N.L. (1988). Renal nerves and renal responses to volume expansion in conscious monkeys. *American Journal of Physiology*, **255**, R388–R394.

Peterson, T.V., Benjamin, B.A., Hurst, N.L. and Euler, C.G. (1991). Renal nerves and postprandial renal excretion in the conscious monkey. *American Journal of Physiology*, **261**, R1197-R1203.

Pettinger, W.A., Umemura, S., Smyth, D.D. and Jeffries, W.B. (1987). Renal α_2-adrenoceptors and the adenylate cyclase-cAMP system: biochemical and physiological interactions. *American Journal of Physiology*, **252**, F199–F208.

Pines, I.U.L. (1959). Electrophysiological investigation on the mechanoreceptors in the intrarenal vessels. *Sechenov Physiological Journal of the USSR (Fiziol zh SSSR)*, **45(11)**, 1339–1347.

Pines, I.U.L. (1960). The electrophysiological characteristics of the afferent connexions of the kidney with the central nervous system. *Sechenov Physiological Journal of the USSR (Fiziol zh SSSR)*, **46(11)**, 1380–1386.

Pomeranz, B.H., Birtch, A.G. and Barger, A.C. (1968). Neural control of intrarenal blood flow. *American Journal of Physiology*, **215**, 1067–1081.

Rankin, A.J., Ashton, N. and Swift, F.V. (1992). The reflex effects of changes in renal perfusion on hindlimb vascular resistance in anaesthetized rabbits. *Pflügers Archiv: European Journal of Physiology*, **421**, 585–590.

Ray, B.S. and Neil, C.L. (1947). Abdominal visceral sensation in man. *Annals of Surgery*, **126**, 709–724.

Recordatti, G.M., Moss, N.G. and Waselkov, L. (1978). Renal chemoreceptors in the rat. *Circulation Research*, **43**, 534–543.

Recordatti, G.M., Moss, N.G., Genovesi, S. and Rogenes, P.R. (1980). Renal receptors in the rat sensitive to alterations of their environment. *Circulation Research*, **46**, 395–405.

Reimann, K.A. and Weaver, L.C. (1980). Contrasting reflex effects evoked by chemical activation of cardiac afferent nerves. *American Journal of Physiology*, **239**, H316–H325.

Reinecke, M. and Forssmann, W.G. (1988). Neuropeptide (neuropeptide Y, neurotensin, vasoactive intestinal polypeptide, substance P, calcitonin gene-related peptide, somatostatin) immunohistochemistry and ultrastructure of renal nerves. *Histochemistry*, **89**, 1–9.

Reinhart, G.A., Lohmeier, T.E. and Hord, C.E. (1993). Role of the renin–angiotensin system in mediating hypertension induced by chronic renal adrenergic stimulation. *Hypertension*, **22**, 442.

Richer, C., Lefevre-Borg, F., Lechaire, J., Gomeni, C., Gomeni, R., Guidicelli, J.F. and Cavero I. (1987). Systemic and regional haemodynamic characterization of α_1 and α_2 adrenoceptor agonists in pithed rats. *Journal of Pharmacology and Experimental Therapeutics*, **240**, 944–953.

Riedel, W. and Peter, W. (1977). Non-uniformity of regional vasomotor activity indicating the existance of 2 different systems in the sympathetic cardiovascular outflow. *Experientia*, **33**, 337–338.

Riedel, W., Kozawa, E. and Iriki, M. (1982). Renal and cutaneous vasomotor and respiratory rate adjustments to peripheral cold and warm stimuli and to bacterial endotoxin in conscious rabbits. *Journal of the Autonomic Nervous System*, **5**, 177–194.

Robins, A. and Sato, Y. (1991). Cardiovascular changes in response to uterine stimulation. *Journal of the Autonomic Nervous System*, **33**, 55–64.

Rogenes, P.R. (1982). Single-unit and multiunit analyses of renorenal reflexes elicited by stimulation of renal chemoreceptors in the rat. *Journal of the Autonomic Nervous System*, **6**, 143–156.

Romson, J.L., Haack, D.W. and Lucchesi, B.R. (1980). Electrical induction of coronary artery thrombosis in the ambulatory canine: a model for *in vivo* evaluation of anti-thrombotic agents. *Thrombosis Research*, **17**, 841–853.

Rudd, M.A., Grippo, R.S. and Arendshorst, W.J. (1986). Acute renal denervation produces a diuresis and natriuresis in young SHR but not WKY rats. *American Journal of Physiology*, **251**, F655–F661.

Ryuzaki, M., Suzuki, H., Kumagai, K., Kumagai, H., Ichikawa, M., Matsukawa, S., et al. (1992). Renal nerves contribute to salt-induced hypertension in sinoaortic-denervated uninephrectomized rabbits. *American Journal of Physiology*, **262**, R733–R737.

Sadowski, J., Kurkus, J. and Gellert, R. (1979). Denervated and intact kidney responses to saline load in awake and anaesthetized dogs. *American Journal of Physiology*, **237**, F262–F267.

Saeki, Y., Terui, N. and Kumada, M. (1988). Physiological characterization of the renal-sympathetic reflex in rabbits. *Japanese Journal of Physiology*, **38**, 251–266.

Salazar, A.E. (1961). Experimental myocardial infarction. Induction of coronary thrombosis in the intact closed-chest dog. *Circulation Research*, **9**, 1351–1356.

Salgado, H.C. and Krieger, E.M. (1973). Reversibility of baroreceptor adaptation in chronic hypertension. *Clinical Science and Molecular Medicine*, **45**, 123s.

Sawyer, P.N., Pate, J.W. and Weldon, C.S. (1953). Relations of abnormal and injury electric potential differences to intravascular thrombosis. *American Journal of Physiology*, **175**, 108–112.

Säynävälammi, P., Vaalasti, A., Pyykönen, M.-L., Ylitalo, P. and Vapaatalo, H. (1982). The effect of renal sympathectomy on blood pressure and plasma renin activity in spontaneously hypertensive and normotensive rats. *Acta Physiologica Scandinavica*, **115**, 289–293.

Schad, H. and Seller, H. (1975). A method for recording autonomic nerve activity in unanaesthetized, freely moving cats. *Brain Research*, **100**, 425–430.

Schnermann, J., Briggs, J.P. and Weber, P.C. (1984). Tubuloglomerular feedback, prostaglandins, and angiotensin in the autoregulation of glomerular filtration rate. *Kidney International*, **25**, 53–64.

Schrier, R.W. (1974). Effects of adrenergic nervous system and catecholamines on systemic and renal haemodynamics, sodium, and water excretion and renin secretion. *Kidney International*, **6**, 291–306.

Schultz, H.D., Fater, D.C., Sundet, W.D., Geer, P.G. and Goetz, K.L. (1982). Reflexes elicited by acute stretch of atrial vs. pulmonary receptors in conscious dogs. *American Journal of Physiology*, **242**, H1065–H1076.

Schuster, V.L., Kokko, J.P. and Jacobson, H.R. (1984). Angiotensin II directly stimulates transport in rabbit proximal convoluted tubules. *Journal of Clinical Investigation*, **73**, 507–515.

Seagard, J.L., Hopp, F.A., Bosnjak, Z.J., Osborn, J.L. and Kampine, J.P. (1984). Sympathetic efferent nerve activity in conscious and isoflurane-anaesthetized dogs. *Anaesthesiology*, **61**, 266–270.

Selkurt, E. (1963). The renal circulation. In *Handbook of Physiology, Circulation, Volume II*, pp. 1456–1516. Washington, D.C.: American Physiological Society.

Shepherd, J.T. and Mancia, G. (1986). Reflex control of the human cardiovascular system. *Reviews of Physiology, Biochemistry, and Pharmacology*, **105**, 1–99.

Shralev, V.N. (1966). Problems in the morphology and nature of renal innervation. Arkhiv Anatomii, Gistologii i Embriologii, vol. 49, p. 54, 1965. In *Federal Proceedings* [Translation Supplement 25], T295–T600.

Simon, O.R. and Schramm, L.P. (1984). The spinal course and medullar termination of myelinated renal afferents in the rat. *Brain Research*, **290**, 239–247.

Simpson, R.U. and Goodfriend, T.L. (1984). Angiotensin and prostaglandin interactions in cultured kidney tubules. *Journal of Laboratory and Clinical Medicine*, **103**, 255–271.

Sit, S.P., Morita, H. and Vatner, S.F. (1984). Responses of renal haemodynamics and function to acute volume expansion in conscious dogs. *Circulation Research*, **54**, 185–195.

Skott, O. and Briggs, J.P. (1987). Direct demonstration of macula densa-mediated renin secretion. *Science*, **237**, 1618–1620.

Smith, H.W. (1939). Physiology of the renal circulation. *Harvey Lectures*, **35**, 166.

Smith, H.W. (1951). *The Kidney. Structure and Function in Health and Disease*. New York: Oxford University Press.

Smith, F.G., Sato, T., McWeeny, O.L., Torres, L. and Robillard, J.E. (1989). Role of renal nerves in response to volume expansion in conscious newborn lambs. *American Journal of Physiology*, **257**, R1519–R1525.

Smits, J.F. and Brody, M.J. (1984). Activation of afferent renal nerves by intrarenal bradykinin in conscious rats. *American Journal of Physiology*, **247**, R1003–R1008.

Sripairojthikoon, W. and Wyss, J.M. (1987). Cells of origin of the sympathetic renal innervation in rat. *American Journal of Physiology*, **252**, F957–F963.

Stein, J.H., Boonjarern, S., Mark, R.C. and Ferris, T.F. (1973). Mechanism of the redistribution of renal cortical blood flow during haemorrhagic hypotension in the dog. *Journal of Clinical Investigation*, **52**, 39–47.

Stein, R.D. and Weaver, L.C. (1988). Multi- and single fibre mesenteric and renal sympathetic responses to chemical stimulation of intestinal receptors in cats. *Journal of Physiology*, **396**, 155–172.

Stella, A. and Zanchetti, A. (1977). Effects of renal denervation on renin release in response to tilting and furosemide. *American Journal of Physiology*, **232**, H500–H507.

Stella, A., Calaresu, F. and Zanchetti, A. (1976). Neural factors contributing to renin release during reduction in renal perfusion pressure and blood flow in cats. *Clinical Science and Molecular Medicine*, **51**, 453–461.

Strandhoy, J.W., Morris, M. and Buckalew, V.M. Jr. (1982). Renal effects of the antihypertensive, guanabenz, in the dog. *Journal of Pharmacology and Experimental Therapeutics*, **221**, 347–352.

Su, H.C., Wharton, J., Polack, J.M., Mulderry, P.K., Ghatel, M.A., Gibson, S.J., *et al.* (1986). Calcitonin gene-related peptide immunoreactivity in afferent neurons supplying the urinary tract: combined retrograde tracing and immunohistochemistry. *Neuroscience*, **18**, 727–747.

Sweet, W.D., Freeman, R.H., Davis, J.O. and Vari, R.C. (1985). Ganglionic blockade in conscious dogs with chronic caval constriction. *American Journal of Physiology*, **249**, H1038–H1044.

Szalay, L., Benscath, P. and Takacs, L. (1977a). Effect of splanchnicotomy on the renal excretion of inorganic phosphate in the anaesthetized dog. *Pflügers Archiv: European Journal of Physiology*, **367**, 283–286.

Szalay, L., Benscath, P. and Takacs, L. (1977b). Effect of splanchnicotomy on the renal excretion of para-aminohippuric acid in the anaesthetized dog. *Pflügers Archiv: European Journal of Physiology*, **367**, 287–290.

Szalay, L., Lang, E., Benscath, P., Mohai, L., Fischer, A. and Takacs, L. (1977). Effect of splanchnicotomy on the renal excretion of uric acid in anaesthetized dogs. *Pflügers Archiv: European Journal of Physiology*, **368**, 185–188.

Takahashi, H., Iyoda, I., Yamasaki, H., Takeda, K., Okajima, H., Sasaki, S., *et al.* (1984). Retardation of the development of hypertension in DOCA-salt rats by renal denervation. *Japanese Circulation Journal*, **48**, 567–574.

Thames, M.D. and Abboud, F.M. (1979). Interaction of somatic and cardiopulmonary receptors in control of renal circulation. *American Journal of Physiology*, **237**, H560–H565.

Thames, M.D. and DiBona, G.F. (1979). Renal nerves modulate the secretion of renin mediated by nonneural mechanisms. *Circulation Research*, **44**, 645–652.

Thames, M.D., Miller, B.D. and Abboud, F.M. (1982). Baroreflex regulation of renal nerve activity during volume expansion. *American Journal of Physiology*, **243**, H810–H814.

Thoren, P. (1979). Role of cardiac vagal C-fibers in cardiovascular control. *Reviews of Physiology, Biochemistry, and Pharmacology*, **86**, 1–94.

Thoren, P. and Ricksten, S.E. (1979). Recordings of renal and splanchnic sympathetic nervous activity in normotensive and spontaneously hypertensive rats. *Clinical Science*, **57**, 197s–199s.

Uchida, Y., Kamisaka, K. and Ueda, H. (1971). Two types of renal mechanoreceptors. *Japanese Heart Journal*, **12**, 233–241.

Van Vliet, B.N., Smith, M.J. and Guyton, A.C. (1991). Time course of renal responses to greater splanchnic nerve stimulation. *American Journal of Physiology*, **260**, R894–R905.

Vander, A.J. (1965). Effect of catecholamines and the renal nerves on renin secretion in anaesthetized dogs. *American Journal of Physiology*, **209**, 659–662.

Vander, A.J. (1967). Control of renin release. *Physiological Reviews*, **47**, 359–382.

Vari, R.C., Zinn, S., Verburg, K.M. and Freeman, R.H. (1987). Renal nerves and the pathogenesis of angiotensin-induced hypertension. *Hypertension*, **9**, 345–349.

Vatner, S.F. (1974). Effects of haemorrhage on regional blood flow distribution in dogs and primates. *Journal of Clinical Investigation*, **54**, 225–235.

Vatner, S.F., Manders, W.T. and Knight, D.R. (1986). Vagally mediated regulation of renal function in conscious primates. *American Journal of Physiology*, **250**, H546–H549.

Villarreal, D., Freeman, R.H., Davis, J.O., Garoutte, G. and Sweet, W.D. (1984). Pathogenesis of one-kidney, one-clip hypertension in rats after renal denervation. *American Journal of Physiology*, **247**, H61–H66.

Wang, W., Chen, J.-S. and Zucker, I.H. (1990). Carotid sinus baroreceptor sensitivity in experimental heart failure. *Circulation*, **81**, 1959–1966.

Weaver, L.C. (1977). Cardiopulmonary sympathetic afferent influences on renal nerve activity. *American Journal of Physiology*, **233**, H592–H599.

Webb, R.L. and Brody, M.J. (1987). Functional identification of the central projections of afferent renal nerves. *Clinical and Experimental Hypertension*, **A9**(Suppl 1), 47–57.

Weinman, E.J., Sansom, S.C., Knight, T.F. and Senekjian, H.O. (1982). α and β-adrenergic agonist stimulated water adsorption in the rat proximal tubule. *Journal of Membrane Biology*, **69**, 107–111.

White, J.C. (1942). Sensory innervation of the viscera. Studies on visceral afferent neurones in man based on neurosurgical procedures for the relief of intractable pain. *Research Publications of the Association for Research of Nervous and Mental Disease*, **23**, 373–390.

Winternitz, S.R., Katholi, R.E. and Oparil, S. (1980). Role of the renal sympathetic nerves in the development and maintenance of hypertension in the spontaneously hypertensive rat. *Journal of Clinical Investigation*, **66**, 971–978.

Wolf, S., Pfeiffer, J.B., Ripley, H.S., Winger, O.S. and Wolf, H.G. (1948). Hypertension as a reaction pattern to stress: Summary of experimental data on variations in blood pressure and renal blood flow. *Annals of Internal Medicine*, **29**, 1056.

Wolff, D.W., Gesek, F.A. and Strandhoy, J.W. (1987). *In vivo* assessment of rat renal α-adrenoceptors. *Journal of Pharmacology and Experimental Therapeutics*, **241**, 472–476.

Wolff, D.W., Colindres, R.E. and Strandhoy, J.W. (1989). Unmasking sensitive α_2-adrenoceptor-mediated renal vasoconstriction in conscious rats. *American Journal of Physiology*, **257**, F1132–F1139.

Wright, F.S. (1984). Intrarenal regulation of glomerular filtration rate. *Journal of Hypertension*, **2**, 105–113.

Wyss, M. and Donovan, M.K. (1984). A direct projection from the kidney to the brainstem. *Brain Research*, **298**, 130–134.

Wyss, J.M., Aboukarsh, N. and Oparil, S. (1986). Sensory denervation of the kidney attenuates renovascular hypertension in the rat. *American Journal of Physiology*, **250**, H82–H86.

Wyss, J.M., Sripairojthikoon, W. and Oparil, S. (1987). Failure of renal denervation to attenuate hypertension in Dahl NaCl-sensitive rats. *Canadian Journal of Physiology and Pharmacology*, **65**, 2428–2432.

Yang, H.M. and Lohmeier, T.E. (1993). Influence of endogenous angiotensin on the renovascular response to noradrenaline. *Hypertension*, **21**, 695–703.

Zambraski, E.J. (1989). Renal nerves in renal sodium retaining states: cirrhotic ascites, congestive heart failure, nephrotic syndrome. *Mineral and Electrolyte Metabolism*, **15**, 5–15.

Zambraski, E.J., DiBona, G.F. and Kaloyanides, G.J. (1976). Effect of sympathetic blocking agents on the antinatriuresis of reflex renal nerve stimulation. *Journal of Pharmacology and Experimental Therapeutics*, **198**, 464–472.

Zimmerman, H.D. (1975). Myelinated nerve fibers in the rat kidney. Light and electron microscopic studies. *Cell and Tissue Research*, **160**, 485–493.

Zimmerman, B.G., Sybertz, E.J. and Wong, P.C. (1984). Interaction between sympathetic and renin–angiotensin system. *Journal of Hypertension*, **2**, 581–588.

Zucker, I.H. (1986). Left ventricular receptors: physiological controllers or pathological curiosities? *Basic Research in Cardiology*, **81**, 539–557.

Zucker, I.H. (1991). Baro and cardiac reflex abnormalities in chronic heart failure. In *Reflex control of the circulation*, edited by I.H. Zucker, and J.P. Gilmore, pp. 849–873. Boca Raton: CRC Press.

Zucker, I.H., Earle, A.M. and Gilmore, J.P. (1977). The mechanism of adaptation of left atrial stretch receptors in dogs with chronic congestive heart failure. *Journal of Clinical Investigation*, **60**, 323–331.

Zucker, I.H., Gorman, A.J., Cornish, K.G. and Lang, M. (1985). Impaired atrial receptor modulation or renal nerve activity in dogs with chronic volume overload. *Cardiovascular Research*, **19**, 411–418.

12 Neural Control of the Gastro-Intestinal Circulation

Christopher J. Mathias[1,2,*], K. Ray Chaudhuri[2,1]
and Thomas Thomaides[1,2]

[1] *Cardiovascular Medicine Unit, Department of Medicine,*
St Mary's Hospital Medical School/Imperial College of Science,
Technology and Medicine, London, UK
[2] *Autonomic Unit, University Department of Clinical Neurology,*
Institute of Neurology and National Hospital for Neurology
and Neurosurgery, Queen Square, London, UK

The gastro-intestinal circulation is unique in having a rich sympathetic and parasympathetic nerve supply and also an "enteric nervous system", with neurons and supporting cells. These secrete neuropeptides and amines along with a wide range of other substances which, either directly or indirectly, affect blood flow. The sympathetic nerves play an important role, which is predominantly mediated through α-adrenoceptors. The gastro-intestinal circulation is particularly sensitive to certain circulating peptides, such as vasopressin and angiotensin II; variable effects are exerted by those substances secreted through the enteric nervous system. The neural control of the gastro-intestinal circulation, during a number of physiological states, which include food ingestion, exposure to exercise and changes in temperature, and the interaction with different humoral substances, is discussed. Examples of how the study of certain diseases have contributed to the understanding of the physiological principles governing control of this large circulatory bed are provided.

KEY WORDS: autonomic nervous system; gastro-intestinal circulation; peptides; autonomic failure; superior mesenteric artery blood flow.

INTRODUCTION

The gastro-intestinal circulation is one of the largest vascular beds in the body. It is the recipient of about 25% of the cardiac output at rest, and may contain up to 30% of the blood

---

*Author for correspondence: Professor C.J. Mathias, Pickering Unit, Department of Medicine, St Mary's Hospital, Imperial College School of Medicine, Praed Street, London W2 1NY, UK.

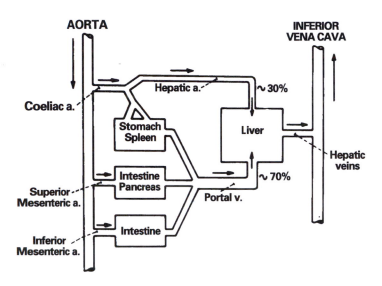

Figure 12.1 Schematic representation of the splanchnic circulation indicating the arterial supply to the stomach and intestine and the venous drainage into the portal vein which supplies the liver with approximately 70% of its flow, the remaining 30% being supplied by the hepatic artery (From Rowell, 1986).

volume. It is involved in digestive and absorptive processes which are critical for energy requirements and for the maintenance of water and electrolyte balance. It also has a major role in cardiovascular homeostasis. In addition to myogenic and neurogenic factors, there is increasing evidence that both circulating and local hormones influence this vascular bed.

In this chapter the neural control of the gastro-intestinal circulation will be described, with an emphasis on factors influencing it under various physiological conditions. The hepatic circulation will not be discussed. Reference also will be made to disease states which have contributed to our understanding of the neural control of this vascular region in man.

VASCULAR ANATOMY

The gastro-intestinal circulation is derived primarily from three major blood vessels which emerge from the abdominal aorta, namely, the coeliac, superior mesenteric and inferior mesenteric artery (Figure 12.1). The coeliac trunk emerges just beneath the diaphragm and branches into the common hepatic artery which divides into the right gastric and gastro-duodenal artery, left gastric artery and splenic artery. The stomach, therefore, has an arterial supply from a number of divisions of the coeliac axis. The superior mesenteric artery leaves the aorta 1 centimetre below the coeliac trunk and supplies the entire small intestine, except for the superior part of the duodenum; it also supplies the caecum, the ascending colon and most of the transverse colon. In 17% of the normal population it may give rise to an accessory right hepatic artery. The major branches of the superior mesenteric artery are the inferior pancreatico-duodenal, jejunal, ileal, ileo-colic, and right and middle colic arteries. The inferior mesenteric artery supplies the rest of the colon and rectum and emerges 4 centimetres above the aortic bifurcation.

The portal system is effectively the gastro-intestinal venous system, and also drains the abdominal viscera. The portal vein begins at the junction of the splenic and superior mesenteric veins, anterior to the inferior vena cava and posterior to the neck of the pancreas. The splenic vein is joined by the inferior mesenteric vein which drains the area supplied by the artery. The superior mesenteric vein drains part of the stomach, the pancreas and the small intestine and colon up to the middle of the transverse colon. The portal vein divides into a right branch which enters the right hepatic lobe and a left branch which divides to supply the other lobes. The portal vein is also directly joined by gastric, cystic and other smaller veins. Its branches divide further into smaller vessels and end in the sinusoids from where vessels converge to form the hepatic veins which join the inferior vena cava.

INNERVATION

The neural supply of the gut consists of both sympathetic and parasympathetic nerves, and the enteric nervous system. The sympathetic supply is from preganglionic fibres from the fifth to the tenth thoracic ganglia which form the greater splanchnic nerve, and from the ninth to the tenth or (eleventh) thoracic ganglia which form the lesser splanchnic nerve. The greater splanchnic nerves on each side supply the coeliac ganglia and the two sides form the coeliac plexus which surround the coeliac artery and the root of the superior mesenteric artery. There are connections to the aortico-renal ganglia, which receive the lesser splanchnic nerves, and to a number of secondary plexuses around the vessels; these plexuses include the superior mesenteric plexus (which contains the superior mesenteric ganglion), and the abdominal aortic plexus, with nerves supplying both blood vessels and the musculature. These contain branches from the coeliac plexus and the 1st and 2nd lumbar nerves.

The parasympathetic supply is mainly from the vagus through its oesophageal, gastric, coeliac and hepatic branches. The coeliac branches of the posterior vagal trunk join the coeliac plexus. The inferior mesenteric ganglion is supplied by the pelvic parasympathetic nerves.

The superior gastric plexus is anterior to the aortic bifurcation and contains both sympathetic fibres and also parasympathetic fibres from the pelvic splanchnic nerves; these are distributed along the inferior mesenteric artery.

The afferent nerves from the viscera, which include vagal afferents from the gastric and intestinal walls and the digestive glands, appear to respond to stretch and contraction. In the distal part of the colon and pelvis they also respond to distension, and travel within the pelvic splanchnic nerves. These afferents end in spinal cord segments from which preganglionic fibres usually innervate the region or the visceral organ concerned.

In addition to the well-defined parasympathetic and sympathetic supply to the gastro-intestinal tract, there is an additional system, the "enteric nervous system", which consists of enteric neurons and supporting cells within the walls of the gastro-intestinal tract and associated organs (Furness and Costa, 1987). Langley (1921), noted that there were differences in histological appearances and anatomical connections, and a disproportion between nerve fibres and numerous enteric nerve cells. Furthermore, there were complete

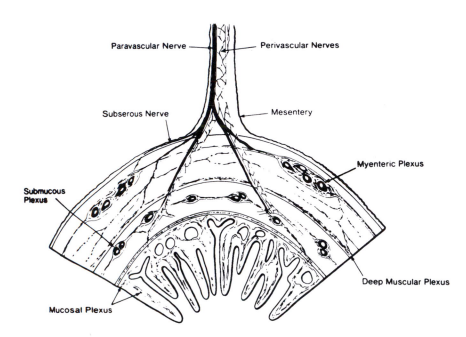

Figure 12.2 Diagrammatic representations of the enteric plexuses as seen in transverse section of the intestine
(From Furness and Costa, 1980).

reflex pathways within the enteric nervous system, which worked independently of other
components of the sympathetic and parasympathetic nervous system, as observed in many
clinical autonomic disorders. The major enteric plexuses, as best seen in the small intestine,
are the myenteric (Auerbach's) plexus and submucosal (Meissner's) plexus (Figure 12.2).
The functions of the enteric nervous system are closely linked to the endocrine cells within
the gastro-intestinal tract which are actively concerned with the secretion of a large number
of hormones, many of which have direct vascular effects, or exert indirect effects through
a multitude of actions, including modulation of activity of autonomic nerves.

The innervation of the gut is closely linked to its arteries, which contain paravascular
and perivascular nerves (Figure 12.2). The former follow the arterial blood supply, and
innervate the gastro-intestinal tract and associated organs en route, including the enteric
ganglia. The perivascular nerves form a fine meshwork or plexus of anastomosing nerves
around the arteries and are actively concerned with dilatation or constriction. The veins in
the mesentery also have a perivascular plexus.

MEASUREMENT OF GASTRO-INTESTINAL BLOOD FLOW

Blood flow measurements may be either invasive as used in animal and some human
studies, or non-invasive, especially in man. These usually measure blood flow in major

vessels supplying different regions of the gut. There are also techniques which measure total splanchnic blood flow, such as that using indocyanine green (ICG) as an indicator.

INVASIVE TECHNIQUES

These can be direct or indirect. In experimental animal studies, the main or branch arteries can be directly cannulated and flow transducers introduced, or the effluent timed. Flow transducers may also be placed around the major vessels and have been particularly useful in chronic instrumentation for the study of conscious animals. The possibility of damage to perivascular nerves, however, cannot be discounted. The levels of flow may vary depending on the circumstances of measurement, whether the animals are conscious or anaesthetised, and in different species.

In man, the invasive techniques employ intra-arterial catheterisation of splanchnic blood vessels, with either a spill-over angiographic reflux (Clark *et al.*, 1980; Anderson and Gianturo, 1981), or a video dilution method (Lanz *et al.*, 1981). The former consists of injection of a contrast medium and assessment of reflux from the mesenteric artery into the aorta. With the latter, superior mesenteric artery blood flow can be expressed as a percentage of cardiac output. Other techniques include the use of inert gases (Hulten *et al.*, 1976), such as 85 Krypton or 133 Xenon, which are injected intra-arterially with the elimination curve of the isotope recorded using a scintillation detector or a Geiger/Muller counting tube.

NON-INVASIVE TECHNIQUES

These have been mainly developed for use in man. With the dye dilution method, non-toxic dyes, such as indocyanine green or bromosulphaphthalein, are infused intravenously at a constant rate, with assessment of flow dependent on the removal of the dye by the liver (Norryd *et al.*, 1974; Rowell, 1975). This technique is probably a better assessment of hepatic clearance, but it provides an overall measure of splanchnic blood flow. The use of technetium 99-labelled red cells and scintigraphy provide a measure of splanchnic blood volume, and also individual organ volume before and after stimulation (Flamm *et al.*, 1990). Measurement of regional blood flow has been considerably aided by the adaptation of transcutaneous, ultrasonic, pulsed Doppler flowmetry for splanchnic blood vessels (Qamar *et al.*, 1986; Moneta *et al.*, 1988; Kooner, Peart and Mathias, 1989a; Nakamura *et al.*, 1989; Chaudhuri *et al.*, 1991) (Figure 12.3). It is dependent on adequate visualisation of the blood vessels to enable measurement of vessel diameter and velocity, from which blood flow can be calculated. This has been successfully used for coeliac and superior mesenteric artery blood flow. The method correlates well with *in vitro* pulsatile systems (Kooner *et al.*, 1989a), is reproducible (Chaudhuri *et al.*, 1991) (Figure 12.4), and provides results similar to those obtained with invasive techniques (Table 12.1).

PHYSIOLOGICAL/PHARMACOLOGICAL ASPECTS

Various aspects of the gastro-intestinal circulation are now described in different situations where neural control is exerted. The initial sections deal with sympathetic control, followed

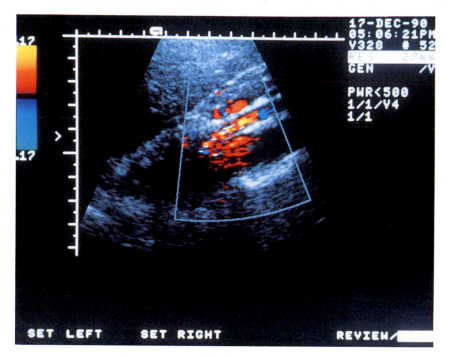

a

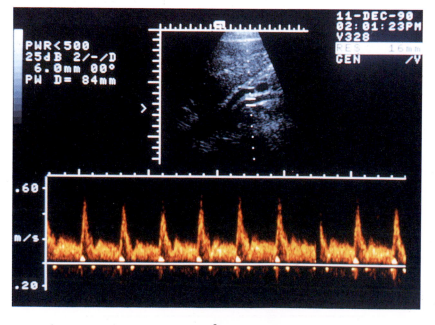

b

Figure 12.3 Real time, two dimensional colour Doppler image showing the superior mesenteric artery and coeliac artery arising from the aorta in longitudinal section. (a) The red colour signifies blood flowing towards the transducer. In (b) the SMA is shown with a cursor placed within its lumen so as to obtain the frequency shift signal (from Chaudhuri *et al.*, 1991).

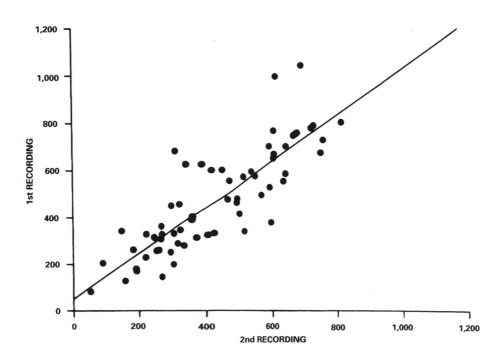

Figure 12.4   Correlation between superior mesenteric artery blood flow values (base line and during stimulation) during the initial (first, 1st) recording and a repeat (second, 2nd) recording under identical circumstances two months later. There is a close correlation ($R = +0.071$, $P < 0.05$) between the two recordings. Measurement with this non-invasive technique within each individual is highly reproducible (From Chaudhuri *et al.*, 1991).

TABLE 12.1

Comparison of superior mesenteric artery blood flow (SMABF) values by invasion and non-invasive methods in man. The mean value is provided with range in brackets, when available or with the ± SEM

	Method	SMABF (ml/min)
Clark *et al.*, 1980 (7)	Spill-over reflux	456 (300–600)
Norryd *et al.*, 1974 (10)	Dye-dilution	708 (620–880)
Hulten *et al.*, 1976 (9)	Inert gas washout	500–600
Qamar *et al.*, 1986 (13)	Doppler ultrasound	517 (250–890)
Nakamura *et al.*, 1989 (14)	Doppler ultrasound	478 ± 166
Moneta *et al.*, 1988 (15)	Doppler ultrasound	538 ± 37
Chaudhuri *et al.*, 1991 (17)	Doppler ultrasound	594 (280–1085)

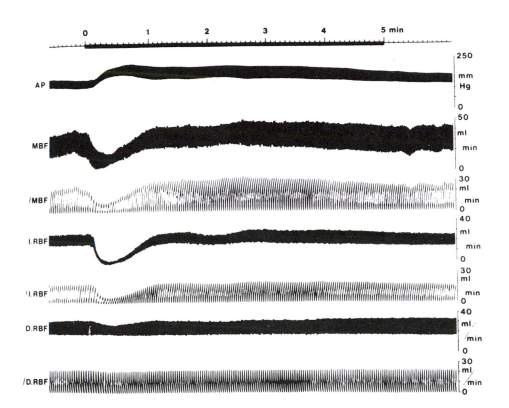

Figure 12.5 Changes in systemic arterial blood pressure (AP) and blood flow in the mesenteric circulation, innervated kidney and denervated kidney, caused by intestinal receptor stimulation in the vagotomised, sino-aortic denervated cat. MBF, i.RBF and D. RBF = mesenteric, innervated renal and denervated renal blood flow, respectively; /MBF, RBF and DRBF = mean mesenteric, innervated kidney and denervated kidney mean renal blood flow, respectively. Stimulation of intestinal receptors by bradykinin causes a greater rise in systemic AP than in normally innervated cats. Mesenteric artery blood flow and conductance decreased during the first minute of stimulation, and then returned to values equal to or greater than controls, despite continuation of stimulation. This provides an example of autoregulatory escape. (From Weaver et al., 1987).

by a brief section on possible cholinergic influences. The role of peptides and autacoids, especially those directly or indirectly concerned with sympathetic stimulation *in vivo*, is discussed.

NEURAL STIMULATION

Sympathetic

Stimulation of the sympathetic nervous system, either directly, reflexly, or by mimicking its action using the neurotransmitter noradrenaline, results in constriction of splanchnic arteries. This was demonstrated by Pfluger in 1855, and has been confirmed on numerous occasions *in vitro*, in both animal and human tissue (Bunch, 1899; Hulten, Lindhagen and Lundgren, 1977; Bohlen *et al.*, 1978; Bell *et al.*, 1990). Unlike vessels in skeletal muscle and adipose tissue (Hadjiminas and Oberg, 1968), however, sympathetically-mediated vasoconstriction does not persist, and is usually followed, within two minutes, by return of flow towards the base line level, despite continuation of stimulation. This was first shown by Folkow *et al.* in 1964 and is referred to as "autoregulatory escape". It results mainly from dilatation in the arterioles and not the precapillary sphincters or venous capacitance vessels (Folkow *et al.*, 1964; Patel, Bose and Greenway, 1981). Autoregulatory escape also occurs during reflex activation (Oberg, 1964; Hadjiminas and Oberg, 1968; Weaver *et al.*, 1987) (Figure 12.5), but is independent of the brain and the autonomic ganglia, as it also occurs during post-ganglionic mesenteric nerve stimulation (Greenway, Scott and Zink, 1976; Fasth, Hulten and Nordgren, 1980). The mechanisms responsible for autoregulatory escape continue to be debated. Whether tachyphylaxis is due to changes in receptors and their effects, or due to the formation and release of other substances, including those which are dependent upon the production of vasodilator substances from the endothelium, is unclear. Developing swine are less capable of autoregulatory escape (Buckley *et al.*, 1987); whether this contributes to intestinal ischaemia, as seen in necrotizing enteritis in the newborn, is unclear.

The neurochemical basis for vasoconstriction induced by sympathetic stimulation has been delineated more clearly. Vasoconstriction is clearly dependent on α-adrenoceptor activation. Both α_1- and α_2-adrenoceptors are present within the vasculature of the mesentery. Noradrenaline causes vasoconstriction (Aviado, 1959), along with other α-adrenoceptor agonists, such as methoxamine (Richardson, 1973; Heyndrickx, Boettcher and Vatner, 1976). The effects are largely dependent on α_1-adrenoceptors, as they are blocked by the α-adrenoceptor antagonists, phentolamine and thymoxamine (Collis and Alps, 1973). Phenoxybenzamine reverses the effects of sympathetic stimulation, revealing a vasodilatation. This may be related to its non-selective α-adrenoceptor blocking effects, as it also inhibits presynaptic α_2-adrenoceptors, which facilitate noradrenaline release, and can be blocked by the α_2-adrenoceptor antagonist, yohimbine (Drew and Whiting, 1979). Effects independent of α-adrenoceptors such as through β-adrenoceptor stimulation may explain the vasodilatation caused by phenoxybenzamine; isoprenaline, for instance, is known to cause intestinal vasodilatation (Taira and Yabuchi, 1977). β-adrenoceptors thus also influence the gastro-intestinal circulation, causing dilatation when stimulated and contributing to constriction when blocked, especially if this may cause a relative increase in α-adrenoceptor stimulation. This probably occurs with the non-selective β-adrenoceptor antagonist, β-blocker propranolol, which increases vascular splanchnic resistance, and has been used beneficially in patients with cirrhosis and portal hypertension.

Stimulation of sympathetic nerves may also result in the release of various co-transmitters, which may act on the vasculature. These include neuropeptide Y (NPY) and adenosine triphosphate (ATP), which also influence the vasculature through post junctional synergism (Ralevic and Burnstock, 1990). Sympathetic stimulation *in vivo* may also result in the release of renin (and formation of angiotensin II), and vasopressin, which have constrictor effects on splanchnic vessels. During situations *in vivo,* such as haemorrhage and hypovolaemia, the changes induced in the splanchnic region (Fell, 1966) may be due to the actions of these

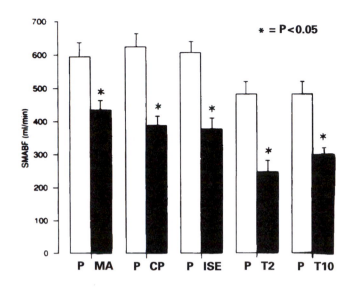

Figure 12.6a Superior mesenteric artery blood flow (SMABF) before (open histograms) and during (filled histograms) a series of pressor tests (mental arithmetic, MA; cold pressor test, CP; isometric exercise, ISE) and head-up tilt to 45 after 2 (T2) and 10 minutes (T10). Each manouevre resulted in stimulation of the sympathetic nervous system (From Chaudhuri et al., 1991).

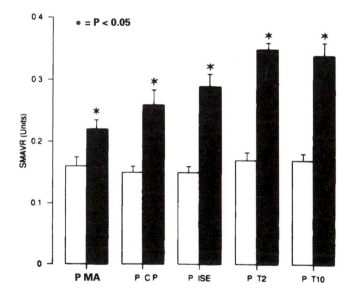

Figure 12.6b Calculated superior mesenteric artery vascular resistance in the same subjects before and during each of the stimuli known to increase sympatho-neural activity, as in 6a (From Chaudhuri et al., 1991).

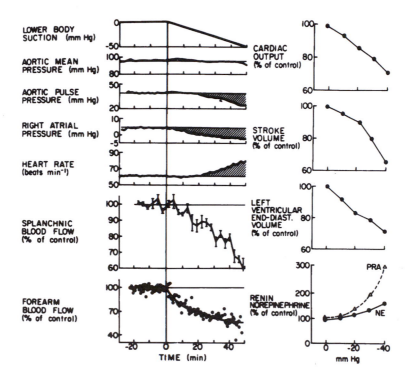

Figure 12.7 Cardiovascular responses to graded lower body suction in normal subjects. Panels on the left show the average responses to negative pressure applied at a continuous rate of minus 1 mm Hg/min (From Johnson *et al.*, 1974). Panels on the right show the central circulatory and hormonal responses to 10 mm Hg steps negative pressure down to −40 mm Hg (Ahmad *et al.*, 1977). Aortic pressure is maintained despite a marked fall in cardiac output, because of readjustments which include an early reduction in blood flow to both muscle and skin followed by a decrease in splanchnic blood flow. (combination figure from Rowell, 1986)

hormones. This has been demonstrated during hypovolaemia, with reversal of constriction by appropriate antagonists (Gardiner, Compton and Bennett, 1989).

In man, the splanchnic circulation is richly supplied by sympathetic efferent nerves, which may be involved in a wide range of reflex activity, from arterial baroreceptors controlling blood pressure homeostasis, to central receptors controlling body temperature. During short-lived stimuli which raise blood pressure by increasing sympathetic neural activity, such as mental arithmetic, the cold pressor test and isometric exercise, there is a reduction in superior mesenteric artery blood flow (SMABF), with a rise in superior mesenteric artery vascular resistance (SMAVR), consistent with active constriction within this major splanchnic artery (Chaudhuri *et al.*, 1991) (Figures 12.6a, b). Whether or not constriction with sympatho-neural stimuli is maintained or reversed by autoregulatory escape, is not known. When reflex sympathetic stimulation through activation of baroreceptors is maintained for longer periods, such as during head-up tilt and lower body negative pressure (Johnson *et al.*, 1974; Chaudhuri *et al.*, 1991) (Figure 12.7) there is also a definite reduction

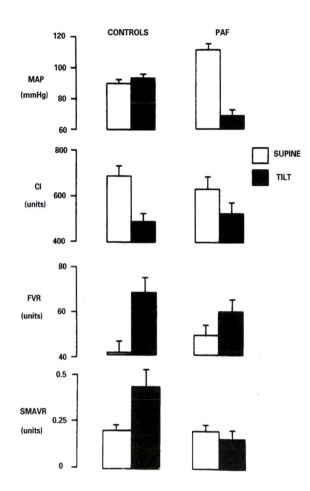

Figure 12.8 Mean arterial blood pressure (MAP), cardiac index (CI), forearm vascular resistance (FVR) and superior mesenteric artery vascular resistance (SMAVR) in normal subjects (controls) and in patients with chronic pure autonomic failure (PAF) while supine (open histograms) and during 10 mins of head-up tilt at 45 (filled histograms). In the normal subjects, there is an increase in FVR and SMAVR, indicating active constriction in skeletal muscle and the splanchnic vascular bed in response to head-up tilt. In the autonomic failure patients who have sympathetic denervation, these changes do not occur. This probably contributed to the marked fall in blood pressure during tilt.

in splanchnic blood flow and rise in SMAVR, which is maintained for 10 min or longer. However, both these stimuli cause a later rise in levels of angiotensin-II and vasopressin, which are potent constrictors of splanchnic blood vessels.

The constriction in the superior mesenteric artery observed during sympathoneural stimulation in normal man, at least in the initial stages, is likely to be neurally-induced, as identical stimuli in patients with sympathetic denervation due to chronic autonomic failure do not change SMABF or raise SMAVR (Chaudhuri *et al.*, 1992) (Figure 12.8). This has been reported in response to mental arithmetic, the cold pressor test and to isometric exercise. During head-up tilt, despite a marked fall in blood pressure, there is no change in SMAVR; this presumably contributes to postural hypotension in such patients. Abnormal neural control probably accounts for the impaired responses in the splanchnic vasculature in patients with diabetic neuropathy (Best *et al.*, 1991; Steven *et al.*, 1991). These observations lend further weight to the importance of neurally-induced vasoconstriction of this large vascular bed in the maintenance of blood pressure in man. It also explains why splanchnic denervation, as previously used for the treatment of severe hypertension (Page and Heuer, 1937), was effective in some patients. It presumably resulted in vasodilatation in this large vascular bed, with a fall in total peripheral vascular resistance. Unfortunately, these effects did not always persist. This may have been due to reinnervation or, as is more likely, to supersensitivity of the denervated splanchnic blood vessels to circulating pressor agents, such as angiotensin-II.

In hypertension, there is increasing experimental and human evidence that the mesenteric vascular bed may play an important role. In Dahl salt-sensitive rats there is evidence of specific sensitivity of the mesenteric vascular bed to noradrenaline and periarterial nerve stimulation; this does not occur with other vasoconstrictors such as angiotensin-II or 5-hydroxytryptamine (5HT) (Kong *et al.*, 1991). Whether this is the result of a change in vascular α_1-adrenoceptors or their coupling to second messenger systems is unclear. In man, there is evidence that SMABF is lower and SMAVR higher in patients with essential hypertension, when compared with age- and sex-matched normotensive controls (Thomaides, Chaudhuri and Mathias, 1991). Moreover, after administration of the centrally acting, α_2-adrenoceptor agonist, clonidine, which lowers blood pressure by a reduction in sympathetic activity, there is an increase in SMABF and a reduction in SMAVR in the hypertensives, which appears to be more prominent in the hypertensives than in the normotensives, and is associated with a substantial fall in blood pressure (Figure 12.9). The rise in SMAVR in the hypertensives may be either neurally-induced or the result of either systemic or local vasoconstrictor substances, although the results with clonidine favour a neural component. It is recognised, however, that hypertrophied vessels, which commonly occur in hypertensives, are more reactive to vasoconstrictor stimuli (Folkow, 1982). This needs consideration when interpreting the effects of clonidine in reversing these changes in vascular resistance.

Parasympathetic

Despite the rich cholinergic supply to the gut there appears to be no direct innervation of gastro-intestinal blood vessels by parasympathetic fibres in mammals. It is unlikely that parasympathetic activity plays a major role in regulating the splanchnic vasculature, except perhaps indirectly. Vagal stimulation, for instance, causes gastric acid secretion and vasodilatation; the latter is more likely to result from an increase in metabolic work load, than to enhanced vasodilator nerve activity (Martinson, 1965). The cholinergic transmitter, acetylcholine has variable effects on the splanchnic vasculature. If given arterially it causes vasodilatation which can be blocked by atropine (Boatman and Brody, 1963; Richardson, 1973). Atropine has the ability to abolish or attenuate superior mesenteric artery vasodilatation induced by food ingestion, whereas phenoxybenzamine or propranolol have

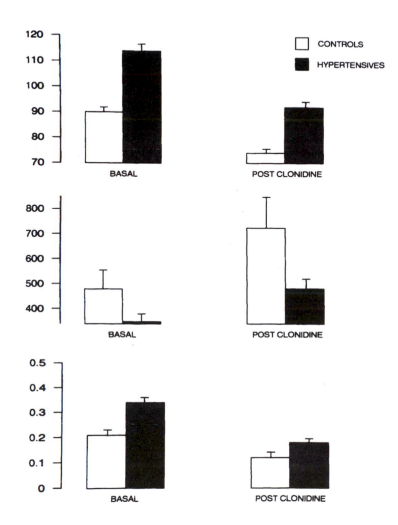

Figure 12.9 Blood pressure (MAP top panels), superior mesenteric artery blood flow (SMABF, middle panels) and calculated superior mesenteric artery vascular resistance (SMAVR, lower panels) in normotensive subjects (open histograms) and hypertensive patients (filled histograms) in the basal state before, and after, intravenous clonidine. The SMABF is lower and SMAVR higher in normotensives. Clonidine increases SMABF and lowers SMAVR in both groups. The bars indicate ± SEM.

no such effect, suggesting that reflex cholinergic mechanisms may contribute to postprandial hyperaemia (Vatner, Franklin and Van Citters, 1970). However, in the cat, neither vagal stimulation (Kewenter, 1965) nor vagotomy (Martinson, 1965) influence intestinal vascular resistance.

In man, there is sparse data on cholinergic influences. Measurement of SMABF in patients with truncal vagotomy and gastric drainage procedures indicate a greater rise in SMABF than in normal subjects (Aldoori et al., 1985). This, however, may be related to the specific problems associated with the dumping syndrome, where the abnormal release of vasodilator gastro-intestinal peptides such as neurotensin, may be involved (Long, Adrian and Bloom, 1985). In situations associated with increased vagal activity, such as carotid sinus hypersensitivity and vasovagal syncope, splanchnic vasodilatation secondary to parasympathetic activation may be expected to contribute. In these situations, cutaneous and skeletal muscle vasodilatation has been demonstrated, but this is more likely to be due to withdrawal of sympathetic tone, as has been demonstrated by microneurography (Wallin and Sundlof, 1982). Atropine may have no effect on the fall in blood pressure despite preventing the fall in heart rate, especially in patients who have the vasodepressor form of carotid sinus hypersensitivity. Furthermore, a role for vasodilatatory peptides associated with cholinergic mechanisms, such as vasoactive intestinal polypeptide (VIP), is less likely as the somatostatin analogue octreotide, which inhibits peptide release, does not prevent the fall in blood pressure in vasodepressor carotid sinus hypersensitivity (Mathias et al., 1991).

PEPTIDES, AMINES AND AUTACOIDS

A variety of substances have effects on the splanchnic vasculature. This may be through endocrine (vasopressin, angiotensin-II, adrenaline), or paracrine/local pathways (VIP, NPY). Reactivity of the splanchnic vascular bed may be different from other vascular beds. Substances linked directly or indirectly to nervous activity are briefly described.

Vasopressin

Vasopressin has powerful effects on the gastro-intestinal vasculature (Gardiner, Bennett and Compton, 1988) (Figure 12.10). It is released during stimuli which activate sympathetic neural pathways, such as during head-up tilt, haemorrhage or hypovolaemia, especially if there is a fall in blood pressure. Its vasoconstrictor effects are the basis of its use in treating oesophageal varices in portal hypertension.

Angiotensin-II

Angiotensin-II formation is dependent on the release of renin, which may occur as a result of sympathetic stimulation in addition to other factors, such as a low renal perfusion pressure. Angiotensin-II has powerful constrictor effects on the gastro-intestinal vasculature. (Figure 12.11). These effects may be either direct, or may result from its ability to interact with the sympathetic nervous system through central or peripheral mechanisms (Zimmerman, 1981).

There are a range of antagonists of the renin-angiotensin system, acting at various stages in the formation of angiotensin II. Inhibition of A-II formation by the A-II converting enzyme inhibitor, captopril, causes both superior mesenteric artery and portal vein dilatation in normal man (Chaudhuri et al., 1993). However, as demonstrated in animals, these effects may be exerted through additional effects, through inhibition of kininase II which increases bradykinin levels (Gardiner, Kemp and Bennett, 1993a), or activation of the vasodilatatory nitric oxide system (Gardiner and Bennett, 1992a). The availability of specific A-II receptor antagonists has extended knowledge of splanchnic vascular effects of A-II in animals (Widdop et al., 1992), and should do so in man.

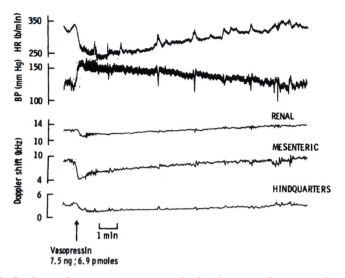

Figure 12.10 Cardiovascular responses to vasopressin given intravenously to a conscious, unrestrained Long Evans rat. HR = heart rate, BP = blood pressure. There is a marked reduction in mesenteric artery blood flow (From Gardiner, Bennett and Compton, 1988).

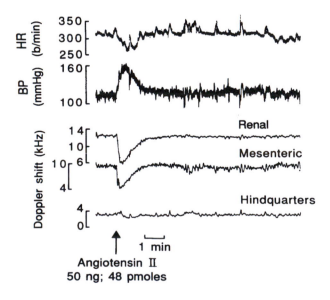

Figure 12.11 Cardiovascular responses to angiotensin-II, given intravenously, in a conscious, unrestrained Long Evans rat. HR = heart rate, BP = blood pressure. There is a marked reduction in both renal and mesenteric artery blood flow. There is minimal change in hindquarters flow (From Gardiner, Bennett and Compton, 1988).

Adrenaline

Adrenaline is released from the adrenal medulla during a range of stimuli which activate the sympatho-adrenal system, such as exercise. Adrenaline constricts the splanchnic vasculature through its α-adrenoceptor agonist effects.

5-Hydroxytryptamine

5-hydroxytryptamine (5HT; serotonin) is present abundantly in the gut. Its role on the gastro-intestinal vasculature, however, is unclear, as it varies under different situations. 5HT acts primarily via classical "D receptors" (Page, 1957) but the vascular effects depend on the dosage, means by which it is administered, species, and the level of sympathetic tone (McCubbin, Kaneko and Page, 1962; Fara, 1976). When given intra-arterially in low doses it causes vasodilatation, but higher doses cause vasoconstriction (Fara, 1976). Sympathetic denervation or blockade of α-adrenoceptors results in a reversal of the vasoconstrictor response to vasodilatation, which is blocked by dihydroergotamine. The constrictor effects may be of relevance to intestinal gangrene which has been observed in the carcinoid syndrome, where 5HT levels are grossly elevated (Adar and Salzman, 1974). Animal studies suggest that parasympathetic activation may influence the release of 5HT from enterochromaffin cells. Whether, or not there is a physiological role for 5HT in man may be determined further by the use of specific 5HT agonists and antagonists, which are now available.

Neuropeptides

Some of the peptides present in the nervous system have marked effects on the splanchnic vasculature. These include corticotropin releasing factor which is a potent vasodilator of the coeliac and superior mesenteric artery (SMA) (MacCannell *et al.*, 1984; Lenz *et al.*, 1985; Gardiner, Compton and Bennett, 1990a). Others, such as neuromedin U-25, cause selective vasoconstriction of the SMA (Gardiner *et al.*, 1990b). NPY is a transmitter co-released with noradrenaline from sympathetic nerve endings. It is capable of vasoconstriction and additionally may exert synergistic effects on the vasculature with noradrenaline. Exogenous NPY, however, has minimal effects on the mesenteric circulation in animal studies (Gardiner, Bennett and Compton, 1988) (Figure 12.12); whether, or not this applies to man is not known. Many neuropeptides are present in high concentrations in the gut and may therefore exert significant local vascular effects.

Gastro-intestinal and pancreatic peptides

A range of these may act at local or distant sites to constrict or dilate the gastro-intestinal vasculature (Granger *et al.*, 1980). For instance glucagon, which is released from the pancreas, may cause a marked increase in splanchnic blood flow (Tibblin, Kock and Schenk, 1970). The release of these peptides may be independent of extrinsic nerves but linked to local reflexes and the intrinsic cholinergic nerve supply of the gut, as in the case of the vasodilator, VIP (Said and Mutt, 1970; Fahrenkrug *et al.*, 1978; Eklund *et al.*, 1979). These peptides appear to play an important role in the regulation of the splanchnic vasculature after food (Mathias, 1990) and alcohol ingestion (Maule *et al.*, 1993; Chaudhuri *et al.*, 1994).

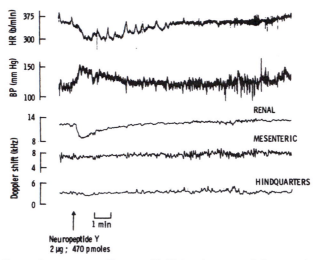

Figure 12.12 Cardiovascular responses to Neuropeptide Y given intravenously in a conscious, unrestrained Long Evans rat. HR = heart rate, BP = blood pressure. There is a pronounced reduction in renal blood flow with little change in mesenteric and hindquarters flow (From Gardiner, Bennett and Compton, 1988).

Endothelium-derived substances

The endothelium contains a number of active substances which are potent dilators or constrictors of blood vessels. Nitric oxide (NO), formed from L-arginine through the action of NO synthetase (NOS), is a key endothelium-derived relaxing factor (EDRF). Experimental evidence indicates that NO has marked effects on the mesenteric circulation, and inhibition of NOS (by N^G-monomethyl-L-arginine, L-NMMA) results in mesenteric vasoconstriction, along with constriction in carotid, renal and skeletal muscle blood vessels (Gardiner *et al.*, 1990c, 1993b). The peptide endothelin, however, has the opposite effects to NO. It is one of the most potent vasoconstrictor peptides known, and causes mesenteric and renal vasoconstriction; there is, however, less marked constriction in the hindquarter bed (Gardiner, Compton and Bennett, 1990d). *In vitro* studies indicate that endothelin causes marked constriction of human mesenteric arteries; this can be specifically reversed by the calcium antagonist nicardipine (Miyauchi, Tomobe and Shiba, 1990) (Figure 12.13). There are a number of different endothelins with differential effects (Gardiner, Kemp and Bennett, 1992b; Gardiner *et al.*, 1992c), and their precise role and their link with neural control of the gastro-intestinal circulation remain unclear.

FOOD INGESTION

The ingestion of food causes marked changes in gastro-intestinal blood flow. In intact animals and man this is due to a combination of neural and hormonal factors. In the cephalic phase of food ingestion, there is a marked increase in gastric mucosal blood flow. Studies in conscious animals indicate that following food ingestion the changes in different segments of the gut depend upon the state of hunger and excitement of the animals and also

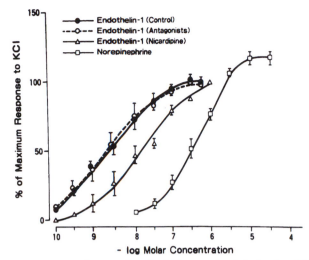

Figure 12.13 Dose response curves for noradrenaline (–□–, norepinephrine) and endothelin-1 in the absence (–●–, control) or in the presence of antagonists (–○–, or 3×10^{-9} M nicardipine (–△–). The responses are maximum vasoconstrictor effects expressed as percents of maximum contraction to 50 mM K^+ in human mesenteric arteries. The antagonists, each 10^{-7} M which included bunazosin, atropine sulphate, diphenhydramine hydrochloride and methysergide hydrogen maleinate, had no effect. Nicardipine however significantly shifted the response to the right. The bars indicate the $\pm$ SEM, (From Miyauchi, Tomobe and Shiba, 1990).

the type of food ingested (Fronek and Stahlgren, 1968; Burns and Schenk, 1969). In the conscious dog, 30 minutes after food ingestion, there is a substantial increase in blood flow to the duodenum, proximal jejunum, and distal jejunum, with little change in the ileum; after 90 minutes however, there is a considerable rise in ileal blood flow (Gallavan *et al.*, 1980) (Figure 12.14). The food-induced increase in splanchnic blood flow and reduction in splanchnic vascular resistance may be largely influenced by release of locally-produced substances (including VIP), and other gastro-intestinal hormones. The vasodilatation is prevented by atropine, but not by α or β-adrenoceptor blockade; it is however, not affected by bilateral thoracic vagotomy (Vatner, Franklin and Van Citters, 1970), suggesting that local cholinergic reflexes, as part of the enteric nervous system, are responsible. These results, however, differ from those in the conscious rat, where atropine has no effect on intestinal hyperaemia, which is reduced by vagotomy (Hernandez, Kvietys and Granger, 1986). The reasons for these differences are unclear and may include species differences and variation in the release of gut hormones, among other factors. There is a developmental and age-related component, as there is less superior mesenteric artery dilatation following a meal in younger, as compared with older, piglets (Yao *et al.*, 1986). The neural and hormonal mechanisms responsible for these differences are unclear.

In man, food ingestion initially increases coeliac artery blood flow (Qamar *et al.*, 1985) and causes a substantial and prolonged (over 60 min) increase in SMABF in normal man (Aldoori *et al.*, 1985; Kooner, Peart and Mathias, 1989a) (Figure 12.15a). There is a fall in SMAVR and an overall fall in peripheral vascular resistance. There are a number of compensatory changes, with an increase in cardiac output and a rise in skeletal muscle

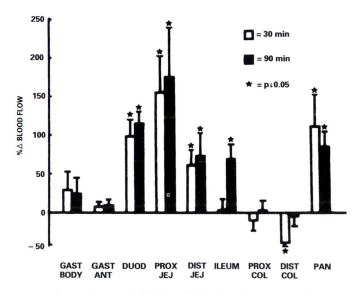

Figure 12.14 Percentage changes (means ± SEM) in blood flow of the gastro-intestinal tract and pancreas 30 and 90 minutes after feeding in conscious dogs. AST = gastric, ANT = antrum, DUOD = duodenum, PROX = proximal, DIST = distal, JEJ = jejunum, COL = colon, PAN = pancreas. (From Gallavan et al., 1980).

vascular resistance, which help maintain blood pressure in normal man (Mathias, 1990) (Figure 12.15b). The importance of these changes is evident in patients with sympathetic denervation due to chronic autonomic failure, in whom food ingestion causes a marked fall in blood pressure (Figure 12.16). In these patients there is a similar post-prandial increase in SMABF, as in normal subjects, but no increase in cardiac output or skeletal muscle vascular resistance, presumably as a result of sympathetic failure (Mathias, 1990). This differs from patients with the early dumping syndrome, after gastric drainage operations and a truncal vagotomy; in these patients food ingestion, especially with a high carbohydrate content, markedly increases SMABF to a greater extent than in normal subjects (Long, Adrian and Bloom, 1985) (Figure 12.17). This accounts for the clinical features which include lightheadedness, palpitations, sweating and occasionally fainting. The sympathetic nervous system is presumably activated and often prevents the blood pressure from falling, unlike patients with sympathetic denervation.

The increase in splanchnic blood flow following food ingestion may be dependent on the type of meal ingested. This is of relevance to patients with primary autonomic failure, in whom the fall in blood pressure after a mixed meal has been compared with that following ingestion of an equivalent caloric load of carbohydrate, lipid or elemental protein (Mathias, 1990). Glucose causes a fall in blood pressure similar to that induced by a mixed meal. With an equivalent load of xylose (an inert sugar administered as a solution at the same osmolality), there is a considerably smaller fall in blood pressure, indicating that the hypertonicity of the glucose solution alone is not responsible. There is a smaller fall for a shorter period after lipid, with virtually no change after protein. The reasons for the

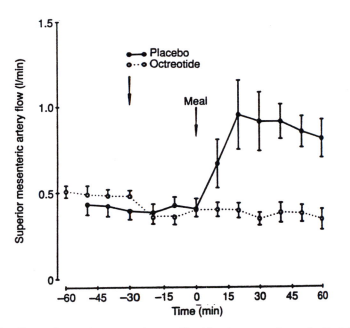

Figure 12.15a Changes in superior mesenteric artery blood flow in a group of normal subjects before and after a balanced liquid meal. After food there is a marked rise in blood flow, which is almost doubled. Flow remains elevated even when measurements are made 60 minutes after food ingestion (From Kooner, Peart and Mathias, 1989a).

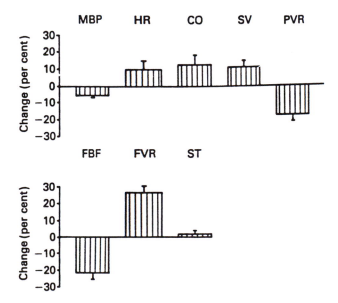

Figure 12.15b Maximum percentage change in mean blood pressure (MBP), heart rate (HR), cardiac output (CO), stroke volume (SV), calculated peripheral vascular resistance (PVR), forearm muscle blood flow (FBF), calculated forearm vascular resistance (FVR) and skin temperature to the index finger (ST) in 6 normal subjects in the first hour after food ingestion. Vertical bars indicate ± SEM (From Mathias and Bannister, 1992).

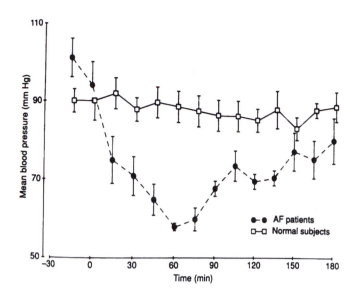

Figure 12.16 Mean blood pressure before (o) and after a standard meal in a group of normal subjects and in patients with autonomic failure and sympathetic denervation. Blood pressure after the meal did not change in the normal subjects. In the patients, however, there was a rapid fall in blood pressure, which remained below baseline over the three hour observation period (from Mathias *et al.*, 1989a).

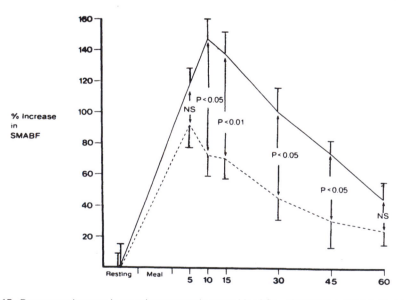

Figure 12.17 Percentage increase in superior mesenteric artery blood flow (SMABF) ± SEM (ml/min) before and after a liquid meal in 9 patients with the dumping syndrome (—), and in 10 control subjects (—). There is a considerably greater increase in the patients (from Aldoori *et al.*, 1985).

difference in composition may relate to the local and gastro-intestinal-pancreatic peptide responses to the different meals.

Insulin also appears to be an important factor in lowering blood pressure and even within two subgroups with primary autonomic failure (pure autonomic failure and multiple system atrophy), there is a positive relationship, as a larger plasma insulin response to a meal is associated with a greater fall in blood pressure (Armstrong and Mathias, 1991). Intravenous administration of insulin, either as a single bolus with ensuing hypoglycaemia (Mathias *et al.*, 1987), or as an infusion with an euglycaemic clamp (Bannister *et al.*, 1987), lowers blood pressure substantially in patients with autonomic denervation. In the latter studies, the fall in blood pressure was not associated with a fall in cardiac output or with peripheral vasodilatation, suggesting a major effect on the splanchnic circulation. Insulin, however, may be one of many other peptides released, including glucagon, which may exert dilatatory effects on the splanchnic circulation.

The role of peptides in causing splanchnic vasodilatation is further emphasised by the efficacy of the somatostatin analogue octreotide, in preventing post-prandial hypotension in autonomic failure (Hoeldtke, O'Dorisio and Boden, 1986; Raimbach *et al.*, 1989) (Figure 12.18). Octreotide prevents peptide release. It, however, exerts its vascular effects rapidly. Part of these actions may be directly on blood vessels and are consistent with *in vitro* studies in human vessels (Tornebrandt, Nobin and Owman, 1987), where somatostatin has been shown to constrict mesenteric veins, rather than arteries. After octreotide, in the autonomic failure patients, there were no changes in cardiac output, or in cutaneous or skeletal muscle blood flow, indicating that a major proportion of its actions were on the splanchnic circulation. The ability of octreotide to prevent mesenteric vasodilatation and the fall in blood pressure induced by food or alcohol (Chaudhuri *et al.*, 1994a), has been confirmed in patients with autonomic failure (Kooner *et al.*, 1989b; Chaudhuri *et al.*, 1994b).

EXERCISE

Dynamic exercise results in a large number of cardiovascular and autonomic adjustments, which maintain blood pressure despite a marked increase in blood flow to exercising muscles (Rowell, 1974). In normal subjects, during upright exercise (when there are additional postural influences on the circulation), there is a marked increase in cardiac output, an increase in systolic blood pressure with a small decrease in diastolic blood pressure, and a decrease in splanchnic blood flow (Wade *et al.*, 1956; Qamar and Read, 1987) (Figure 12.19). During upright exercise, there is a fall in splanchnic blood volume (as indicated by studies utilising labelling of red cells with technetium 99M, Flamm *et al.*, 1990), with mobilisation of blood from the splanchnic region into the thorax; this redistribution helps increase blood flow to exercising muscles while maintaining a reasonable perfusion pressure. Superior mesenteric artery blood flow has also been studied after exercise performed before and after a meal; the food induced increase in superior mesenteric artery blood flow was reduced by exercise (Qamar and Read, 1987).

A combination of neural and hormonal factors is probably responsible for the constriction in splanchnic blood vessels after exercise. During isometric exercise, impulses from contracting muscles and through the central nervous system increase sympathoneural activity and result in a marked reduction in SMABF (Chaudhuri *et al.*, 1991). During

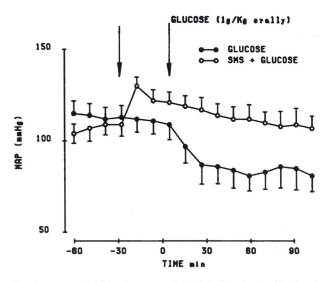

Figure 12.18 Levels of mean arterial blood pressure (MAP) in 7 patients with chronic primary autonomic failure before and after oral glucose at time given after pretreatment with either a placebo (●—●) or the somatostatin analogue, octreotide (SMS), 50umc sc (○—○), given at −30 minutes. After placebo, oral glucose caused a substantial fall in blood pressure. This was reversed with the peptide release inhibitor, octreotide (From Mathias *et al.*, 1989).

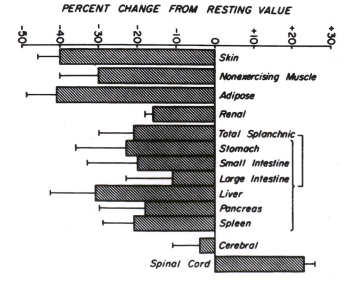

Figure 12.19 Redistribution of blood flow during mild dynamic exercise induced by cycling in conscious baboons. Measurements are from the distribution of radioactive microspheres. During the 4 min period of exercise oxygen uptake rose from 6.7 to 17.2 ml/kg/min; cardiac output tram 2.75 to 4.14 litres/min, heart rate from 118 to 157 beats per min. and arterial blood pressure from 106 to 117 mm Hg. There is a fall in blood flow in all the tissues where measurements are recorded, including non-exercising muscle. The only inactive region where blood flow rose was the spinal cord (Data from Hohimer *et al.*, 1983 and adapted by Rowell, 1986).

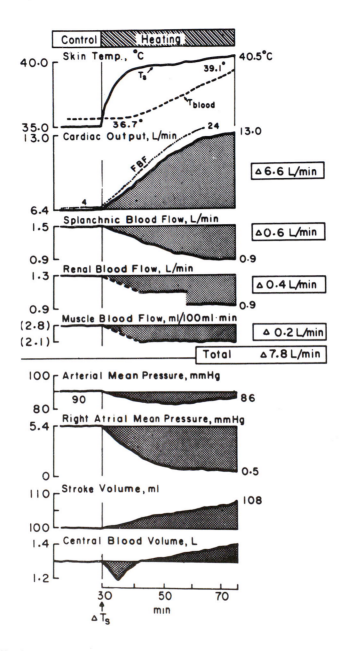

Figure 12.20   Circulatory responses to direct whole body heating, clamped close to 40°C by water perfused suits. The initial values for each variable are shown on the left with final values on the right. Right atrial blood temperature (T blood) rose from 36.7 to 39.1°C, while cardiac output rose from 6.4 to 13.0 litres/min (averages from 12 subjects) reductions in splanchnic, renal and skeletal muscle blood flow could add 1.21 litres/min totals to the 6.6 litres/min increase in cardiac output to give total skin blood flow of approximately 7.8 litres/min. These changes (△) are shown in boxes on the right (From Rowell, 1974).

dynamic exercise, in addition to these factors, there is a rise in circulating adrenaline levels which, through its α-adrenoceptor-mediated effects, also contribute to splanchnic vasoconstriction. It is possible that other substances such as vasopressin, angiotensin-II and other vasoconstrictor peptides contribute.

The importance of the splanchnic region in vascular readjustments during exercise are probably of major importance to patients with autonomic failure. These patients have severe exercise-induced hypotension, which also occurs in the supine position, indicating that the mechanisms causing such hypotension are in addition to, or separate from, those causing posturally-induced hypotension (Marshall, Schirger and Shepherd, 1961; Smith, Matteoda and Mathias, 1993). Although the regional haemodynamic changes during supine exercise are not currently known, it is possible that the inability of these sympathetically denervated patients to neurally constrict the splanchnic blood vessels may contribute to the lack of readjustment, and thus the fall in blood pressure.

THERMAL STRESS

As with food and exercise, changes in body temperature result in a number of cardiovascular and autonomic responses (Rowell, 1974, 1986). A rise in body temperature, induced by either increasing environmental temperature or by radiant heat, results in marked cutaneous dilatation. There is an increase in cardiac output and redistribution of blood flow (Figure 12.20), which is either unchanged or falls in skeletal muscle, and is reduced in the splanchnic region. This is associated with an increase in splanchnic nerve activity. These changes help to maintain blood pressure. The reverse, a decrease in temperature, results in a reduction in splanchnic neural activity and an increase in splanhnic blood flow.

ACKNOWLEDGEMENTS

We thank the Wellcome Trust, the Charles Wolfson Charitable Trust and the Brain Research Trust for their support.

REFERENCES

Adar, R. and Salzman, E.W. (1974). Serotonin and the mesenteric circulation. *British Medical Journal*, **2**, 444.

Ahmad, M., Blomquist, C.G., Mullins, C.B. and Willerson, J.T. (1977). Left ventricular function during lower body negative pressure. *Aviation, Space and Environmental Medicine*, **48**, 512–515.

Aldoori, M.I., Qamar, M.I. Read, A.E. and Williamson, R.C.N. (1985). Increased flow in superior mesenteric artery in dumping syndrome. *British Journal of Surgery*, **72**, 389–390.

Anderson, J.H. and Gianturo, C. (1981). Angiographic spillover technique for estimating blood flow. In *Measurement of blood flow in applications to the Splanchnic Circulation*. Edited by D. Granger and G. Bilkey, pp. 401–424. Baltimore: Williams and Wilkins.

Armstrong, E. and Mathias, C.J. (1991). The effects of the somatostatin analogue, octreotide, on postural hypotension, before and after food ingestion, in primary autonomic failure. *Clinical Autonomic Research*, **2**, 135–140.

Aviado, D.M. (1959). Cardiovascular effects of some commonly-used pressor amines. *Anaesthesiology*, **20**, 71–97.

Bannister, R., Da Costa, D.F., Kooner, J.S., MacDonald, I.A. and Mathias, C.J. (1987). Insulin induced hypotension in autonomic failure in euglycaemia in man. *Journal of Physiology*, **382**, 36P.

Bell, L., Hennecken, J., Zaret, B.L. and Rutlen, D.L. (1990). α-adrenergic regulation of splanchnic volume and cardiac output in the dog. *Acta Physiologica Scandinavica*, **138**, 321–329.

Best, I.M., Pitzele, A., Green, A., Halperin, J. Mason, R. and Giron, F. (1991). Mesenteric blood flow in patients with diabetic neuropathy. *Journal of Vascular Surgery*, **13**, 84–90.

Boatman, D.L. and Brody, M.J. (1963). Effects of acetylcholine on the intestinal vasculature of the dog. *Journal of Pharmacology and Experimental Therapeutics*, **7**, 185–191.

Bohlen, H.G., Henrich, H., Gore, R.W. and Johnson P.C. (1978). Intestinal muscle and mucosal blood flow during direct sympathetic stimulation. *American Journal of Physiology*, **235**(1), H40–H45.

Buckley, N.M., Jarenwattananon, M., Gootman, P.M. and Frasier, I.D. (1987). Autoregulatory escape from vasoconstriction of intestinal circulation in developing swine. *American Journal of Physiology*, **252**, H118–H124.

Bunch, J.L. (1899). On the vaso-motor nerves of the small intestine. *Journal of Physiology*, **24**, 72–98.

Burns, G.P. and Schenk, W.G. (1969). Effect of digestion and exercise on intestinal blood flow and cardiac output. *Archives of Surgery*, **98**, 790–794.

Chaudhuri, K.R., Thomaides, T., Hernandez, P., Alam, N. and Mathias, C.J. (1991). Non-invasive quantification of superior mesenteric artery blood flow during sympathoneural activation in man. *Clinical Autonomic Research*, **1**, 37–42.

Chaudhuri, K.R., Thomaides, T., Hernandez, P. and Mathias, C.J. (1992). Abnormality of superior mesenteric artery blood flow response in human sympathetic failure. *Journal of Physiology (London)*, **457**, 477–489.

Chaudhuri, K.R., Thomaides, T., Maule, S., Watson, L., Lowe, S., Mathias, C.J. (1993). The effect of captopril on the superior mesenteric artery and portal venous blood flow in normal man. *British Journal of Clinical Pharmacology*, **35**, 517–542.

Chaudhuri, K.R., Maule, S., Thomaides, T., Pavitt, D. and Mathias, C.J. (1994a). Alcohol ingestion lowers supine blood pressure, causes splanchnic vasodilatation and worsens postural hypotension in primary autonomic failure. *Journal of Neurology*, **241**, 145–152.

Chaudhuri, K.R., Thomaides, T., Pavitt, D., and Mathias, C.J. (1994b). Octreotide prevents alcohol induced hypotension and mesenteric vasodilatation in primary autonomic failure. *Clinical Autonomic Research*, **4**, 77–78.

Clark, R., Colley, D., Jacobson, E., Herman, R., Tyler, G. and Stahl, D. (1980). Superior mesenteric angiography and blood flow measurement following intra-arterial injection of prostaglandin E1. *Radiology*, **134**, 327–333.

Collis, M.G. and Alps, B.J. (1973). The evaluation of the α-adrenoceptor blocking action of indoramin, phentolamine, thymoxamine on rat and guinea-pig isolated mesenteric vascular and aortic spiral preparations. *Journal of Pharmacology and Therapeutics*, **25**, 621–628.

Drew, G.M. and Whiting, S.B. (1979). Evidence for two distinct types of postsynaptic α-adrenoceptors in vascular smooth muscle *in vivo*. *British Journal of Pharmacology*, **67**, 207–215.

Eklund, S., Jodal, M., Lundgren, O. and Sjoqvist, A. (1979). Effects of vasoactive intestinal polypeptide on blood flow, motility and fluid transport in the gastrointestinal tract of the cat. *Acta Physiologica Scandinavica*, **73**, 461–468.

Fahrenkrug, J., Haglund, U., Jodal, M., Lundgren, O., Olbe, L. and Schaffalitzky de Muckadell, O.B. (1978). Nervous release of vasoactive intestinal polypeptide in the gastrointestinal tract of cats: possible physiological implications. *Journal of Physiology*, **284**, 291–305.

Fara, J. (1976). Mesenteric vasodilator effect of 5-hydroxytryptamine: possible enteric neuron mediation. *Archives of International Pharmacodynamics*, **221**, 235–249.

Fasth, S., Hulten L. and Nordgren, S. (1980). Adjustments of hepatic and small intestine blood flow on selective vasoconstrictor fibre stimulation. *Acta Physiologica Scandinavica*, **110**, 343–350.

Fell, C. (1966). Changes in distribution of blood flow in irreversible hemorrhagic shock. *American Journal of Physiology*, **210**(4), 863–868.

Flamm, S.D., Taki, J. Moore, R. *et al.* (1990). Redistribution of regional and organ blood volumes and effect on cardiac function in relation to upright exercise intensity in healthy human subjects. *Circulation*, **81**, 1550–1559.

Folkow, B., Lewis, D.H., Lundgren, O., Mellander, S. and Wallentin I. (1964). The effect of graded vasoconstrictor fibre stimulation on the intestinal resistance and capacitance vessels. *Acta Physiologica Scandinavica*, **61**, 445–457.

Folkow, B. (1982). Physiological aspects of primary hypertension. *Physiological Reviews*, **62**, 347–503.

Fronek, K. and Stahlgren, L.H. (1968). Systemic and regional haemodynamic changes during food intake and digestion in nonanaesthetized dogs. *Circulation Research*, **6**, 687–692.

Furness, J.B. and Costa, M. (1987). The enteric nervous system. Melbourne: Churchill Livingstone.

Furness, J.B. and Costa, M. (1980). Types of nerves in the enteric nervous system. *Neuroscience*, **5**, 1–20.

Gallavan, R.H., Chou, C.C., Kvietys, P.R. and Sit, S.P. (1980). Regional blood flow during digestion in the conscious dog. *American Journal of Physiology*, **238**, H220–H225.

Gardiner, S.M., Bennett, T. and Compton, A.M. (1988). Regional haemodynamic effects of neuropetide Y, vasopressin and angiotensin-II in conscious, unrestrained, Long Evans and Brattleboro rats. *Journal of the Autonomic Nervous System*, **24**, 15–27.

Gardiner, S.M., Compton, A.M. and Bennett, T. (1989). Regional haemodynamic changes following hypovolemia in conscious rats. *American Journal of Physiology*, **256**, R1076–R1083.

Gardiner, S.M., Compton, A.M. and Bennett, T. (1990a). Differential effects of neuropeptides on coeliac and superior mesenteric blood flows in conscious rats. *Regulatory Peptides*, **29**, 215–227.

Gardiner, S.M., Compton, A.M., Bennett, T., Domin, J. and Bloom S.R. (1990b). Regional haemodynamic effects of neuromedin U in conscious rats. *American Journal of Physiology*, **258**, R32–R38.

Gardiner, S.M., Compton, A.M., Bennett, T., Palmer, R.M.J. and Moncada, S. (1990c). Control of regional blood flow by endothelium-derived nitric oxide. *Hypertension*, **15**, 486–492.

Gardiner, S.M., Compton, A.M. and Bennett, T. (1990d). Regional haemodynamic effects of endothelin-2 and sarafotoxin-S6b in conscious rats. *American Journal of Physiology*, **258**, R912–R917.

Gardiner, S.M., and Bennett, T. (1992a). Involvement of nitric oxide in the regional haemodynamic effects of perindoprilat and captopril in hypovolaemic Brattleboro rats. *British Journal of Pharmacology*, **107**, 1181–1191.

Gardiner, S.M., Kemp, P.A., and Bennett, T. (1992b). Inhibition by phosphoramidon of the regional haemodynamic effects of proendothelin-2 and -3 in conscious rats. *British Journal of Pharmacology*, **107**, 584–590.

Gardiner, S.M., Kemp, P.A., Compton, A.M., and Bennett, T. (1992c). Coeliac haemodynamic effects of endothelin-1, endothelin-3, proendothelin-1 (1–38) and proendothelin-3 (1–41) in conscious rats. *British Journal of Pharmacology*, **106**, 483–488.

Gardiner, S.M., Kemp, P.A., and Bennett, T. (1993a). Differential effects of captopril on regional haemodynamic responses to angiotensin I and bradykinin in conscious rat. *British Journal of Pharmacology*, **108**, 769–775.

Gardiner, S.M., Kemp, P.A., Bennett, T., Palmer, R.M.J. and Moncada, S. (1993b). Regional and cardiac haemodynmic effects of NG, N^G-dimethyl-L-arginine and their reversibility by vasodilators in conscious rats. *British Journal of Pharmacology*, **110**, 1457–1464.

Granger, D.N., Richardson, P.D.I., Kvietys, P.R. and Mortillaro, N.A. (1980). Intestinal blood flow. *Gastroenterology*, **78**, 837–863.

Greenway, C.V., Scott, G.D. and Zink, J. (1976). Sites of autoregulatory escape of blood flow in the mesenteric vascular bed. *Journal of Physiology*, **259**, 1–12.

Hadjiminas, J. and Oberg, B. (1968). Effects of carotid baroreceptor reflexes on venous tone in skeletal muscle and intestine of the cat. *Acta Physiologica Scandinavica*, **72**, 518–532.

Hernandez, L.A., Kvietys, P.R. and Granger, D.N. (1986). Postprandial haemodynamics in the conscious rat. *American Journal of Physiology*, **251**, G117–G123.

Heyndrickx, G.R., Boettcher, D.H. and Vatner, S.F. (1976). Effects of angiotensin, vasopressin and methoxamine on cardiac function and blood flow distribution in conscious dogs. *American Journal of Physiology*, **231**, 1579–1587.

Hoeldtke, R.D., O'Dorisio, T.M. and Boden, G. (1986). Treatment of autonomic neuropathy with somatostatin analogue, SMS 201–995. *Lancet*, **ii**, 602–605.

Hohimer, A.R., Hales, J.R., Rowell, L.B. and Smith, O.A. (1983). Regional distribution of blood flow during mild dynamic leg exercise in the baboon. *Journal of Applied Physiology, Respiratory, Enviromental and Exercise Physiology*, **55**, 1173–1177.

Hulten, L., Jodal, M., Lindhagen, J. and Lundgren, O. (1976). Blood flow in small intestine of cat and man as analysed by an inert gas washout technique. *Gastroenterology*, **70**, 45–51.

Hulten, L., Lindhagen, J. and Lundgren, O. (1977). Sympathetic nervous control of intramural blood flow in the feline and human intestines. *Gastroenterology*, **72**, 41–48.

Johnson, J.M., Rowell, L.B., Niederberger, M. and Eisman, M.N. (1974). Human splanchnic and forearm vasoconstrictor responses of right arterial and aortic pressure. *Circulation Research*, **34**, 515–524.

Kewenter, J. (1965). The vagal control of the jejunal and ileal motility and blood flow. *Acta Physiologica Scandinavica*, (Suppl.), **251**, 1–68.

Kong, J.Q., Taylor, D.A., Fleming, W.W. and Kotchen, T.A. (1991). Specific supersensitivity of the mesenteric vascular bed of dahl salt-sensitive rats. *Hypertension*, **17**, 349–356.

Kooner, J.S., Peart, W.S. and Mathias, C.J. (1989a). The peptide release inhibitor, octeotide (SMS 201–995) prevents the haemodynamic changes following food ingestion in normal human subjects. *Quarterly Journal of Experimental Physiology*, **74**, 569–572.

Kooner, J.S., Armstrong, E., Peart, W.S., Bannister, R. and Mathias, C.J. (1989b). Octreotide (SMS 201–995) prevents superior msenteric artery vasodilatation and postprandial hypotension in human autonomic failure. *British Journal of Clinical Pharmacology*, **29**, 154P.

Langley, J.N. (1921). The autonomic nervous system, part 1. Herfer: Cambridge.

Lanz, M., Link, D., Holcroft, J. and Foerster, J. (1981). Video dilution technique angiographic determination of splanchnic blood flow in application to the splanchnic circulation. Baltimore: Williams and Wilkins, 425–437.

Lenz, H.J., Fisher, L.A., Vale, W.W. and Brown, M.R. (1985). Corticotropin-releasing factor, sauagine, and urotensin I: effects on blood flow. *American Journal of Physiology*, **249**, R85–R90.

Long, R.G., Adrian, T.E. and Bloom, S.R. (1985). Somatostatin and the dumping syndrome. *British Medical Journal*, **290**, 886–888.

MacCannell, K.L., Hamilton, P.L., Lederis, K., Newton, C.A. and Rivier, J. (1984). Corticotropin releasing factor-like peptides produce selective dilatation of the dog mesenteric circulation. *Gastroenterology*, **87**, 94–102.

Marshall, R.J., Schirger, A. and Shepherd, J.T. (1961). Blood pressure during supine exercise in idiopathic orthostatic hypotension. *Circulation Research*, **24**, 76–81.

Martinson, J. (1965). The effect of graded vagal stimulation on gastric motility, secretion and blood flow in the cat. *Acta Physiologica Scandinavica*, **65**, 300–309.

Mathias, C.J., Da Costa, D.F., Fosbraey, P., Christensen, N.J. and Bannister, R. (1987). Hypotensive and sedative effects of insulin in autonomic failure. *British Medical Journal*, **295**, 161–163.

Mathias, C.J., da Costa, D.F., Fosbraey, P., Bannister, R., Wood, S.M., Bloom, S.R. and Christensen, N.J. (1989a). Cardiovascular, biochemical and hormonal changes during food induced hypotension in chronic autonomic failure. *Journal of the Neurological Sciences*, **94**, 255–269.

Mathias, C.J., Bannister, R., Bloom, S.R., Cortelli, P., da Costa, D.F., Kooner, J.S., Raimbach, S.J. and Wood, S.M. (1989b). Food-induced hypotension in human subjects with impaired autonomic nervous function — pathophysiological changes and therapeutic strategies. In *Nerves and the Gastrointestinal Tract. Falk Symposium No. 50*, edited by M.V. Singer, H. Goebell, pp. 787–796. Lancaster: MTP Press Ltd.

Mathias C.J. (1990). Effect of food intake on cardiovascular control in patients with impaired autonomic function. *Journal of Neuroscience Methods*, **34**, 193–200.

Mathias, C.J., Armstrong, E., Browse, N., Chaudhuri, K.R., Enevoldson, P. and Ross Russell, R.W. (1991). Value of non-invasive continuous blood pressure monitoring in the detection of carotid sinus hypersensitivity. *Clinical Autonomic Research*, **2**, 157–159.

Mathias, C.J. and Bannister, R. (1992). Postcibal hypotension in autonomic disorders. In *Autonomic Failure. A Textbook of Disorders of the Autonomic Nervous System. 3rd ed.*, edited R. Bannister and C.J. Mathias, pp. 367–380. Oxford: Oxford University Press.

Maule, S., Chaudhuri, K.R., Thomaides, T., Pavitt, D.V., McCleery, J., Mathias, C.J. (1993). Effects of oral alcohol on superior mesenteric artery blood flow in normal man, supine and tilted. *Clinical Science*, **84**, 419–423.

McCubbin, J.W., Kaneko, Y. and Page, I.H. (1962). Inhibition of neurogenic vasoconstriction by serotonin. *Circulation Research*, **11**, 74–83.

Miyauchi, T., Tomobe, Y. and Shiba, R. (1990). Involvement of endothelin in the regulation of human vascular tonus: potent vasoconstrictor effect and existance in endothelial cells. *Circulation*, **81**, 1874–1880.

Moneta, G.L., Taylor, D.C., Helton, W.S., Mulholland, M.W. and Strandess, Jr. D.E. (1988). Duplex ultrasound measurement of postprandial intestinal blood flow: effect of meal composition. *Gastroenterology*, **95**, 1294–1301.

Nakamura, T., Moriyasu, F., Ban, N. *et al.* (1989). Quantitative image of abdominal arterial blood flow using image directed doppler ultrasonography. Superior mesenteric splenic and common hepatic arterial blood flow in normal adults. *Journal of Clinical Ultrasound*, **17**, 261–268.

Norryd, C., Deneken, H., Lundenquist, A. and Olin, T. (1974). Superior mesenteric artery blood flow in man studied with a dye-dilution technique. *Acta Scandinavica*, **141**, 109–118.

Oberg, B. (1964). Effects of cardiovascular reflexes on net capillary fluid transfer. *Acta Physiologica Scandinavica (suppl)*, **6(222)**, 1–98.

Page, I.H. and Heuer, G.J. (1937). Effect on splanchnic nerve section on patients suffering from hypertension. *American Journal of Medical Society*, **193**, 820–841.

Page, I.H. (1957). Cardiovascular actions of serotonin (5-hydroxy-tryptamine). In: Lewis, G.P. ed. 5-Hydroxytryptamine. London: Pergamon, 93–108.

Patel, P., Bose, D. and Greenway, C.V. (1981). Effects of prazosin and phenoxybenzamine on α and β receptor mediated responses in intestinal resistance and capacitance vessels. *Journal of Cardiovascular Pharmacology*, **3**, 1050–1059.

Pfluger, E. (1855). Zweite vorlaufige Mittheilung uber die Einwirkung der vorderen Ruckenmarkswurzeln auf das Lumen der Gefeasse. *Allgemeine Medicinische Central-Zeitung*, **24**, 601.

Qamar, M.I., Read, A.E., Skidmore, R., Evans, J.M. and Williamson, R.C.N. (1985). Transcutaneous Doppler ultrasound measurement of coeliac axis blood flow in man. *British Journal of Surgery*, **72**, 391–393.

Qamar, M.I. and Read, A.E. (1987). Effects of exercise on mesenteric blood flow in man. *Gut*, **28**, 583–587.

Qamar, M.I., Read, J., Skidmore, R., Evans, J.M. and Wells, P.N.T. (1986). Transcutaneous Doppler ultrasound measurement of superior mesenteric artery blood flow in man. *Gut*, **27**, 100–105.

Raimbach, S.J., Cortelli, P., Kooner, J.S., Bannister, R., Bloom, S.R. and Mathias, C.J. (1989). Prevention of glucose-induced hypotension by the somatostatin analogue Octreotide (SMS 201–995) in chronic autonomic failure — Haemodynamic and hormonal changes. *Clinical Science*, **77**, 623–628.

Ralevic, V. and Burnstock, G. (1990). Postjunctional synergism of noradrenaline and adenosine 5′-tryphosphate in the mesenteric arterial bed of the rat. *European Journal of Pharmacology*, **175**, 291–299.

Richardson, P.D.I. (1973). Pharmacological responses of the vasculature of the mammalian small intestine, with particular regard to the responses of the microcirculation. PhD Thesis, University of London.

Rowell, L.B. (1974). Human cardiovascular adjustments to exercise and thermal stress. *Physiological Reviews*, **54**, 75–159.

Rowell, L.B. (1975). The splanchnic circulation. In *The peripheral circulations*, edited by R. Zelis, pp. 163–192. Grune and Stratton Inc.

Rowell, L.B. (1986). Human circulation regulation during physical stress. Oxford: Oxford University Press.

Said, S.I. and Mutt, V. (1970). Potent peripheral and splanchic vasodilator peptide from normal gut. *Nature*, **225**, 863–844.

Smith, G.D.P., Watson, L.P., Pavitt, D.V. and Mathias, C.J. (1995). Abnormal cardiovascular and catecholamine responses to supine exercise in human subjects with sympathetic dysfunction. *Journal of Physiology (London)*, **485**, 255–265.

Stevens, M.J., Edmonds, M.E., Meire, H. and Watkins, P.J. (1991). Failure of vasoconstriction of the splanchnic vascular bed may contribute to postural hypotension in diabetic autonomic neuropathy. *Clinical Autonomic Research*, **1**, 87.

Taira, N. and Yabuchi, Y. (1977). Profile of β-adrenoceptors on femoral, superior mesenteric and renal vascular beds of dogs. *British Journal of Pharmacology*, **59**, 577–583.

Thomaides, T.N., Chaudhuri, K.R. and Mathias, C.J. (1991). Superior mesenteric artery vascular resistance is higher in hypertensives and is lowered by clonidine, unlike in normal subjects. *Journal of Hypertension*, **9**, (Suppl. 6), 582–583.

Tibblin, S., Kock, N.G. and Schenk, Jr. W.G. (1970). Splanchnic haemodynamic responses to glucagon. *Archives of Surgery*, **100**, 84–89.

Tornebrandt, K., Nobin, A. and Owman, C.H. (1987). Contractile and dilatory action of neuropeptides on isolated human mesenteric blood vessels. *Peptides*, **8(2)**, 251–256.

Vatner, S.F., Franklin, D. and Van Citters, R.L. (1970). Mesenteric vasoactivity associated with eating and digestion in the conscious dog. *American Journal of Physiology*, **219(1)**, 170–174.

Wade, O.L., Combes, B., Childs, A.W., Wheeler, H.O., Cournand, A. and Bradley, S.E. (1956). The effect of exercise on the splanchnic blood volume in normal man. *Clinical Science*, **15**, 457–463.

Wallin, B.G. and Sundlof, G. (1982). Sympathetic outflow to muscles during vasovagal syncope. *Journal of Autonomic Nervous System*, **6**, 287–291.

Weaver, L.C., Genovesi, S., Stella, A. and Zanchetti, A. (1987). Neural, haemodynamic and renal responses to stimulation of intestinal receptors. *American Journal of Physiology*, **253**, H1167–H1176.

Widdop, R.E., Gardiner, S.M., Kemp, P.A. and Bennett, T. (1992). Inhibition of the haemodynamic effects of angiotensin II in conscious rats by AT_2-receptor antagonists given after the AT_1-receptor antagonist, EXP 3174. *British Journal of Pharmacology*, **107**, 873–880.

Yao, A.C., Gootman, P.M., Frankfurt, P.P. and Di Russo, S.M. (1986). Age-related superior mesenteric arterial flow changes in piglets: effects of feeding and haemorrhage. *American Journal of Physiology*, **251**, G718–G723.

Zimmerman, B.G. (1981). Adrenergic facilitation by angiotensin: does it serve a physiological function? *Clinical Science*, **60**, 343–348.

13 Hepatic Circulation

W. Wayne Lautt

Department of Pharmacology & Therapeutics, Faculty of Medicine, University of Manitoba, Winnipeg, Manitoba, Canada, R3E OW3

Only the sympathetic nerves appear to play any significant role in neural regulation of the hepatic circulation. These nerves result in constriction of the *hepatic artery* with maximal responses (Rmax) being equivalent to conductance decreasing to zero; the stimulation frequency required to produce 50% of the maximal response (Hz_{50}) is 2.4 Hz. Arterial responses *in vivo* are best measured using vascular conductance rather than resistance as the index of vascular tone. Vascular escape occurs in the cat and rat but not in the dog.

Active contractile responses of the *venous resistance* system does not cause blood flow to change, rather pressure changes. The nerves lead to presinusoidal portal venous constriction that also shows vascular escape in contrast to the well maintained constriction of hepatic venous resistance sites. Presinusoidal resistance leads to elevated portal but not intrahepatic pressure; postsinusoidal constriction occurs across a sphinter-like zone of the hepatic veins and leads to equal elevation of intrahepatic and portal venous pressure. Calculated resistance (R) is a poor index of active vascular responses since venous resistance is dramatically altered passively in response to the distending pressure (Pd) caused by changes in portal, intrahepatic, or central venous pressure. A new 'Index of Contractility' is unaffected by passive distension and dramatically affected by active contractile reactions ($IC = R \cdot Pd^3$).

Hepatic *capacitance vessels* represent an important venous reservoir where blood is stored, 60% as stressed volume and 40% as unstressed volume at normal portal pressure (8 mmHg). Stressed volume is the product of hepatic vascular compliance and distending blood pressure; unstressed volume is a theoretical volume that would exist at zero distending pressure. Active constriction appears to result in reduced volume by reducing unstressed volume. The Rmax is equivalent to expulsion of about 50% of total liver volume and the Hz_{50} is 1.7–3.4 Hz, similar to the Hz_{50} range for the hepatic arterial conductance response. Net fluid filtration is not notably altered by nerve stimulation, however the rate of filtration is considerably less than what would be expected based solely on the rise in intrahepatic pressure indicating some mechanism to reduce filtration is activated by nerve stimulation.

The *transmitter* is noradrenaline with the suggestion that ecosanoids or ATP may play a modulating role. α_1 receptors appear to predominate in the arterial responses with α_2 prejunctional receptors playing a role in suppressing noradrenaline release. The hepatic capacitance receptors are α_2 and the venous resistance vessels are constricted by both α_1 and α_2 stimulation but the responses have not been specified as to the receptor involvement at pre- versus postsinusoidal resistance sites. Adenosine suppresses arterial but not portal contractions and reduces capacitance responses only at high doses. The effect of blood-borne factors in the portal blood on hepatic nerve-induced responses has not been studied except for glucagon which earlier studies reported to suppress contraction but later studies find has very modest potentiating effects and suppresses arterial vascular escape at high doses as well as elevating the Hz_{50} for the capacitance responses. Little is known about modified nerve functions in disease states.

KEY WORDS: hepatic artery; portal vein; capacitance; blood flow; stressed volume; unstressed volume.

VASCULAR BACKGROUND

At every level of vascular organization from microscopic to macroscopic, the liver is unique. This brief overview is intended to provide the basis for discussion of the effect of nerves in the regulation of this vascular bed. Recent reviews (Lautt and Greenway, 1987; Greenway and Lautt, 1989; Ballet, 1990) provide more detailed information and references.

The liver receives 25% of the cardiac output even though it constitutes only 2.5% of body weight. The hepatic parenchymal cells are the most richly perfused of any of the organs, with each cell on average being in contact with perfusate on two sides. Of the total hepatic blood flow, 100 to 130 ml per min per 100 gm liver (30 ml per min per kg body weight), 20 to 33% is supplied by the hepatic artery, the remainder by the portal vein. The liver sits astride a massive river of portal venous blood that flows out of the highlands of the intestine (60%), stomach (20%), spleen (10%), and pancreas (10%) carrying blood of low oxygenation but rich in nutrients, hormones, and ingested toxins.

The portal vein and hepatic artery subdivide within the liver and the terminal branches of each vessel travel in intimate contact to the center of each of the 100,000 hepatic functional units, the acinus (Figure 13.1). The acinus is a cluster of parenchymal cells about 2 mm in diameter that is supplied with portal and arterial blood that enters into the central zone (Rappaport's zone 1) where the blood is well mixed (Rappaport, 1981).

Blood flows outward to the periphery of the acinus with concurrent flow in adjacent sinusoids. All exit points from terminal hepatic venules are at the periphery (zone 3) of the acinus and diffusion from zone 3 to zone 1 is not possible. This vascular arrangement allows the activity of the parenchymal cells to develop strong gradients from zones 1 to 3 including the ability to extract selected compounds with virtually 100% efficiency. Blood passing the full length of a sinusoid ($220–480\mu$) is sequentially distributed to approximately 20 hepatocytes (Gumucio and Miller, 1981). There is substantial evidence that the microvascular environment of the hepatocyte regulates hepatocyte function. Heterogeneity of hepatic enzyme distribution across the acinus has been reviewed (Gumucio, 1983; Goresky and Groom, 1984; Thurman, Kauffman and Jungermann, 1986) and the classification of chemically induced injury has been discussed relative to the acinus and its zones (Plaa, 1975).

The portal vein supplies the majority of hepatic blood flow; however, the liver is unable to regulate portal blood flow. Intrahepatic vascular resistance can be altered either by the passive distensibility of the resistance sites or active vasoconstriction. Active vasoconstriction can result in elevation of portal pressure up to three times normal levels. Despite this large elevation in intrahepatic resistance, portal flow is not altered by this manoeuvre. Portal flow is regulated by the outflow of the splanchnic organs and the liver must accommodate whatever portal flow is sent to it. Since the liver cannot regulate portal flow, the only control of flow within the liver is via the hepatic artery.

Extrinsic factors such as hepatic nerves can markedly influence hepatic arterial flow, however the primary regulation of arterial flow is via an intrinsic regulatory mechanism that appears to be unique for the liver. The first unique feature of intrinsic regulation of hepatic arterial flow is that this flow is not regulated by metabolic demands of the hepatic parenchymal cells. Alterations in overall hepatic metabolism can lead to considerable changes in oxygen demand without altering hepatic arterial blood flow. The details of

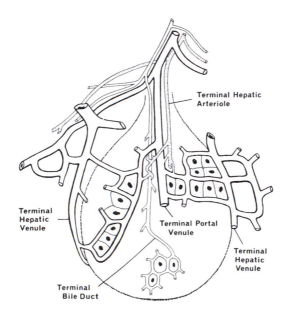

Figure 13.1   The acinus is the functional unit of the liver (Rappaport, 1981). There are about 100,000 acini per human liver; each is about 2 mm in diameter. Acini cluster like grapes at the end of vascular stalks comprising the terminal branch of portal veins, hepatic arteries and bile ducts. Blood flows into the center (zone 1) of the acinus and flows outward to drain into terminal venules at the periphery (zone 3). Zone 1 is well oxygenated and rich in nutrients, hormones and toxins. Because flow in adjacent sinusoids is concurrent, zone 3 has the lowest oxygenation and short-circuiting of substances across the vascular system does not occur nor do vasoactive substances in zone 3 diffuse back upstream to zone 1 where the hepatic arterial resistance vessels exist. Based on the acinar concept of Rappaport (1981). Reprinted with permission from Lautt and Greenway (1987).

intrinsic blood flow regulation are covered in previous reviews (Lautt and Greenway, 1987; Greenway and Lautt, 1989). The two forms of intrinsic regulation appear to be mediated by the same adenosine-washout mechanism. The most dramatic form of intrinsic regulation is referred to as the hepatic arterial buffer response (Lautt, 1981a), which is the inverse hepatic arterial response to changes in portal venous flow. When portal flow decreases, the hepatic arterial flow instantly increases to compensate for the flow change, thus tending to buffer the net effect of changes in portal flow. The hepatic artery undergoes essentially complete vasoconstriction at very high portal flows and full vasodilation at very low portal flows (Lautt, Legare and Ezzat, 1990). The impact of the hepatic arterial buffer response on liver functions and the criteria that have been fulfilled to support this hypothesis have been reviewed. Figure 13.2 briefly outlines the mechanism of the buffer response. A similar adenosine-mediated washout mechanism operates to account for the second intrinsic regulatory mechanism of the hepatic artery, that is, autoregulation. Autoregulation of the hepatic artery is not of a myogenic nature as was previously thought but rather is dependent upon local production of adenosine (oxygen independent). This mechanism is also described in Figure 13.2.

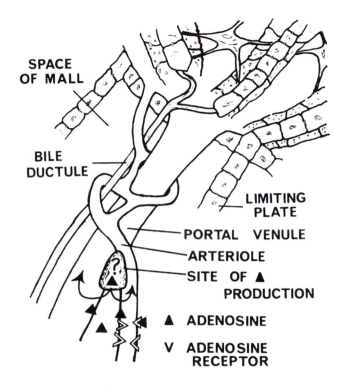

Figure 13.2 Adenosine washout hypothesis: The area shown is the portal triad which represents the vascular stalk leading into the center of each acinus. The terminal branches of the hepatic arteriole, portal venule and bile ductule lie within an enclosed space delimited by a limiting plate of cells. The fluid surrounding these vessels and contained within the limiting plate comprises the space of Mall. The data are consistent with the hypothesis that adenosine is continuously secreted into the space of Mall (independent of general parenchymal cell oxygen supply or demand) and that the local concentration of adenosine determines the tone of the hepatic artery. The adenosine can be washed away into the portal vein and hepatic arterial flow. The hepatic arterial buffer response is accounted for by, for example, reduced portal blood flow washing away less adenosine and the accumulated adenosine leading to dilation of the hepatic artery (Lautt, 1985). The mechanism of classical autoregulation is explained by the same hypothesis, for example, increased arterial blood pressure leads to increased arterial blood flow and a subsequent washout of adenosine. The reduced adenosine concentration accounts for the resultant arterial constriction (Ezzat and Lautt, 1987). Reprinted with permission from Lautt, Legare and d'Almeida (1985).

About 30% of hepatic volume is blood (12% of total body blood volume). This total capacitance consists of stressed and unstressed volumes. Stressed volume depends upon intrahepatic pressure and vascular compliance (distensibility). Unstressed volume is the theoretical volume remaining in an organ at zero pressure. Pressures and flows would not be altered in the cardiovascular system if unstressed volume was absent. Active constriction of the capacitance vessels results in transfer of unstressed volume to stressed volume, which maintains or increases venous pressure and venous return. Changes in passive volume, secondary to flow changes, and thus intrahepatic pressure, are also dramatic in the liver and represent changes in stressed volume.

HEPATIC INNERVATION

The liver is an extremely richly innervated organ, the functions of which have managed to remain ignored even when they are reasonably clearly understood. The hepatic sympathetic and parasympathetic nerves play important roles in regulating a wide variety of hepatic metabolic functions (previously reviewed by Lautt, 1980, 1983). The sympathetic nerves affect all aspects of the hepatic circulation and the impact on the overall cardiovascular system is considerable. In addition, the liver may well be the richest sensory organ in the body with afferent nerves that play largely unknown integrative roles as sensors of blood temperature, pressure, and the ionic and nutrient content of portal blood. Implications of the hepatic sensory system have been suggested for internal homeostasis, including control of the kidneys, as well as behavioural control of feeding and thirst (reviewed by Lautt, 1980; Friedman, 1982; Lautt, 1983).

EXTRINSIC NERVE SUPPLY

Previous reviews have summarized the early anatomical studies (Sawchenko and Friedman, 1979; Lautt, 1980). Sympathetic nerves (T7–10) reach the liver via the celiac plexus and intermingle with parasympathetic nerves in the right and left vagus and perhaps the right phrenic nerve (Alexander, 1940; Rappaport, 1975). The posterior hepatic plexus ramifies around the bile duct and portal vein and freely communicates with the anterior plexus. The anterior plexus receives nerves from the left and right celiac ganglion and the left vagus nerve. The anterior plexus supplies the cystic duct, gallbladder, and the pancreatico-choledochus nerve. The anterior plexus forms a sheath around the hepatic artery which can be conveniently prepared for stimulation in physiological preparations in most species. The posterior plexus derives from the right celiac ganglion and the right vagus (Alexander, 1940). The majority of nerves enter the liver in association with the blood vessels and bile duct, branching and communicating in the connective tissue of the perivascular spaces (Sutherland, 1964, 1965). Some parasympathetic branches from the left vagus may pass directly to the liver outside of the two major plexuses (Alexander, 1940). The gallbladder and bile ducts and the hepatic parenchymal cells (metabolic control) receive both sympathetic and parasympathetic nerves but the blood vessels appear to receive only sympathetic nerves (Rappaport, 1975).

The fact that the liver is supplied by two plexuses and perhaps other nerve branches reaching the liver via other routes makes surgical denervation difficult and may complicate nerve stimulation experiments. Variability in nerve distribution to the liver has been reported for humans and lower species. A study in the human showed a marked variability in distribution of the branches of the vagus to the stomach and liver in 100 cadavers (Skandalakis et al., 1980). They found no constant pattern and concluded that many descriptions in the literature are misleading at best, with many surgical selective vagotomies having resulted in incomplete or erroneous denervations. Variable distribution of sympathetic nerves to the liver through the anterior and posterior plexus has been shown by studying the effects of selective surgical denervation on reflexly mediated sympathetic vasoconstriction in the cat (Lautt, 1981b). The arterial constriction produced by unloading the carotid baroreceptors was affected from 0–100% by anterior plexus denervation. The mean data showed 59% of the constriction being eliminated by cutting the anterior plexus with the remaining 41% being abolished by cutting the posterior plexus and hepatic ligaments. Comparisons of metabolic and portal resistance responses have been made in the perfused rat liver indicating more marked effects with anterior plexus stimulation. The metabolic responses of stimulation of the anterior and posterior plexus were additive but this was not true for the hemodynamic responses. The arterial responses were similar with either plexus but the portal responses were greater with anterior plexus stimulation (Gardemann, Strulik and Jungermann, 1987). In the dog, tyrosine caused release of noradrenaline and induced vascular responses when injected into the hepatic artery but not into the portal vein (Garceau and Yamaguchi, 1982). The microvascular responses of all vessels visible on the surface of the rat liver were more dramatically affected by stimulation of the nerves around the hepatic artery than around the portal vein (Reilly, McCuskey and Cilento, 1981).

Full denervation can be assured surgically by tedious and lengthy procedure or by complete removal of the liver and replacement; both methods result in formation of adhesions (Cucchiaro *et al.*, 1990). Surgical denervation can be somewhat simplified by applying a few drops of 1% toluidine blue solution to identify nerve fibres (Holmin *et al.*, 1984). A simpler and more reliable method of producing denervation is demonstrated using phenol (85%) applied on a swab and painted around each of the vessels. This form of denervation produces full functional denervation within 20 minutes of application (Lautt and Carroll, 1984) that is still complete by 8 weeks post-application with no obvious untoward effects (Cucchiaro *et al.*, 1990). Both surgical and phenol denervation are non-selective. Selective hepatic denervation of afferent nerves may be possible using capsaicin but functional demonstration of selectivity and effectiveness of this approach has not been reported in the liver.

Selective *sympathectomy* of the liver can be produced using intraportal injections of 6-hydroxydopamine. Methods have been developed to demonstrate effectiveness and selectivity of such sympathectomy in the cat (Lautt and Cote, 1976) and rat (Lautt and Cote, 1977; Cucchiaro *et al.*, 1990). Stimulation of the remaining nerve fibers following chronic 6-hydroxydopamine exposure results in a parasympathetically-induced reduction in glucose output (Lautt and Wong, 1978) which is taken as evidence of selectivity. Some authors (Allman *et al.*, 1982) have preferred to pretreat animals with phentolamine and propranolol to protect against the severe hypertension that was seen with systemic administration of 6-hydroxydopamine. This type of pretreatment does not appear to affect the denervation potential. The effectiveness of 6-hydroxydopamine is dose-dependent with doses of 50–100 mg/kg producing low levels of noradrenaline after one week but the lower doses resulting in more rapid re-innervation (Cucchiaro *et al.*, 1990). Although a few researchers (eg. Louis-Sylvester *et al.*, 1980) are scrupulous in their demonstration of functional denervation, the vast majority of publications that are reported to have produced a denervation offer no evidence of effective denervation. This is especially critical when reporting a lack of effect of a presumed denervation procedure. One advantage of the use of either 6-hydroxydopamine or phenol denervation is that a functional test for sympathectomy is readily available by electrical stimulation of the anterior plexus and monitoring such responses as elevation in portal venous pressure or release of glucose from the liver.

The human liver has *cholinergic* nerve fibres in contact with the intrahepatic branches of the hepatic artery, portal and hepatic veins (Amenta *et al.*, 1981). Koo and Liang (1979) reported sinusoidal dilation with vagal nerve stimulation and intraportal acetylcholine infusion, however others have not seen dilator responses to parasympathetic stimulation (reviewed by Greenway and Stark, 1971) and topical application of ACh produced constrictions attributable to mast cell degranulation and adrenergic activation (Reilly *et al.*, 1982). If the parasympathetic nerves play any role in hepatic vascular responses it is completely unclear. Certainly these nerves play a role in hepatic metabolic regulation (reviewed by Lautt, 1980).

INTRINSIC NERVES

Intrahepatic distribution of nerves shows considerable species variation. The rat and mouse liver have the least extensive adrenergic innervation of hepatocytes, with fibers contacting cells only in zone 1 of the acinus (periportal region). The rat shows nerves mainly restricted to the portal space of the hilus, with both cholinergic and adrenergic fibers following the preterminal hepatic artery and, to a lesser extent, the portal venules. The guinea-pig and primate livers show more dense innervation where nerves penetrate the acinus right to the central venules (Reilly, McCuskey and McCuskey, 1978; Metz and Forssmann, 1980; Burt *et al.*, 1989). Earlier studies and controversies have been reviewed (Lautt, 1983). The human liver shows a rich hepatocyte innervation and catecholaminergic nerves contact Kupffer cells, endothelial lining cells, and the fat storing cells of Ito.

In those livers with sparse innervation, electrical contact between hepatocytes may occur via gap junctions. The gap junctions appear the most numerous in the areas of the liver that are the least heavily innervated leading Forssmann and Ito (1977) to speculate on their role in electrotonic coupling. This is supported by the observation that the responses to nerve stimulation are similar in the rat, guinea-pig, and tree shrew, yet the density of innervation and catecholamine content is remarkably different, the guinea-pig having six times and the tree shrew twenty-four times the noradrenaline content of the rat liver (Beckh *et al.*, 1990).

DEVELOPMENTAL ASPECTS

Noradrenergic innervation in rats is seen in large portal tracts one day after birth and shows final distribution after five days. Although nerve development occurs over the same time that acinar heterogeneity of enzyme distribution occurs, the normal development of nerve pattern is only coincident since enzyme heterogeneity develops in the 6-hydroxydopamine sympathectomized animal (Lamers *et al.*, 1988). The liver has unique regenerative capacity; after removal of 70% of the liver mass, recovery of mass is essentially complete within 7–10 days. The newly regenerated areas show intensive re-innervation at 10 days, however, if the liver is deprived of either the hepatic arterial or portal venous flow, nerve regeneration is reduced (Pietroletti *et al.*, 1987).

VASCULAR RESPONSES

THE HEPATIC ARTERY

Electrical stimulation of the hepatic nerves leads to a marked decrease in hepatic arterial conductance, with blood flow and conductance reaching a minimum level approaching zero

HEPATIC ARTERY — NERVE STIMULATION

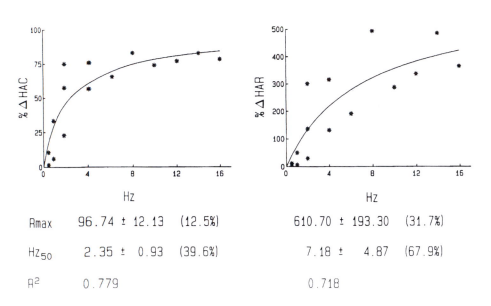

Rmax	96.74 ± 12.13	(12.5%)	610.70 ± 193.30	(31.7%)
Hz$_{50}$	2.35 ± 0.93	(39.6%)	7.18 ± 4.87	(67.9%)
R^2	0.779		0.718	

Figure 13.3 The peak vasoconstrictions to hepatic nerve stimulation expressed as percent change in hepatic arterial conductance (HAC, note this is negative indicating constriction) and resistance (HAR) in one cat. The dynamic parameters of the frequency-response curve are based on non-linear regression to estimate the maximal response (Rmax) and the nerve frequency required to produce 50% of the Rmax (Hz$_{50}$). Results are mean ± SEM with variance in brackets. The line is best fit to the rectangular hyperbolic curve with regression values shown (R^2) for data based on HAC and HAR. The HAC is the appropriate index (see text section on Resistance or Conductance). Legare and Lautt, unpublished.

at approximately 1–2 min at nerve frequencies of 6–12 Hz in cats and dogs (Greenway and Oshiro, 1972). The nerve frequency required to produce 50% of the maximal conductance response occurs at 2.4±0.9 Hz (Figure 13.3). The first observations of the response of the hepatic artery to nerve stimulation appear to have been made by Burton-Opitz (1910). Since that time many people have stimulated the nerves and noted arterial constriction. The pattern of response appears to be of two varieties. The first is typified by the reactions of the dog where the hepatic arterial flow and conductance decreases and remains low for the duration of nerve stimulation (Greenway and Oshiro, 1972). The second pattern is typified by the response in the cat where hepatic arterial flow and conductance decrease but return toward control levels in spite of continued nerve stimulation. This vascular escape from neurogenic stimulation can be distinguished from mere nerve exhaustion.

The extent of vascular escape is not dependent upon the intensity of initial vasoconstriction (Lautt, Legare and Lockhart, 1988). Previous statements to the contrary are artifacts created by the use of vascular resistance as the index of vascular responses (Lautt, 1989). The error in quantification of escape by the use of resistance (escape appears greater from more intense constrictions) is of serious consequence if one is attempting to study factors that may modulate the degree of escape. By the use of resistance, escape will artifactually appear to be reduced by any substance that decreases the initial vasoconstriction (see arguments below under "Resistance or Conductance?"). Conductance begins to escape from the peak vasoconstriction at 1–2 minutes of stimulation and reaches a plateau of about an 80% escape by 4–5 minutes with the time to three-quarters of full escape being 3.4 ± 0.5 minutes (Lautt, 1977). Vascular escape is a phenomenon not exclusive to cat livers and is reported to occur in a variety of organs and species in response to nerve stimulation and noradrenaline infusion (Lautt, 1980; Greenway, 1984a,b).

The *mechanism of vascular escape* from neurogenic constriction is unknown but a variety of possibilities have been excluded. Escape is not due to failure of the nerves since the capacitance vessel constriction is well maintained (Greenway, Stark and Lautt, 1969) and hepatic venous resistance remains elevated throughout the stimulation (Lautt and Legare, 1992a). The escape also occurs in response to infusions of noradrenaline, thereby eliminating the possibility of nerve fatigue being the mechanism. Escape is not modified by β adrenergic blocking agents; it is not modified by atropine, antihistamines or prostaglandin synthetase inhibitors. It occurs in preparations with constant arterial perfusion thereby eliminating flow-dependent accumulation of metabolites as a likely means of producing dilation of the constricted vessels. Comprehensive reviews of vascular escape provide details of the organs and species showing vascular escape and discussion of data leading to elimination of many suggested mechanisms of escape (Greenway, 1984a, 1984b). The most likely vascular involvement is that those vessels initially constricted are later partially relaxed. This is supported principally by the lack of redistribution seen with microspheres as well as the lack of interference with drug clearance (Lautt and Skelton, 1976) and oxygen uptake (Lautt, 1977).

Glucagon has recently been shown to be able to produce a complete suppression of vascular escape in the cat hepatic artery in response to initial vasoconstriction induced by either nerves or noradrenaline infusion (d'Almeida and Lautt, 1989a,b). This is the only report of any manipulation that has been able to modulate the extent of hepatic arterial vascular escape. Unpublished observations in my laboratory indicate that there is no role for adenosine or oxygen supply in modulation of the extent of escape. Capsaicin pretreatment was able to prevent escape in the small intestine of the rat (Remak, Hottenstein and Jacobson, 1990). Recently a hypothesis has been presented (Chen and Shepherd, 1991) that relates generation of hydrogen ions during nerve stimulation to inhibition of postjunctional α_2 adrenergic receptor-induced constriction in canine gut. The hydrogen ion theory requires testing in the liver. However, whether the mechanism of escape is the same in the liver and small intestine appears unlikely since glucagon, in doses that completely blocked escape in the hepatic artery, was without effect in the superior mesenteric artery of the cat (d'Almeida and Lautt, 1991).

On cessation of nerve stimulation a brief hyperemic period is usually seen. The mechanism of the *post-stimulatory hyperemia* is unknown, but it is not necessarily associated with escape as it occurs in both cats and dogs. Unpublished results from my lab indicate no role for adenosine or β-adrenergic receptors.

The amount of tonic *sympathetic tone* on the hepatic arterial resistance vessels is not clear but several lines of evidence indicate that it is probably very minor in the anaesthetized animal. Acute denervation produced no significant hemodynamic effects in the cat (Lautt, 1977), dog (Cohn and Kountz, 1963; Mundschau et al., 1966), rat, or rabbit (Ginsburg, Grayson and Johnson, 1952). These forms of denervation however, may not have produced effective physiological denervation if nerves from the posterior plexus were left intact.

Reflex activation

Bilateral carotid occlusion or carotid pressure manipulation leads to reflex constriction of the hepatic artery (Greenway, Lawson and Mellander, 1967; Carneiro and Donald, 1977; Tyden, Samnegard and Thulin, 1979; Lautt, 1982). Whether or not vascular escape occurs to the reflex stimulation is complicated by the fact that such reflex activation is not selective for the liver. In the dog, where escape does not occur to direct stimulation, Mundschau et al. (1966) found that reflex activation resulted in an initial constriction but the hepatic artery showed normal tone by 5 minutes. It seems highly likely that this sort of response does not represent a true vascular escape but rather represents an interaction between the direct constrictor effect of the hepatic nerve activation and the indirect vasodilator influence of the hepatic arterial buffer response. In this situation the buffer response would be activated secondary to a reflex-induced reduction of blood flow that supplies the portal vein. A reduction in portal venous flow will activate the hepatic arterial buffer response (see Figure 13.2) and lead to a dilation of the hepatic artery. Note that the buffer response is an extremely powerful mechanism that can lead to nearly full vasodilation if portal venous flow decreases sufficiently. The interaction between the buffer response and direct nerve or drug-induced effects on the hepatic artery represent an extremely severe and almost universally ignored complication in hepatic vascular studies. Examples of confusion in the literature are shown by the interactions between the buffer response and intravenously infused vasoactive compounds where direct acting dilators can cause hepatic arterial constriction if the drugs are administered intravenously (Lautt et al., 1988).

Systemic hypercapnia or hypoxia result in reflex hepatic arterial vasoconstriction in the dog that is eliminated or reversed by selective hepatic denervation (Mathie and Blumgart, 1983). In these studies there was no indication of functional buffer response since after hepatic arterial denervation, portal flow showed a normal increase to hypercapnia but the hepatic artery did not constrict. The direct effect of hypercapnia on the hepatic artery may, however, have confounded these responses.

Resistance or conductance?

Studies requiring quantification of vascular responses require appropriate selection of indices of active vascular responses. Because nerve stimulation results in effects on perfusion pressure as well as blood flow, simply reporting results as changes in blood flow is unacceptable and, for that reason, a calculated index of vascular tone has been used. The traditional index of vascular tone is resistance (driving pressure gradient ÷ blood flow). This index incorporates both the changes in pressure and flow and offers considerable advantage. I have previously argued and provided a number of examples to indicate, however, that the inverse of resistance, conductance, should be used in preference for *in vivo* studies (Lautt, 1989). Conductance is a more useful index of vascular tone because the parameter that is changing (blood flow) appears in the numerator of the calculation. Thus, changes in vascular tone produce linearly related changes in both blood flow and conductance but non-linearly related changes in resistance. This non-linear relationship between changes in resistance and changes in blood flow results in severe distortion of many vascular responses. Consider, for example, that intense nerve stimulation will lead to a decrease in blood flow so that as flow and conductance approach zero, vascular resistance approaches infinity. A pharmacological antagonist that reduces this constriction by 50% will produce a response in resistance that is essentially meaningless, whereas the same data expressed as conductance will show a 50% decrease in blood flow response and vascular conductance response. Thus, the use of vascular resistance precludes even taking simple average responses. Examples of distortion of data have been demonstrated. Expressing vascular escape in terms of resistance is one clear example. If the initial vasoconstriction reduces blood flow by 90 ml/min from a control level of 100 ml/min to 10 ml/min and subsequently escapes by 45 ml/min to plateau flow of 55 ml/min, the calculated blood flow escape would be 50% (45 ml ÷ 90 ml). If blood pressure remains relatively constant at 100 mmHg, vascular conductance would also show a 50% escape but resistance would show a 91% escape. If the initial constriction only reduced blood flow by 10 ml/min from the control level of 100 ml/min and flow undergoes a 50% escape (5 ml/min), conductance shows a 50% escape but resistance shows a 54% escape. Thus, not only does escape calculated from resistance produce responses that are not related to the flow responses but escape measured using resistance suggests a degree of escape that becomes more intense as the level of vasoconstriction is increased, data clearly in contrast to reported data using conductance measurements (Lautt et al., 1988). Recently this theoretical argument has been supported by comparative analysis of actual escape responses (d'Almeida and Lautt, 1991). Further details of this argument are provided (Lautt, Legare and Lockhart, 1988; Lautt, 1989).

It is important to note that vascular conductance is the appropriate index of vascular tone only in situations where blood flow is the parameter that is primarily affected by the relevant stimulus. In situations where arterial long circuits are used to hold flow steady or in other situations where flow does not alter but active vascular tone results in changes in pressure, then resistance becomes the appropriate calculation since the changing parameter should always be in the numerator in order that the index be linearly related to the primary changing parameter.

Pharmacodynamic approach in vivo

With the realization that the use of vascular conductance would allow classical pharmacodynamic approaches to be used for in vivo studies of intact vascular beds, a powerful research tool has been added to these studies. The first in vivo study to use arterial conductance responses to calculate maximal vascular responses (Rmax) and the doses of drugs required to produce 50% of the maximal response (ED_{50}) was reported in 1985 (Lautt and Legare, 1985), when 8-phenyltheophylline was shown to be a competitive antagonist of adenosine's vasodilator effect on the hepatic artery. In that study the Rmax and ED_{50} were estimated by linearizing the dose-response curve using the Eadie Hofstee transformation. Other forms of linearization such as the Lineweaver Burke method have also been used, but the recent ready availability of non-linear regression solving capacities from commercial software packages (eg. Graphpad, ISI Software) makes the older methods largely of historical interest. We have recently used the non-linear regression of the rectangular hyperbolic dose-response curves for a variety of studies. Of relevance to this chapter, we have also found that the nerve frequency-response relationship can also be analyzed using this non-linear regression approach to estimate the maximum response and the nerve frequency required to produce 50% of the maximum response (Hz_{50}). Figure 13.3 shows this relationship analyzed for the hepatic artery contrasting the use of resistance and conductance. This method thus allows for direct comparisons of responsiveness to nerve stimulation in various disease states and in the presence of various neuromodulators. This classical pharmacodynamic approach has allowed the demonstration that adenosine is able to produce a dose-related suppression of Rmax with no effect on the Hz_{50} (classical non-competitive type antagonism) in the superior mesenteric artery (Lockhart, Legare and Lautt, 1988). This is a potentially very powerful tool but it must be cautioned that the technical limitations and interpretations of these *in vivo* responses have not been fully evaluated. Many of the technical limitations involved with pharmacological studies (recirculation of drugs, for example) are not of consequence for analysis of the nerve responses. However, the complexity of the nerve-induced responses may prove a limitation in some settings. In this regard, it should be noted, however, that a similar pharmacodynamic approach can also be used to analyze frequency-response relationships for hepatic volume responses to nerve stimulation and the effect of modulators of this response have been reported using this methodology (see capacitance responses below).

BLOOD FLOW DISTRIBUTION

Stimulation of hepatic nerves in an isolated perfused liver preparation led to a marked and well-maintained decrease in oxygen uptake correspondent with a reversible gross heterogeneity of flow, as shown by surface appearance following injection of trypan blue. About 30% of the tissue was estimated to be without flow during stimulation but flow appeared normal 10 minutes after cessation of stimulation (Ji, Beckh and Jungermann, 1984). Similar heterogeneity was produced in this type of preparation in response to noradrenaline infusion (Beckh *et al.*, 1985). It was concluded that the mechanism of the reduced oxygen uptake is related to the circulatory changes rather than a metabolic effect (Ji, Beckh and Jungermann, 1984). In contrast, flow distribution is not altered *in vivo* in response to noradrenaline infusion (Krarup, 1973) or hepatic nerve stimulation (3–5 minutes) as shown by distribution of radioactive microspheres (Greenway and Oshiro, 1972) and unaltered uptake of lidocaine (Lautt and Skelton, 1976) and oxygen (Lautt, 1977). In the cat, oxygen uptake decreased transiently but as vascular escape proceeded, oxygen uptake returned to control levels suggesting that some redistribution of flow may have occurred at the onset of stimulation secondary to arterial sphincter-like constriction (Lautt, 1978). Indicator-dilution methodology confirmed that, despite a 40% reduction in vascular volume induced reflexly by carotid arterial occlusion, the interstitial space and accessible cell water space were unchanged indicating that there were no significant zones of no-flow (Cousineau *et al.*, 1985).

   The major regions of unperfused tissue that are generated by nerve stimulation in the isolated liver must surely have metabolic consequences and, in view of the recently proposed oxygen-dependent eicosanoid mediation, some of the vascular and metabolic responses to nerves may be artifacts of regional hypoxia (see section on Neurotransmitters and Neuromodulation). The dramatic contrast between the isolated, *in situ* perfused rat liver and the responses of cat and dog livers *in vivo* reinforces the concerns previously raised by Greenway and Stark (1971) that "conclusions from isolated perfused liver preparations cannot be extrapolated to the intact liver and such preparations have proven of limited value in vascular studies".

VENOUS RESISTANCE

Knowledge of the regulation and importance of the venous system in the liver has undergone intense development and controversy. In this section of the chapter I will focus on recent developments regarding the low pressure side of the hepatic circulation. This work focuses on studies carried out over the past five years. Reference to earlier work can be obtained from some classical reviews or books (Child, 1954: Brauer, 1963; Greenway and Stark, 1971).

Overview

The portal blood flows in massive quantity (20% of the cardiac output) through an organ that weighs approximately 1.5 kilograms in an adult male. The portal blood has had its hydrostatic pressure fall from approximately 120 mmHg to 7 mmHg as the blood has passed through the vascular beds of the splanchnic organs (spleen, stomach, intestine, pancreas, omentum). The combined portal flow surges through the subdividing portal venules, through the syncytium of sinusoids (passing approximately 20 hepatocytes and perfusing the muralium of liver cell plates with blood on both sides of the plate), then hence flowing through the collecting hepatic veins and the large conducting veins to flood into the inferior vena cava. The portal blood is rich with hormones and bioactive chemicals derived from a variety of organs. The liver interacts with the portal blood by mixing it evenly with arterial blood and performing a multitude of chemical interactions with the bloodstream. The inferior vena cava collects "used blood" from the lower regions and this blood, along with purified blood from the kidneys, meets the blood flowing from the hepatic veins and passes a short distance through the chest and into the right atrium. The pressures along this venous system are astonishingly low. The regulation of pressures at the various points is of hemodynamic and homeostatic importance and is determined by the passive distensibility of the blood vessels and by active control through the sympathetic nervous system and hormones.

The resistance to blood flow through the liver is extremely low with pressure gradients between the portal venous inflow and hepatic venous outflow of the liver being in the range of 5 mmHg or less. Considering that the pressure gradient across all other organs is in the range of 115 mmHg, the vascular resistance within the hepatic portal system might erroneously appear to be trivial and of no consequence. In fact, the pressures are regulated at precise regions of the venous circuit at pre- and postsinusoidal sites, and the proportion of pressure drop across the two sites and the total resistance determines intrahepatic and portal venous pressure and volumes. In diseases of the liver, the most common cause of death is directly related to the vascular consequences of increased resistance to portal blood flow. If the pressure gradient becomes elevated by as little as 15 mmHg, hemodynamic and homeostatic instability can lead to the demise of the patient. Portal venous pressure reaches approximately 25 mmHg in the most severely cirrhotic conditions (Van Leeuwen et al., 1989).

The adjustment of pressure in the normal state is achieved by changes of vascular resistance within the presinusoidal portal venules and the postsinusoidal hepatic veins. These sites of resistance have three important characteristics: they offer very low resistance; the resistance is able to be more than doubled by active vascular constriction; the resistance sites are passively distensible. To understand the vascular responses to sympathetic nerve stimulation, it must first be appreciated that the active responses interact with and are severely modulated by the passive distensibility of the resistance sites. The ability to describe this interaction is dependent upon being able to measure resistance at the key regulatory locations.

Essential assumptions

The description of active and passive regulation of pre- and postsinusoidal resistance sites is dependent upon the assumption that the pressures measured are valid and not subject to significant artifact. The pressures of relevance are the portal venous pressure prior to entry into the liver, the central venous pressure at the exit of the hepatic veins, and the intrahepatic pressure representing sinusoidal blood pressure. With these three pressures, the presinusoidal and postsinusoidal resistance can be quantified. The portal and vena caval pressures are technically easily measured and validated because of ready access to these vessels under experimental conditions. The intrahepatic pressure is the contentious pressure.

As a pressure catheter is advanced via the vena cava into the hepatic veins, pressure is similar to central venous pressure until the catheter tip passes through a narrow length of hepatic vein. This region has the characteristics of a smooth muscle sphincter and morphological studies support the existence of sphincter-like regions in large hepatic veins (Child, 1954). These sphincters are localized to third-order branches (ramuli, according to the nomenclature of Elias and Petty, 1952) of the hepatic veins in cats (Lautt et al., 1986) and in the terminal 2 cm of the lobar hepatic vein proper in dogs (Legare and Lautt, 1987). Physiological sphincters have not been proven in other species and morphological data directly correlating functional and structural evidence are missing. The sudden rise of pressure from central venous pressure to portal pressure as a catheter is advanced has usually been assumed to represent wedging of the catheter and the pressure readings were assumed to be via a static column. Several factors indicate that this measurement is not a "wedged" pressure. First, the catheter need not be wedged and can often be advanced at least an additional 1–2 cm beyond the sphincter even in cats (Lautt et al., 1986). Second, the catheters we have used have the tips sealed and pressure is recorded via side-holes cut 3 and 7 mm back from the tip. We assume that the ability to record a valid pressure beyond the sphincter, but distal to the sealed catheter tip, is dependent upon the existence of collaterals between the veins proximal to the sphincters. The sphincters are contracted by neural and pharmacological stimuli and the site of the sphincter is not altered by catheter size or state of contraction (Lautt et al., 1986; Lautt, Greenway and Legare, 1987; Legare and Lautt, 1987) as would be expected if the "sphincter" really represented an artifact of wedging in the vein. Finally, in the dog, an unusual species in that the hepatic resistance site is located in the terminal portion of the hepatic vein, it is possible to position a catheter in the hepatic vein proximal to the sphincter site via an incision in the surface of the liver. By locating a small hepatic venous tributary and passing a catheter downstream into the hepatic vein; (the catheter thus does not pass through the putative sphincter zone) pressure similar to portal pressure can be demonstrated. With the catheter thus placed, histamine-induced sphincter contraction led to equal and parallel elevations in portal venous pressure and in hepatic venous pressure proximal to the hepatic veins in a position where it is impossible to be measuring a "wedged" pressure (Legare and Lautt, 1987). Other arguments have been presented (Lautt and Greenway, 1987; Greenway and Lautt, 1989; Lautt and Legare, 1992a) to support the view that measurement of lobar venous pressure (LVP) using a catheter that is passed proximal to the hepatic venous resistance site is representative of a true pressure measured at that site.

Thus, LVP is assumed to be representative of sinusoidal pressure. The pressure gradient between LVP and central venous pressure (CVP) is the pressure gradient primarily regulated by a sphincter-like zone in the hepatic veins. In the basal state, this pressure gradient usually represents virtually the entire pressure gradient across the liver. Therefore, in the basal state, the vascular resistance of the portal venules and sinusoids is normally trivial with sinusoidal pressure and portal pressure being insignificantly different. The observation that equal reductions in arterial and portal flow lead to the same changes in hepatic volume (Bennett, MacAnespie and Rothe, 1982) also supports the contention that virtually all the resistance to venous flow is in the hepatic veins. The pressure gradient between the portal vein (PVP) and the pressure measured just proximal to the hepatic venous sphincters (LVP) is assumed to represent primarily resistance within the portal venules. Note, however, that the pressure gradient represents pressure lost across the large and small portal tributaries and the sinusoidal bed as well as the small hepatic venules proximal to the LVP catheter. Active vasoconstriction results in a very significant increase in the PVP to LVP gradient. I will refer to this pressure gradient as being due to presinusoidal or portal venous resistance; the primary observation that supports this assumption is described elsewhere (Lautt and Legare, 1992a) and is more fully discussed below under the section of Presinusoidal Resistance Responses. The essential argument, however, is that after 5 minutes of nerve stimulation the hepatic blood volume is reduced by up to 50% while the PVP to LVP pressure gradient and the calculated vascular resistance of this segment has escaped and is trivial (Lautt and Legare, 1992a) (Figure 13.4). At this stage the maintained 50% reduction in hepatic blood volume has not contributed significantly to vascular resistance suggesting that the sinusoidal cross-sectional area is so vast as to offer trivial resistance, and that very large changes in this cross-sectional area can be achieved without adding significantly to overall resistance. Therefore, the assumption is that the primary active resistance site proximal to the LVP catheter in the normal liver is restricted to inlet vessels of the portal vein.

In summary, the principle assumptions here are that the LVP measurement is a valid pressure measurement representative of pressures proximal to the hepatic venous sphincter-like zone and that the PVP-LVP gradient represents largely presinusoidal or portal venous resistance and the LVP-CVP gradient represents primarily resistance across the hepatic venous sphincter-like zones.

EFFECTS OF DISTENDING PRESSURE ON RESISTANCE

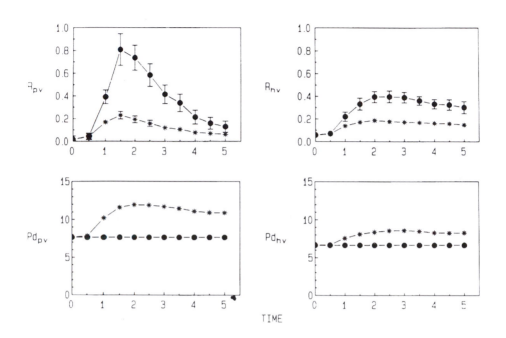

Figure 13.4   Resistance of the portal vein (R_{pv}) and hepatic venous segment (R_{hv}) contrasting actual measured resistance (*) during 5 minutes of nerve stimulation with calculated resistance (•) that would have been determined if the distending blood pressure (Pd) had not risen from control level. This calculation is based on the theory that the index of contractility (IC) would be the same, for example at the peak response, regardless of whether Pd changed; IC is independent of passive changes in Pd. The calculated R at constant Pd exactly parallels the IC curve in terms of percentage change. IC and R are equally useful indexes of active vascular tone change only if Pd does not change. Differences in change in IC and R are due to the distending effects of Pd on R. The rise in Pd causes the actively contracting sphincters to passively distend thus minimizing the net change in R. Data are means ± S.E.M. The calculated R at unaltered Pd are means of individual curves rather than being taken from the mean data (n=8). Reprinted from Lautt and Legare, 1992a.

Passive distensibility

In order to understand the effects of active contraction of the pre- and postsinusoidal hepatic resistance sites, some further background is required. The large passive distensibility of these resistance sites has been quantified and studied under a variety of conditions (Lautt, Greenway and Legare, 1991; Lautt and Legare, 1991a,b). Vascular resistance is reduced by 75% in response to an elevation of vena caval pressure of roughly 3 mmHg (Lautt, Greenway and Legare, 1991). The small rise in distending pressure produces very large decreases in vascular resistance that has been quantified as having a constant relationship under basal condition and under conditions of actively increased basal tone. The distending pressure (Pd) has been found to be able to be estimated from the average value of the pressures measured on either side of the resistance site (Greenway and Lautt, 1988). Resistance (R) is inversely linearly related to the distending pressure cubed (Pd^3) and the slope of this linear relationship is referred to as the "*index of contractility*" (IC) where $IC = R \cdot Pd^3$. This index of contractility is affected acutely only by active vascular responses and is independent of passive alterations in the distending blood pressure. Thus, active vascular responses can be measured using the IC whereas the use of calculated vascular resistance provides a measure that is the result of interaction between active and passive influences. The importance of this differentiation will become more clear in the next section.

RESISTANCE VESSEL RESPONSES TO SYMPATHETIC NERVE STIMULATION

Presinusoidal or portal responses

There are literally hundreds of reports in the literature, beginning with Bayliss and Starling in 1894, indicating that stimulation of hepatic sympathetic nerves leads to elevation in portal venous pressure. The specific intrahepatic sites of resistance had not, however, been determined until recently and the introduction of the new index of contractility allows quantification to be done at a more refined level. Previous studies can be found in the following reviews (Child, 1954; Greenway and Stark, 1971; Lautt, 1980; Richardson and Withrington, 1981a; Lautt, 1983; Lautt and Greenway, 1987; Greenway and Lautt, 1989). Figure 13.5 shows the response to a 5 min stimulation of the hepatic nerves at a frequency of 8 Hz. The presinusoidal resistance increases from insignificant levels in the basal state to account for 50% of the total venous resistance at the peak measured at 2 min. By 5 min extensive escape of the presinusoidal component had occurred despite the well maintained constriction of the hepatic venous site. This amount of vasoconstriction resulted in the presinusoidal pressure gradient rising from an insignificant level (0.2 ± 0.5 mmHg) to account for 39% of the total elevated gradient of 7.2 ± 0.6 mmHg at the peak of the response. After 5 minutes of stimulation the pressure gradient had decreased and was only 0.9 ± 0.4 mmHg. In contrast, the hepatic venous pressure gradient remained steady (4.4 ± 0.6 mmHg at 2 min, 4.4 ± 0.8 mmHg at 5 min). This *presinusoidal vascular escape* is also clearly seen using the index of contractility (Figure 13.5). The mechanism of the vascular escape is unknown but it is of interest to note that both the hepatic arterial and the portal venous resistance sites undergo escape. Escape is also seen in the isolated rat liver responses to nerve stimulation but whether this represents true escape or nerve fatigue is unclear since the vascular response and noradrenaline overflow both declined to basal levels by 6 minutes (Sannemann, Beckh and Jungermann, 1986). The vascular response was measured as blood flow change in a constant pressure system so the return to basal flow indicated that contraction of all vascular resistance segments (pre- and postsinusoidal) was absent by 6 minutes. In contrast, the blood volume and hepatic venous sphincter responses do not show escape *in vivo* (Figure 13.5).

The index of contractility has a similar qualitative appearance to the calculated responses using resistance as the vascular index (Figure 13.5). However, the resistance calculation grossly quantitatively underestimates the constriction as a result of the interaction between the active vascular constriction and the passive distending effect of the elevated intrahepatic pressures. Figure 13.4 makes this point graphically where the calculated resistance is

HEPATIC VENOUS AND PORTAL VENOUS RESPONSES TO NERVE STIMULATION

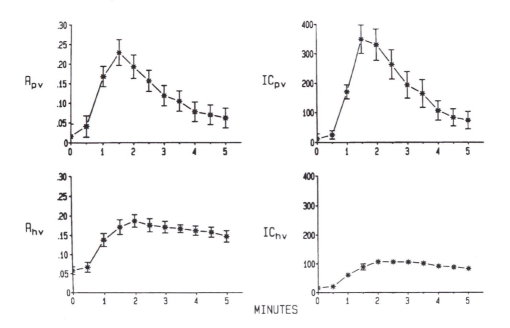

Figure 13.5   Mean (± SE) responses of portal venous resistance (R_{pv} = (PVP – LVP)/portal flow, mmHg/ml·min^{-1}kg^{-1}) and index of contractility (IC_{pv} = R_{pv} × Pd^3_{pv}, mmHg^4/ml·min^{-1}kg^{-1}; Pd_{pv} = (PVP + LVP)/2) and hepatic venous resistance (R_{hv} = (LVP – IVCP)/total hepatic flow) and IC (IC_{hv} = R_{hv} × Pd^3_{hv}; Pd_{hv} = (LVP + IVCP)/2) to 8 Hz stimulation of the anterior plexus of the hepatic nerve for 5 minutes measured at 30 sec intervals (n = 8). PVP = portal venous pressure, LVP = lobar venous pressure = sinusoidal pressure, IVCP = inferior vena caval pressure. Note the different impression of relative pre- versus post-sinusoidal constrictions dependent upon use of R or IC. Reprinted from Lautt and Legare, 1992a.

shown along with the measured distending pressure. Because the index of contractility is not affected by distending pressure (Lautt, Greenway and Legare, 1991), the index of contractility would be identical regardless of whether distending pressure had remained steady or was elevated. Therefore, vascular resistance can be calculated from the equation, $IC = R \cdot Pd^3$, for any distending pressure. In Figure 13.4 resistance has been recalculated for the situation where the distending pressure had not changed. That is, the impact of active constriction and the interaction between active and passive forces has been separated. This exercise indicates that the simultaneous elevation of active vascular tone and distending blood pressure led to a much smaller rise in resistance than would have occurred had the distending pressure not changed. The error that is incurred by using vascular resistance as an index of the active vascular tone is in the range of 400%. The change in resistance will accurately reflect active vascular responses only if Pd does not change; the underestimate in the active contractile response by using calculated vascular resistance is magnified as the Pd change is increased.

The selection of the index of vascular reactions must be made rationally and with a clear understanding of the implications of each index. For therapeutic purposes, dealing with amelioration of portal hypertension, the pressure gradient is probably the most important concern for the physician. The effect of various drugs on the intrahepatic pressures is best understood using vascular resistance because the resistance is both affected by the pressure and affects the pressure and this index thus focuses on the net interaction between active and passive forces. To study purely active responses, however, the index of contractility must be used. Thus, this index would be the appropriate index to use to determine the effect of modulators of nerve-induced responses or for studies where the mechanism of changes of resistance is to be determined.

Hepatic venous resistance responses

Calculation of vascular resistance across the hepatic veins is done using the pressure gradient LVP to CVP and total hepatic blood flow. This is in contrast to the calculations for presinusoidal resistance that uses only portal venous flow. In the basal state the vascular resistance to the hepatic veins, which is primarily localized to a sphincter-like zone, accounts for almost all of the resistance to blood flow. Depending upon the index of vascular tone used, however, the proportion of pre- versus postsinusoidal involvement appears quite different. For example, in the data shown in Figure 13.5, the presinusoidal component of the total pressure gradient across the liver was insignificant with 90% of the gradient being accounted for by the hepatic veins. The hepatic veins accounted for about 78% of the total calculated resistance and only about 57% of the calculated index of contractility. Thus, the higher distending pressure at the presinusoidal site produces a passive distention of the presinusoidal vessels that gives the impression that there is no significant vascular tone unless the index of contractility is used. The active vasoconstriction produced by 8 Hz nerve stimulation is shown in Figure 13.5 where the hepatic venous IC rose by 563% from 16.7 to 110.8 IC units. The distending pressure had also increased over this time (from 6.6 to 8.4 mmHg) and this increase in distending pressure produced a passive dilation of the hepatic venous resistance sites. The net effect on resistance was that it increased by only 222% (from 0.058 to 0.187). The underestimate of active vascular tone responses using resistance in contrast to the new index of contractility is shown in Figure 13.4. Note that the constriction of the hepatic veins is well maintained for the entire 5 minutes nerve stimulation, in contrast to the very dramatic vascular escape from neurogenic stimulation seen for the presinusoidal portal venous and hepatic arterial sites. As with the hepatic artery and portal venous responses, appropriate selection of the index of vascular responses is important.

HEPATIC BLOOD VOLUME

Overview

Blood volume in mammals is 60–85 ml/kg body weight with about 70% of this volume located in the veins (Rothe, 1983). The capacitance function of the venous system controls distribution of blood volumes and cardiac filling pressures (Greenway and Lautt, 1986). To serve as a blood reservoir an organ must be able to adjust the contained blood volume.

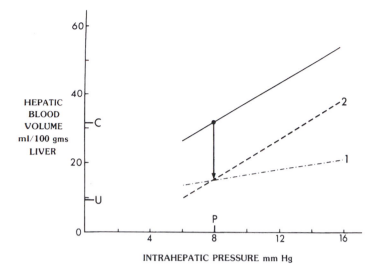

Figure 13.6   Pressure-volume relationship in hepatic venous bed (solid line). At transmural pressure P, hepatic blood volume or capacitance is C, [unstressed volume (U) plus stressed volume]. Slope of solid line, compliance. Venoconstriction (arrow) could result from a change in compliance with no change in unstressed volume (line 1), a change in unstressed volume with no change in compliance (line 2), or a combination of changes in both compliance and unstressed volume. Reprinted with permission from Greenway and Lautt (1989).

The *capacitance* is the total blood volume and is 37 ml/100 g liver (8.2 ml/kg body weight) in denervated cat liver at a portal blood pressure of 8 mmHg (Greenway, Seaman and Innes, 1985) with somewhat lesser volume in innervated livers. This is equal to about 12% of total blood volume, a value similar to that reported for humans (Cohn, Khatry and Groszmann, 1972).

Capacitance is the total volume which consists of *stressed volume* and unstressed volume. Stressed volume is determined by vascular compliance and the intrahepatic blood pressure. *Compliance* refers to the distensibility of the vascular bed and is defined as the change in volume per unit change in distending blood pressure. Many publications incorrectly interchange the terms compliance and capacitance. There is a linear relationship between distending pressure and volume over a wide physiological range; the slope of the line is the compliance. Compliance is about 2.8 ml/mmHg (per 100 g tissue or 0.6 per kg body weight) and at a pressure of 8 mmHg the stressed volume is 22 ml/100 g or roughly 60% of total liver capacitance. Extrapolation of the linear pressure-volume curve to zero gives the *unstressed volume*, a theoretical volume that would exist at zero distending pressure (Figure 13.6).

Stressed and unstressed volume

Liver volume could decrease in response to sympathetic nerve stimulation either by a reduction in compliance or by a reduction in unstressed volume (Figure 13.6). All available evidence indicates that active venous contraction occurs mainly by a change in unstressed volume (Rothe, 1983). The responses to noradrenaline infusions were studied in the cat liver (Greenway, Seaman and Innes, 1985). Intrahepatic pressure was varied by changing portal flow and by changing outflow pressure, and pressure-volume curves were determined before, during, and after noradrenaline infusion. It was shown that the volume response was entirely due to a reduction in unstressed volume (the pressure-volume curves underwent a parallel shift indicating that compliance was unchanged). When these data are evaluated in conjunction with other data (Rothe, 1983), it seems reasonable to conclude that active venoconstriction in the liver and other organs involves a decrease in unstressed volume. Direct support for a similar mechanism of contraction in response to sympathetic nerves has been technically difficult to produce. Only two studies have attempted to address the question of mechanism of hepatic volume change in response to nerve stimulation; both studies have acknowledged technical problems that make interpretation difficult. Bennett, MacAnespie and Rothe (1982) found an apparent decrease in hepatic compliance and Greenway (1987) found an apparent increase in compliance. Bennett's group measured the volume response to a single one min, 5 mmHg step elevation in venous pressure with the assumption that the pressure was transmitted similarly to the capacitance vessels in control and stimulated state. This is the same assumption that Dr. Clive Greenway and I previously erroneously made for compliance measurements (1976). Pressure transmission of a rise in hepatic outflow pressure beyond the hepatic venous resistance sites is dependent upon venous resistance and is reduced by nerve stimulation (Lautt, Greenway and Legare, 1987). This reduced pressure transmission would create an apparent reduced compliance. Recalculation of data from recent study confirms this interpretation. Risoe, Hall and Smiseth (1991) calculated hepatic compliance from two different degrees of hepatic venous pressure elevation. The elevations in hepatic venous pressure resulted in elevation of portal venous pressure with 63% of the low hepatic venous pressure increment (4.9 mmHg) being transmitted to the portal vein and a greater percentage transmission (70%) occurring in response to the higher pressure increment (7.3 mmHg). This is predictable from the venous distensibility model (Lautt, Legare and Greenway, 1987; Lautt, Greenway and Legare, 1991). If the venous compliance is calculated by dividing the change in volume by the change in blood pressure, it is seen that using the hepatic venous pressure results in a greater apparent compliance for the higher pressure elevation. If, however, one makes the assumption that the pressure gradient PVP-HVP is mainly due to postsinusoidal resistance and uses PVP as the distending pressure, the compliance is the same for both degrees of pressure elevation. This study is thus compatible with the notion that virtually all of the venous resistance is postsinusoidal; that the stressed volume is primarily proximal to the hepatic veins and that portal pressure is a better estimate of the sinusoidal blood pressure than is hepatic venous pressure. The use of hepatic venous pressure will underestimate hepatic compliance and make it appear to be non-linearly related to pressure, as we saw in our earlier study (Lautt and Greenway, 1976).

In contrast, Greenway's recent study attempted to determine the slope of a pressure-volume line to graded elevation in venous pressure during sympathetic nerve stimulation. Although intrahepatic pressures were measured, the data are inconclusive because nerve responses were progressively impaired at higher venous pressures (Karim and Hainsworth, 1976; Greenway, 1981) so that apparent compliance increased progressively. Greenway

(1987) concluded that "These results suggest that this approach of measuring hepatic volume-pressure relationships cannot be used to determine compliance and unstressed volume in innervated livers, owing to the presence of an unknown degree of venoconstrictor tone which may, or may not, be mediated by sympathetic nerves". Because of the difficulty with these studies and in consideration of the clear lack of compliance effects of noradrenaline on the liver (Greenway, Seaman and Innes, 1985) where capacitance responses are well maintained at elevated venous pressure (Lautt, Brown and Durham, 1980), we tentatively conclude that compliance probably does not change in response to nerve stimulation. Recent studies based on mean circulatory filling pressure have indicated that splanchnic nerve stimulation raises MCFP but probably does so by reducing unstressed volume without affecting compliance (Bower and O'Donnell, 1991).

The concept of venoconstriction as a change in unstressed volume rather than a change in venous compliance has interesting physiological consequences (Greenway and Lautt, 1989). If venoconstriction occurred by a decrease in compliance, the amount of blood actively mobilized would become progressively smaller as the intrahepatic pressure decreased (see Figure 13.6, line 1). This would mean that in those situations where mobilization of blood was most vital, for example during haemorrhage, the amount that could be mobilized by the sympathetic nervous system would become smaller as the hemodynamic status deteriorated. In contrast, when venoconstriction causes a change in unstressed volume with no change in compliance, the amount of blood mobilized by the sympathetic nervous system is independent of intrahepatic pressure (Figure 13.6, line 2). In this case, the volume mobilized actively by the change in unstressed volume and passively by the decline in intrahepatic pressure are additive. This would give the animal the best chance of survival.

Although the net capacitance response of the liver superficially appears quite straight-forward, the interaction between stressed and unstressed volume during sympathetic nerve-induced contraction becomes quite complex. Figure 13.7 shows conceptually the interactions that probably occur during nerve stimulation. Nerve stimulation does not likely alter compliance but, because of constriction of the hepatic venous sphincters, intrahepatic pressure increases thus leading to an increase in the stressed volume. Unstressed volume is decreased with a net effect being a reduction in total capacitance, but an increase in the stressed volume. This also would appear to have survival advantage in permitting further additional reduction in capacitance that might occur secondary to passive hemodynamic reactions such as the reduction in portal pressure that would occur with the reduction in cardiac output during haemorrhage.

Unstressed volume is hemodynamically inactive but when venoconstriction changes unstressed volume into stressed volume, it is equivalent to a transfusion of a significant amount of blood. Sympathetic nerve stimulation can expel up to 50% of the total blood volume of the liver within 90 seconds and thus provide an effective transfusion equal to approximately 6% of the total blood volume of the body.

Responses to direct nerve stimulation

Early studies have previously been reviewed (Greenway and Stark, 1971; Greenway and Lautt, 1989). Cats and dogs show frequency-response relationships that are very similar. Maximal expulsion of blood volume occurs between 6–8 Hz with maximum volumes of

HEPATIC VOLUMES AND RESISTANCE SITES

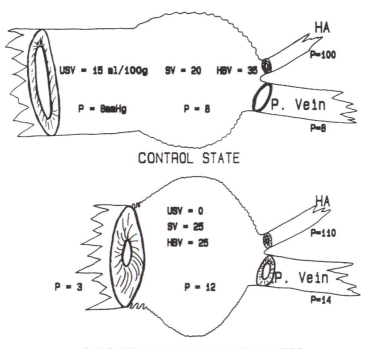

Figure 13.7 Model of hepatic capacitance and resistance vessel responses to sympathetic nerves. Unstressed volume (USV) is dramatically reduced. The compliance is probably not altered (see text) but the hepatic venous sphincters constrict thus raising pressure (P) in the sinusoids and elevating stressed volume (SV). Total hepatic blood volume (HBV) is decreased. In basal state the presinusoidal resistance is trivial and no significant pressure gradient exists between the portal vein and sinusoids; nerve stimulation constricts this site and creates a gradient.

expulsion being equivalent to roughly 50% of the total blood volume (Greenway and Oshiro, 1972). The nerve responses are mediated by α_2 adrenoreceptors (Segstro and Greenway, 1986). The use of non-linear regression of the frequency-response curves allows quantitative assessment of the maximal response (Rmax) and the nerve frequency required to produce 50% of this response (Hz$_{50}$). The use of such dynamic parameters allows for well-defined quantification that can be used to assess the impact of neuromodulators or diseased states on the capacitance responses. If a diseased liver, for example, had a reduced responsiveness to one frequency of nerve stimulation, it would be impossible to determine whether the sensitivity to the stimulation was decreased or whether the overall ability of the liver to develop a capacitance response was diminished. Figure 13.8 shows non-linear regression best fit to the frequency-response curve indicating a Hz$_{50}$ of 3.2±1.0. A separate series of cats reported in the same study had a Hz$_{50}$ of 1.7±0.3 (Lautt, Schafer and Legare, 1991).

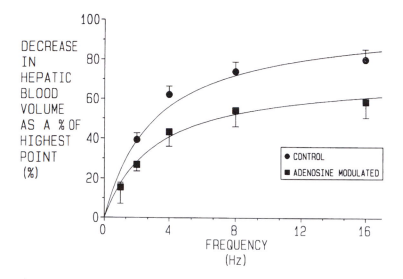

Figure 13.8 Frequency-response curve for change in hepatic blood volume *in vivo* measured using a plethysmo-graph in control state and during intra-arterial infusion of adenosine (2.0 mg·kg^{-1}·min^{-1}). Dynamic parameters were estimated from non-liner regression of the rectangular hyperbolic frequency-response curve and best fit lines are shown. The maximal response (Rmax) was suppressed (100.5±10.7% for control and 72.6±4.3% during adeno-sine) but the frequency that produced 50% of the Rmax (Hz$_{50}$) was not altered (3.2±1 and 3.1±0.5 Hz respectively). This type of antagonism has the appearance of a classical non-competitive nature. Reprinted with permission from Lautt, Schafer and Legare (1991).

These values are in the same range as those that can be determined by visual inspection of frequency-response curves for dogs and cats (Greenway and Oshiro, 1972) where the Hz$_{50}$ is in the range of 2 Hz. This is in the same range as the responsiveness of the hepatic arterial resistance vessels (2.4±0.9, see Figure 13.3). The Hz$_{50}$ for volume responses of the large, extrahepatic portal vein is 3.4 Hz (Takeuchi, Horiuchi and Terada, 1989). Thus, the resistance vessel responses and capacitance responses appear to show similar intensity of constriction at each nerve frequency. This is in contrast to previous implications that indicated that capacitance responses reached a greater effect at comparable nerve frequencies relative to the maximum response that is seen with the resistance vessels. The impression of a less sensitive resistance response is probably because the responses were calculated according to vascular resistance rather than conductance (Stark, 1968). This interpretation is supported by comparing the Hz$_{50}$ based on conductance (2.4 Hz) to that estimated from calculated resistance (7.2 Hz) shown in Figure 13.3.

Reflex control of hepatic capacitance

Reflex control of the venous system has been previously reviewed (Rothe, 1983). Despite the large and clearly demonstrable capacitance responses to direct electrical stimulation of the nerves, physiological involvement of reflex control has been more difficult to convincingly demonstrate. Partly the problem is related to the fact that most reflexes produce complex interacting responses in many vascular beds. In addition, it is clear that in order to differentiate direct nerve effects from indirect effects on stressed volume secondary to reduced splanchnic blood flow, it is necessary to monitor intrahepatic pressures. Perhaps the most severe limitation is that hepatic capacitance responses cannot yet be studied in conscious animals. A number of observations indicate that the presence of anaesthesia blunts the central nervous mechanisms that control the venous system including the liver (Greenway and Lautt, 1989).

Bilateral carotid occlusion had no effect on hepatic blood volume in cats (Lautt and Greenway, 1972; Lautt, 1982; Maass-Moreno and Rothe, 1991). Lack of effect was also confirmed using perfusion of the carotid vessels (Lautt, 1982; Maass-Moreno and Rothe, 1991). The arterial baroreceptors did, however, produce changes in hepatic arterial and other resistance vessels. Either reflex responses of the venous system are blocked by anaesthesia or the major reflex mechanisms have not yet been discovered. However, responses to haemorrhage have also shown no evidence of active reflex hepatic venous responses (Lautt, Brown and Durham, 1980; Greenway, 1987). The entire large capacitance response to haemorrhage could be accounted for by the effects of reduced blood flow acting through changes in stressed volume (Greenway, 1987).

A variety of studies in the dog have quite consistently demonstrated reductions in hepatic and splanchnic volume upon reducing blood pressure at the carotid sinus. Carneiro and Donald (1977) found a carotid sinus pressure-related hepatic volume response that led to about a 25% reduction of hepatic volume at sinus pressure reduction of 80 mmHg. Portal and arterial resistance rose at the same time. The responses were potentiated by removal of vagal tone. Since portal pressure rose significantly, the reduced volume would likely represent reduced unstressed volume. Several related studies report total splanchnic volume responses which does not differentiate liver from the other organs; portal pressure is often, and intrahepatic pressure is never measured so mechanisms of volume response are unclear. This work has been reviewed (Donald, 1981: Greenway and Lautt, 1989). Cousineau, Goresky and Rose (1983) used indicator dilution techniques to measure hepatic blood volume in response to bilateral carotid occlusion. Although hepatic blood flow was not altered by this manoeuvre, hepatic blood volume decreased by 40%. Mild acidosis (pH 7.2) prevented the carotid occlusion-induced hepatic capacitance effect in dogs (Goresky et al., 1986) but it is not clear if this may have been because systemic acidosis (pH 6.9) had already produced active capacitance constriction (Rothe et al., 1985).

Cerebral ischemia led to a neurogenic reduction of volume of the portal vein by up to 26% in rabbits (Takeuchi, Horiuchi and Terada, 1989) that was equivalent to the volume response produced by 10 Hz transmural electrical field stimulation. Frequency-response curves were presented and indicate a Hz_{50} of about 3.4 Hz. The methodology of using in vivo plethysmography on a segment of portal vein is a novel approach that may prove to be a valuable tool for studying venous responses.

The role of the venous system in cardiovascular reflexes is controversial and has been discussed (Rothe, 1983; Rowell, 1984; Greenway and Lautt, 1986; Greenway and Lautt, 1989). There is a large body of circumstantial evidence in favor of reflex control of the venous system and of the splanchnic and hepatic venous beds in particular, but studies directed to unravelling the reflex control of these capacitance beds are inconclusive.

HEPATIC FLUID EXCHANGE

The major physiological variable controlling net fluid exchange in the liver is sinusoidal hydrostatic pressure. Elevation of hepatic venous pressure results in partial transmission of this pressure to the sinusoid and produces a constant filtration rate that is maintained for at least 8 h, provided plasma volume is maintained (Greenway and Lautt, 1970). The filtered fluid does not represent pooling in an interstitial fluid compartment, since this filtered fluid could be quantitatively collected from a plethysmograph in which the intact liver with ligated lymphatics was contained. The liver thus clearly lacks the protective mechanisms which limit filtration in the intestine and skeletal muscle. Increase in filtration across the porous endothelial cells results in fluid passing into the space of Disse. The hepatic sinusoids are perforated by fenestrae of 1–3 mm (Granger et al., 1979) and these fenestrae are of the appropriate size to exclude certain of the large molecular weight lipoproteins from the space of Disse (Fraser, Day and Fernando, 1986). The physiological importance of the fenestrae in regulation of lipoprotein metabolism is not clear, but there is evidence to suggest that enlargement of the fenestrae size leads to increased cholesterol and lipid uptake by the hepatocytes (Fraser, Bowler and Day, 1980).

Increased intrahepatic pressure results in increased filtration from the blood compartment into hepatic lymphatics and, if the lymphatic system becomes overloaded, filtration across the capsule of the liver. Fluid filters readily across the liver capsule and has approximately the same protein content as the plasma (Greenway and Lautt, 1970). In diseased livers with elevated intrahepatic pressure this fluid is referred to as ascites and can expand to as much as 20 litres in volume.

Sympathetic nerve stimulation produces very perplexing responses. Intrahepatic and sinusoidal pressure is clearly elevated (see previous sections), however fluid filtration does not occur and liver volume remains stable for long periods of nerve stimulation (Greenway, Stark and Lautt, 1969). When filtration is induced by elevation of the hepatic venous pressure, nerve stimulation results in no further increase in filtration and, in fact, results in a small decrease (Greenway, 1981). Since the intrahepatic pressure has increased, it appears that the ability of fluid to exit the plasma compartment has been decreased. Similarly, the intrahepatic pressure at which exudate appears is higher in innervated livers than in denervated livers (Greenway, 1987). The nerve-induced reductions in filtration could occur secondary to reduction in size of endothelial fenestrae. Alternatively, the site of restriction could be the small gaps that lead from the space of Disse into the space of Mall from where the lymphatics arise. Reduced fenestrae size is shown to occur in response to noradrenaline and serotonin infusion (Wisse et al., 1980) but effects of nerves have not been studied. In a constant flow preparation, nerve stimulation led to large increases in portal pressure and elevated fluid filtration estimated from hematocrit changes (Bennett, MacAnespie and Rothe, 1982). The reason for this difference from Greenway's data is not clear but the methodologies are dramatically different. Considering the possible physiological and patho-physiological relevance of changes in fenestrae size and the potential for fenestrae to regulate the access of plasma-borne lipoproteins to hepatocyte surfaces, this area requires intensive investigation.

NORADRENALINE OVERFLOW

Data on noradrenaline overflow into the hepatic venous effluent of the liver are of limited value because of lack of information as to the source of the released noradrenaline (arterial, portal, sinusoidal, venous sites?). In addition, noradrenaline that is released upstream from the region of the arterial or portal venous resistance sites must pass through the sinusoids and past the parenchymal cells, through the hepatic venous sphincters and into the venous effluent prior to being sampled. Noradrenaline that might be released from the hepatic veins, on the other hand, passes none of these other potential uptake sites.

The importance of the amount of noradrenaline released may be highly species-dependent, with those species such as the rat, which have sparse innervation releasing less noradrenaline, in contrast to species such as the guinea-pig and tree shrew that release substantially more noradrenaline while producing vascular and metabolic responses that are similar to that of the rat (Beckh *et al.*, 1990). The rat liver contains few nerves and low levels of noradrenaline compared to the guinea-pig and tree shrew but the kinetics of release on stimulation are similar, reaching a peak at 60 seconds. The maximal levels of release were 6–7 fold higher in guinea-pig and tree shrew compared to the rat. It was estimated from these data that a 5 min stimulation period led to release of about 26% of the total hepatic content of noradrenaline in the guinea-pig, 6% in the tree shrew, and 22% from the rat liver (Beckh *et al.*, 1990). Similar data from other species are not available.

Beckh, Balks and Jungermann (1982) found no correlation of hemodynamic effects of sympathetic nerve stimulation with noradrenaline overflow in the rat liver perfusion preparation, whereas a good correlation is seen *in vivo* in the dog (Yamaguchi and Garceau, 1980). The reason for the different results is unclear and may relate to the fact that many *in vivo* responses are different from results obtained in isolated perfusion systems or the vascular response used as the index might determine the degree of correlation. For example, Yamaguchi and Garceau (1980) showed that changes in arterial conductance correlated better than changes in resistance (see previous section on Resistance or Conductance) or portal pressure; the hemodynamic response quantified in the rat preparation was the decrease in portal blood flow. Other possibilities have been discussed (Lautt, 1983).

NEUROTRANSMITTERS AND NEUROMODULATION

The arterial and portal constrictor effects of nerve stimulation are prevented by α receptor blockade (Greenway, Lawson and Mellander, 1967; Greenway and Lawson, 1969; Lautt, 1979). On complete blockade by α adrenergic antagonists, a small β adrenergic vasodilation can be produced which is blocked by propranolol (Greenway and Lawson, 1969).

Adenosine is able to suppress the arterial but not portal venous constriction to nerve stimulation, but the response to noradrenaline is equally well suppressed, suggesting postjunctional antagonism (Lautt and Legare, 1986). Unpublished observations suggest that such modulation probably does not occur in physiological conditions in the liver. Adenosine receptor blockade does not alter initial vasoconstriction, the extent of escape or post-stimulatory hyperemia. Glucagon was reported to antagonize the arterial but not portal venous constrictor response to nerve stimulation and the response to noradrenaline and other constrictors in dogs (Richardson and Withrington, 1976, 1977, 1978, 1981a,b), but later studies (d'Almeida and Lautt, 1989a,b) failed to confirm this in cats and found that at some doses constriction was actually enhanced to a small extent. Vascular escape was suppressed by glucagon but the doses required to affect the arterial responses to nerve stimulation were well outside of even pathological levels. Whether the different observations are due to the species studied is not clear and further studies are required to clarify the possible role of glucagon as a neuromodulator. The ecosanoids, discussed later, appear to be a possible family of physiological modulators of hepatic arterial responses to sympathetic nerves.

The foregoing discussion of the differences between vascular resistance and index of contractility indicates clearly that modulation studies of the venous resistance sites should be done using the index of contractility. Such studies have not yet been done. However, certain tentative conclusions can be made. The neurotransmitter appears to be noradrenaline which may or may not be co-released with ATP and other transmitters. The rise in portal pressure in response to sympathetic nerve stimulation can, however, be eliminated by the use of the non-selective α adrenergic receptor antagonist, phenoxybenzamine (Greenway and Lawson, 1969) or phentolamine (Lautt, 1979). Portal pressure appears to be under the control of both α_1 and α_2 receptors (Segstro and Greenway, 1986), however the relative contribution of receptor types at the pre- and postsinusoidal site is completely unknown. The question of modulation of sympathetic nerve responses is extremely important in view of the controversial involvement of the sympathetic nervous system in contributing to elevated portal pressure in the cirrhotic patient (Henriksen *et al.*, 1990).

Only a few studies of neuromodulation have been done related to the hepatic capacitance vessels. The blood volume responses to sympathetic nerve stimulation are mediated by α_2 adrenoreceptors (Segstro and Greenway, 1986). The direct effect of infused noradrenaline was not affected by the calcium channel blocker, nifedipine, but the response to sympathetic nerve stimulation was reduced by 33% and increasing the dose produced no further impairment. Nifedipine may have acted presynaptically to reduce the release of noradrenaline from the sympathetic terminals in the hepatic venous bed (Segstro *et al.*, 1986). Similarly, bromocryptine, a dopamine (DA$_2$ receptor) agonist that is reported to cause presynaptic inhibition of noradrenaline release, resulted in impaired volume responses to sympathetic nerve stimulation but not portal pressure responses nor responses to direct infusions of noradrenaline (Greenway, Burczynski and Innes, 1986). Elevations in intrahepatic pressure also produce selective inhibition of the capacitance responses to nerve stimulation such that volume responses are almost eliminated at intrahepatic pressures of 16 mmHg (Greenway, 1981, 1987) whereas the response to direct infusions of noradrenaline is well maintained (Lautt, Brown and Durham, 1980). Systemic acidosis (pH 7.2) has been reported to virtually eliminate the hepatic capacitance response to bilateral carotid occlusion in the dog liver. Noradrenaline overflow into the portal and hepatic veins was reduced despite normal arterial pressure responses to the carotid occlusion (Goresky *et al.*, 1986). Adenosine suppresses the Rmax but does not alter the Hz$_{50}$, whereas glucagon increases the Hz$_{50}$ from 3.4 to 5.6 Hz (Lautt, Schafer and Legare, 1991). Although these compounds showed the ability to modulate the nerve responses, the doses needed were non-physiological.

Iwai and Jungermann (1987) found that inhibitors of eicosanoid synthesis reduced the vasoconstriction induced by ATP and nerve stimulation and noradrenaline infusion. Noradrenaline overflow was not altered, leading to the conclusion that the eicosanoids might be released from parenchymal cells to cause a portion of the vasoconstriction. A role for leukotriene C_4 and D_4 in this regard has been eliminated (Iwai and Jungermann, 1989) and prostaglandin F_{2a} and D_2, based largely on their ability to mimic the metabolic and hemodynamic effects of nerve stimulation, are implicated (Iwai et al., 1988). PGE_2 is released from the liver by nerve stimulation (Tran Thi et al., 1988). Hypoxia reduced the constrictor effects of noradrenaline, PGF_{2a} and sympathetic nerves and reduced the metabolic effects of the nerves but not noradrenaline and PGF_{2a}. The suggestion was made that oxygen-dependent eicosanoid production is involved with mediating those responses that were suppressed by hypoxia (Becker, Beuers and Jungermann, 1990). A similar role for prostaglandin mediation of nerve responses was suggested not only for the rat, where the sparse innervation and low noradrenaline content indicate a need for some sort of cell-to-cell propagation, but also in the guinea-pig with its much more dense innervation and 6-fold higher noradrenaline content and noradrenaline overflow upon stimulation (Beckh et al., 1990). The oxygen dependence of the eicosanoid involvement in sympathetic nerve responses is potentially very problematic since it appears clear that sympathetic nerve stimulation in the perfused rat preparation leads to markedly heterogeneous flow, with as much as 30% of the liver sinusoids being unperfused during the stimulation (Ji, Beckh and Jungermann, 1984), in contrast to the lack of heterogeneity induced in vivo in the cat and dog (see previous section on Distribution of Blood Flow). It would appear that in order to supply adequate oxygen to allow normal oxygen uptake using blood cell-free perfusate, hyper-physiological levels of oxygen (75%) and blood flow (4.6 ml/min/g of tissue) are required (Becker, Beuers and Jungermann, 1990).

Some degree of presynaptic modulation of transmitter release (from unknown sites) appears to occur in both the dog (Yamaguchi, 1982) and rat (Beckh, Balks and Jungermann, 1982). α_2 adrenergic receptor antagonism by yohimbine results in a greater transmitter overflow into the hepatic veins of the dog and clonidine (an α_2 agonist) reduced overflow (Yamaguchi, 1982). Noradrenaline infusion reduced noradrenaline overflow and phentolamine increased overflow in the rat (Beckh, Balks and Jungermann, 1982). Thus, there is evidence for α_2 postsynaptic receptors mediating the capacitance responses and α_2 receptors mediating presynaptic noradrenaline release in the resistance vessels. The metabolic, portal, and arterial constrictions in response to nerve stimulation were inhibited by the α_1 adrenergic antagonist, prazosin, in the rat liver (Gardemann, Strulik and Jungermann, 1987).

Co-release of neurotransmitters other than noradrenaline is unclear in the liver. The distribution of noradrenergic and neuropeptide Y regulating enzymes suggests co-localization (Burt et al., 1989). In both human and rat liver there is a rich distribution of several peptides in association with nerve fibers and ganglion cells mainly localized to the arterial vessels. Immunoreactivity was shown for neuron-specific enolase, neuropeptide Y, substance P, and vasoactive intestinal polypeptide (Carlei et al., 1988). Co-release of ATP may also occur based on studies of isolated blood vessels.

In vitro pharmacological studies of isolated hepatic blood vessels will not be extensively reviewed here. The portal veins are large, thin walled vessels that offer virtually no resistance to flow except for the small intrahepatic tributaries. They have, inexplicably, been used as models of resistance vessels in some studies. Recent reports of *in vivo* plethysmographic recording of extrahepatic portal vein volume indicate a clear capacitance function with reflex activation being produced by cerebral ischemia (Takeuchi, Horiuchi and Terada, 1989). This preparation may prove quite useful for studies of neuromodulators *in vivo*. The isolated large veins are responsive to nerve and drug-induced contractions but there are quite remarkable species differences. The isolated rabbit portal vein, but not that of the guinea-pig, shows ATP co-localized and released from sympathetic nerves. A non-adrenergic, non-cholinergic inhibitory response resistant to combined α and β adrenergic blockade and 6-hydroxydopamine-induced sympathectomy is a classical purinergic nerve relationship that is seen in the rabbit, but not the guinea-pig, portal venous muscle (Burnstock, Crowe and Wong, 1979; Burnstock *et al.*, 1984). In the isolated rat portal vein, adenosine serves as a prejunctional inhibitor of noradrenergic neurotransmission (Brown and Collis, 1983; Kennedy and Burnstock, 1984). Adenosine is a potent dilator of the hepatic artery of the cat *in vivo* but does not affect portal pressure or portal responses to nerve stimulation (Lautt and Legare, 1986). The isolated rabbit hepatic artery also shows evidence of ATP cotransmission with noradrenaline (Brizzolara and Burnstock, 1990). The physiological relevance of the responses in these large conducting arteries is unclear. The frequency-response relationships in the isolated hepatic artery are grossly dissimilar from those seen in the cat, dog, and rat where the nerve frequency response that produces 50% of the maximal response is 1.7–3 Hz, and maximal responses are reached between 6 and 20 Hz in all of these preparations. This is in contrast to the responses of the isolated hepatic artery where responses were rarely evoked at a stimulation frequency of less than 8 Hz, never below 4 Hz and frequency dependency was still seen up to 64 Hz.

DISEASE STATES

The contractility of isolated portal veins is enhanced in spontaneously hypertensive rats in response to noradrenaline and nerve stimulation. The prejunctional modulatory effects of purines is not altered. The intensity of response was increased at all doses and frequencies but the EC_{50} for noradrenaline and Hz_{50} for nerve stimulation were not altered (Reilly, Saville and Burnstock, 1989).

Cirrhotic patients have elevated levels of circulating catecholamines of neural origin (Henriksen, Ring-Larsen and Christensen, 1990) and the levels correlate with the severity and prognosis of the disease and the extent of portal hypertension. The decrease in circulating noradrenaline and reduction in portal pressure with no change in hepatic blood flow following clonidine treatment (Willet *et al.*, 1986; Moreau *et al.*, 1987) is compatible with the possibility that portal pressure elevation may be partly under sympathetic control in alcoholic cirrhosis. The adrenergic innervation appears grossly normal in diseased livers (Kyosola *et al.*, 1985) but the normally dense catecholamine-specific fluorescence and AChE-positive terminals are reported to be absent after 4 days of bile duct ligation in the guinea-pig; after 2 weeks the nerve fibers could again be detected (Ungvary and Donath, 1975). No functional studies in diseased livers appear to have been done and the status of autonomic hepatic innervation in diabetes mellitus, where autonomic neuropathy is very common and can be severe, is unknown (Reichel, Bruns and Rabending, 1982).

TECHNICAL CONSIDERATIONS

Throughout this review there is a strong emphasis on the fact that vascular reactions to passive influences may be as large as those that occur to active stimuli and that both active and passive influences occur simultaneously and interactively. Therefore, the technical procedures used to record vascular responses become extremely important. Each of the vascular responses have technical concerns that must be addressed. The hepatic artery, presinusoidal venous resistance, hepatic venous resistance, and hepatic capacitance responses are all subject to serious technical artifact.

The *hepatic artery* is affected by sympathetic nerves and by the hepatic arterial buffer response. Details of both responses have been previously discussed. It is important to note that in the *in vivo* preparation, direct electrical stimulation of the hepatic nerve plexus results in no significant blood flow change through the portal vein. Thus, the hepatic arterial response is a direct response to the nerve stimulation and is not complicated by a simultaneously activated buffer response. The use of vascular perfusion circuits to supply blood to the portal vein should be done in a physiological manner. If the increase in venous resistance leads to no flow change in the venous circuit, this represents the *in vivo* situation. However, in many isolated liver perfusion preparations, the portal circuit is perfused using a constant pressure perfusion, where active vasomotion leads to changes in portal flow. These changes in portal flow will be expected to produce a hepatic arterial buffer response which will complicate interpretation of the direct effects of the stimulus on the hepatic artery. This type of problem is dramatically shown with responses to intravenously administered vasoactive compounds where the buffer response can overwhelm the direct effect of the drug and, in fact, produce the opposite change in vascular tone to what the drug produces on direct intra-arterial administration. The vasodilators glucagon, isoproterenol, and adenosine have been shown to elevate portal blood flow and reduce hepatic arterial flow at certain doses. When the portal blood flow change is prevented, only the direct dilator effect on the hepatic artery is revealed (Lautt *et al.*, 1988). Similar complications would be anticipated to distort the response to nerve stimulation. The other major technical concern is that the changes in vascular tone of the hepatic artery should be estimated using calculated vascular conductance rather than resistance (see previous section on "Resistance or Conductance").

The *portal venous resistance site* is strongly influenced by sympathetic nerves but also the high distensibility of these resistance sites leads to them being dramatically influenced by the distending blood pressure. Changes in active tone can be determined using the calculated index of contractility as opposed to calculated vascular resistance (see previous section on "Passive Distensibility"). However, for many situations, the net interaction between active and passive responses may be of importance and interest and the calculated resistance might be the most relevant measurement. In such cases it is important to duplicate the most physiological condition so that the changes in distending pressure that occur in response to the active vascular tone adjustments will lead to appropriate passive effects on distension. For example, the effect on resistance could be dramatically different depending on whether blood flow is held constant or allowed to decrease. Nerve stimulation *in vivo* leads to marked elevation in intrahepatic pressure whereas in a portal perfusion with pressure held steady, the reduced flow that ensues could be anticipated to result in increased heterogeneity of flow across the very low pressure gradient of the venous system.

Similarly, the interaction between stressed and unstressed volume within the liver and the net effect on *capacitance* must be carefully considered. Presumably the effects on unstressed volume will be identical whether the blood flow or perfusion pressure is held steady. The consequences to stressed volume will, however, be quite different since the constant flow preparation will result in higher intrahepatic pressures. Reducing blood flow to the liver leads to large decreases in stressed volume.

Despite the fact that sympathetic nerve stimulation decreases hepatic arterial blood flow, it is not appropriate to attempt to assess the impact of this reduced arterial blood flow on the capacitance response using a mechanical occlusion of the blood flow to duplicate the flow pattern. Although the flow pattern would be similar in this situation, the intrahepatic pressure will decrease with the mechanical occlusion and result in a reduction of stressed volume, whereas in response to sympathetic nerve stimulation the intrahepatic pressure rises and stressed volume will be increased.

Another technical concern that must be addressed when attempting to measure stressed volume of the liver is related to the intrahepatic pressure measurements. Hepatic compliance is the measurement of the change in liver volume per unit change in the appropriate distending blood pressure. In earlier studies, we made the erroneous assumption that most of the resistance to blood flow resided in the portal veins and that the transmission of an elevation in central venous pressure to the compliant vasculature was virtually complete over a wide physiological range (Lautt and Greenway, 1976). Subsequent studies have convinced us that the earlier interpretation was in error and that the primary resistance site is postsinusoidal and that the transmission of an elevation in central venous pressure is incomplete and dependent upon the magnitude of the vascular resistance (Lautt, Legare and Greenway, 1987). The lobar venous pressure measurement (see previous section) appears to be an acceptable estimate of intrahepatic distending pressure acting on the compliant capacitance vessels (Greenway, Seaman and Innes, 1985). The use of portal venous pressure as an estimate of lobar venous pressure is accurate in basal situations where there is an insignificant pressure gradient between these two sites, however it becomes inaccurate under situations of active vasoconstriction where presinusoidal resistance can become significantly elevated and a pressure gradient develops between PVP and LVP.

FUTURE PERSPECTIVES

In assembling the literature for this review, certain areas of controversy and important gaps in knowledge became obvious. The following list includes some of the more obvious areas that require resolution.

THE HEPATIC ARTERY

To what extent and in what species does vascular escape occur *in vivo* in response to reflex activation; what is the mechanism of escape; what blood borne factors in the portal venous effluent can modulate the intensity of constriction and the extent of escape; what degree of interaction between the hepatic arterial buffer response and nerve stimulation occurs; what physiological and pathological role do co-localized transmitters (e.g. ATP and neuropeptides) and intrahepatic modulators (e.g. arachidonic acid metabolites) play?

THE PRESINUSOIDAL PORTAL RESISTANCE

Is this a discreet resistance site or does it comprise significant sinusoidal resistance as well; what is the role of sympathetic nerves as a physiological regulator; what is the mechanism and role of the presinusoidal escape from neurogenic stimulation and does it occur in the human; what receptors mediate the constriction and what blood borne factors modify it; is the passive distensibility and the index of contractility quantitatively and qualitatively similar in all species and in the diseased state?

THE SINUSOIDAL VESSELS

Is their resistance to flow insignificant in basal and other states including diseased states; does vasoconstriction lead to heterogeneity of flow; is there active regulation of flow distribution; does the venous resistance serve to maintain intrahepatic pressure and prevent regions of stagnation and vascular collapse during reduced flow states; is the hepatic arterial buffer response important to prevent local sinusoidal stagnation; are the sinusoids the major site of capacitance responses and is the volume response due to stressed or unstressed volume; is the sinusoidal capacitance response due to active contraction of the parenchymal muralium or secondary to larger vessel smooth muscle contraction; are the sinusoidal endothelial fenestrations under nerve and other active control and how does this impact on plasma — hepatocyte interactions (e.g. albumin and lipoproteins); are Kupffer cells controlled by nerves; is there a regulatory "pore" between the space of Disse and the space of Mall that regulates lymph formation?

THE POSTSINUSOIDAL VENOUS RESISTANCE

What proportion of total venous resistance is accounted for by the hepatic veins in the various species; is the distensibility similar in various species and in disease; is the resistance localized to discrete sphincter-like zones and do the sites of resistance vary with species and disease; what is the role of nervous control in health and disease especially in portal hypertension; do intrahepatic modulators of nerve action exist; can the action of the venous resistance be shown to play a role in regulating sinusoidal pressure and homogeneity of flow distribution and exchange across the endothelial cells?

CAPACITANCE VESSELS

Where are they; are the stressed and unstressed volume located in different anatomical regions (e.g. sinusoids versus hepatic veins); do the nerves produce their effects in the unstressed volume; why are venous reflexes not readily produced in anaesthetized cats and only modestly in dogs: why does elevated intrahepatic pressure block sympathetic nerve but not noradrenaline-induced contraction; does a diseased liver show altered compliance and altered capacitance responses; are there endogenous modulators of nerve-induced responses?

ACKNOWLEDGEMENTS

My own work related to neural roles and the liver has been funded for two decades by the Medical Research Council of Canada. The work could not have been done without the dedication of my technicians, students, and colleagues. I am especially grateful for the scientific interaction with Dr. Clive V. Greenway and Mr. Dallas J. Legare. This manuscript was prepared by Karen Sanders.

REFERENCES

Alexander, W.F. (1940). The innervation of the biliary system. *Journal of Comparative Neurology*, **73**, 357–370.

Allman, F.D., Rogers, E.L., Caniano, D.A., Jacobowitz, D.M. and Rogers, M.C. (1982). Selective chemical hepatic sympathectomy in the dog. *Critical Care Medicine*, **10**, 100–103.

Amenta, F., Cavallotti, C., Ferrante, F. and Tonelli, F. (1981). Cholinergic nerves in the human liver. *Histochemical Journal*, **13**, 419–424.

Ballet, F. (1990). Hepatic circulation: potential for therapeutic intervention. *Pharmacology and Therapeutics*, **47**, 281–328.

Bayliss, W.M. and Starling, E.H. (1894). Observations on venous pressures and their relationship to capillary pressures. *Journal of Physiology*, **16**, 159–202.

Becker, G., Beuers, U. and Jungermann, K. (1990). Modulation by oxygen of the actions of noradrenaline, sympathetic nerve stimulation and prostaglandin F_{2a} on carbohydrate metabolism and hemodynamics in perfused rat liver. *Biological Chemistry Hoppe-Seyler*, **371**, 983–990.

Beckh, H., Balks, H.J. and Jungermann, K. (1982). Activation of glycogenolysis, and noradrenaline overflow in the perfused rat liver during repetitive perivascular nerve stimulation. *FEBS Letters*, **149**, 261–265.

Beckh, K., Fuchs, E., Balle, C. and Jungermann, K. (1990). Activation of glycogenolysis by stimulation of the hepatic nerves in perfused livers of guinea-pig and tree shrew as compared to rat: differences in the mode of action. *Biological Chemistry Hoppe-Seyler*, **371**, 153–158.

Beckh, K., Otto, R., Ji, S. and Jungermann, K. (1985). Control of oxygen uptake, microcirculation and glucose release by circulating noradrenaline in perfused rat liver. *Biological Chemistry Hoppe-Seyler*, **366**, 671–678.

Bennett, T.D., MacAnespie, C.L. and Rothe, C.F. (1982). Active hepatic capacitance responses to neural and humoral stimuli in dogs. *American Journal of Physiology*, **242**, H1000–H1009.

Bower, E.A. and O'Donnell, C.P. (1991). Mean circulatory filling pressure duing splanchnic nerve stimulation and whole-body hypoxia in the anaesthetized cat. *Journal of Physiology*, **432**, 543–556.

Brauer, R.W. (1963). Liver circulation and function. *Physiological Reviews*, **43**, 115–213.

Brizzolara, A.L. and Burnstock, G. (1990). Evidence for noradrenergic-purinergic cotransmission in the hepatic artery of the rabbit. *British Journal of Pharmacology*, **99**, 835–839.

Brown, C.M. and Collis, M.G. (1983). Adenosine α_1 receptor mediated inhibition of nerve stimulation-induced contractions of the rabbit portal vein. *European Journal of Pharmacology*, **93**, 277–282.

Burnstock, G., Crowe, R. and Wong, H.K. (1979). Comparative pharmacological and histochemical evidence for purinergic inhibitory innervation of the portal vein of the rabbit, but not guinea-pig. *British Journal of Pharmacology*, **65**, 377–388.

Burnstock, G., Crowe, R., Kennedy, C. and Torok, J. (1984). Indirect evidence that purinergic modulation of perivascular adrenergic neurotransmission in the portal vein is a physiological process. *British Journal of Pharmacology*, **81**, 533.

Burt, A.D., Tiniakos, D., MacSween, R.N.M., Griffiths, M.R., Wisse, E. and Polak, J.M. (1989). Localization of adrenergic and neuropeptide tyrosine-containing nerves in the mammalian liver. *Hepatology*, **9**, 839–845.

Burton-Opitz, R. (1910). The vascularity of the liver: I. The flow of the blood in the hepatic artery. *Quarterly Journal of Experimental Physiology*, **3**, 297–313.

Carlei, F., Lygidakis, N.J., Speranza, V., Brummelkamp, W.H., McGurrin, J.F., Peitroletti, R., *et al.* (1988). Neuroendocrine innervation of the hepatic vessels in the rat and in man. *Journal of Surgical Research*, **45**, 417–426.

Carneiro, J.J. and Donald, D.E. (1977). Change in liver blood flow and blood content in dogs during direct and reflex alteration of hepatic sympathetic nerve activity. *Circulation Research*, **40**, 150–157.

Chen, L.Q. and Shepherd, A.P. (1991). Role of H^+ and α_2 receptors in escape from sympathetic vasoconstriction. *American Journal of Physiology*, **261**, H868–H873.

Child, C.G. (1954). *The Hepatic Circulation and Portal Hypertension.* Philadelphia, Pennsylvania: W.B. Saunders Co.

Cohn, J.N., Khatry, I.M. and Groszmann, R.J. (1972). Hepatic blood flow in alcoholic liver disease measured by an indicator dilution technique. *American Journal of Medicine*, **53**, 704–714.

Cohn, R. and Kountz, S. (1963). Factors influencing control of arterial circulation in the liver of the dog. *American Journal of Physiology*, **205**, 1260–1264.

Cousineau, D., Goresky, C.A. and Rose, C.P. (1983). Blood flow and noradrenaline effects on liver vascular and extravascular volumes. *American Journal of Physiology*, **244**, H495–H504.

Cousineau, D., Goresky, C.A., Rose, C.P. and Lee, S. (1985). Reflex sympathetic effects on liver vascular space and liver perfusion in dogs. *American Journal of Physiology*, **248**, H186–H192.

Cucchiaro, G., Yamaguchi, Y., Mills, E., Kuhn, C.M., Anthony, D.C., Branum, G.D., *et al.* (1990). Evaluation of selective liver denervation methods. *American Journal of Physiology*, **259**, G781–G785.

d'Almeida, M.S. and Lautt, W.W. (1989a). The effect of glucagon on vasoconstriction and vascular escape from nerve and noradrenaline-induced constriction of the hepatic artery of the cat. *Canadian Journal of Physiology and Pharmacology*, **67**, 1418–1425.

d'Almeida, M.S. and Lautt, W.W. (1989b). The effect of glucagon on autoregulatory escape from hepatic arterial vasoconstriction in the cat. *Proceedings of the Western Pharmacology Society*, **32**, 265–267.

d'Almeida, M.S. and Lautt, W.W. (1991). Glucagon pharmacodynamics and modulation of sympathetic nerve and noradrenaline-induced constrictor responses in the superior mesenteric artery of the cat. *Journal of Pharmacology and Experimental Therapeutics*, **259**, 118–123.

Donald, D.E. (1981). Mobilization of blood from the splanchnic circulation. In *Hepatic Circulation in Health and Disease*, edited by W.W. Lautt, pp. 193–201. New York: Raven Press.

Elias, H. and Petty, D. (1952). Gross anatomy of the blood vessels and ducts within the human liver. *American Journal of Anatomy*, **90**, 59–111.

Ezzat, W.R. and Lautt, W.W. (1987). Hepatic arterial pressure-flow autoregulation is adenosine mediated. *American Journal of Physiology*, **252**, H836–H845.

Forssmann, W.F. and Ito, S. (1977). Hepatocyte innervation in primates. *Journal of Cellular Biology*, **74**, 299–313.

Fraser, F., Bowler, L.M. and Day, W.A. (1980). Damage of rat liver sinusoidal endothelium by ethanol. *Pathology*, **12**, 371–376.

Fraser, R., Day, W.A. and Fernando, N.S. (1986). Atherosclerosis and the liver sieve. In *Cells of the Hepatic Sinusoid, Volume 1*, edited by A. Kirn, D.L. Knook, and E. Wisse, pp. 317–322. Kupffer Cell Foundation.

Friedman, M.I. (1982). Hepatic nerve function. In *The Liver: Biology and Pathobiology*, edited by I. Arias *et al.*, pp. 663–673. New York: Raven Press.

Garceau, D. and Yamaguchi, N. (1982). Pharmacological evidence for the existence of a neuronal amine uptake mechanism in the dog liver *in vivo*. *Canadian Journal of Physiology and Pharmacology*, **60**, 755–762.

Gardemann, A., Strulik, H. and Jungermann, K. (1987). Nervous control of glycogenolysis and blood flow in arterially and portally perfused liver. *American Journal of Physiology*, **253**, E238–E245.

Ginsburg, M., Grayson, J. and Johnson, D.H. (1952). The nervous regulation of liver blood flow. *Proceedings of the Physiological Society of London*, **17**, 74P–75P.

Goresky, C.A., Cousineau, D., Rose, C.P. and Lee, S. (1986). Lack of liver vascular response to carotid occlusion in mildly acidotic dogs. *American Journal of Physiology*, **251**, H991–H999.

Goresky, C.A. and Groom, A.C. (1984). Microcirculatory events in the liver and spleen. In *Handbook of Physiology. Section 2. Cardiovascular System*, pp. 689–780. Baltimore: Williams & Wilkins.

Granger, D.N., Miller, T., Allen, R., *et al.* (1979). Permselectivity of cat liver blood-lymph barrier to endogenous macromolecules. *Gastroenterology*, **77**, 103–109.

Greenway, C.V. (1981). Hepatic plethysmography. In *Hepatic Circulation in Health and Disease*, edited by W.W. Lautt, pp. 41–56. New York: Raven Press.

Greenway, C.V. (1984a). Neural control and autoregulatory escape. In *Physiology of the Intestinal Circulation*, edited by A.P. Shepherd and D.N. Granger, pp. 61–71. New York: Raven Press.

Greenway, C.V. (1984b). Autoregulatory escape in arteriolar resistance vessels. In *Smooth Muscle Contraction*, edited by N.L. Stephens, pp. 473–484. New York: Marcel Dekker Inc.

Greenway, C.V. (1987). Effects of haemorrhage and hepatic nerve stimulation on venous compliance and unstressed volume in cat liver. *Canadian Journal of Physiology and Pharmacology*, **65**, 2168–2174.

Greenway, C.V. and Lautt, W.W. (1970). Effects of hepatic venous pressure on transsinusoidal fluid transfer in the liver of the anaesthetized cat. *Circulation Research*, **26**, 697–703.

Greenway, C.V. and Lautt, W.W. (1986). Blood volume the venous system, preload, and cardiac output. *Canadian Journal of Physiology and Pharmacology*, **64**, 383–387.

Greenway, C.V. and Lautt, W.W. (1988). Distensibility of hepatic venous resistance sites and consequences on portal pressure. *American Journal of Physiology*, **254**, H452–H458.

Greenway, C.V. and Lautt, W.W. (1989). Hepatic circulation. In *Handbook of Physiology — The Gastrointestinal System I*, Volume 1, Part 2, Chapter 41, edited by S.G. Schultz, J.D. Wood, and B.B. Rauner, pp. 1519–1564. New York: Oxford University Press.

Greenway, C.V. and Lawson, A.E. (1969). β-adrenergic receptors in the hepatic arterial bed of the anaesthetized cat. *Canadian Journal of Physiology and Pharmacology*, **47**, 415–419.

Greenway, C.V. and Oshiro, G. (1972). Comparison of the effects of hepatic nerve stimulation on arterial flow, distribution of arterial and portal flows and blood content in the livers of anaesthetized cats and dogs. *Journal of Physiology (London)*, **227**, 487–501.

Greenway, C.V. and Stark, R.D. (1971). Hepatic vascular bed. *Physiology Reviews*, **51**, 23–65.

Greenway, C.V., Burczynski, F. and Innes, I.R. (1986). Effects of bromocryptine on hepatic blood volume responses to hepatic nerve stimulation in cats. *Canadian Journal of Physiology and Pharmacology*, **64**, 621–624.

Greenway, C.V., Lawson, A.E. and Mellander, S. (1967). The effects of stimulation of the hepatic nerves, infusions of noradrenaline and occlusion of the carotid arteries on liver blood flow in the anaesthetized cat. *Journal of Physiology (London)*, **192**, 21–41.

Greenway, C.V., Seaman, K.L. and Innes, I.R. (1985). Noradrenaline on venous compliance and unstressed volume in cat liver. *American Journal of Physiology*, **248**, H468–H476.

Greenway, C.V., Stark, R.D. and Lautt, W.W. (1969). Capacitance responses and fluid exchange in the cat liver during stimulation of the hepatic nerves. *Circulation Research*, **25**, 277–284.

Gumucio, D.L. (1983). Functional and anatomic heterogeneity in the liver acinus: impact on transport. *American Journal of Physiology*, **244**, G578–G582.

Gumucio, J.J. and Miller, D.L. (1981). Functional implications of liver cell heterogeneity. *Gastroenterology*, **80**, 393–403.

Henriksen, J.H., Ring-Larsen, H. and Christensen, N.J. (1990). Autonomic nervous function in liver disease. In *Cardiovascular Complications in Liver Disease*, edited by A. Bomzon and L.M. Blendis, pp. 63–79. Boston: CRC Press.

Holmin, T., Ekelund, M., Kullendorff, C.-M. and Lindfeldt, J. (1984). A microsurgical method for denervation of the liver in the rat. *European Journal of Surgical Research*, **16**, 288–293.

Iwai, M. and Jungermann, K. (1987). Possible involvement of eicosanoids in the actions of sympathetic hepatic nerves on carbohydrate metabolism and hemodynamics in perfused rat liver. *FEBS Letters*, **221**, 155–160.

Iwai, M. and Jungermann, K. (1989). Mechanism of action of cysteinyl leukotrienes on glucose and lactate balance and on flow in perfused rat liver. *European Journal of Biochemistry*, **180**, 273–281.

Iwai, M., Gardemann, A., Puschel, G. and Jungermann, K. (1988). Potential role for prostaglandin F_{2a}, D_2, E_2 and thromboxane A_2 in mediating the metabolic and hemodynamic actions of sympathetic nerves in perfused rat liver. *European Journal of Biochemistry*, **175**, 45–50.

Ji, S., Beckh, K. and Jungermann, K. (1984). Regulation of oxygen consumption and microcirculation by α-sympathetic nerves in isolated perfused rat liver. *FEBS Letters*, **167**, 117–122.

Karim, F. and Hainsworth, R. (1976). Responses of abdominal vascular capacitance to stimulation of splanchnic nerves. *American Journal of Physiology*, **231**, 434–440.

Kennedy, C. and Burnstock, G. (1984). Evidence for an inhibitory prejunctional P_1-purinoceptor in the rat portal vein with characteristics of the A_2 rather than of the A_1 subtype. *European Journal of Pharmacology*, **100**, 363–368.

Koo, A. and Liang, I.Y.S. (1979). Parasympathetic cholinergic vasodilator mechanism in the terminal liver microcirculation in rats. *Quarterly Journal of Experimental Physiology*, **64**, 149–159.

Krarup, N. (1973). The effects of noradrenaline and adrenaline on hepatosplanchnic hemodynamics, functional capacity of the liver and hepatic metabolism. *Acta Physiological Scandinavica*, **87**, 307–319.

Kyosola, K., Pentitila, O., Ihamaki, T., Varis, K. and Salaspuro, M. (1985). Adrenergic innervation of the human liver. *Scandinavian Journal of Gastroenterology*, **20**, 254–256.

Lamers, W.H., Hoynes, K.E., Zonneveld, D., Moorman, A.F.M. and Charles, R. (1988). Noradrenergic innervation of developing rat and spiny mouse liver: its relation to the development of the liver architecture and enzymic zonation. *Anatomical Embryology*, **178**, 175–181.

Lautt, W.W. (1977). Effect of stimulation of hepatic nerves on hepatic O_2 uptake and blood flow. *American Journal of Physiology*, **232**, H652–H656.

Lautt, W.W. (1978). Hepatic presinusoidal sphincters affected by altered arterial pressure and flow, venous pressure and nerve stimulation. *Microvascular Research*, **15**, 309–317.

Lautt, W.W. (1979). Neural activation of α-adrenoreceptors in glucose mobilization from liver. *Canadian Journal of Physiology and Pharmacology*, **57**, 1037–1039.

Lautt, W.W. (1980). Hepatic nerves — a review of their functions and effects. *Canadian Journal of Physiology and Pharmacology*, **58**, 105–123.

Lautt, W.W. (1981a). Role and control of the hepatic artery. In *Hepatic Circulation in Health and Disease*, edited by W.W. Lautt, pp. 203–226, New York: Raven Press.

Lautt, W.W. (1981b). Evaluation of surgical denervation of the liver in cats. *Canadian Journal of Physiology and Pharmacology*, **59**, 1013–1016.

Lautt, W.W. (1982). Carotid sinus baroreceptor effects on cat livers in control and haemorrhaged states. *Canadian Journal of Physiology and Pharmacology*, **60**, 1592–1602.

Lautt, W.W. (1983). Afferent and efferent neural roles in liver function. *Progress in Neurobiology*, **21**, 323–348.

Lautt, W.W. (1985). Mechanism and role of intrinsic regulation of hepatic arterial blood flow: the hepatic arterial buffer response. *American Journal of Physiology*, **249**, G549–G556.

Lautt, W.W. (1989). Resistance or conductance for expression of arterial vascular tone. *Microvascular Research*, **37**, 230–236.

Lautt, W.W. and Carroll, A.N. (1984). Evaluation of topical phenol as a means of producing autonomic denervation of the liver. *Canadian Journal of Physiology and Pharmacology*, **62**, 849–853.

Lautt, W.W. and Cote, M.G. (1976). Functional evaluation of 6-hydroxydopamine-induced hepatic sympathectomy in the liver of the cat. *Journal of Pharmacology and Experimental Therapeutics*, **198**, 562–567.

Lautt, W.W. and Cote, M.G. (1977). The effect of 6-hydroxydopamine-induced hepatic sympathectomy on the early hyperglyaemic response to surgical trauma under anaesthesia. *Journal of Trauma*, **17**, 270–274.

Lautt, W.W. and Greenway, C.V. (1972). Hepatic capacitance vessel responses to bilateral carotid occlusion in anaesthetized cats. *Canadian Journal of Physiology and Pharmacology*, **50**, 244–247.

Lautt, W.W. and Greenway, C.V. (1976). Hepatic venous compliance and role of liver as a blood reservoir. *American Journal of Physiology*, **231**, 292–295.

Lautt, W.W. and Greenway, C.V. (1987). Conceptual review of the hepatic vascular bed. *Hepatology*, **7**, 952–963.

Lautt, W.W. and Legare, D.J. (1985). The use of 8-phenyltheophylline as a competitive antagonist of adenosine and an inhibitor of the intrinsic regulatory mechanism of the hepatic artery. *Canadian Journal of Physiology and Pharmacology*, **63**, 717–722.

Lautt, W.W. and Legare, D.J. (1986). Adenosine modulation of hepatic arterial but not portal venous constriction induced by sympathetic nerves, noradrenaline, angiotensin, and vasopressin in the cat. *Canadian Journal of Physiology and Pharmacology*, **64**, 449–454.

Lautt, W.W. and Legare, D.J. (1992a). Evaluation of hepatic venous resistance responses using index of contractility (IC). *American Journal of Physiology*, **262**, G510–G516.

Lautt, W.W. and Legare, D.J. (1992b). Passive autoregulation of a portal venous pressure: distensible hepatic resistance. *Hepatology*, **263**, G702–G708.

Lautt, W.W. and Skelton, F.S. (1976). Effect of hepatic nerve stimulation on hepatic uptake of lidocaine in the cat. *Life Sciences*, **19**, 433–436.

Lautt, W.W. and Wong, C. (1978). Hepatic parasympathetic neural effect on glucose balance in the intact liver. *Canadian Journal of Physiology and Pharmacology*, **56**, 679–682.

Lautt, W.W., Brown, L.C. and Durham, J.S. (1980). Active and passive control of hepatic blood volume responses to haemorrhage at normal and raised hepatic venous pressures in cats. *Canadian Journal of Physiology and Pharmacology*, **58**, 1049–1057.

Lautt, W.W., Greenway, C.V. and Legare, D.J. (1987). Effect of hepatic nerves, noradrenaline, angiotensin, elevated central venous pressure on postsinusoidal resistance sites and intrahepatic pressures. *Microvascular Research*, **33**, 50–61.

Lautt, W.W., Greenway, C.V. and Legare, D.J. (1991). Index of contractility: quantitative analysis of hepatic venous distensibility. *American Journal of Physiology*, **260**, G325–G332.

Lautt, W.W., Legare, D.J. and d'Almeida, M.S. (1985). Adenosine as putative regulator of hepatic arterial flow (the buffer response). *American Journal of Physiology*, **248**, H331–H338.

Lautt, W.W., Legare, D.J. and Ezzat, W.R. (1990). Quantitation of the hepatic arterial buffer response to graded changes in portal blood flow. *Gastroenterology*, **98**, 1024–1028.

Lautt, W.W., Legare, D.J. and Greenway, C.V. (1987). Effect of hepatic venous sphincter contraction on transmission of central venous pressure to lobar and portal pressure. *Canadian Journal of Physiology and Pharmacology*, **65**, 2235–2243.

Lautt, W.W., Legare, D.J. and Lockhart, L.K. (1988). Vascular escape from vasoconstriction and post-stimulatory hyperemia in the superior mesenteric artery of the cat. *Canadian Journal of Physiology and Pharmacology*, **66**, 1174–1180.

Lautt, W.W., Lockhart, L.K. and Legare, D.J. (1988). Adenosine modulation of vasoconstrictor responses to sympathetic nerves and noradrenaline infusion in the superior mesenteric artery of the cat. *Canadian Journal of Physiology and Pharmacology*, **66**, 937–941.

Lautt, W.W., Schafer, J. and Legare, D.J. (1991). Effect of adenosine and glucagon on hepatic blood volume responses to sympathetic nerves. *Canadian Journal of Physiology and Pharmacology*, **69**, 43–48.

Lautt, W.W., d'Almeida, M.S., McQuaker, J. and D'Aleo, L. (1988). Impact of the hepatic arterial buffer response on splanchnic vascular responses to intravenous adenosine, isoproterenol and glucagon. *Canadian Journal of Physiology and Pharmacology*, **66**, 937–941.

Lautt, W.W., Greenway, C.V., Legare, D.J. and Weisman, H. (1986). Localization of intrahepatic portal vascular resistance. *American Journal of Physiology*, **14**, G375–G381.

Legare, D.J. and Lautt, W.W. (1987). Hepatic venous resistance site in the dog: localization and validation of intrahepatic pressure measurements. *Canadian Journal of Physiology and Pharmacology*, **65**, 352–359.

Lockhart, L.K., Legare, D.J. and Lautt, W.W. (1988). Kinetics of adenosine antagonism of sympathetic nerve-induced vasoconstriction. *Proceedings of the Western Pharmacology Society*, **31**, 105–107.

Louis-Sylvester, J., Servant, J.M., Molimard, R. and Le Magnen, J. (1980). Effect of liver denervation on the feeding pattern of rats. *American Journal of Physiology*, **239**, R66–R70.

Maass-Moreno, R. and Rothe, C.F. (1991). Carotid baroreceptor control of liver and spleen volume in cats. *American Journal of Physiology*, **260**, H254–H259.

Mathie, R.T. and Blumgart, L.H. (1983). Effect of denervation on the hepatic hemodynamic response to hypercapnia and hypoxia in the dog. *Pflügers Archives*, **397**, 152–157.

Metz, W. and Forssmann, W.G. (1980). Innervation of the liver in guinea-pig and rat. *Anatomical Embryology*, **160**, 239–252.

Moreau, R., Lee, S.S., Hadengue, A., Braillon, A. and Lebrec, D. (1987). Hemodynamic effects of a clonidine-induced decrease in sympathetic tone in patients with cirrhosis. *Hepatology*, **7**, 149–154.

Mundschau, G.A., Zimmerman, S.W., Gildersleeve, J.W. and Murphy, Q.R. (1966). Hepatic and mesenteric artery resistances after sinoaortic denervation and haemorrhage. *American Journal of Physiology*, **211**, 77–82.

Pietroletti, R., Chamuleau, R.A.F.M., Speranza, V. and Lygidakis, N.J. (1987). Immunocytochemical study of the hepatic innervation in the rat after partial hepatectomy. *Histochemical Journal*, **19**, 327–332.

Plaa, G.L. (1975). Toxicology of the liver. In *Toxicology: The Basic Science of Poisons*, edited by L.J. Casarett and J. Doull, pp. 170–189. New York: Macmillan.

Rappaport, A.M. (1975). Anatomic considerations. In *Diseases of the Liver*, edited by L. Schiff, pp. 1–50. Toronto: J.B. Lippincott.

Rappaport, A.M. (1981). Microvascular methods — the transilluminated liver. In *Hepatic Circulation in Health and Disease*, edited by W.W. Lautt, pp. 1–12. New York: Raven Press.

Reichel, G., Bruns, W. and Rabending, G. (1982). Classification of diabetic neuropathy from pathogenetic aspects. *Endokrinologic*, **79**, 321–336.

Reilly, F.D., McCuskey, R.S. and Cilento, E.V. (1981). Hepatic microvascular regulatory mechanisms. I. Adrenergic mechanisms. *Microvascular Research*, **21**, 103–116.

Reilly, F.D., McCuskey, P.A. and McCuskey, R.S. (1978). Intrahepatic distribution of nerves in the rat. *Anatomical Record*, **191**, 55–67.

Reilly, W.M., Saville, V.L. and Burnstock, G. (1989). Vessel reactivity and prejunctional modulatory changes in the portal vein of mature spontaneously hypertensive rats. *European Journal of Pharmacology*, **160**, 283–289.

Reilly, F.D., Dimlich, R.V.W., Cilento, E.V. and McCuskey, R.S. (1982). Hepatic microvascular regulatory mechanisms. II. Cholinergic mechanisms. *Hepatology*, **2**, 230–235.

Remak, G., Hottenstein, O.D. and Jacobson, E.D. (1990). Sensory nerves mediate neurogenic escape in rat gut. *American Journal of Physiology*, **258**, H778–H786.

Richardson, P.D.I. and Withrington, P.G. (1976). The inhibition of glucagon of the vasoconstrictor actions of noradrenaline, angiotensin, and vasopressin on the hepatic arterial vascular bed of the dog. *British Journal of Pharmacology*, **57**, 93–102.

Richardson, P.D.I. and Withrington, P.G. (1977). Glucagon inhibition of hepatic arterial responses to hepatic nerve stimulation. *American Journal of Physiology*, **233**, H647–H654.

Richardson, P.D.I. and Withrington, P.G. (1978). The effects of intraportal infusions of glucagon on the hepatic arterial and portal venous vascular beds of the dog: inhibition of hepatic arterial vasoconstrictor responses to noradrenaline. *Pflügers Archives*, **378**, 135–140.

Richardson, P.D.I. and Withrington, P.G. (1981a). Liver blood flow. I. Intrinsic and nervous control of liver blood flow. *Gastroenterology*, **81**, 159–173.

Richardson, P.D.I. and Withrington, P.G. (1981b). Liver blood flow. II. Effects of drugs and hormones on liver blood flow. *Gastroenterology*, **81**, 356–375.

Risoe, C., Hall, C. and Smiseth, O.A. (1991). Splanchnic vascular capacitance and positive end-expiratory pressure in dogs. *Journal of Applied Physiology*, **70**, 818–824.

Rothe, C.F. (1983). Reflex control of veins and vascular capacitance. *Physiological Reviews*, **63**, 1281–1342.

Rothe, C.F., Stein, P.M., MacAnespie, C.L. and Gaddis, M.L. (1985). Vascular capacitance responses to severe systemic hypercapnia and hypoxia in dogs. *American Journal of Physiology*, **249**, H1061–H1069.

Rowell, L.B. (1984). Reflex control of regional circulation in humans. *Journal of the Autonomic Nervous System*, **11**, 101–114.

Sannemann, J., Beckh, K. and Jungermann, K. (1986). Control of glycogenolysis and hemodynamics in perfused rat liver by the sympathetic innervation. *Biological Chemistry Hoppe-Seyler*, **367**, 401–409.

Sawchenko, P.E. and Friedman, M.I. (1979). Sensory functions of the liver — a review. *American Journal of Physiology*, **236**, R5–R20.

Segstro, R. and Greenway, C.V. (1986). α adrenoceptor subtype mediating sympathetic mobilization of blood from the hepatic venous system in anaesthetized cats. *Journal of Pharmacology and Experimental Therapeutics*, **236**, 224–229.

Segstro, R., Seaman, K.L., Innes, I.R. and Greenway, C.V. (1986). Effects of nifedipine on hepatic blood volume in cats: indirect venoconstriction and absence of inhibition of post synaptic α_2-adrenoceptor responses. *Canadian Journal of Physiology and Pharmacology*, **64**, 615–620.

Skandalakis, J.E., Gray, S.W., Soria, R.E., Sorg, J.L. and Rowe, J.S. (1980). Distribution of the vagus nerve to the stomach. *The American Surgeon*, **46**, 130–139.

Stark, R.D. (1968). Conductance or resistance? *Nature (London)*, **217**, 779.

Sutherland, S.D. (1964). An evaluation of cholinesterase techniques in the study of the intrinsic innervion of the liver. *Journal of Anatomy*, **98**, 321–326.

Sutherland, S.D. (1965). The intrinsic innervation of the liver. *Reviews of International Hepatology*, **15**, 569–578.

Takeuchi, T., Horiuchi, J. and Terada, N. (1989). Central vasomotor control of the rabbit portal vein. *Pflügers Archives*, **413**, 348–353.

Thurman, R.G., Kauffman, F.C. and Jungermann, K. (1986). *Regulation of Hepatic Metabolism*. New York: Plenum Press.

Tran Thi, T.A., Haussinger, D., Gyufko, K. and Decker, K. (1988). Stimulation of prostaglandin release by Ca^2-mobilizing agents from the perfused rat liver. *Biological Chemistry Hoppe-Seyler*, **369**, 65–68.

Tyden, G., Samnegard, H. and Thulin, L. (1979). The effects of changes in the carotid sinus baroreceptor activity on splanchnic blood flow in anaesthetized man. *Acta Physiological Scandinavica*, **106**, 187–189.

Ungvary, G. and Donath, T. (1975). Neurohistochemical changes in the liver of guinea pigs following ligation of the common bile duct. *Experimental and Molecular Pathology*, **22**, 29–34.

Van Leeuwen, D.J., Sherlock, S., Scheuer, P.J. and Dick, R. (1989). Wedged hepatic venous pressure recording and venography for the assessment of pre-cirrhotic and cirrhotic liver disease. *Scandinavian Journal of Gastroenterology*, **24**, 65–73.

Willet, I.R., Jennings, G., Esler, M. and Dudley, F.J. (1986). Sympathetic tone modulates portal venous pressure in alcoholic cirrhosis. *The Lancet*, **II**, 939–943.

Wisse, E., Van Dierendonck, J.H., De Zanger, R.B., Fraser, R. and McCuskey, R.S. (1980). On the role of the liver endothelial filter in the transport of particulate fat (chylomicrons and their remnants) to parenchymal cells and the influence of certain hormones on the endothelial fenestrae. *Communications of Liver Cells*, edited by H. Popper, L. Bianchi, F. Gudat, and W. Reutter, pp. 195–200. England: MTP Press Ltd.

Yamaguchi, N. (1982). Evidence supporting the existence of presynaptic α-adrenoceptors in the regulation of endogenous noradrenaline release upon hepatic sympathetic nerve stimulation in the dog liver *in vivo*. *Archives of Pharmacology*, **321**, 177–184.

Yamaguchi, N. and Garceau, D. (1980). Correlations between hemodynamic parameters of the liver and noradrenaline release upon hepatic nerve stimulation in the dog. *Canadian Journal of Physiology and Pharmacology*, **58**, 1347–1355.

14 Adipose Tissue Circulation

K.N. Frayn[1] and I.A. Macdonald[2]

[1] *Oxford Lipid Metabolism Group,*
   Radcliffe Infirmary, Oxford, OX2 6HE
[2] *Department of Physiology and Pharmacology,*
   University of Nottingham Medical School,
   Nottingham, NG7 2UH

This chapter considers adipose tissue blood flow in terms of direct neural control of the vasculature and the link between adipose tissue metabolism and blood flow. The two distinct types of adipose tissue, namely white and brown, are considered separately (although many aspects of vascular control are similar for the two tissues), and the review is restricted to intact tissue rather than the isolated vasculature. The methods available to study adipose tissue flow and metabolism are reviewed critically. In particular, the limitations and possible errors in using the techniques of xenon washout and of microdialysis to estimate blood flow are discussed.

There is good histochemical evidence that the vasculature in white adipose tissue has a rich sympathetic innervation, but innervation of the adipocytes is much less common. Nevertheless, the adipocytes do have adrenoceptors on their surface, which respond to circulating catecholamines to produce metabolic responses. These metabolic responses, in particular lipolysis (breakdown of the stored triacylglycerol), are accompanied by increases in tissue blood flow — presumably due to vascular effects of some metabolic products. There is marked species variation in the type of adrenoceptor present on the adipose tissue vasculature, with α-adrenoceptors being predominant in some species and β-adrenoceptors in others. In addition to effects of sympathetic nerves and plasma catecholamines, adenosine may have a role in controlling adipose tissue blood flow, either via direct effects on the vascular smooth muscle, or indirect effects on adipocyte metabolism. The effects on white adipose tissue blood flow of a variety of metabolic disturbances (including feeding, starvation, hypoglycaemia) provide evidence of the important link between tissue metabolism and perfusion.

By contrast to white adipose tissue, brown adipose tissue has a higher vascular density and larger number of very active mitochondria, which combine to give it the characteristic brown colour. This tissue has a dense sympathetic innervation to the blood vessels and adipocytes. However, the vascular nerves appear to be entirely vasoconstrictor in nature, the profound vasodilation seen on stimulation of the adipocytes being secondary to the metabolic response. An important feature of the brown adipocyte is the presence on its surface of a β_3-adrenoceptor, which is responsible for stimulating lipolysis and thermogenesis. This thermogenesis is a major function of brown adipose tissue, and its role in thermoregulation is discussed.

KEY WORDS: white adipose tissue; brown adipose tissue; lipolysis; adrenoceptors; adenosine; thermogenesis.

INTRODUCTION

ADIPOSE TISSUE AS A SPECIAL EXAMPLE OF LINKS BETWEEN METABOLISM AND BLOOD FLOW

In adipose tissue, more than in most other tissues, there is an intimate relationship between blood flow and metabolism. The primary role of white adipose tissue, as will be developed further below, is one of nutrient storage and release. Although this also happens in brown adipose tissue, its major role is as a site of non-shivering heat production (thermogenesis). These roles depend upon exchange of materials or heat with the blood. The ability to store excess substrate depends upon the blood-borne carriage of that substrate; the ability to deliver substrate or heat to the rest of the body depends upon delivery in the blood. The relationship with blood flow is strengthened by the fact that the substrates with which adipose tissue primarily deals with are not simple water-soluble compounds but are for the most part hydrophobic lipid compounds. These compounds are highly dependent upon specialized blood-borne carrier systems for their delivery to and removal from the tissue. This intimate relationship between blood flow and metabolism is highlighted also by the fact that a key enzyme in adipose tissue metabolism, lipoprotein lipase (EC 3.1.1.34), which is synthesized within the adipocytes, acts not in or on those cells but attached to the luminal surface of the capillary endothelium, to which site it is transported by mechanisms as yet unidentified. Probably in no other tissue do catecholamines, either locally released at sympathetic nerve terminals or delivered systemically, have such intimately related effects on both circulation and metabolism. Adipose tissue is also the site of metabolic action of a variety of vasoactive agents, both endogenous and exogenous, such as adenosine and nicotinic acid.

The writing of this review has been enormously helped by the appearance, at intervals, of some extremely comprehensive reviews on adipose tissue blood flow and, in some cases, of its relationship to metabolic events. The following have been used extensively in preparing this review: Rosell and Belfrage (1979); Roddie (1983); Fredholm (1985); Trayhurn and Nicholls (1986); Crandall and DiGirolamo (1990).

EXPERIMENTAL TECHNIQUES

Any reviewer of this field is also acutely aware of the enormous body of work on adipose tissue circulation which has come from Scandinavia, and in particular from a group at the Karolinska Institute in Stockholm (reviewed by Rosell, 1969). In one specific respect, however, this body of work has had a restricting influence, in that it is based largely upon studies in the dog. A point to be made in this chapter is that the nervous regulation of adipose tissue blood flow is to a certain extent species specific, and the dog is not, in some ways, a good model for man (Hjemdahl and Linde, 1983; Hjemdahl *et al.*, 1983).

The introduction by Rosell and colleagues of a system for perfusion of the innervated subcutaneous abdominal adipose tissue with defibrinated blood was the starting point for this work (Oro, Wallenberg and Rosell, 1965; Rosell, 1966). The sympathetic innervation could be stimulated and the circulatory and metabolic responses studied, the former by perfusion at a constant flow rate and monitoring of pressure. Variations on this technique have formed the basis of much of the Scandinavian work. The tissue may be autoperfused, diverting blood from the femoral artery via a drop counter for measuring blood flow directly (Ngai, Rosell and Wallenberg, 1966; Ballard, Cobb and Rosell, 1971). Alternatively, samples of arterial and venous blood from this depot may be collected and the blood flow measured by xenon washout, as described below, allowing the study of physiological states such as exercise (Bülow, 1982; Bülow and Madsen, 1986). This allows the study of both metabolism and circulation in conditions close to those obtaining *in vivo*. Very similar studies have been performed in the rabbit (again with direct measurement of blood flow) (Lewis and Matthews, 1968), the sheep (Thompson, 1984) and, more recently, in humans (Frayn *et al.*, 1989; Coppack *et al.*, 1990a).

The study of adipose tissue blood flow in man (and smaller animals) has been facilitated by the introduction of the xenon-washout technique (Larsen, Lassen and Quaade, 1966). This is based on the idea of washout of a marker such as ^{22}Na, first introduced by Kety for muscle and skin (Kety, 1949). Xenon has the advantage of considerable fat-solubility and thus longer retention in the tissue. ^{133}Xenon, a γ-emitting isotope, is usually injected into the tissue in a small volume of isotonic saline and the disappearance of radioactivity from the site monitored externally. Knowledge of the partition coefficient for xenon between adipose tissue and blood (Andersen and Ladefoged, 1967; Jelnes, Rasmussen and Eickhoff, 1984; Jelnes, Astrup and Bülow, 1985) allows calculation of blood flow in, for example, ml·min^{-1}·(100 g tissue)$^{-1}$, on the assumption that a diffusion equilibrium is maintained between fat-dissolved and blood xenon; there is some evidence that this holds from comparison of different markers (Lindbjerg, 1967) and from studies of the diffusion coefficient for xenon in tissues (Evans *et al.*, 1974). It should be noted, however, that the partition coefficient for xenon may not be as clearly known as is sometimes assumed; Bülow, Jelnes and colleagues have shown different values in different sites and with different degrees of obesity (Jelnes *et al.*, 1984; Bülow *et al.*, 1987b). It has been pointed out previously (Rosell and Belfrage, 1979; Roddie, 1983) that estimates of the resting blood flow through white adipose tissue in humans (usually around 2–3 ml·min^{-1}·(100 g)$^{-1}$) are substantially lower than values measured more directly in experimental animals (typically 7–12 ml·min^{-1}·(100 g)$^{-1}$) (Table 14.1). Whether this reflects problems with the inert gas technique or species differences is not clear. Uncertainty over the partition coefficient for xenon should not affect relative changes in blood flow during an experiment, but might affect comparisons between, for instance, different groups of subjects (e.g. normal vs obese). xenon is quantitatively exhaled during passage through the lung and so recirculation is not a problem. Other tracers have been used, notably ^{99m}Tc in the form of pertechnetate (^{99m}TcO$_4^-$) (Linde and Hjemdahl, 1982; Linde, Rosell and Rökaeus, 1982; Hjemdahl and Linde, 1983); this has the advantage over xenon of a lesser residence time in the tissue, allowing greater resolution of rapid changes, but the disadvantages that for a long experiment further injections may then have to be given, and of recirculation, so that radioactivity returning in arterial blood must be corrected for. Whilst the xenon-washout technique can be applied even to the rat (Madsen, Malchow-Møller and Waldorff, 1975; Madsen and Malchow-Møller, 1983), in small animals the microsphere method has found most favour, in particular for the measurement of brown adipose tissue blood flow. Microspheres can be, and have been, used in larger species such as the pig (Mersmann, 1989), sheep (Gregory, Christopherson and Lister, 1986) and dog (Smiseth *et al.*, 1983), but cannot, for obvious reasons, be applied to man.

TABLE 14.1

Blood flow rates through white adipose tissue in different species, measured by various techniques

Species	Method	Mean resting flow $ml \cdot min^{-1} \cdot (100\ g)^{-1}$	Reference
Rat	^{14}C-DDT uptake	10–16	Herd, Goodman and Grose, 1968
	[86]Rb uptake	7–18[a]	Mayerle and Havel, 1969
	[133]Xe washout	10–12[a]	Madsen, Malchow-Møller and Waldorff, 1975
	microspheres	9	Larsen et al., 1981
	microspheres	19 ⎫	Crandall et al., 1986
Obese (Zucker) rat	microspheres	10 ⎭	
Dog	Direct (drop-counter)	8.5	Ngai, Rosell and Wallenberg, 1966
	Direct (drop-counter)	3	Linde and Hjemdahl, 1982
	[133]Xe washout	5	Bülow, 1982
Sheep	Microspheres	5	Barnes, Comline and Dobson, 1983
Rabbit	Direct collection	8	Lewis and Matthews, 1968
Human	[133]Xe washout	2.6	Larsen, Lassen and Quaade, 1966
	[133]Xe washout	2 ⎫	Nielsen et al., 1968
Obese humans	[133]Xe washout	1.3 ⎭	

Where a range is given, it covers more than one adipose depot. [a]Intra-abdominal fat depots. DDT – Dichlorodiphenyltrichloroethane. Based in part on Vernon and Clegg (1985).

A new technique that can be applied in humans makes use of the technique of microdialysis. A fine fibre of dialysis tubing is placed in the adipose tissue and perfused with a salt solution. At the flow rates normally used, substances only partially equilibrate across the membrane, between the dialysate and the interstitial fluid. The extent of equilibration depends partly upon the rate of removal of the substance from the interstitial fluid. If a relatively metabolically inert, water-soluble substance such as ethanol is added to the perfusate, then the concentration in the solution leaving the dialysis tubing will be less than that entering by an amount which depends upon the tissue blood flow (the greater the blood flow, the lower the concentration in the dialysis effluent). The ratio of inflowing to outflowing ethanol concentration has been proposed as an indicator of tissue blood flow, initially in muscle (Hickner et al., 1991, 1992), but now applied to adipose tissue (Galitzky et al., 1993). At present this method cannot be said to give an absolute measure of blood flow, but it may be useful for estimating relative changes during an experiment.

BASIC FEATURES OF CIRCULATION AND INNERVATION IN WHITE ADIPOSE TISSUE

VASCULATURE OF WHITE ADIPOSE TISSUE

The histology of adipose tissue began to receive attention in the 19th Century (reviewed in Lewis and Matthews, 1970; Ryan and Curri, 1989a). Modern interest in the vasculature of adipose tissue was kindled by the work of Gersh and Still (1945), who commented upon "the close topographic and functional relationship of fat to blood vessels", and made quantitative estimates of capillary density in adipose tissue and muscle. They showed that

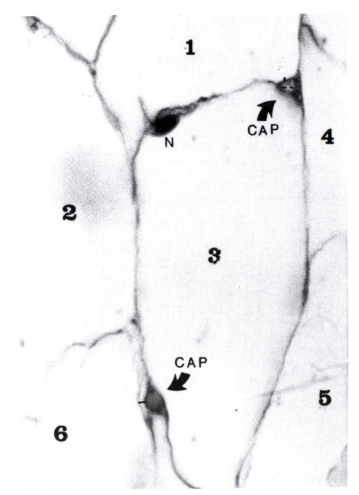

Figure 14.1 White adipose tissue lobule showing six adipocytes, nucleus (N) and capillaries (CAP); the capillaries have a lumen 3–4 μm in diameter. Reproduced from Ryan and Curri (1989b) with permission of J.B. Lippincott Co.

the capillary density of adipose tissue was less (per unit volume of tissue) than that of even the most poorly supplied muscle. When expressed per unit volume of cytoplasm, however, the picture was reversed, adipose tissue having a "much richer" capillary bed than muscle. Subsequent studies, using a variety of techniques, confirmed the existence of an extensive capillary network, such that each cell appears to be in close contact with more than one capillary (Ballard, Malmfors and Rosell, 1974; Ryan and Curri, 1989b) (Figure 14.1).

SYMPATHETIC INNERVATION

The innervation of adipose tissue has also been the subject of histological attention (early studies reviewed by Wirsén, 1965). Specific study of the noradrenergic innervation became possible with the introduction by Falck of a fluorescence microscopic technique (Falck, 1962). Most authors who have used this technique agree that, whilst the tissue is in some respects richly supplied with sympathetic nerves, these make contact more consistently with the vasculature than with the parenchymal cells themselves. Thus, Wirsén (1964) claimed the existence of sympathetic fibres "in the walls of arteries down to precapillary level", but "no fibres around the capillaries or veins, nor could any be seen around the fat cells". He believed these nerves to be mainly vasoregulatory. Ballantyne (1968) and Daniel and Derry (1969) likewise showed dense networks of fibres around the arterial blood vessels, but found no innervation of parenchymal cells. Ballard, Malmfors and Rosell (1974), on the other hand, whilst agreeing about the "rich perivascular plexus of . . . nerves" (around arteries and veins), found areas in which there were apparent contacts between nerve fibres and adipocytes, but other areas in which no such innervation occurred. They postulated two pools of adipocytes, some cells being innervated and responding directly to sympathetic activity and some not. A contrasting view came from Diculescu and Stoica (1970), who claimed both intertwining of nerve fibres and capillaries (the nerve fibres running "like 'puttees' around the capillaries") and close contacts between nerve fibres and fat cells. This controversy has not been fully resolved.

A consensus would be that there is a dense capillary network in white adipose tissue such that each cell is in close contact with at least one vessel, and that the vasculature is highly sympathetically innervated. The presence of nerve endings making contact with the fat cells themselves and thus exerting direct metabolic effects is more controversial, although the results of studies on the metabolic effects of sympathetic stimulation (reviewed below), imply at least some such contact. One way of resolving this apparent discrepancy has been proposed by Slavin (1985), who claims the existence of "gap-like junctions" between adipocytes, and suggests a form of electrical coupling between cells such that action potentials arriving at innervated cells may be passed on, electrically, to non-innervated cells.

It should be noted that, whatever the true status of the innervation of fat cells, there is no doubt that adipocytes have adrenoceptors on their surfaces, and respond to adrenergic stimuli. The question of whether these stimuli are predominantly local (i.e. noradrenaline release from nerve endings) or systemic (i.e. circulating adrenaline and noradrenaline) will be discussed in more detail below.

CHOLINERGIC INNERVATION

Although most studies of the innervation of adipose tissue have concentrated on the sympathetic system, there were early reports that cholinergic innervation might be present or that cholinergic agonists or antagonists could influence lipolysis (reviewed in Salvador and Kuntzman, 1965; Rosell and Belfrage, 1979; Roddie, 1983). Thus, cholinesterase activity was found in homogenates of adipose tissue from various species (Salvador and Kuntzman, 1965). Ballantyne, however, has shown histochemically that this cholinesterase activity is present in the adipocytes rather than the nerves, and concludes that the innervation of white adipose tissue is postganglionic sympathetic in type (Ballantyne, 1968). In support of this, acetylcholine has very weak vasoactivity in adipose tissue (Fredholm, Öberg and Rosell, 1970) and atropine has no effect on the response to sympathetic nerve stimulation (Ngai, Rosell and Wallenberg, 1966).

VASCULAR EXCHANGE

It might be considered that a tissue such as white adipose tissue, whose physiological function involves exchange of substances with the blood, would have a high ability to transfer substrates across the capillary endothelium, and this is so. The resting capillary filtration coefficient (CFC) in white adipose tissue is typically around twice that of skeletal muscle (Öberg and Rosell, 1967; Rosell and Belfrage, 1979; Roddie, 1983). The CFC is a measure of both capillary surface area and capillary permeability. The former can be studied by histological measurements of surface area, and by studies of the transport of small molecules. The work of Gersh and Still (1945), reviewed earlier, provided evidence that the capillary surface area (per unit weight of tissue) is rather less than that of muscle, and this is borne out by a relatively poor exchange of small molecules (reviewed in Rosell and Belfrage, 1979). This suggests a high capillary permeability, for which there is indirect evidence from the relatively high colloid osmotic pressure in adipose tissue interstitial fluid compared with that of skeletal muscle (Aukland and Johnsen, 1974; Johnsen, 1974).

GENERAL FEATURES OF THE REGULATION OF BLOOD FLOW IN WHITE ADIPOSE TISSUE

SYMPATHETIC NERVOUS/ADRENERGIC EFFECTS

On the circulation

In an early study, Oro, Wallenberg and Rosell (1965) showed that stimulation of the sympathetic nerves supplying canine subcutaneous adipose tissue caused vasoconstriction. This has been an almost universal finding (Oro, Wallenberg and Rosell, 1965; Rosell, 1966; Ballard and Rosell, 1971; Hjemdahl and Fredholm, 1974) (Figure 14.2), but requires some provisos. The vasoconstriction is frequency dependent and more pronounced at higher stimulation frequencies (Ngai, Rosell and Wallenberg, 1966; Rosell, 1966). It may be transient and "autoregulatory escape" may convert it to vasodilatation (Ballard and Rosell, 1971; Hjemdahl and Sollevi, 1978). Whilst the response may appear uniform at a macroscopic level, at the level of the microcirculation it is somewhat heterogeneous, with some vessels failing to respond or displaying vasodilatation (Rosell, Intaglietta and Chisholm, 1974), perhaps reflecting the "patchy" pattern of innervation remarked upon by some observers (Ballard, Malmfors and Rosell, 1974). One other proviso is that in most of these studies the sympathetic fibres have been transected and the distal end stimulated. In sheep, the response of adipose tissue to sympathetic stimulation (vasodilation or constriction) depends upon whether the tissue is innervated (Thompson, 1986); in tissue with intact innervation, dilatation is the favoured response, whereas after acute or chronic denervation, constriction is seen.

In general, it is clear that α-adrenoceptor stimulation causes vasoconstriction, whilst β-adrenoceptor stimulation causes dilatation. Thus, sympathetic stimulation during α-adrenoceptor blockade results in dilatation (Ngai, Rosell and Wallenberg, 1966; Fredholm and Rosell, 1968; Rosell, 1969; Ballard and Rosell, 1971), whereas β-adrenoceptor blockade removes the dilatatory response or the autoregulatory escape (Rosell, 1969; Ballard

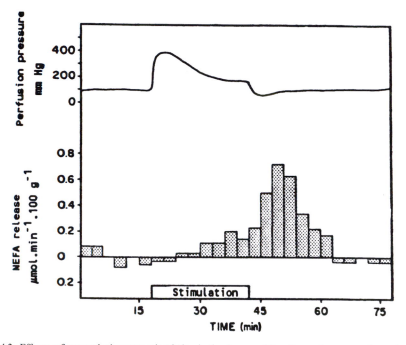

Figure 14.2 Effects of sympathetic nerve stimulation in the dog on white adipose tissue vascular resistance and metabolism. Blood flow was constant at 6 ml/min·(100 g). Nerve stimulation was at 8 V, 10 Hz, for 24 min. Stimulation caused some increase in lipolysis (reflected in free fatty acid release), but with vasoconstriction, as shown by the increase in perfusion pressure. At the end of the stimulation, there is transient rebound vasodilatation with considerable release of free fatty acids, possibly from a pool of fatty acids mobilized during stimulation, but trapped by the vasoconstriction. Reproduced from Rosell (1966) with permission of the publishers.

and Rosell, 1971). Infusion of β-adrenoceptor agonists (e.g. isoprenaline) will increase adipose tissue blood flow (Mersmann, 1989), and systemic β-adrenoceptor blockade will decrease it (Risberg, Hordnes and Tyssebotn, 1987).

What is not so clear is the relative roles, *in vivo*, of the sympathetic system and of circulating catecholamines. When catecholamines are supplied in the blood, the responses observed are not always consistent. "Close intra-arterial injection" of catecholamines, in which the agent under test is added to the arterial supply to a perfused adipose depot, might be considered to mimic nerve stimulation most closely. Noradrenaline under these conditions may cause either constriction (Ballard, Cobb and Rosell, 1971) or vasodilatation (Ballard, Cobb and Rosell, 1971; Belfrage, 1978; Thompson, 1986), sometimes either response being reported in the same paper (Ballard, Cobb and Rosell, 1971). Adrenaline (in the dog) causes constriction when infused to produce levels well above those reached physiologically (Ballard, Cobb and Rosell, 1971; Belfrage, 1978). The intravenous infusion of catecholamines generally, but not always, bears out these findings. Thus, noradrenaline infusion (in dogs) may cause either vasoconstriction or vasodilatation in adipose tissue (Ballard, 1973). As expected, the constrictor response is blocked by α-adrenoceptor

TABLE 14.2
Reported effects of exogenous catecholamines on white adipose tissue blood flow in humans

Reference	C'pound infused	Rate $nmol \cdot min^{-1}$ $(kg\ body\ weight)^{-1}$ and duration	Route	Plasma concentration reached	How flow measured?	Result
Nielsen et al., 1968	NA	0.4–0.8 30–40 min	i.v.	30+ nmol/l[a]	^{133}Xe	Resistance down ~50%
Hjemdahl and Linde, 1983	NA	0.2–0.5 30 min	i.v.	8–20 nmol/l	^{133}Xe and ^{99}Tc	Resistance up ~80%
	A	0.1–0.2 30 min	i.v.	3–6 nmol/l	^{133}Xe and ^{99}Tc	Resistance down 20–30%
Freyschuss et al., 1986	A	0.05–0.30 45 min	i.v.	0.3–6 nmol/l	^{133}Xe	Resistance down ~50%
Fernqvist, Gunnarsson and Linde, 1988	A	0.1–0.3 40 min	i.v.	2–6 nmol/l	^{133}Xe	Resistance down ~40% at lower infusion rate; little change at higher rate

Note that because of changes in blood pressure, some authors have reported results in terms of vascular resistance (= mean arterial pressure/blood flow). For other studies this has been calculated from data in the paper. A, adrenaline; NA, noradrenaline. [a] Estimated from infusion rate, by comparison with Hjemdahl and Linde (1983).

blockade and the dilator response by β-adrenoceptor blockade (Ballard, 1973). The results in humans are summarized in Table 14.2.

The situation is undoubtedly complicated by species differences, particularly in adrenoceptor subtypes. These have only emerged relatively recent, as much of the early work used catecholamines at high, unphysiological concentrations at which responses may be more consistent. Adrenaline is a more potent β_2- than β_1-adrenoceptor agonist (Lands et al., 1967; Belfrage, 1978), but also, in general terms, a more potent α-adrenoceptor agonist than noradrenaline. Noradrenaline is a more effective β_1- than β_2-adrenoceptor agonist (Lands et al., 1967; Hjemdahl, Belfrage and Daleskog, 1979). In canine adipose tissue, the β-adrenoceptor-mediated dilatation appears to occur via β_1-adrenoceptors (Belfrage, 1978) (whereas in canine skeletal muscle β_2-adrenoceptors appear to predominate). Thus, in the dog, intravenous infusion of noradrenaline at physiological concentrations is less effective at causing vasoconstriction in adipose tissue than is adrenaline (Hjemdahl, Belfrage and Daleskog, 1979), perhaps reflecting the preponderance of β_1-adrenoceptors mediating dilatation in canine adipose tissue. In humans, however, intravenous adrenaline will cause dilatation (Table 14.2; Hjemdahl and Linde, 1983; Freyschuss et al., 1986; Fernqvist, Gunnarsson and Linde, 1988); noradrenaline at low concentrations will cause constriction (Hjemdahl and Linde, 1983), but noradrenaline infusion at higher rates in humans causes vasodilatation (Nielsen et al., 1968). This different pattern of responses from that seen in the dog may reflect a preponderance of vascular β_2-adrenoceptors in humans (Hjemdahl and Linde, 1983); it seems that at higher concentrations, noradrenaline will also activate these β_2-adrenoceptors and cause dilatation (Nielsen et al., 1968). In humans, vasoconstriction is mediated by α_2-adrenoceptors (Galitzky et al., 1993).

The apparent discrepancies between responses to adrenaline and noradrenaline and between nerve stimulation and infused catecholamines may relate also to the location of adrenoceptors. Noradrenaline locally released at sympathetic nerve terminals may have readier access to certain adrenoceptors than will circulating catecholamines. Thus, α-adrenoceptors may predominate around sympathetic nerve terminals and be responsible for vasoconstriction. β-adrenoceptors may play more of a role in controlling metabolic responses (discussed later) and be less readily accessible to neuronally released agonists, but perhaps more so to circulating agonists (Fredholm, 1985).

The central connections responsible for eliciting these changes in adipose tissue are not clear. Electrical stimulation of the posterior hypothalamus in dogs will produce changes in adipose tissue vascular resistance: whereas stimulation of the medial hypothalamus produces dilatation (which is reversed to vasoconstriction by propranolol), stimulation of the lateral hypothalamus produces vasoconstriction (which is abolished by α-adrenoceptor blockade) (Parker et al., 1979). This implies that separate vasodilator and constrictor fibres supply adipose tissue, rather than the balance between neurally discharged and circulating catecholamines being the deciding factor between dilatation and constriction. None of these treatments caused stimulation of lipolysis, suggesting that separate fibres yet again (or circulating catecholamines) are responsible for metabolic effects (Parker et al., 1979).

A resume of this somewhat conflicting picture might be along these lines. Studies by microscopy, reviewed earlier, show that the vasculature of white adipose tissue is densely innervated by sympathetic fibres. Adipocytes themselves have adrenoceptors, but these will be concerned with metabolic, rather than circulatory, responses. They may in some cases be supplied by sympathetic fibres, but perhaps more commonly are accessible to circulating catecholamines. Sympathetic stimulation, acting via release of noradrenaline at the vascular α-adrenoceptors, will have a mainly vasoconstrictive effect. Circulating catecholamines, on the other hand, may have more access to the smooth muscle β-adrenoceptors which mediate vasodilatation, as well as to the adipocyte "metabolic" adrenoceptors. The diversity of β-adrenoceptor subtypes is responsible for at least some of the species differences. In the dog, β_1-adrenoceptors predominate, and circulating noradrenaline is thus a more potent vasoactive agent than is adrenaline. In humans, β_2-adrenoceptors predominate, and the reverse is true.

On filtration

It was mentioned earlier that the washout of a marker from adipose tissue may be used as an indicator of the rate of blood flow. In early experiments on canine adipose tissue perfused at a constant flow rate, however, it was noted that the disappearance of both water-soluble iodide and fat-soluble xenon decreased during sympathetic nerve stimulation (Rosell, 1969; Ballard and Rosell, 1971), implying decreased transcapillary transport. [This finding is still somewhat difficult to reconcile with studies on naturally perfused adipose tissue in vivo, which show that the "diffusion equilibrium" for xenon is maintained, and transcapillary exchange should not affect the rate of washout (Lindbjerg, 1967; Evans et al., 1974)]. These studies led to the direct measurement, by a hydrostatic technique, of the CFC of adipose tissue, which showed that it unexpectedly rose during sympathetic stimulation (Öberg and Rosell, 1967; Rosell, 1969; Fredholm, Öberg and Rosell, 1970; Ballard and Rosell, 1971).

In other tissues, the CFC falls or is unchanged by this treatment (reviewed in Rosell, 1969). The rise in adipose tissue CFC on nerve stimulation is an α-adrenoceptor-mediated effect (Öberg and Rosell, 1967). Studies of the exchange of other small molecules (such as ^{86}Rb) have shown that the increase in CFC does not reflect an increase in capillary surface area during sympathetic stimulation (Linde and Gainer, 1974), leading to the conclusion that sympathetic stimulation must increase the intrinsic permeability of the capillaries of white adipose tissue (Rosell, 1969; Rosell, Intaglietta and Chisholm, 1974). In indirect support of this view, substances such as histamine and bradykinin, which are known to increase permeability in other tissues, will mimic the increase in CFC seen with nerve stimulation, whereas other vasoactive substances do not (Fredholm, Öberg and Rosell, 1970).

OTHER ENDOGENOUS REGULATORS

Adenosine

Adenosine is a breakdown product of the adenine nucleotide AMP. It is not a direct intermediate in the normal biosynthetic pathway of these compounds, although an enzyme, adenosine kinase, can reconvert adenosine into AMP, and it has been argued that a cycle thus exists giving precise control of the adenosine concentration in tissues (Arch and Newsholme, 1978). It has a very short half-life in blood (less than 10 s; Ontyd and Schrader, 1984), making it a potential "local regulator" (Arch and Newsholme, 1978). In adipose tissue, as in some other tissues, adenosine has potent properties both in the regulation of metabolism and of circulation. Its possible involvement in the integrated regulation of metabolism and circulation will be considered in more detail below. In the kidney and liver, adenosine has vasoconstrictor effects, but in most other tissues it acts as a vasodilator (reviewed by Haddy and Scott, 1968; Arch and Newsholme, 1978). Adenosine may be an activator or an inhibitor of adenylate cyclase. There are two generic types of adenosine-binding site. These have been termed the P-site (recognizing the purine group), which is part of the catalytic subunit of adenylate cyclase on the cytoplasmic face of the cell membrane and responsive to micromolar concentrations, and the R-site (recognizing the ribose moiety), which is on the extracellular side and responsive to nanomolar concentrations (Fain and Malbon, 1979; Lafontan and Berlan, 1985). The latter has the properties of a true receptor (Lafontan and Berlan, 1985). More recently, R-sites have been termed adenosine receptors and the nomenclature of A receptors has become accepted (Williams, 1987). These receptors are themselves divided into at least two groups (van Calker, Muller and Hamprecht, 1979): A_1, formerly known as R_i, which inhibit adenylate cyclase, and A_2, formerly known as R_a, which activate it. The A_2 receptors appear to predominate in vascular smooth muscle, whereas the A_1 are found on adipocytes (Lafontan and Berlan, 1985; Kennedy, Gurden and Strong, 1992). The relaxing action of adenosine on vascular smooth muscle may be mediated via activation of adenylate cyclase as are the effects of β-adrenoceptor stimulation (Fain and Malbon, 1979), although this is disputed by others (Arch and Newsholme, 1978).

The role of adenosine in the normal regulation of adipose tissue blood flow has been studied in several ways. Most directly, adenosine has been infused, intra-arterially in dogs (Sollevi and Fredholm, 1983) and into a central vein in man (Edlund, Sollevi and Linde, 1990). In the former study, adenosine reduced the resting vascular resistance of adipose tissue and diminished the constrictor effect of sympathetic stimulation. Perhaps paradoxically, it also reduced the dilator response to sympathetic stimulation in the presence of α-adrenoceptor blockade (Sollevi and Fredholm, 1983). In man, adenosine is present in adipose tissue interstitial fluid at concentrations high enough to affect metabolism (Lönnroth et al., 1989), but systemic infusion of adenosine causes little change in adipose tissue blood flow (or in the mean arterial pressure, implying no change in vascular resistance) (Edlund, Sollevi and Linde, 1990).

Infusion of adenosine inevitably raises the plasma concentration well above that normally occurring. An alternative technique is to use the adenosine uptake inhibitor dipyridamole, or the non-selective adenosine receptor antagonist theophylline. These compounds have no effect on resting flow in human adipose tissue, although the former potentiates the hyperaemia following arterial occlusion, suggesting a role for adenosine in this phenomenon (Linde and Sollevi, 1987). The reactive hyperaemia following nerve stimulation in dogs, however, is not significantly affected either by dipyrimadole or by adenosine infusion (Sollevi and Fredholm, 1983). Again, it might be argued that dipyrimadole is raising local adenosine concentrations into the "pharmacological" range. The enzyme adenosine deaminase is responsible for adenosine breakdown, and has been infused intra-arterially into fat pads of dogs, where it increased resting vascular resistance and blocked the vasodilator effect of noradrenaline (Martin and Bockman, 1986); the latter was taken as evidence that adrenergically induced vasodilatation in adipose tissue may be mediated via adenosine release.

In summary, although adenosine is undoubtedly a potent vasoactive compound in many tissues, evidence that it plays a major role in the regulation of resting blood flow, particularly in human adipose tissue, is not strong.

Nicotinic acid, although an exogenous compound, is an analogue of adenosine and is thought to act via the same receptors. Although a well-known vasodilator in skin, nicotinic acid has little effect on adipose tissue blood flow in the rat (Madsen and Malchow-Møller, 1983) or dog (Fredholm, 1985), and it has been suggested that what effect it does have is secondary to reduced cyclic-AMP formation in, and adenosine release from, adipocytes (Madsen and Malchow-Møller, 1983).

Thyroid hormones

Chronic treatment with T_3 in the rat increases white adipose tissue blood flow considerably ($>100\%$), suggesting that this tissue may even make a contribution to thyroid-induced thermogenesis (Rothwell and Stock, 1984). In a study of hypo- and hyperthyroid patients and their responses to treatment, adipose tissue blood flow was found to be increased in hyperthyroidism, decreased in hypothyroidism, and to return towards normal with treatment (Wennlund and Linde, 1984). There was a strong positive correlation between adipose tissue blood flow and blood levels of both T_3 and T_4 (Wennlund and Linde, 1984).

Dopamine

Infusion of dopamine at high (pharmacological) concentrations in canine adipose tissue causes lipolysis but not circulatory effects; injection of large single doses causes both lipolysis and α-adrenoceptor-mediated vasoconstriction (Fredholm, 1972). It seems unlikely that these represent physiological effects (Fredholm, 1985). In the sheep, however, large quantities of dopamine are present in the tissue and may have a physiological role (Thompson, 1984). Infusion of dopamine into sheep will increase adipose tissue blood flow and lipolysis (Thompson, 1984).

Other regulators

Interleukin-1β appears not to regulate adipose tissue blood flow (Dascombe et al., 1989). Vasopressin may do so: in the rabbit and rat, injection or infusion of vasopressin causes a marked decrease in white adipose tissue blood flow (Lewis and Matthews, 1968; Rofe and Williamson, 1983); whether this applies to humans is not known.

The importance of endogenous prostaglandins in the regulation of adipose tissue blood flow has not been clarified. Exogenous PGE_1 is a potent vasodilator in rabbit and canine adipose tissue (Lewis and Matthews, 1968; Fredholm, Öberg and Rosell, 1970). Both prostaglandin I_2 (prostacyclin) and prostaglandin E_2 are produced by rat adipocytes during lipolysis and may be responsible for the accompanying vasodilatation (discussed below) (Axelrod and Levine, 1981; Lafanton and Berlan, 1985; Richelsen, 1992). [There has been some controversy about whether the prostaglandins are produced by adipocytes themselves or by other cell types: it seems that in intact adipose tissue, an interaction between different cell types increases production of these compounds (Richelsen, 1992).] In animals, indomethacin or aspirin abolish the functional vasodilatation associated with lipolysis (Bowery and Lewis, 1973). In humans, however, indomethacin has no effect on basal adipose tissue blood flow or on the vasodilation following release of arterial occlusion (reactive hyperaemia) (Carlsson, Linde and Wennmalm, 1983), suggesting that prostaglandins play little role in the regulation of human adipose tissue blood flow.

INTERACTIONS BETWEEN BLOOD FLOW AND METABOLISM

BASIC FEATURES OF THE METABOLISM OF WHITE ADIPOSE TISSUE

The metabolism of white adipose tissue has been reviewed several times in recent years (Saggerson, 1985; Vernon and Clegg, 1985; Frayn, 1989, 1992) and here will only be outlined in so far as it is relevant to the blood circulation through the tissue. The place of adipose tissue in whole-body lipid metabolism is outlined in Figure 14.3.

Fat storage

Fat is stored in adipocytes in the form of triacylglycerol (TAG; also called triglyceride). In the mature white fat cell this takes the form of a single lipid droplet occupying the bulk of the cell, with the cytoplasm, mitochondria and nucleus occupying a thin "crust" around the droplet. Fat may be deposited via two major routes: synthesis from non-lipid precursors, amino acids or glucose (lipogenesis) within the adipocytes, or uptake of preformed TAG from circulating lipoproteins. Although extracellular fatty acids are taken up and esterified in experimental situations, this is not thought to play a significant role physiologically. It is now

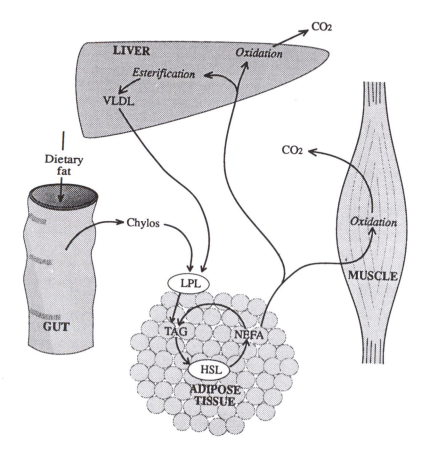

Figure 14.3   The place of white adipose tissue in lipid metabolism. Stored triacylglycerol (TAG) is derived mainly by the uptake of circulating TAG, either in the form of chylomicrons postprandially, or very-low-density lipoprotein (VLDL) secreted from the liver. TAG uptake occurs via the action of the enzyme lipoprotein lipase (LPL) within the capillary lumen. Stored TAG is hydrolysed by the intracellular enzyme "hormone-sensitive lipase" (HSL) to release non-esterified fatty acids (NEFA) for use by other tissues. Since the major substrates of white adipose tissue metabolism (NEFA, TAG) are hydrophobic, control of adipose tissue perfusion may play a particularly important role in the regulation of its metabolism. Reproduced from Frayn (1989) with permission of J.B. Lippincott Co.

clear that adipose tissue lipogenesis is of little importance in man (reviewed in Frayn, 1989) and may not be in the rat, the species in which it has been most studied (Williamson, 1990). Most of the fat in our adipose tissue comes from lipoprotein–TAG, which is taken up into the adipocytes after hydrolysis by the enzyme lipoprotein lipase (LPL); the fatty acids thus liberated enter the adipocytes, where they are reesterified. Lipoprotein lipase is synthesized within the adipocytes, modified there by post-translational processing (thought to involve progressive N-glycosylation), and then exported in some manner not yet understood to its site of action, the luminal surface of the capillary endothelium. There it is bound by heparan sulphate chains forming part of the endothelial glycocalyx. The relative dimensions of the enzyme, the capillary and a typical lipoprotein particle, together with data on maximal rates of hydrolysis of lipoprotein–TAG, suggest that several LPL molecules act simultaneously on an individual lipoprotein particle (Cryer, 1981; Eckel, 1989).

Like most of the metabolic transactions in adipose tissue, the major participants in this scheme are highly hydrophobic. TAG itself is able to circulate only by incorporation into lipoprotein particles (where it is "protected" by a less hydrophobic outer shell of proteins, phospholipids and free cholesterol). The fatty acids released by the action of LPL are also virtually insoluble, and are transported in plasma by binding to albumin. The means by which they are transferred into the adipocytes after liberation by LPL is not certain, although one model envisages that there is a continuous membrane-like lipid layer from the lipoprotein particle to the adipocyte cell membrane in which the fatty acids move by diffusion (Scow, Blanchette-Mackie and Smith, 1976). Because of the hydrophobic nature of the participants, there is no free diffusion of substances in plasma or extracellular fluid. Regulation of the rate of perfusion of the tissue is thus essential to proper functioning of the process of fat deposition.

Fat mobilization

The stored TAG is "mobilized" when required as an energy source for other tissues by hydrolysis to form non-esterified fatty acids (NEFA) and glycerol; these NEFA are the form in which "lipid energy" is transferred from adipose tissue to other tissues. Hydrolysis is brought about by the intracellular enzyme known as hormone-sensitive lipase (HSL; EC 3.1.1.3). This is an unfortunate name in that LPL is also hormone sensitive, and both are responsive to insulin: insulin activates LPL whilst suppressing HSL, thus leading to fat storage and sparing fat mobilization. Not all the NEFA released by the action of HSL are liberated into the plasma (where they will be bound by albumin). A proportion (around 20% in the overnight fasted state; Coppack *et al.*, 1990b) will be reesterified and remain within the tissue. The extent of reesterification can conveniently be assessed by a comparison of the molar rates of release of NEFA and glycerol (which would be 3:1 if no reesterification occurred), since adipose tissue almost entirely lacks the enzyme glycerol kinase necessary for reutilization of the glycerol. The glycerol 3-phosphate required for reesterification is produced from glucose via the pathway of glycolysis, as discussed in more detail below. The release of fatty acids is completely dependent upon adipose tissue perfusion; the fatty acids are not able to leave the tissue by diffusion in the absence of a supply of albumin in the plasma. Glycerol release, on the other hand, is not dependent upon plasma flow; glycerol is a small, water-soluble molecule and appears to be able to diffuse out of the tissue to some extent, even in conditions of severely reduced perfusion. One of the characteristics of states of reduced blood flow in adipose tissue is thus an increase in the ratio of glycerol to NEFA in the plasma.

Fat mobilization is stimulated by circulating catecholamines and, under many experimental conditions, by sympathetic stimulation. It is also stimulated by a range of other humoral factors including glucagon, adrenocorticotrophic hormone (at high concentrations), growth hormone and cortisol. (The last two act via induction of enzyme protein and are thus slow responses; the others act rapidly via a cyclic $3',5'$-AMP (cAMP)-linked system which phosphorylates and activates HSL). It is inhibited by insulin which both inactivates HSL and increases reesterification (at least in part by increasing the provision of glycerol 3-phosphate). Fat mobilization is also inhibited by some potential modulators of adipose tissue blood flow: adenosine, acting via the A_1 receptors, nicotinic acid (acting via the same receptor) and prostaglandin E_2.

WAYS IN WHICH METABOLISM MAY AFFECT CIRCULATION

The above discussion would make it reasonable to suppose that changes in adipose tissue perfusion and metabolism would be closely linked. This appears to be so in a number of situations. For instance, infusion of adrenaline into normal subjects at various rates produces increases in adipose tissue blood flow and in systemic plasma glycerol (an index of adipose tissue lipolysis) which are highly correlated (Freyschuss *et al.*, 1986). During the infusion of various fat-mobilizing substances into rabbits, increases in adipose tissue blood flow always accompany the increased lipolysis (Lewis and Matthews, 1970). The linkage appears to operate in both "feed-forward" and "feedback" directions. The mechanisms behind it are only partially understood.

Feed-forward mechanisms

The close link between stimulation of lipolysis and increases in adipose tissue blood flow led Lewis and Matthews (1970) to test for vasodilator activity in adipose tissue venous effluent, and in extracts of adipose tissue. The former was negative, but extraction of lipolytically stimulated adipose tissue with acid–ether produced an unidentified vasodilator substance.

Feedback mechanisms

Evidence for the involvement of adenosine in the regulation of adipose tissue blood flow has been reviewed above. There has been considerable speculation that adenosine production during stimulation of lipolysis provides the link between blood flow and metabolism. The stimulation of lipolysis involves an increase in the cellular concentration of cAMP, which is then broken down through the action of phosphodiesterase to AMP and potentially to adenosine. The evidence for such a link is at present only indirect. Thus, changes in adipose tissue lipolysis induced by insulin, glucose and nicotinic acid are associated with reductions in blood flow in a manner which would correlate with the expected reductions in cellular cAMP and thus adenosine production (Madsen and Malchow-Møller, 1983). Adenosine, acting via the A_1 receptors (Lafontan and Berlan, 1985), is an inhibitor of adipocyte lipolysis, and so the possibility exists for a feedback loop: when lipolysis is stimulated, adenosine is released and acts both to increase local blood flow and to restrain the rate of fat mobilization (Fredholm, 1985).

The idea that flow limitation can restrict NEFA release from adipose tissue was mentioned above. The reverse also appears to be true. When the NEFA/albumin ratio in the perfusing blood rises (above a molar ratio of about 3:1), so there is an increase in adipose tissue vascular resistance (Madsen, Bülow and Nielsen, 1986). This finding has been confirmed in intact adipose tissue *in vivo*, the plasma NEFA/albumin ratio being raised by administration of a lipid emulsion (Bülow *et al.*, 1985). The mechanism for this link has not been established: changes in flow do not, for instance, relate to changes in catecholamine concentrations (Bülow *et al.*, 1985). Again it might be seen as part of a feedback loop restricting the rate of NEFA release under conditions of lipolytic stimulation.

WAYS IN WHICH CIRCULATION MAY AFFECT METABOLISM

Albumin delivery and fatty acid removal

The main product of adipocyte metabolism is the release of NEFA into the circulation. These NEFA are not water soluble, and are carried in the plasma bound to albumin. The albumin molecule has two to three high-affinity binding sites for NEFA, and more binding sites with progressively decreasing affinities (Spector, 1975). In perfused adipose tissue preparations, the rate of delivery of albumin (i.e. the product of plasma flow and albumin concentration) determines the maximum rate at which NEFA can leave the adipose tissue (Scow, 1965; Bülow and Madsen, 1981; Madsen, Bülow and Nielsen, 1986). Excess NEFA accumulate within the tissue and their presence may stimulate intracellular reesterification (Scow, 1965; Madsen, Bülow and Nielsen, 1986). There is thus good reason for believing that high rates of lipolysis should be accompanied by an increase in adipose tissue perfusion, and this appears to be the case in "physiological states" such as exercise and fasting, although not in "pathophysiological states" such as hypovolaemia or hypotension.

A further way in which flow may affect fatty acid release has recently been proposed. There is evidence that the fatty acid reesterification pathway (which serves to restrict the rate of NEFA release) may involve an extracellular step. Thus, NEFA released by the action of HSL and those forming the substrates for esterification may be separated (compartmentalized), and a NEFA molecule may have to leave the cell and re-enter it in order to be reesterified rather than exported from the tissue (Edens, Leibel and Hirsch, 1990). In this case, a low flow rate would tend to favour reesterification, whereas a high flow would tend to remove NEFA from the tissue (Edens, Leibel and Hirsch, 1990).

Cellular redox potential

The reesterification of fatty acids within the adipocyte requires the provision of glycerol 3-phosphate. This is a product of glycolysis, formed from dihydroxy-acetone phosphate (DHAP), a glycolytic intermediate, via the enzyme glycerol 3-phosphate dehydrogenase:

$$DHAP + NADH \longrightarrow glycerol\ 3\text{-phosphate} + NAD^+$$

This reaction is at near-equilibrium, and a change in the cytosolic $NADH/NAD^+$ ratio or a change in the DHAP concentration will affect the concentration of glycerol 3-phosphate. The stimulatory effect of insulin on reesterification is thought to involve in part increased glucose uptake, glycolysis, and thus DHAP and glycerol 3-phosphate production. The $NADH/NAD^+$ ratio is, in turn, a reflection of the cytosolic redox state. In hypoxia, the ratio will rise in part through lack of oxygen to reoxidise the NADH, in part through the accompanying rise in lactate concentration. Lactate affects the cytosolic redox state through another near-equilibrium reaction, that catalysed by lactate dehydrogenase (Fredholm, 1970):

$$\text{Lactate} + \text{NAD}^+ \longrightarrow \text{Pyruvate} + \text{NADH}$$

Thus, either systemic or local hypoxia (perhaps reflecting vasoconstriction in adipose tissue) may increase the reesterification of fatty acids within adipose tissue, and decrease NEFA release (Bülow and Madsen, 1981).

BLOOD FLOW AND METABOLISM OF WHITE ADIPOSE TISSUE IN DIFFERENT STATES

REGULATION OF BASAL ADIPOSE TISSUE BLOOD FLOW

In the rat, administration of the β_1-adrenoceptor antagonist, atenolol, causes a marked fall (67%) in adipose tissue blood flow (Risberg, Hordnes and Tyssebotn, 1987), suggesting a high degree of "tonic" β_1-adrenoceptor stimulation. In humans, this does not appear to be the case. After sympathectomy, subcutaneous adipose tissue blood flow returns (after a few days) to its previous value (Henriksen, 1977), and in intact subjects propranolol infusion does not change resting adipose tissue blood flow (Simonsen et al., 1990).

NUTRIENT PROVISION AND HYPOGLYCAEMIA

The delivery of nutrients to adipose tissue, largely in the form of water-insoluble lipoprotein–TAG, might be expected to involve changes in blood flow. Less is known, however, about such changes than about those occurring in situations of fat mobilization. Infusion of glucose in the rat causes a fall in adipose tissue blood flow, which appears to be secondary to insulin release since it is abolished by anti-insulin serum (Madsen and Malchow-Møller, 1983). It was suggested that reductions in adenosine production provided the link. Also in rats, eating a single meal produced a fall in white adipose tissue blood flow in a number of depots (Glick et al., 1984; West, Prinz and Greenwood, 1989). In sheep, there is little change (a tendency to decrease) in subcutaneous adipose tissue blood flow after a meal (Barnes, Comline and Dobson, 1983). In humans, the opposite appears to be true: blood flow through subcutaneous adipose tissue increases after an oral glucose load (Bülow et al., 1987a) or a single meal (Coppack et al., 1990a; Simonsen et al., 1990). These changes in blood flow were not obviously related to changes in plasma catecholamine concentrations, although the rise after a meal was partially abolished by continuous propranolol infusion (Simonsen et al., 1990), suggesting an adrenergic component. It should be noted that in one other study in humans, intravenous glucose administration caused a rise in adipose tissue blood flow, but oral glucose a fall (Quaade et al., 1967); there is no obvious reason for this discrepancy with other work.

The deficiency of nutrient represented by insulin-induced hypoglycaemia is not, of course, an exact opposite of feeding since a "counter-regulatory" response, with activation of the sympatho-adrenal system in particular, will occur. Adipose tissue blood flow has been studied in this condition in part because of interest in the absorption of subcutaneously injected insulin. In dogs and rats, hypoglycaemia produces an increase in adipose tissue blood flow (at thermoneutrality), but a less marked decrease in flow in rats below thermoneutrality (Benzi and Girardier, 1986). In humans, there are reports of an increase of around 100% in adipose tissue blood flow (Fernqvist-Forbes, Linde and Gunnarsson, 1988; Fernqvist-Forbes, Gunnarsson and Linde, 1989) or of little change (Hilsted *et al.*, 1985) during hypoglycaemia, with a plasma adrenaline concentration of 5–6 nmol/l at the nadir of blood glucose (Hilsted *et al.*, 1985; Fernqvist-Forbes, Linde and Gunnarsson, 1988; Fernqvist-Forbes, Gunnarsson and Linde, 1989). This variability of responses between and even within species is reminiscent of the variable responses to catecholamines reviewed earlier, and suggests that adrenergic mechanisms are involved.

STARVATION AND OBESITY

Starvation is a state in which lipid mobilization is important, and by the arguments advanced above, adipose blood flow might be expected to increase. In the only study of adipose blood flow during acute starvation in humans, there was a doubling during four days of total starvation in four obese women (Nielsen *et al.*, 1968). In rats, 24 or 48 h starvation also caused a rise in blood flow per unit weight of adipose tissue (Mayerle and Havel, 1969; Madsen, Malchow-Møller and Waldorff, 1975). More is known about the changes that occur with prolonged changes in body weight. Here a difficulty arises, however, because adipocytes more than any other cell type change in volume during weight gain or loss as the amount of stored lipid changes. Most measurements of adipose tissue blood flow are made on the basis of tissue wet weight. This can give a different picture from measurements made on a "per cell" basis (Crandall and DiGirolamo, 1990). In general, blood flow per unit weight or per unit cell surface area decreases with increasing obesity in both rats and sheep (Crandall *et al.*, 1986; Gregory, Christopherson and Lister, 1986; West *et al.*, 1987; Crandall and DiGirolamo, 1990), whereas blood flow per cell is unaltered or even increased (depending on the depot studied) (Crandall *et al.*, 1984b; Crandall *et al.*, 1986; West *et al.*, 1987; Crandall and DiGirolamo, 1990). With 30% body weight reduction in rats, blood flow per unit weight of adipose tissue stays approximately constant (calculated from data in Crandall *et al.*, 1984a). Since adipose tissue weight decreases considerably, the total "organ flow" through individual adipose depots falls markedly, and the proportion of cardiac output to adipose tissue decreases (Crandall *et al.*, 1984a). It should be borne in mind when interpreting these results that the weight of adipose tissue increases much more, proportionately, than that of other tissues during the development of obesity (and *vice versa* during weight loss). Whether adipose cell number also changes is a point of considerable controversy (Björntorp and Sjöström, 1985; Julien, Despres and Angel, 1989). It has been suggested, however, that the expansion of adipose tissue mass in obesity places an increased demand on the cardiovascular system, with elevation of blood volume and of cardiac output (Crandall and DiGirolamo, 1990).

EXERCISE

The body's fat stores are called upon at a higher rate during strenuous exercise than in any other state. It would thus be expected that adipose tissue blood flow would increase to allow

TABLE 14.3

Adipose tissue blood flow and plasma non-esterified fatty acid (NEFA) and glycerol concentrations during exercise in humans

	Rest	1	2	3	4	5	6
Adipose tissue blood flow ml·100 g^{-1}·min^{-1}	3.9	5.1	8.1	9.3	10.0	11.5	11.0
Plasma concentration of							
NEFA, mmol/l	0.78	1.98	3.75	3.57	4.70	5.37	5.95
glycerol, μmol/l	42	154	273	382	447	413	458

Taken from data in Bülow and Madsen, 1976. Exercise consisted of six periods each of 50 min on a bicycle ergometer at around 50% $\dot{V}O_{2\ max}$, with 10 min rest periods between. There were eight physically fit, male subjects; one did not complete the last period.

the release of NEFA, and this is indeed the case, although there is considerable evidence that the rate of blood flow still limits the rate of fatty acid entry into the systemic circulation.

Increased adipose tissue blood flow during prolonged exercise has been demonstrated in humans, rats and dogs (Bülow and Madsen, 1976; Larsen *et al.*, 1981; Bülow, 1982; Bülow and Tøndevold, 1982; reviewed in Bülow, 1983, 1988) (Table 14.3). The mechanism for this increase in flow is not certain; it occurs even in a denervated adipose depot (Bülow and Madsen, 1986), and may represent the "feed-forward" regulation by some product of lipolysis discussed earlier. Although it has been claimed that adenosine is the mediator of the increased flow in exercise (Bülow, 1988), mainly on the basis of experiments with adenosine deaminase reviewed earlier (Martin and Bockman, 1986), there is no firm evidence for this during exercise. Since strenuous exercise is characterized by intense sympathetic activity, there is a paradox, in that this might be expected to decrease adipose tissue blood flow.

During strenuous exercise, the NEFA:albumin molar ratio in the adipose venous drainage will exceed the usual "maximum" of around 3 (Hodgetts *et al.*, 1991). This would be expected to produce a decrease in adipose tissue blood flow as discussed earlier (Bülow *et al.*, 1985; Madsen, Bülow and Nielsen, 1986). This may work against whatever mechanism is increasing adipose tissue perfusion and would also be expected to stimulate reesterification of fatty acids within the tissue, thus restraining the rate of NEFA release. Reesterification may also be stimulated by the increased systemic lactate concentration (Fredholm, 1970). There is evidence for increased reesterification during exercise in the dog (Bülow, 1982), although not in humans (Hodgetts *et al.*, 1991), and also evidence that with cessation of exercise there is a sudden "washout" of NEFA presumably physically trapped in the tissue by lack of albumin delivery (Larsen *et al.*, 1981; Hodgetts *et al.*, 1991). It could well be argued that inhibitory feedback on adipose tissue blood flow is inappropriate in this situation, and limits the capacity for exercise when there is usually no shortage of substrate (stored lipid). One hypothesis is that high levels of circulating NEFA can have deleterious effects on blood vessels and on tissues, and that these mechanisms evolved to limit the plasma concentration of NEFA (reviewed in Newhsolme and Leech, 1983).

STRESS, TRAUMA AND HYPOVOLAEMIA

Perhaps the mildest form of stress is the physiological adjustment to a change in posture; but it induces a surprisingly large fall (30–50%) in adipose tissue blood flow due to vasoconstriction (Linde and Hjemdahl, 1982; Skagen, 1983; Hildebrandt *et al.*, 1985). This response is thought to be mediated by sympathetic activation (Linde and Hjemdahl, 1982), and is abolished (at least in the arm, although not in the leg) by proximal nervous blockade with lignocaine (Skagen, 1983).

In contrast, mental stress, induced by the colour/word conflict test, caused an increase in adipose tissue blood flow (up 60–90%; vascular resistance down 25–40%) (Linde *et al.*, 1989) accompanied by moderate increases in plasma concentrations of adrenaline and noradrenaline; in other, similar experiments in which the rise in plasma noradrenaline was slightly less, the response of adipose tissue blood flow was even greater (up 100%) (Fernqvist and Linde, 1988). The usual picture of conflicting α-adrenoceptor-mediated vasoconstriction moderating β-adrenoceptor-mediated vasodilatation is thus seen, and confirmed by the use of propranolol which converted the decrease in vascular resistance to an increase (Linde *et al.*, 1989).

With physical trauma and hypovolaemia, much greater changes in adipose tissue blood flow are seen. This is an interesting situation for many reasons. In shock or trauma, there is an intense lipolytic drive, which might be expected, by mechanisms discussed earlier, to increase adipose tissue blood flow. On the other hand, there are factors that would be expected to increase adipose tissue perfusion: marked sympathetic activation, elevation of vasopressin, elevation of the NEFA/albumin ratio and, in severe hypovolaemia, decreased cardiac output. The organism in severe shock or trauma appears to be mobilizing fuel stores, but meeting restraint imposed by a number of mechanisms (Frayn, 1986). It has been suggested that a failure to mobilize fatty acids from adipose tissue may be deleterious in terms of "internal starvation", since the carbohydrate stores are rapidly depleted in such conditions (Rosell, Sándor and Kovách, 1973). The usual outcome, as judged by the appearance of NEFA in the systemic plasma, is that there is a rise, but not such a large rise as might be expected from the lipolytic stimulus (reviewed in Frayn, 1986).

The dog has been the subject for much of this work, and appears to be a misleadingly susceptible model. (This apparent susceptibility may, however, simply represent the fact that dogs seem to be subjected to more severe forms of trauma than other species). Thus, during haemorrhagic hypotension, canine adipose tissue blood flow falls to very low levels and this is accompanied by a surprising fall (in view of the lipolytic stimulus) in systemic plasma NEFA concentrations (Kovách *et al.*, 1970). Pretreatment with the α-adrenoceptor blocker phenoxybenzamine results in a much lesser change in adipose tissue blood flow and a rise in the systemic plasma NEFA concentration (Kovách *et al.*, 1970). Treatment with β_2-adrenoceptor blockade (in cats subjected to haemorrhage), in contrast, further increased adipose tissue vascular resistance (Gustafsson *et al.*, 1984). A very similar picture has been observed in dogs during acute ischaemic left ventricular failure (Smiseth *et al.*, 1983). In these experiments, the typical picture of an increase to plasma glycerol unaccompanied by an elevation of NEFA concentration reflected the "trapping" of fatty acids in adipose tissue because of inadequate perfusion. Other treatments including ventricular fibrillation, systemic hypoxaemia, hyperinflation of the lungs and coronary artery occlusion also increase vascular resistance in canine adipose tissue (Hanley, Sachs and Skinner, 1971).

In humans, we lack direct measurements of adipose tissue blood flow in acute shock or trauma. Some inferences can, however, be made. Plasma catecholamine concentrations in the severely injured will rise many-fold above those observed in the "stress" experiments (tilting or colour–word conflict) described above (Frayn, 1986). These seem likely to cause adipose tissue vasoconstriction. The vasopressin response to acute trauma may be marked (reviewed in Barton, Frayn and Little, 1990) and (based on work in small animals reviewed earlier) might further impair adipose tissue perfusion. Although the sympatho-adrenal response to injury is directly related to the severity of injury (Frayn *et al.*, 1985), the resulting plasma NEFA concentration is not so: in the severely injured patient, plasma NEFA concentrations may be raised less than in patients with less severe injuries (Stoner *et al.*, 1979). Plasma glycerol concentrations show a more direct relationship with severity of injury, again arguing for a retention of fatty acids in adipose tissue by restriction of flow after severe injury. Trials of adrenoceptor blockade have not been carried out in this situation, and would almost certainly be unethical.

BASIC FEATURES OF CIRCULATION AND INNERVATION OF BROWN ADIPOSE TISSUE

Interest in brown adipose tissue as being separate to white adipose tissue was increased substantially in the 1960s with the emergence of interest in thermoregulation during cold exposure. There have been many reviews published on the morphological and biochemical characteristics of brown adipose tissue since then, with the most recent and one of the broadest being that edited by Trayhurn and Nicholls (1986). The present review will focus on the role of the sympathetic nervous system in controlling the metabolism and blood flow of brown adipose tissue. More detailed discussion of the biochemical features of the tissue is beyond the scope of this chapter.

The majority of the factors described earlier that regulate white adipose tissue, are also of importance in the control of brown adipose tissue. The following sections will describe the major differences between the tissues and focus on the specialized function of brown adipose tissue (namely non-shivering thermogenesis) and how this relates to the control of the tissue's blood flow.

MORPHOLOGY AND LOCATION

An anatomical/histological distinction between white and brown adipose tissue has been recognized for several centuries. Brown adipose tissue receives its name from its red–brown appearance, resulting from the combination of its high degree of vascularization (giving a high blood content) and the large cytochrome content of the mitochondria. In the rat, brown adipose tissue has a vascular density four to six times greater than that of white adipose tissue (Fawcett, 1952; Hauberger and Widelitz, 1963). This gives rise to each cell in brown adipose tissue being in contact with at least two capillaries (Nechad, 1986).

The other major distinguishing feature of the tissue is that it is normally composed of cells containing multilocular TAG droplets, whereas white adipocytes contain a single droplet (being unilocular). There has been some discussion as to whether there were in fact two distinct tissues, but the balance of evidence now favours the brown and white tissues being distinct. There is still the potential for confusion in this area because many of the major locations of brown adipose tissue in the neonate are sites of white adipose tissue depots in adults. However, this is not because of brown adipose tissue turning into white, but rather a regression of the brown adipose tissue due to aging, with the remaining cells taking on a unilocular appearance, followed by an expansion of the white adipose tissue into those areas. This process is not necessarily irreversible, as cold exposure in adult rats is accompanied by the development of new brown adipocytes (Himms-Hagen, Traindafillou and Gwilliam, 1981) and in adult guinea-pigs leads to reactivation of existing tissue which had taken on the appearance of white adipose tissue (Holloway et al., 1984).

Brown adipose tissue is present in characteristic locations in the newborn of most mammalian species, the most common sites being the interscapular, cervical, perirenal and periaortic (Hull and Segall, 1965). The proximity of the tissue to the major organs or arteries supplying them, subserves the tissue's role in thermoregulation. The most widely studied site of mammalian brown adipose tissue is the interscapular, especially from the rat. There are undoubtedly some metabolic differences between the tissue from different sites (as there are for white adipose tissue) but little is known as to whether there are any regional differences in the innervation or vascularization of the tissue. The consequence of this is that the majority of the work considered in this review will be concerned with interscapular brown adipose tissue. The interscapular brown adipose tissue depot comprises two lobes, which receive separate arterial supplies and have separate venous drainage. There is also a third vein (Sulzer's vein) draining both lobes simultaneously. The bilateral venous drainage passes close to the arterial inflow and so offers the possibility of some counter-current heat exchange (Smith and Roberts, 1964) which would lead to progressive warming of the depot of brown adipose tissue. However, if the venous drainage is directed via Sulzer's vein, the heat generated within the interscapular brown adipose tissue will be transferred away to the tissues of the back and into the central circulation (Girardier and Seydoux, 1986).

There has been recent anatomical (Nnodim and Lever, 1988) and physiological (Woods and Stock, 1990) evidence of the existence of arteriovenous anastomoses in interscapular brown adipose tissue in the rat. These shunt vessels receive a sympathetic innervation, and seem to dilate during intense stimulation of the tissue. This is accompanied by reduced capillary flow and tissue oxygen consumption. Cessation of stimulation is accompanied by increased capillary and decreased anastomotic flow, with stimulation of non-shivering thermogenesis.

INNERVATION

Whilst there is still some uncertainty as to the extent of innervation of white adipocytes, it is clear that there is a direct sympathetic innervation of the cells in brown adipose tissue. In addition, the vasculature in brown adipose tissue has a sympathetic innervation which is mainly to the arterial side (Thureson-Klein, Lagercrantz and Barnard, 1976). Most of the information on the innervation of brown adipose tissue is from studies of interscapular brown adipose tissue. This tissue receives numerous sympathetic fibres, five or six distinct nerves to each lobe, arising from intercostal nerves and synapsing on the adipocytes (with some nerves continuing through to subcutaneous tissue), plus some perivascular nerves which also seem to innervate the adipocytes (Thureson-Klein, Lagercrantz and Barnard, 1976). Cannon *et al.* (1986) observed the coexistence of neuropeptide Y in the perivascular nerves, but not in the sympathetic innervation of the adipocytes, but it is not clear what the functional significance is of these observations. Nnodim and Lever (1988) confirmed the presence of non-adrenergic nerve fibres around the blood vessels in the interscapular brown adipose tissue of the rat. The overall density of the sympathetic innervation of brown adipose tissue is much greater than of white adipose tissue; in fact, the noradrenaline concentration per unit weight of brown adipose tissue is similar to that of the myocardium (Young *et al.*, 1982). The specific area of interscapular brown adipose tissue innervated by each nerve is markedly heterogeneous between animals, so functional studies of the effects of nerve stimulation are only meaningful and reproducible if all of the nerves are stimulated.

It was originally thought that the brown adipocytes were innervated by postganglionic nerves arising from intrinsic ganglia within the depots of brown adipose tissue, as the fibres remained intact after denervation (Derry, Schonbaum and Steiner, 1969). However, subsequent investigations have failed to demonstrate such ganglia morphologically (Barnard, Mory and Nechad, 1980; Mory, Combes-George and Nechad, 1983). Further confusion and disagreement concerning the innervation of brown adipose tissue arises from the demonstration by Seydoux *et al.* (1977) that some of the perivascular nerves in interscapular brown adipose tissue supply both ipsilateral and contralateral lobes, which Foster, Depocas and Zaror-Behrens (1982) were unable to confirm.

BLOOD FLOW

Some of the earlier confusion regarding the quantitative importance of brown adipose tissue in non-shivering thermogenesis arose from the inaccurate measurement of blood flow. This was resolved by Foster and Frydman (1978a), who demonstrated that the earlier ^{86}Rb methods seriously underestimated blood flow in interscapular brown adipose tissue compared to the results obtained with radioactive microspheres. Most of the information now available on blood flow in brown adipose tissue is based on the microsphere technique described by Foster and Frydman. The main exceptions are the original work on brown adipose tissue neonatal rabbit from Hull and colleagues, which collected the venous drainage from the tissue in anaesthetized animals (Hull and Segall, 1965), and the study by Astrup and colleagues in man, which used the xenon washout technique described earlier (Astrup *et al.*, 1984).

The main physiological function of brown adipose tissue is to mediate non-shivering thermogenesis and export the heat to the vital organs. The activation of brown adipose tissue thermogenesis is closely linked to an increase in blood flow through the tissue, e.g. at rest the flow is 0.1–1.0 ml/g/min, whilst on maximal stimulation the values are 5–28 ml/g/min (Foster, 1986). It was originally thought that the sympathetic innervation directly mediated the vasodilatation. However, this does not seem to be the case as there do not appear to be any β-adrenoceptors in the vasculature, and vasodilator doses of isoprenaline do not increase blood flow in interscapular brown adipose tissue (Foster, 1984). Furthermore, in the anaesthetized rat, electrical stimulation of the sympathetic nerves leads to an initial vasoconstriction (which can be prevented by phentolamine) in interscapular brown adipose tissue before an eventual vasodilatation (Flaim, Horwitz and Horowitz, 1977). Thus, it would appear that the sympathetic innervation of the vasculature of brown adipose tissue produces α-adrenoceptor mediated vasoconstriction, although it is not known if this is the case in humans. It has been reported that α-adrenoceptor antagonists actually reduce noradrenaline-induced thermogenesis and hyperaemia in interscapular brown adipose tissue in rat (Foster, 1984), even though the direct stimulation of adipocytes is due to β-adrenoceptor activation. This is somewhat complex, and may differ between species, as α-adrenoceptor stimulation in the lamb causes vasoconstriction in brown adipose tissue and reduces the thermogenic response (Alexander and Stevens, 1980).

The observation that stimulation of α-adrenoceptors is important in the production of the full thermogenic response is consistent with the effects of the α_1-adrenoceptor antagonist, prazosin, in reducing whole body, noradrenaline-induced thermogenesis in the rat (Siyamak, 1991). This effect of α-adrenoceptor blockade in reducing catecholamine-induced thermogenesis may be due to less oxygen consumption by vascular smooth muscle, which would be a result of a diminished vasoconstrictor response (Ye et al., 1990).

The absence of direct vasodilator responses to nerve stimulation in brown adipose tissue would indicate that the increased blood flow seen when thermogenesis is stimulated is secondary to a metabolic event. This was first suggested by Heim and Hull (1966), and has been confirmed subsequently. Foster and Depocas (1980) showed that the plasma noradrenaline concentration had no direct impact on the magnitude of the hyperaemia. By altering the haematocrit and arterial pO_2 values and keeping plasma noradrenaline constant, they found that blood flow varied to maintain oxygen supply. The candidates for the metabolic mediators of vasodilatation in brown adipose tissue are similar to those described above for white adipose tissue, although the most likely mechanism would involve some feature of tissue oxygen tension or redox state. Girardier (1983) suggested that the vasodilatation was mediated through H^+, K^+, and changes in osmolality, but this would not explain the importance of oxygen availability shown by Foster and Depocas (1980). Ma and Foster (1984) have shown that the cytosolic $NAD^+/NADH$ or redox state was related to the hyperaemic response; the mechanisms linking intra-adipocyte metabolism to relaxation of the vascular smooth muscle have not been elucidated. It is also possible that the rise in temperature in brown adipose tissue reduces the affinity of the α-adrenoceptors (in the opposite way to the effect of cold on skin vessels) (Janssens and Vanhoutte, 1978) and thus lessens any noradrenaline-induced vasoconstriction. However, this would not produce marked vasodilatation unless there was a high degree of resting vasoconstrictor tone.

The other aspect of the control of the vasculature of brown adipose tissue relates to the regulation of the venous drainage from interscapular brown adipose tissue mentioned earlier. In theory, neural regulation of the route of venous outflow would determine whether tissue thermogenesis affected the tissue itself, or the rest of the body (including spinal cord thermoreceptors). However, the extent of any sympathetic control of these veins is not known.

BROWN ADIPOSE TISSUE FUNCTION

Although the major function of brown adipose tissue is as a site of non-shivering thermogenesis, the tissue can also act as a site of TAG storage. For example, during arousal from hibernation, brown adipose tissue may release NEFA, which then act as a substrate for shivering in skeletal muscle (Joel, 1965). One interesting feature of the metabolism of brown adipose tissue related to the storage of TAG is that in the rat the endothelial LPL responsible for hydrolysis of plasma TAG, enabling NEFA uptake into the tissue, is stimulated by noradrenaline (Carneheim, Nedergaard and Cannon, 1984) which is opposite to the effect in white adipose tissue.

The mechanisms of non-shivering thermogenesis operating in brown adipose tissue involve the uncoupling of oxidative phosphorylation so that oxygen consumption and heat production are not closely tied to the generation of ATP. It seems most likely that this mitochondrial uncoupling is linked to the presence in the inner mitochondrial membranes of brown adipose tissue of a specific 32,000 dalton protein which has been termed "thermogenin" (Cannon, Nedergaard and Sundin, 1981), or "GDP-binding protein". This protein forms an ion channel which is capable of conducting small anions (e.g. OH^-, Cl^-, Br^-), but is normally inoperative due to binding of purine nucleotides (e.g. ATP, GDP) to the protein. Activation of lipolysis within the brown adipocyte is thought to lead to displacement of the nucleotide from the binding site (probably by NEFA or fatty acyl CoA), thus allowing OH^- ions to move through the mitochondrial membrane. This will eliminate the H^+ gradient produced by the respiratory chain, consuming oxygen and liberating heat without producing ATP.

It is well established that this physiological uncoupling of mitochondria in brown adipose tissue is an important mechanism of thermogenesis in the newborn of most species and in the cold adaptation of mammals such as the rat. A possible role for brown adipose tissue in the regulation of energy balance is somewhat more contentious.

NEONATAL THERMOREGULATION

The early studies by Hull and colleagues on anaesthetized newborn rabbits showed that brown adipose tissue made a substantial contribution to overall heat production — in some cases accounting for more than 50% of the total heat production (Hull and Segall, 1965). The profound increase in the blood flow in brown adipose tissue needed to support this thermogenesis was illustrated by Heim and Hull (1966), who showed that injected noradrenaline increased the blood flow in brown adipose tissue nearly four-fold, and that the tissue received approximately 25% of the cardiac output. (The choice of the neonatal rabbit for these studies was particularly apposite, as this species has one of the highest contents of brown adipose tissue per unit body weight in the neonatal period). This group also showed that neonatal humans have extensive brown adipose tissue stores (Aherne and Hull, 1966), and it is now established that most mammalian species (including sheep, pigs and cattle) have substantial amounts of brown adipose tissue as neonates (Alexander, Bennett and Gemmell, 1975).

COLD ACCLIMATION

Until the definitive studies of Foster and Frydman (1978b), there was disagreement as to the quantitative significance of brown adipose tissue as a site of non-shivering thermogenesis in cold-adapted rats. However, Foster and Frydman showed that the earlier studies that suggested a trivial role for brown adipose tissue were flawed by the use of an unreliable technique for measuring blood flow. Their studies with radioactive microspheres showed a high blood flow in the brown adipose tissue of cold-adapted rodents. Furthermore, they sampled venous blood (from Sulzer's vein) in the brown adipose tissue of anaesthetized rats during infusion of noradrenaline and showed very high rates of oxygen extraction. Thus, brown adipose tissue is an important site of non-shivering thermogenesis in cold-adapted rats, and also in other rodent species.

DIETARY AND METABOLIC ALTERATIONS

Rothwell and Stock (1979) showed that growing rats offered a highly palatable (cafeteria) diet had a marked elevation of energy intake, but did not become obese. These rats had a substantial hypertrophy of interscapular brown adipose tissue and showed enhanced whole-body thermogenic responses to noradrenaline. Subsequent studies confirmed that such animals adapted to the increased energy intake by increasing energy expenditure, at least partly through activation of thermogenesis in brown adipose tissue. This effect on the brown adipose tissue was very similar to that seen in rats during adaptation to cold exposure. By contrast, underfeeding is accompanied by a reduced mass of brown adipose tissue and thermogenic responsiveness, whilst hypoglycaemia in rats is accompanied by a decrease in the blood flow in brown adipose tissue when the rats are adapted to cool environmental conditions (Benzi and Girardier, 1986). Thus, the regulation of thermogenesis in brown adipose tissue (and by inference blood flow) is closely related to the control of metabolism in the rat.

BROWN ADIPOSE TISSUE IN ADULT MAN

The demonstration of a role for brown adipose tissue in the regulation of energy expenditure in rodents led to the speculation that the tissue may be of importance in the control of energy balance in man. However, normal adults have very little identifiable brown adipose tissue, thus raising doubts as to its quantitative importance. Furthermore, Astrup et al. (1984) investigated heat production in perirenal adipose tissue (which has a marked content of brown adipose tissue) in adult men during the administration of the sympathomimetic ephedrine. Whole-body thermogenesis increased by approximately 20%, but there were no changes in perirenal blood flow (measured by xenon washout) or temperature (measured with a thermocouple), thus indicating no increase in heat production in the tissue.

β-ADRENOCEPTORS IN BROWN ADIPOSE TISSUE

It is well established that catecholamine- and sympathetic nerve-stimulated lipolysis and thermogenesis in brown adipose tissue are mediated via activation of β-adrenoceptors. Arch *et al.* (1984) have shown that the receptors involved do not fall into the classical β_1- or β_2-categories and should be regarded as atypical, or β_3-adrenoceptors. Although this is the main mechanism by which catecholamines stimulate thermogenesis in brown adipose tissue, there is some evidence that stimulation of adipocyte α-adrenoceptors is also involved in mediating thermogenesis in hamsters (Mohell, 1984).

REFERENCES

Aherne, W. and Hull, D. (1966). Brown adipose tissue and heat production in the newborn infant. *Journal of Pathology and Bacteriology*, **91**, 223–234.

Alexander, G. and Stevens, D. (1980). Sympathetic innervation and the development of structure and function of brown adipose tissue: studies on lambs chemically sympathectomised *in utero* with 6-hydroxydopamine. *Journal of Developmental Physiology*, **2**, 119–137.

Alexander, G., Bennett, J.W. and Gemmell, R.T. (1975). Brown adipose tissue in the newborn calf (Bos taurus). *Journal of Physiology (London)*, **244**, 223–239.

Andersen, A.M. and Ladefoged, J. (1967). Partition coefficient of ^{133}xenon between various tissues and blood *in vivo*. *Scandinavian Journal of Clinical and Laboratory Investigation*, **19**, 72–78.

Arch, J.R.S. and Newsholme, E.A. (1978). The control of the metabolism and the hormonal role of adenosine. *Essays in Biochemistry*, **14**, 82–123.

Arch, J.R.S., Ainsworth, A.T., Cawthorne, M.A., Piercy, V., Sennitt, M.V., Thody, V.E., *et al.* (1984). Atypical β-adrenoceptors on brown adipocytes as target of antiobesity drugs. *Nature*, **309**, 163–165.

Astrup, A.V., Bülow, J., Christensen, N.J. and Madsen, J. (1984). Ephedrine induced thermogenesis in man: no role for interscapular brown adipose tissue. *Clinical Science*, **66**, 179–186.

Aukland, K. and Johnsen, H.M. (1974). Protein concentrations and colloid osmotic pressure of rat skeletal muscle interstitial fluid. *Acta Physiologica Scandinavica*, **91**, 354–364.

Axelrod, L. and Levine, L. (1981). Prostacyclin production by isolated adipocytes. *Diabetes*, **30**, 163–167.

Ballantyne, B. (1968). Histochemical and biochemical aspects of cholinesterase activity of adipose tissue. *Archives Internationales de Pharmacodynamie*, **173**, 343–350.

Ballard, K. (1973). Blood flow in canine adipose tissue during intravenous infusion of norepinephrine. *American Journal of Physiology*, **225**, 1026–1031.

Ballard, K. and Rosell, S. (1971). Adrenergic neurohumoral influences on circulation and lipolysis in canine omental adipose tissue. *Circulation Research*, **28**, 389–396.

Ballard, K., Cobb, C.A. and Rosell, S. (1971). Vascular and lipolytic responses in canine subcutaneous adipose tissue following infusion of catecholamines. *Acta Physiologica Scandinavica*, **81**, 246–253.

Ballard, K., Malmfors, T. and Rosell, S. (1974). Adrenergic innervation and vascular patterns in canine adipose tissue. *Microvascular Research*, **8**, 164–171.

Barnard, T., Mory, G. and Nechad, M. (1980). Biogenic amines and the trophic response of brown adipose tissue. In *Biogenic Amines and Development*, edited by S. Parvez and H. Parvez, pp. 391–439. Amsterdam, Elsevier.

Barnes, R.J., Comline, R.S. and Dobson, A. (1983). Changes in the blood flow to the digestive organs of sheep induced by feeding. *Quarterly Journal of Experimental Physiology*, **68**, 77–88.

Barton, R.N., Frayn, K.N. and Little, R.A. (1990). Trauma, burns and surgery. In *The Metabolic and Molecular Basis of Acquired Disease*, edited by R.D. Cohen, B. Lewis, K.G.M.M. Alberti and A.M. Denman, pp. 684–717. London: Baillière Tindall.

Belfrage, E. (1978). Comparison of β-adrenoceptors mediating vasodilatation in canine subcutaneous adipose tissue and skeletal muscle. *Acta Physiologica Scandinavica*, **102**, 469–476.

Benzi, R.H. and Girardier, L. (1986). The response of adipose tissue blood flow to insulin-induced hypoglycemia in conscious dogs and rats. *Pflügers Archiv: European Journal of Physiology*, **406**, 37–44.

Björntorp, P. and Sjöström, L. (1985). Adipose tissue dysfunction and its consequences. In *New Perspectives in Adipose Tissue: Structure, Function and Development*, edited by A. Cryer and R.L.R. Van, pp. 447–458. London: Butterworths.

Bowery, B. and Lewis, G.P. (1973). Inhibition of functional vasodilatation and prostaglandin formation in rabbit adipose tissue by indomethacin and aspirin. *British Journal of Pharmacology*, **47**, 305–314.

Bülow, J. (1982). Subcutaneous adipose tissue blood flow and triacylglycerol-mobilization during prolonged exercise in dogs. *Pflügers Archiv: European Journal of Physiology*, **392**, 230–234.

Bülow, J. (1983). Adipose tissue blood flow during exercise. *Danish Medical Bulletin*, **30**, 85–100.

Bülow, J. (1993). Lipid mobilization and utilization. *Medicine and Sport Science*, **38**, 158–185.

Bülow, J. and Madsen, J. (1976). Adipose tissue blood flow during prolonged, heavy exercise. *Pflügers Archiv: European Journal of Physiology*, **363**, 231–234.

Bülow, J. and Madsen, J. (1981). Influence of blood flow on fatty acid mobilization from lipolytically active adipose tissue. *Pflügers Archiv: European Journal of Physiology*, **390**, 169–174.

Bülow, J. and Madsen, J. (1986). Exercise-induced increase in dog adipose tissue blood flow before and after denervation. *Acta Physiologica Scandinavica*, **128**, 471–474.

Bülow, J. and Tøndevold, E. (1982). Blood flow in different adipose tissue depots during prolonged exercise in dogs. *Pflügers Archiv: European Journal of Physiology*, **392**, 235–238.

Bülow, J., Madsen, J., Astrup, A. and Christensen, N.J. (1985). Vasoconstrictor effect of high FFA/albumin ratios in adipose tissue *in vivo*. *Acta Physiologica Scandinavica*, **125**, 661–667.

Bülow, J., Astrup, A., Christensen, N.J. and Kastrup, J. (1987a). Blood flow in skin, subcutaneous adipose tissue and skeletal muscle in the forearm of normal man during an oral glucose load. *Acta Physiologica Scandinavica*, **130**, 657–661.

Bülow, J., Jelnes, R., Astrup, A., Madsen, J. and Vilmann, P. (1987b). Tissue/blood partition coefficients for xenon in various adipose tissue depots in man. *Scandinavian Journal of Clinical and Laboratory Investigation*, **47**, 1–3.

Cannon, B., Nedergaard, J. and Sundin, U. (1981). Thermogenesis, brown fat and thermogenin. In *Survival in Cold*, edited by X.S. Musacchia and L. Jansky, pp. 99–120. Amsterdam: Elsevier.

Cannon, B., Nedergaard, J., Lundberg, J.M., Hökfelt, T., Terenius, L. and Goldstein, M. (1986). Neuropeptide tyrosine (NPY) is costored with noradrenaline in vascular but not in parenchymal sympathetic nerves of brown adipose tissue. *Experimental Cell Research*, **164**, 546–550.

Carlsson, I., Linde, B. and Wennmalm, A. (1983). Arachidonic acid metabolism and regulation of blood flow: effect of indomethacin on cutaneous and subcutaneous reactive hyperaemia in humans. *Clinical Physiology*, **3**, 365–373.

Carneheim, C., Nedergaard, J. and Cannon, B. (1984). β-adrenergic stimulation of lipoprotein lipase activity in rat brown adipose tissue during cold acclimation. *American Journal of Physiology*, **246**, E327–E333.

Coppack, S.W., Fisher, R.M., Gibbons, G.F., Humphreys, S.M., McDonough, M.J., Potts, J.L. and Frayn, K.N. (1990a). Postprandial substrate deposition in human forearm and adipose tissues *in vivo*. *Clinical Science*, **79**, 339–348.

Coppack, S.W., Frayn, K.N., Humphreys, S.M., Whyte, P.L. and Hockaday, T.D.R. (1990b). Arteriovenous differences across human adipose and forearm tissues after overnight fast. *Metabolism*, **39**, 384–390.

Crandall, D.L. and DiGirolamo, M. (1990). Hemodynamic and metabolic correlates in adipose tissue: pathophysiologic considerations. *FASEB Journal*, **4**, 141–147.

Crandall, D.L., Goldstein, B.M., Huggins, F. and Cervoni, P. (1984a). Adipocyte blood flow: influence of age, anatomic location, and dietary manipulation. *American Journal of Physiology*, **247**, R46–R51.

Crandall, D.L., Goldstein, B.M., Gabel, R.A. and Cervoni, P. (1984b). Hemodynamic effects of weight reduction in the obese rat. *American Journal of Physiology*, **247**, R266–R271.

Crandall, D.L., Goldstein, B.M., Lizzo, F.H., Gabel, R.A. and Cervoni, P. (1986). Hemodynamics of obesity: influence of pattern of adipose tissue cellularity. *American Journal of Physiology*, **251**, R314–R319.

Cryer, A. (1981). Tissue lipoprotein lipase activity and its action in lipoprotein metabolism. *International Journal of Biochemistry*, **13**, 525–541.

Daniel, H. and Derry, D.M. (1969). Criteria for differentiation of brown and white fat in the rat. *Canadian Journal of Physiology and Pharmacology*, **47**, 941–945.

Dascombe, M.J., Rothwell, N.J., Sagay, B.O. and Stock, M.J. (1989). Pyrogenic and thermogenic effects of interleukin 1β in the rat. *American Journal of Physiology*, **256**, E7–E11.

Derry, D.N., Schonbaum, E. and Steiner, G. (1969). Two sympathetic nerve supplies to brown adipose tissue of the rat. *Canadian Journal of Physiology and Pharmacology*, **47**, 57–63.

Diculescu, I. and Stoica, M. (1970). Fluorescence histochemical investigation on the adrenergic innervation of the white adipose tissue in the rat. *Journal of Neuro-Visceral Relations*, **32**, 25–36.

Eckel, R.H. (1989). Lipoprotein lipase. A multifunctional enzyme relevant to common metabolic diseases. *New England Journal of Medicine*, **320**, 1060–1068.

Edens, N.K., Leibel, R.L. and Hirsch, J. (1990). Mechanism of free fatty acid re-esterification in human adipocytes *in vitro*. *Journal of Lipid Research*, **31**, 1423–1431.

Edlund, A., Sollevi, A. and Linde, B. (1990). Haemodynamic and metabolic effects of infused adenosine in man. *Clinical Science*, **79**, 131–138.

Evans, A.L., Busuttil, A., Gillespie, F.C. and Unsworth, J. (1974). The rate of clearance of xenon from rat liver sections *in vitro* and its significance in relation to intracellular diffusion rates. *Physics in Medicine and Biology*, **19**, 303–316.

Fain, J.N. and Malbon, C.C. (1979). Regulation of adenylate cyclase by adenosine. *Molecular and Cellular Biochemistry*, **25**, 143–169.

Falck, B. (1962). Observations on the possibilities of the cellular localization of monoamines by a fluorescence method. *Acta Physiologica Scandinavica*, **56**, Supplement 197.

Fawcett, D.W. (1952). A comparison of the histological organisation and histochemical reactions of brown fat and ordinary adipose tissue. *Journal of Morphology*, **90**, 363–405.

Fernqvist, E. and Linde, B. (1988). Potent mental stress and insulin absorption in normal subjects. *Diabetes Care*, **11**, 650–655.

Fernqvist, E., Gunnarsson, R. and Linde, B. (1988). Influence of circulating epinephrine on absorption of subcutaneously injected insulin. *Diabetes*, **37**, 694–701.

Fernqvist-Forbes, E., Linde, B. and Gunnarsson, R. (1986). Insulin absorption and subcutaneous blood flow in normal subjects during insulin-induced hypoglycemia. *Journal of Clinical Endocrinology and Metabolism*, **67**, 619–623.

Fernqvist-Forbes, E., Gunnarsson, R. and Linde, B. (1989). Insulin-induced hypoglycaemia and absorption of injected insulin in diabetic patients. *Diabetic Medicine*, **6**, 621–626.

Flaim, K.E., Horwitz, B.A. and Horowitz, J.M. (1977). Coupling of signals to brown fat: α and β-adrenergic responses in intact rats. *American Journal of Physiology*, **232**, R101–R109.

Foster, D.O. (1984). Auxiliary role of α-adrenoceptors in brown adipose tissue thermogenesis. In *Thermal Physiology*, edited by J.R.S. Hales, pp. 201–204. New York: Raven Press.

Foster, D.O. (1986). Quantitative role of brown adipose tissue in thermogenesis. In *Brown Adipose Tissue*, edited by P. Trayhurn and D.G. Nicholls, pp. 31–51. London: Edward Arnold.

Foster, D.O. and Depocas, F. (1980). Evidence against noradrenergic regulation of vasodilatation in rat brown adipose tissue. *Canadian Journal of Physiology and Pharmacology*, **58**, 1418–1425.

Foster, D.O. and Frydman, M.L. (1978a). Comparison of microspheres and $^{86}Rb^{+}$ as tracers of the distribution of cardiac output in rats indicates invalidity of $^{86}Rb^{+}$ based measurements. *Canadian Journal of Physiology and Pharmacology*, **56**, 97–109.

Foster, D.O. and Frydman, M.L. (1978b). Non-shivering thermogenesis in the rat: II Measurements of blood flow with microspheres point to brown adipose tissue as the dominant site of calorigenesis induced by noradrenaline. *Canadian Journal of Physiology and Pharmacology*, **56**, 110–112.

Foster, D.O., Depocas, F. and Zaror-Behrens, C. (1982). Unilaterality of the sympathetic innervation of each pad of rat interscapular brown adipose tissue. *Canadian Journal of Physiology and Pharmacology*, **60**, 107–113.

Frayn, K.N. (1986). Hormonal control of metabolism in trauma and sepsis. *Clinical Endocrinology*, **24**, 577–599.

Frayn, K.N. (1989). Adipose tissue metabolism. *Clinics in Dermatology*, **7**, 48–61.

Frayn, K.N. (1992). Studies of human adipose tissue *in vivo*. In *Energy Metabolism: Tissue Determinants and Cellular Corollaries*, edited by J.M. Kinney and H.N. Tucker, pp. 267–295. New York: Raven Press.

Frayn, K.N., Little, R.A., Maycock, P.F. and Stoner, H.B. (1985). The relationship of plasma catecholamines to acute metabolic and hormonal responses to injury in man. *Circulatory Shock*, **16**, 229–240.

Frayn, K.N., Coppack, S.W., Humphreys, S.M. and Whyte, P.L. (1989). Metabolic characteristics of human adipose tissue *in vivo*. *Clinical Science*, **76**, 509–516.

Fredholm, B.B. (1970). The effect of lactate in canine subcutaneous adipose tissue *in situ*. *Acta Physiologica Scandinavica*, **81**, 110–123.

Fredholm, B.B. (1972). Actions of dopamine in canine subcutaneous adipose tissue. *Naunyn-Schmiedeberg's Archives of Pharmacology*, **274**, 315–324.

Fredholm, B. (1985). Nervous control of circulation and metabolism in white adipose tissue. In *New Perspectives in Adipose Tissue: Structure, Function and Development*, edited by A. Cryer and R.L.R. Van, pp. 45–64. London: Butterworths.

Fredholm, B. and Rosell, S. (1968). Effects of adrenergic blocking agents on lipid mobilization from canine subcutaneous adipose tissue after sympathetic nerve stimulation. *Journal of Pharmacology and Experimental Therapeutics*, **159**, 1–7.

Fredholm, B.B., Öberg, B. and Rosell, S. (1970). Effects of vasoactive drugs on circulation in canine subcutaneous adipose tissue. *Acta Physiologica Scandinavica*, **79**, 564–574.

Freyschuss, U., Hjemdahl, P., Juhlin-Dannfelt, A. and Linde, B. (1986). Cardiovascular and metabolic responses to low dose adrenaline infusion: an invasive study in humans. *Clinical Science*, **70**, 199–206.

Galitzky, J., Lafontan, M., Nordenström, J. and Arner, P. (1993). Role of vascular α_2-adrenoceptors in regulating lipid mobilization from human adipose tissue. *Journal of Clinical Investigation*, **91**, 1997–2003.

Gersh, I. and Still, M.A. (1945). Blood vessels in fat tissue. Relation to problems of gas exchange. *Journal of Experimental Medicine*, **81**, 219–232.

Girardier, L. (1983). Brown Fat: An energy dissipating tissue. In *Mammalian Thermogenesis*, edited by L. Girardier and M.J. Stock, pp. 50–98. London and New York: Chapman and Hall.

Girardier, L. and Seydoux, J. (1986). Neural control of brown adipose tissue. In *Brown Adipose Tissue*, edited by P. Trayhurn and D.G. Nicholls, pp. 122–151. London: Edward Arnold.

Glick, Z., Wicklet, S.J., Stern, J.S. and Horwitz, B.A. (1984). Regional blood flow in rats after a single low-protein, high-carbohydrate test meal. *American Journal of Physiology*, **247**, R160–R166.

Gregory, N.G., Christopherson, R.J. and Lister, D. (1986). Adipose tissue capillary blood flow in relation to fatness in sheep. *Research in Veterinary Science*, **40**, 352–356.

Gustafsson, D., Andersson, L., Martensson, L. and Lundvall, J. (1984). Microsphere analysis of β_2-adrenergic control of resistance in different vascular areas after haemorrhage. *Acta Physiologica Scandinavica*, **121**, 119–126.

Haddy, F.J. and Scott, J.B. (1968). Metabolically linked vasoactive chemicals in local regulation of blood flow. *Physiological Reviews*, **48**, 688–707.

Hanley, H.G., Sachs, R.G. and Skinner, N.S. (1971). Reflex responsiveness of vascular bed of dog subcutaneous adipose tissue. *American Journal of Physiology*, **220**, 993–999.

Hausberger, F.X. and Widelitz, M.M. (1963). Distribution of labeled erythrocytes in adipose tissue and muscle in the rat. *American Journal of Physiology*, **204**, 649–652.

Heim, T. and Hull, D. (1966). The effect of propranolol on the calorigenic response in brown adipose tissue of newborn rabbits to catecholamines, glucagon, corticotrophin and cold exposure. *Journal of Physiology (London)*, **187**, 271–286.

Henriksen, O. (1977). Local sympathetic reflex mechanism in regulation of blood flow in human subcutaneous adipose tissue. *Acta Physiologica Scandinavica*, Supplement 450.

Herd, J.A., Goodman, H.M. and Grose, S.A. (1968). Blood flow through adipose tissue of anaesthetized rats. *American Journal of Physiology*, **214**, 263–268.

Hickner, R.C., Rosdahl, H., Borg, I., Ungerstedt, U., Jorfeldt, L. and Henriksson, J. (1991). Ethanol may be used with the microdialysis technique to monitor blood flow changes in skeletal muscle: dialysate glucose concentration is blood-flow-dependent. *Acta Physiological Scandinavica*, **143**, 355–356.

Hickner, R.C., Rosdahl, H., Borg, I., Ungerstedt, U., Jorfeldt, L. and Henriksson, J. (1992). The ethanol technique of monitoring local blood flow changes in rat skeletal muscle: implications for microdialysis. *Acta Physiologica Scandinavica*, **146**, 87–97.

Hildebrandt, P., Birch, K., Sestoft, L. and Nielsen, S.L. (1985). Orthostatic changes in subcutaneous blood flow and insulin absorption. *Diabetes Research*, **2**, 187–190.

Hilsted, J., Bonde-Petersen, F., Madsbad, S., Parving, H.-H., Christensen, N.J., Adelhøj, B., *et al.* (1985). Changes in plasma volume, in transcapillary escape rate of albumin and in subcutaneous blood flow during hypoglycaemia in man. *Clinical Science*, **69**, 273–277.

Himms-Hagen, J., Traindafillou, J. and Gwilliam, C. (1981). Brown adipose tissue of cafeteria fed rats. *American Journal of Physiology*, **241**, E116–E120.

Hjemdahl, P. and Fredholm, B.B. (1974). Comparison of the lipolytic activity of circulating and locally released noradrenaline during acidosis. *Acta Physiologica Scandinavica*, **92**, 1–11.

Hjemdahl, P. and Linde, B. (1983). Influence of circulating NE and Epi on adipose tissue vascular resistance and lipolysis in humans. *American Journal of Physiology*, **245**, H447–H452.

Hjemdahl, P. and Sollevi, A. (1978). Vascular and metabolic responses to adrenergic stimulation in isolated canine subcutaneous adipose tissue at normal and reduced temperature. *Journal of Physiology*, **281**, 325–338.

Hjemdahl, P., Belfrage, E. and Daleskog, M. (1979). Vascular and metabolic effects of circulating epinephrine and norepinephrine. Concentration-effect study in dogs. *Journal of Clinical Investigation*, **64**, 1221–1228.

Hjemdahl, P., Linde, B., Daleskog, M. and Belfrage, E. (1983). Sympatho-adrenal regulation of adipose tissue blood flow in dog and man. *General Pharmacology*, **14**, 175–177.

Hodgetts, V., Coppack, S.W., Frayn, K.N. and Hockaday, T.D.R. (1991). Factors controlling fat mobilization from human subcutaneous adipose tissue during exercise. *Journal of Applied Physiology*, **71**, 445–451.

Holloway, B.R., Davidson, R.G., Freeman, S., Wheeler, H. and Stribling, D. (1984). Post-natal development of interscapular (brown) adipose tissue in the guinea pig: Effect of environmental temperature. *International Journal of Obesity*, **8**, 295–303.

Hull, D. and Segall, M.M. (1965). The contribution of brown adipose tissue to heat production in the newborn rabbit. *Journal of Physiology*, **181**, 449–457.

Janssens, W.J. and Vanhoutte, P.M. (1978). Instantaneous changes of α-adrenoceptor affinity caused by moderate cooling in canine cutaneous veins. *American Journal of Physiology*, **234**, H330–H337.

Jelnes, R., Rasmussen, L.B. and Eickhoff, J.H. (1984). Direct determination of the tissue-to-blood partition coefficient for xenon in human subcutaneous adipose tissue. *Scandinavian Journal of Clinical and Laboratory Investigation*, **44**, 643–647.

Jelnes, R., Astrup, A. and Bülow, J. (1985). The double isotope technique for *in vivo* determination of the tissue-to-blood partition coefficient for xenon in human subcutaneous adipose tissue — an evaluation. *Scandinavian Journal of Clinical and Laboratory Investigation*, **45**, 565–568.

Joel, C.D. (1965). The physiological role of brown adipose tissue. In *Handbook of Physiology, Section 5 Adipose Tissue*, edited by A. Renold and G.F. Cahill, pp. 59–85. Washington: American Physiological Society.

Johnsen, H.M. (1974). Measurement of colloid osmotic pressure of interstitial fluid. *Acta Physiologica Scandinavica*, **91**, 142–144.

Julien, P., Despres, J.-P. and Angel, A. (1989). Scanning electron microscopy of very small fat cells and mature fat cells in human obesity. *Journal of Lipid Research*, **30**, 293–299.

Kennedy, I., Gurden, M. and Strong, P. (1992). Do adenosine A_3 receptors exist? *General Pharmacology*, **23**, 303–307.

Kety, S.S. (1949). Measurement of regional circulation by the local clearance of radioactive sodium. *American Heart Journal*, **38**, 321–328.

Kovách, A.G.B., Rosell, S., Sándor, P., Koltay, E., Kovách, E. and Tomka, N. (1970). Blood flow, oxygen consumption, and free fatty acid release in subcutaneous adipose tissue during haemorrhagic shock in control and phenoxybenzamine-treated dogs. *Circulation Research*, **26**, 733–741.

Lafontan, M. and Berlan, M. (1985). Plasma membrane properties and receptors in white adipose tissue. In *New Perspectives in Adipose Tissue: Structure, Function and Development*, edited by A. Cryer and R.L.R. Van, pp. 145–182. London: Butterworths.

Lands, A.M., Arnold, A., McAuliff, J.P., Luduena, F.P. and Brown, T.G., Jr. (1967). Differentiation of receptor systems activated by sympathomimetic amines. *Nature*, **214**, 597–598.

Larsen, O.A., Lassen, N.A. and Quaade, F. (1966). Blood flow through human adipose tissue determined with radioactive xenon. *Acta Physiologica Scandinavica*, **66**, 337–345.

Larsen, T., Myhre, K., Vik-Mo, H. and Mjøs, O.D. (1981). Adipose tissue perfusion and fatty acid release in exercising rats. *Acta Physiologica Scandinavica*, **113**, 111–116.

Lewis, G.P. and Matthews, J. (1968). The mobilization of free fatty acids from rabbit adipose tissue *in situ*. *British Journal of Pharmacology*, **34**, 564–578.

Lewis, G.P. and Matthews, J. (1970). The mechanism of functional vasodilatation in rabbit epigastric adipose tissue. *Journal of Physiology*, **207**, 15–30.

Lindbjerg, I.F. (1967). Disappearance rate of [133]xenon, 4-Iodo-antipyrine-^{131}I and [131]I[-] from human skeletal muscles and adipose tissue. *Scandinavian Journal of Clinical and Laboratory Investigation*, **19**, 120–128.

Linde, B. and Gainer, J.L. (1974). Disappearance of [133]xenon and [125]Iodide and extraction of [86]Rubidium in subcutaneous adipose tissue during sympathetic nerve stimulation. *Acta Physiologica Scandinavica*, **91**, 172–179.

Linde, B. and Hjemdahl, P. (1982). Effect of tilting on adipose tissue vascular resistance and sympathetic activity in humans. *American Journal of Physiology*, **242**, H161–H167.

Linde, B. and Sollevi, A. (1987). Effects of dipyridamole and theophylline on reactive hyperaemia in subcutaneous adipose in humans. *Clinical Physiology*, **7**, 319–327.

Linde, B., Rosell, S. and Rökaeus, Å. (1982). Blood flow in human adipose tissue after infusion of (Gln[4])-neurotensin. *Acta Physiologica Scandinavica*, **115**, 311–315.

Linde, B., Hjemdahl, P., Freyschuss, U. and Juhlin-Dannfelt, A. (1989). Adipose tissue and skeletal muscle blood flow during mental stress. *American Journal of Physiology*, **256**, E12–E18.

Lönnroth, P., Jansson, P.-A., Fredholm, B.B. and Smith, U. (1989). Microdialysis of intercellular adenosine concentration in subcutaneous tissue in humans. *American Journal of Physiology*, **256**, E250–E255.

Ma, S.W.Y. and Foster, D.O. (1984). Redox state of brown adipose tissue as a possible determinant of its blood flow. *Canadian Journal of Physiology and Pharmacology*, **62**, 949–956.

Madsen, J. and Malchow-Møller, A. (1983). Effects of glucose, insulin and nicotinic acid on adipose tissue blood flow in rats. *Acta Physiologica Scandinavica*, **118**, 175–180.

Madsen, J., Malchow-Møller, A. and Waldorff, S. (1975). Continuous estimation of adipose tissue blood flow in rats by ^{133}Xe elimination. *Journal of Applied Physiology*, **39**, 851–856.

Madsen, J., Bülow, J. and Nielsen, N.E. (1986). Inhibition of fatty acid mobilization by arterial free fatty acid concentration. *Acta Physiologica Scandinavica*, **127**, 161–166.

Martin, S.E. and Bockman, E.L. (1986). Adenosine regulates blood flow and glucose uptake in adipose tissue of dogs. *American Journal of Physiology*, **250**, H1127–H1135.

Mayerle, J.A. and Havel, R.J. (1969). Nutritional effects on blood flow in adipose tissue of unanaesthetized rats. *American Journal of Physiology*, **217**, 1694–1698.

Mersmann, H.J. (1989). Acute changes in blood flow in pigs infused with β-adrenergic agonists. *Journal of Animal Science*, **67**, 2913–2920.

Mohell, N. (1984). α-adrenergic receptors in brown adipose tissue. Thermogenic significance and mode of action. *Acta Physiologica Scandinavica*, **530**, Supplement.

Mory, G., Combes-George, M. and Nechad, M. (1983). Localisation of serotonin and dopamine in the brown adipose tissue of the rat and their variations during cold exposure. *Biology of the Cell*, **48**, 159–166.

Nechad, M. (1986). Structure and development of brown adipose tissue. In *Brown Adipose Tissue*, edited by P. Trayhurn and D.G. Nicholls, pp. 1–30. London: Edward Arnold.

Newsholme, E.A. and Leech, A.R. (1983). *Biochemistry for the Medical Sciences*, pp. 286–299. Chichester: John Wiley.

Ngai, S.H., Rosell, S. and Wallenberg, L.R. (1966). Nervous regulation of blood flow in the subcutaneous adipose tissue in dogs. *Acta Physiologica Scandinavica*, **68**, 397–403.

Nielsen, S.L., Bitsch, V., Larsen, O.A., Lassen, N.A. and Quaade, F. (1968). Blood flow through human adipose tissue during lipolysis. *Scandinavian Journal of Clinical and Laboratory Investigation*, **22**, 124–130.

Nnodim, J.O. and Lever, J.D. (1988). Neural and vascular provisions of rat IBAT. *American Journal of Anatomy*, **182**, 283–293.

Öberg, B. and Rosell, S. (1967). Sympathetic control of consecutive vascular sections in canine subcutaneous adipose tissue. *Acta Physiologica Scandinavica*, **71**, 47–56.

Ontyd, J. and Schrader, J. (1984). Measurement of adenosine, inosine, and hypoxanthine in human plasma. *Journal of Chromatography*, **307**, 404–409.

Oro, L., Wallenberg, L. and Rosell, S. (1965). Circulatory and metabolic processes in adipose tissue *in vivo*. *Nature*, **205**, 178–179.

Parker, R.E., Hall, R.E., Marr, H.B. and Skinner, N.S. (1979). Vascular responses in canine subcutaneous adipose tissue to hypothalamic stimulation. *American Journal of Physiology*, **237**, H386–H391.

Quaade, F., Larsen, O.A., Lassen, N.A. and Nielsen, S.L. (1967). Observation on the influence of glucose upon subcutaneous adipose tissue blood flow. *Acta Medica Scandinavica*, (Suppl. 476), 85–90.

Richelsen, B. (1992). Release and effects of prostaglandins in adipose tissue. *Prostaglandins, leukotrienes and essential fatty acids*, **47**, 171–182.

Risberg, J., Hordnes, C. and Tyssebotn, I. (1987). The effect of $β_1$-adrenoceptor blockade on cardiac output and organ blood flow in conscious rats. *Scandinavian Journal of Clinical and Laboratory Investigation*, **47**, 521–527.

Roddie, I.C. (1983). Circulation to skin and adipose tissue. In *Handbook of Physiology Section 2: The Cardiovascular System Volume III*, edited by J.T. Shepherd and F.M. Abboud, pp. 285–317. Bethesda: American Physiological Society.

Rofe, A.M. and Williamson, D.H. (1983). Mechanism for the 'anti-lipolytic' action of vasopressin in the starved rat. *Biochemical Journal*, **212**, 899–902.

Rosell, S. (1966). Release of free fatty acids from subcutaneous adipose tissue in dogs following sympathetic nerve stimulation. *Acta Physiologica Scandinavica*, **67**, 343–351.

Rosell, S. (1969). Nervous and pharmacological regulation of vascular reactions in adipose tissue. *Advances in Experimental Medicine and Biology*, **4**, 25–34.

Rosell, S. and Belfrage, E. (1979). Blood circulation in adipose tissue. *Physiological Reviews*, **59**, 1078–1104.

Rosell, S., Sándor, P. and Kovách, A.G.B. (1973). Adipose tissue and haemorrhagic shock. *Advances in Experimental Medicine and Biology*, **33**, 323–336.

Rosell, S., Intaglietta, M. and Chisholm, G.M. (1974). Adrenergic influence on isovolumetric capillary pressure in canine adipose tissue. *American Journal of Physiology*, **227**, 692–696.

Rothwell, N.J. and Stock, M.J. (1979). A role for brown adipose tissue in diet-induced thermogenesis. *Nature*, **281**, 31–35.

Rothwell, N.J. and Stock, M.J. (1984). Tissue blood flow in control and cold-adapted hyperthyroid rats. *Canadian Journal of Physiology and Pharmacology*, **62**, 928–933.

Ryan, T.J. and Curri, S.B. (1989a). The development of adipose tissue and its relationship to the vascular system. *Clinics in Dermatology*, **7**, 1–8.

Ryan, T.J. and Curri, S.B. (1989b). Blood vessels and lymphatics. *Clinics in Dermatology*, **7**, 25–36.

Saggerson, E.D. (1985). Hormonal regulation of biosynthetic activities in white adipose tissue. In *New Perspectives in Adipose Tissue: Structure, Function and Development*, edited by A. Cryer and R.L.R. Van, pp. 87–120. London: Butterworths.

Salvador, R.A. and Kuntzman, R. (1965). Cholinesterase of adipose tissue. *Journal of Pharmacology and Experimental Therapeutics*, **150**, 84–91.

Scow, R.O. (1965). Perfusion of isolated adipose tissue: FFA release and blood flow in rat parametrial fat body. In *Handbook of Physiology Section 5: Adipose Tissue*, edited by A.E. Renold and G.F. Cahill, pp. 437–453. Washington, DC: American Physiological Society.

Scow, R.O., Blanchette-Mackie, E.J. and Smith, L.C. (1976). Role of capillary endothelium in the clearance of chylomicrons. A model for lipid transport from blood by lateral diffusion in cell membranes. *Circulation Research*, **39**, 149–162.

Seydoux, J., Constantinidis, J., Tsacopoulos, M. and Girardier, L. (1977). *In vitro* study of the control of the metabolic activity of brown adipose tissue by the sympathetic nervous system. *Journale de Physiologie (Paris)*, **73**, 985–986.

Simonsen, L., Bülow, J., Astrup, A., Madsen, J. and Christensen, N.J. (1990). Diet-induced changes in subcutaneous adipose tissue blood flow in man: effect of β-adrenoceptor inhibition. *Acta Physiologica Scandinavica*, **139**, 341–346.

Siyamak, A.Y. (1991). The effect of nutritional state on catecholamine induced thermogenesis. *Ph.D. Thesis*. University of Nottingham.

Skagen, K. (1983). Sympathetic reflex control of blood flow in human subcutaneous tissue during orthostatic maneuvres. *Danish Medical Bulletin*, **30**, 229–241.

Slavin, B. (1985). The morphology of adipose tissue. In *New Perspectives in Adipose Tissue: Structure, Function and Development*, edited by A. Cryer and R.L.R. Van, pp. 23–43. London: Butterworths.

Smiseth, O.A., Riemersma, R.A., Steinnes, K. and Mjos, O.D. (1983). Regional blood flow during acute heart failure in dogs. Role of adipose tissue perfusion in regulating plasma-free fatty acids. *Scandinavian Journal of Clinical and Laboratory Investigation*, **43**, 285–292.

Smith, R.E. and Roberts, J.C. (1964). Thermogenesis of brown adipose tissue in cold-acclimated rats. *American Journal of Physiology*, **206**, 143–148.

Sollevi, A. and Fredholm, B.B. (1983). Influence of adenosine on the vascular responses to sympathetic nerve stimulation in the canine subcutaneous adipose tissue. *Acta Physiologica Scandinavica*, **119**, 15–24.

Spector, A.A. (1975). Fatty acid binding to plasma albumin. *Journal of Lipid Research*, **16**, 165–179.

Stoner, H.B., Frayn, K.N., Barton, R.N., Threlfall, C.J. and Little, R.A. (1979). The relationships between plasma substrates and hormones and the severity of injury in 277 recently injured patients. *Clinical Science*, **56**, 563–573.

Thompson, G.E. (1984). Dopamine and lipolysis in adipose tissue of the sheep. *Quarterly Journal of Experimental Physiology*, **69**, 155–159.

Thompson, G.E. (1986). Vascular and lipolytic responses of the inguinal fat pad of the sheep to adrenergic stimulation, and the effects of denervation and autotransplantation. *Quarterly Journal of Experimental Physiology*, **71**, 559–567.

Thureson-Klein, A., Lagercrantz H. and Barnard, T. (1976). Chemical sympathectomy of interscapular brown adipose tissue. *Acta Physiologica Scandinavica*, **98**, 8–18.

Trayhurn, P. and Nicholls, D.G. (Editors) (1986). *Brown Adipose Tissue*, London: Edward Arnold.

van Calker, D., Muller, M. and Hamprecht, B. (1979). Adenosine regulates via two different types of receptors the accumulation of cyclic AMP in cultured brain cells. *Journal of Neurochemistry*, **33**, 999–1005.

Vernon, R.G. and Clegg, R.A. (1985). The metabolism of white adipose tissue *in vivo* and *in vitro*. In *New Perspectives in Adipose Tissue: Structure, Function and Development*, edited by A. Cryer and R.L.R Van, pp. 65–86. London: Butterworths.

Wennlund, A. and Linde, B. (1984). Influence of hyper- and hypothyroidism on subcutaneous adipose tissue blood flow in man. *Journal of Clinical Endocrinology and Metabolism*, **59**, 258–262.

West, D.B., Prinz, W.A. and Greenwood, M.R. (1989). Regional changes in adipose tissue blood flow and metabolism in rats after a meal. *American Journal of Physiology*, **257**, R711–R716.

West, D.B., Prinz, W.A., Francendese, A.A. and Greenwood, M.R. (1987). Adipocyte blood flow is decreased in obese Zucker rats. *American Journal of Physiology*, **253**, R228–R233.

West, D.B., Prinz, W.A. and Greenwood, M.R. (1989). Regional change in adipose blood flow and metabolism in rats after a meal. *American Journal of Physiology*, **257**, R711–R716.

Williams, M. (1987). Purine receptors in mammalian tissues: pharmacology and functional significance. *Annual Review of Pharmacology and Toxicology*, **27**, 315–345.

Williamson, D.H. (1990). The endocrine control of adipose tissue metabolism and the changes associated with lactation and cancer. In *The Control of Body Fat Content*, edited by J.M. Forbes and G.R. Hervey, pp. 43–61. London: Smith-Gordon.

Wirsén, C. (1964). Adrenergic innervation of adipose tissue examined by fluorescence microscopy. *Nature*, **202**, 913.

Wirsén, C. (1965). Distribution of adrenergic nerve fibers in brown and white adipose tissue. In *Handbook of Physiology, Section 5. Adipose Tissue*, edited by A.E. Renold and G.F. Cahill, pp. 197–199. Washington, DC: American Physiological Society.

Woods, A.F. and Stock, M.J. (1990). A novel role for arteriovenous anastomoses in regulating brown fat metabolism. *International Journal of Obesity*, **14**, 906A.

Ye, J.M., Colquhoun, E.Q., Hettiarachchi, M. and Clark, M.G. (1990). Flow induced oxygen uptake by the perfused rat hindlimb is inhibited by vasodilators and augmented by norepinephrine — A possible role for the microvasculature in hindlimb thermogenesis. *Canadian Journal of Physiology and Pharmacology*, **68**, 119–125.

Young, J.B., Saville, E., Rothwell, N.J., Stock, M.J. and Landsberg, L. (1982). Effect of diet and cold exposure on norepinephrine turnover in brown adipose tissue of the rat. *Journal of Clinical Investigation*, **69**, 1061–1071.

15 Thyroid Circulation

Linda J. Huffman, Mieczyslaw Michalkiewicz, Malay Dey
and George A. Hedge

Department of Physiology, West Virginia University
Health Sciences Center, Morgantown, West Virginia, 26506, USA

The vascular system of the thyroid is extensive and capable of undergoing marked changes in response to demands made upon this organ during different functional states. Thyroid blood vessels are well innervated and blood flow can be altered by stimulation of the major sympathetic and parasympathetic neural inputs to this gland. The substances which are involved in the mediation of these effects appear to include the established neurotransmitters, noradrenaline and acetylcholine, as well as more recently discovered neuropeptides, such as vasoactive intestinal peptide and neuropeptide Y. Although the functional significance of the neural control of the thyroid circulation has not been firmly established, it is likely that such effects are important in modulating the rate of iodine delivery and uptake within the thyroid, and thus contribute to the overall regulation of thyroid hormone biosynthesis.

KEY WORDS: thyroid; blood flow; neurotransmitters; neuropeptides.

INTRODUCTION

Since the mid-1800's, the existence, distribution and functional aspects of nerve fibres within the thyroid gland have been subjects of scientific inquiry (see Cannon and Cattell, 1916; Soderberg, 1959 for review and citation of the early literature). The majority of these investigations have focused primarily upon the neural control of the secretory activity of this endocrine organ and the consensus of evidence to date suggests that nerves can directly influence hormone release from thyroid follicular tissue (Ahren, 1986; Melander, 1986; Green, 1987). However, the possibility that intrathyroidal nerves may also play a significant role in the control of blood flow to this gland has not gone unnoticed. As we will discuss, the vascular network in the thyroid is extensive. Furthermore, thyroid blood vessels are well innervated and nerve stimulation or the administration of neurotransmitters, neuropeptides, or other vasoactive substances can markedly influence the thyroid circulation. These aspects and the significance of the neural control of the thyroid vasculature in the overall functioning of this gland are the primary issues addressed in this chapter.

STRUCTURAL ASPECTS OF THE THYROID CIRCULATION

THYROIDAL VASCULATURE

Blood flow per unit weight of thyroid tissue is very high relative to that of other organs in the body (Shinaberger and Bruner, 1956; Soderberg, 1959; Kapitola, 1973). Complementary to this high rate of perfusion is an extensive vascular system in which each thyroid follicle is enclosed within a complex capillary network. This network does not form a static framework, rather, it is capable of dramatic structural responses to demands made upon the thyroid during different functional states.

Arterial supply

The arterial input to the thyroid gland is generally similar across mammalian species and is bilaterally symmetrical (Soderberg, 1958a; Sloan, 1971; Laurberg, 1976; Tzinas *et al.*, 1976; Johanson, Ofverholm and Ericson, 1987). The primary arterial supply is to the superior pole of the thyroid via the superior thyroid artery. This artery arises from either the external carotid artery just cephalad to the carotid bifurcation or from the common carotid artery. Branches of this artery supply the isthmus of the thyroid and anastomose with the contralateral artery in this region. In many species (e.g., rat, mice, humans but not dogs), the thyroid also receives arterial blood from an inferior thyroid artery which arises from the thyrocervical trunk off the subclavian artery and enters the inferior pole of the thyroid. Significant anastomoses and communication between the superior and inferior thyroid arteries occur in the medial aspects of the thyroid. As indicated above, the primary arterial supply is derived from the superior thyroid artery. If the blood supply to a thyroid lobe is disrupted by coagulating the small inferior thyroid artery in the rat or mouse, then no obvious impairment of blood flow to any part of the lobe can be noted (Johanson, Ofverholm and Ericson, 1987). In humans, an accessory artery to this gland, the thyroid ima artery, has been described as occurring in a small percentage of patients studied. This vessel, if present, usually arises from the aortic arch and supplies the inferior, isthmic, portion of the gland (Sloan, 1971; Tzinas *et al.*, 1976). Arteries from the larynx, trachea, and oesophagus also provide collateral branches to the thyroid. Thus, even if the superior and inferior arteries are ligated and sectioned during partial surgical removal of thyroid gland, there can still be functional survival of thyroid remnants (Sloan, 1971).

Venous drainage

The venous drainage of the thyroid is much more diffuse and variable than the arterial supply to this gland (Soderberg, 1958a; Sloan, 1971; Laurberg, 1976; Tzinas *et al.*, 1976; Johanson, Ofverholm and Ericson, 1987). However, the most common pattern described across species is the presence of two large veins emanating from each thyroid lobe. These are, in general, parallel to the arterial supply in that a superior thyroid vein projects laterally from the superior pole of the thyroid and an inferior thyroid vein runs alongside the inferior thyroid artery. In some humans, a third thyroid vein, arising from the middle of the gland, has also been described. The internal jugular vein receives most of the thyroidal venous return, although the inferior thyroid vein empties into the bracheocephalic vein in man.

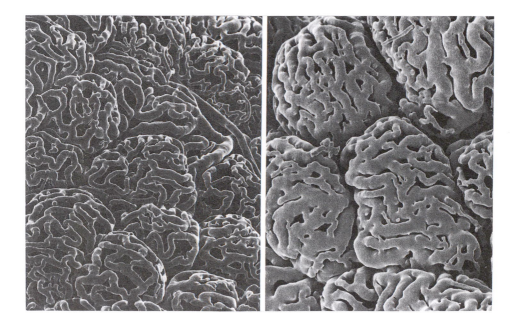

Figure 15.1   Scanning electron micrographs of a vascular cast of a thyroid from a normal rat (left panel; ×450) and of a thyroid from a rat fed a low iodine diet (right panel; ×640). Reproduced with permission; from Imada, Kurosumi and Fujita, 1986b.

Capillary perfusion

Within the thyroid, the main arterial supply ramifies into interlobular and interfollicular arteries and finally forms an extensive blood capillary system. Dense networks of sinusoidal capillaries surround each follicle in a basket-like arrangement and appear optimally arranged for the provision of raw materials to, and transport of hormonal products from, thyroid follicular cells (Figure 15.1). In some species, such as the monkey, the capillary baskets of individual follicles are totally independent. However, in the dog and rat, a common capillary wall often occurs between adjacent follicles. Two basement membrane layers and a connective tissue space are interposed between the follicular epithelial cell basal plasma membrane and the capillary endothelial cell. As in other endocrine glands, the endothelial wall has numerous fenestrations which are covered by a thin diaphram (Hansen and Skaaring, 1973; Fujita and Murakami, 1974; Fujita, 1975).

Function-induced alterations in the thyroidal vasculature

The thyroidal vascular network can undergo significant remodeling during alterations in the functional status of this gland. For instance, during thyroxine treatment, decreases in the density of the capillary network and diameter of individual capillaries, as well as a reduction in the number of anastomoses occurs (Imada, Kurosumi and Fujita, 1986a). In contrast, challenge with thiouracil or thyrotropin, or low iodine diet treatment results in an increased diameter of thyroidal blood vessels and endothelial cell proliferation (Figure 15.1; Thomas, 1945; Wollman et al., 1978; Smeds and Wollman, 1983; Imada, Kurosumi and Fujita, 1986b). The striking nature of this phenomenon is indicated by the observation that the vascular volume can increase to seventy-times its normal value during prolonged goitrogenic stimulation (Herveg and Wollman, 1977). These changes are specific to blood vessels supplying follicular areas of the thyroid in that the structure of capillaries within the parathyroid glands is not altered during these treatments (Wollman et al., 1978; Smeds and Wollman, 1983). Wollman et al. (1978) proposed that the structural remodeling might be a consequence of a direct action of thyrotropin on endothelial cells or reflect the effect of a paracrine factor of epithelial cell origin on the vascular network. A number of angiogenic factors have recently been purified (Folkman and Klagsbrun, 1987). The operation of such a factor under conditions of structural remodeling of the thyroid gland is supported by observations that (1) transplanted thyroid tissue induces the formation of vascular sprouts in surrounding host connective tissue (Molne et al., 1987), (2) thyroid follicular cells produce an endotheliotropic chemoattractant that is distinct from thyroid hormones and thyroglobulin (Goodman and Rone, 1987), and (3) cultured porcine thyroid follicles release an endothelial cell growth factor which has properties similar to that of known angiogenic agents (Greil et al., 1989). The possible involvement of neural factors in this remodeling has not received much attention. A modulatory role for neuropeptides on cell growth is suggested by the finding that substance P and neurokinin A can stimulate the growth of smooth muscle cells derived from aortic media (Nilsson, von Euler and Dalsgaard, 1985), whereas vasoactive intestinal peptide can inhibit DNA synthesis in these cells (Hultgardh-Nilsson et al., 1988). Whether neural factors participate in the structural adaptations of the thyroid vasculature to changes in the functional status of this gland remains an open question.

THYROIDAL NEUROANATOMY

The innervation of the thyroid gland has been a subject of study since the early observation that nerve fibres are abundant in this gland (see Cannon and Cattell, 1916, for citation of the early literature). The recent introduction of fluorescence and immunohistochemical methods have more precisely identified the fibre distribution and neurotransmitter specificity of the extrinsic and intrinsic thyroid nerves. However, our knowledge in this field is still incomplete, and there is great need for further structural electron-microscopic studies, neurotransmitter receptor analysis, and examination of the electrical characteristics of the thyroidal nerves.

Gross innervation

Relative to its size, the thyroid receives an extensive and complex innervation. The thyroid nerves are composed of sympathetic and parasympathetic fibres. Predominantly, they are considered to be efferent nerves; sensory innervation of the gland has been suggested (Nonidez, 1931b; Lewinski, 1981), but not yet studied in detail. Thyroid nerves are

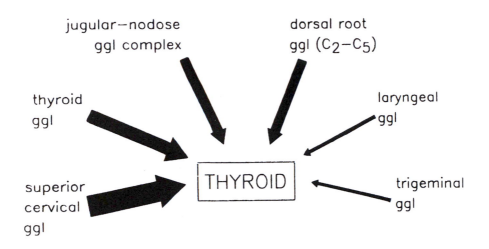

Figure 15.2   Schematic presentation of the contributions made by different ganglia (ggl) to the innervation of the rat thyroid gland. The thickness of the arrow represents the approximate extent of each contribution. Adapted from Grunditz *et al.*, 1988b.

composed of fibres originating from widely varying sources, namely from the superior cervical ganglion (SCG), nodose ganglion, jugular ganglion, laryngeal ganglion, trigeminal ganglion, dorsal root ganglia (C2–C5), local thyroid ganglia, directly from the vagus nerve, and probably also from the middle and/or inferior cervical ganglion (Figure 15.2; Nonidez, 1931b; Holmgren and Naumann, 1949; Romeo *et al.*, 1986; Grunditz *et al.*, 1988b). Sympathetic postganglionic nerve fibres appear to derive from cell bodies in the middle and inferior cervical ganglia as well as the SCG; these fibres then course through the external carotid nerve to the thyroid (Romeo *et al.*, 1986; Grunditz *et al.*, 1988b). Ramifications of the superior laryngeal nerve and inferior laryngeal (recurrent) nerve constitute the main source of thyroid parasympathetic innervation. These are chiefly preganglionic fibres which enter the gland along with the superior and inferior thyroid arteries. The location of the ganglionic synapse is not clear; some preganglionic fibres may synapse in the nodose ganglia, in the trunk of superior laryngeal nerves, or in the local ganglia (Nonidez, 1931a; Grunditz *et al.*, 1988b). There is also a possibility that ganglionic synapses of parasympathetic preganglionic fibres occur within the thyroid gland, since intrinsic thyroid neurons have been described in some species (Nonidez, 1931a; Grunditz *et al.*, 1984).

Intrinsic thyroidal innervation

The application of specific histochemical and fluorescent techniques for the identification of adrenergic and cholinergic nerve fibres has revealed the detailed characteristics of the distribution and neurotransmitter specificity of the intrathyroidal nerve fibres. The conclusion from these findings was that the thyroid nerves, both adrenergic and cholinergic, were distributed to the blood vessels as well as to the thyroidal parenchymal structures

(Melander, 1986). These observations seem to be confirmed by recent electronmicroscopic studies (Tice and Creveling, 1975; Uchiyama, Murakami and Ohno, 1985). The recent introduction of immunohistochemical techniques using specific antibodies to various neuropeptides has disclosed that the thyroid nerve fibres also contain a great variety of peptides such as vasoactive intestinal peptide (VIP), peptide histidine-isoleucine (PHI), neuropeptide Y (NPY), substance P and calcitonin gene-related peptide (CGRP) (Hedge *et al.*, 1984; Grunditz *et al.*, 1988b).

Intrathyroidal noradrenergic nerve fibres: The integral characteristics of the thyroidal noradrenergic innervation have been described in the elegant studies of Melander, Sundler and colleagues (Melander, Sundler and Westgren, 1973; Melander, Ericson and Ljunggren, 1974; Melander *et al.*, 1974; Melander *et al.*, 1975a; Melander, Sundler and Westgren, 1975). Using a combination of catecholamine fluorescence histochemistry and autoradiography for localization of exogenously-administered tritiated noradrenaline to identify adrenergic nerves, they have demonstrated the presence of noradrenergic nerve fibres in the thyroids of all species studied. They are distributed in close spatial association with the arterioles, characteristically appearing around the vessels. Some fibres also appear to innervate the thyroidal follicles. This pattern of innervation is similar in the thyroid glands of human, mouse and sheep, but is in contrast to that of rats, dogs, and pigs, where the nerve bundles are thinner and the density of innervation is less pronounced. The thyroids from younger animals have more noradrenergic terminals than those from older animals.

Studies with electron microscopy (Tice and Creveling, 1975; Uchiyama, Murakami and Ohno, 1985) have disclosed that the noradrenergic nerves are composed of axons that are partially, or totally, surrounded by Schwann cells. The axons display dilated segments (varicosities) which contain mitochondria and characteristic small-core vesicles. The varicosities establish close contact with both blood vessels and epithelial cells. This type of morphological configuration meets the criteria of a nerve terminal synaptic (neuroeffector) junction. In the mouse, electron-microscopy was used to examine the localization of exogenous false noradrenergic neurotransmitters (Tice and Creveling, 1975). Accumulations of the tracers were observed in axonal varicosities packed with small vesicles which were in direct contact with vascular smooth muscle and basal membranes of thyroid epithelial cells. Neuroeffector junctions were identified as 250–400 Å gaps separating the plasma membrane of the smooth muscle or epithelial cell from the membrane of the axolemma.

Intrathyroidal cholinergic nerve fibres: Information on the intrinsic cholinergic innervation of the thyroid gland is largely based on the results of histochemical studies by Amenta *et al.* (1978), Melander and Sundler (1979) and Van Sande *et al.* (1980). These studies have shown that acetylcholine esterase-containing (i.e. cholinergic) nerve fibres are present in thyroids of all species studied: calf, mouse and human. The cholinergic fibres are distributed as a dense network around small blood vessels and also as "fibres running between and around follicles." In the species studied, it appears that both the spatial configuration and the density of the cholinergic nerve fibres are similar to those of the noradrenergic nerve endings in this gland.

TABLE 15.1
Source of thyroidal neurotransmitters and neuropeptides in the rat.
Adapted from Grunditz *et al.*, 1988b

Neurotransmitters and/or neuropeptides	Thyroid	Laryngeal	Ganglion Superior cervical	Nodose	Jugular	Dorsal root	Trigeminal
NA	0^a	0	+	0	0	0	0
VIP	++	+	(+)	+	0	0	0
Galanin	0	+	0	+	+	+	+
Substance P	0	+	0	+	+	+	+
CGRP	0	+	0	+	++	++	++
NA + NPY	0	0	+++	0	0	0	0
VIP + NPY	++	++	0	0	0	0	0
VIP + Galanin	+	++	0	+++	0	0	0
Substance P + CGRP	0	+	0	+	++	++	++
Galanin + Substance P + CGRP	0	0	0	0	+	+	+

[a] The relative frequency of cell bodies was graded arbitrarily: 0, none; (+), very few; +, few; ++, moderate in number; +++, numerous.

Intrathyroidal peptidergic nerve fibres: The thyroid gland is also richly innervated with nerves which contain numerous neuropeptides (Table 15.1). VIP was the first peptide to be discovered in intrathyroidal nerve fibres (Ahren *et al.*, 1980) and subsequently such fibres have also been found to contain a variety of other peptides as well (Ahren *et al.*, 1983; Grunditz *et al.*, 1984; Hedge *et al.*, 1984; Grunditz *et al.*, 1986a, 1986b, 1987, 1988a). Because of the rapid development of this field, it is very likely that still more neuropeptides will be added to this list in the near future. It is not clear whether some of these peptidergic fibres constitute a distinct neural arrangement, i.e., — "a peptidergic nervous system" — or whether the peptides are exclusively co-localized with the classical neurotransmitters.

VIP immunoreactive fibres have been observed in the thyroids of all species studied: human, mouse, rat, cat, guinea pig and pig (Ahren *et al.*, 1980, Hedge *et al.*, 1984; Grunditz *et al.*, 1988a, 1988b). They were most frequent in the rat and cat, but rather sparse in the pig and human. With the light microscope, the VIP-positive nerve fibres were observed as fine filaments with many varicosities running in close apposition to small blood vessels and between thyroid follicles. They were more numerous around arterioles than around venules (Grunditz *et al.*, 1988a). In the mouse, VIP immunoreactivity was also seen in nerve cell bodies forming a ganglionic structure located on the external surface of the thyroid capsule (Ahren *et al.*, 1980). It has been reported (Grunditz *et al.*, 1988a, 1988b) that such immunoreactive fibres project from this local ganglion into the thyroid gland. However, detailed immunohistochemical studies on neuronal pathways have revealed that nerve cell bodies showing VIP immunoreactivity are also located in various parasympathetic ganglia projecting to the thyroid, for example, the nodose ganglion, laryngeal ganglion and jugular ganglion (Grunditz *et al.*, 1988b). These observations suggest that this peptide may be associated with cholinergic nerves. Indeed, transection of the superior laryngeal nerve resulted in a 60% decrease in the thyroidal content of VIP (Michalkiewicz, Huffman and Hedge, 1990). Whether VIP coexists with acetylcholine within the same nerve terminals

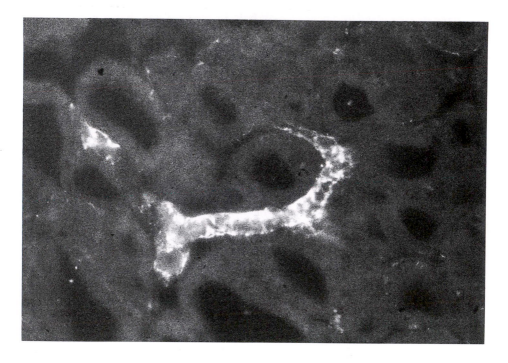

Figure 15.3   Rat thyroid section immunostained for NPY. Dense networks of NPY-containing nerve fibres occur around blood vessels (×200).

and may thus be co-secreted, as has been shown in the salivary gland (Lundberg, 1981), remains to be established. It has been shown, however, that other neuropeptides, such as PHI or NPY, coexist with VIP in thyroid nerve fibres (Grunditz *et al.*, 1986b, 1988a). On the other hand, VIP immunoreactivity, although sparse, has been demonstrated in the SCG which is known to provide most of the noradrenergic fibres to the thyroid (Grunditz *et al.*, 1988b). An age-dependent difference in the quantity of VIP-containing fibres in the thyroid has also been observed and such fibres are more numerous in the glands of younger than of older rats (Grunditz *et al.*, 1988a).

NPY has also been shown to be present in numerous intrathyroidal nerve fibres (Grunditz *et al.*, 1984; Hedge *et al.*, 1984; Grunditz *et al.*, 1988a, 1988b). Thyroid specimens of several mammals, including man, mouse, rat and calf, display dense networks of NPY fibres (Figure 15.3) with varicosities surrounding small blood vessels which penetrate the adventitia and extend close to the media. Retrograde tracing studies indicate that NPY-containing cell bodies in the SCG project to the thyroid gland and removal of SCG results in a drastic reduction of NPY fibres, clearly indicating that the majority of the intrathyroidal NPY fibres originate in this ganglion (Grunditz *et al.*, 1988b). However, a small ganglion containing NPY immunoreactive cell bodies has also been demonstrated in a single specimen of the calf thyroid indicating that, in some species, at least a few of these thyroidal fibres are of intrinsic origin (Grunditz *et al.*, 1984). Most of the NPY fibres in the thyroid gland also appear to contain noradrenaline on the basis of sequential immunostaining for dopamine-β-hydroxylase. However, NPY may also coexist with VIP in some thyroid nerve fibres (Grunditz *et al.*, 1988a, 1988b). Similar to the distribution of VIP-immunoreactive fibres, intrathyroidal NPY-immunoreactive fibres are more numerous around arterioles than around venules. They are also more frequently seen in thyroids of younger animals (Grunditz *et al.*, 1988a).

Results of specific immunohistochemical staining of thyroid slices from many species have demonstrated that intrathyroidal nerve fibres may also contain substance P, neurokinin A, galanin and CGRP (Ahren *et al.*, 1983; Hedge *et al.*, 1984; Grunditz *et al.*, 1986a, 1987, 1988b). Such fibres were observed in all species studied. They were seen as thin beaded fibres running around blood vessels and often found penetrating the vascular walls into the adventitia or to the adventitia-media border of the small thyroidal arteries. The results of immunohistological examination of the neighboring ganglia, together with studies using a retrograde tracer applied to the thyroid, or local denervation, indicate that these thyroidal peptidergic nerve fibres derive from several locations. Immunopositive peptidergic cell bodies projecting to the thyroid have been found in jugular ganglia, cervical dorsal root ganglia (C2–C5), or trigeminal ganglia. These neural formations are known to harbour primarily sensory neurons. Therefore, it can be suggested that the above mentioned peptidergic nerve fibres participate in relaying sensory information from the thyroid gland to the higher centers of the autonomic nervous system.

NEURAL CONTROL OF THE THYROID CIRCULATION

EFFERENT AUTONOMIC CONTROL

Based upon extensive morphological studies of the distribution of nerve fibres within the thyroid, Nonidez (1935) predicted that blood flow within this gland would be under close neural control since dense plexuses of nerve fibres terminate in arteriolar walls within the thyroid. Subsequent studies which have examined the effects of nerve stimulation on thyroid activity support this hypothesis. In general, stimulation of the sympathetic neural input to the thyroid is associated with decreases in thyroid blood flow, whereas parasympathetic nerve stimulation is accompanied by increases in thyroid blood flow. However, the neurotransmitters and/or neuropeptides which effect these responses, and how such neural influences contribute to the physiological regulation of thyroidal function, have not been fully studied.

Noradrenergic mechanisms

Thyroid vasomotor tone can be influenced by the sympathetic neural input to this gland. Electrical stimulation of the cervical sympathetic trunk causes thyroidal vasoconstriction, thereby decreasing blood flow to this gland (Watts, 1915; Soderberg, 1958a; Ito *et al.*, 1987). However, the extent of this decrease in thyroid blood flow appears to be much less than that of the increase in blood flow which can be elicited by parasympathetic stimulation (Ito *et al.*, 1987). When measured by venous drop counter, thyroid blood flow decreases gradually as the stimulus frequency to the cervical sympathetic trunk increases, approaching a plateau at 10 Hz (Ito *et al.*, 1987). On the other hand, when measured by laser Doppler flowmetry, thyroid blood flow decreases with increasing stimulus frequency to this trunk before reaching a plateau at 60 Hz (Dey *et al.*, unpublished observations). Differences in the method used to monitor thyroid blood flow or the anaesthetic agents used may account for these observations; however, collectively these results indicate that sympathetic stimulation will decrease thyroid blood flow. Thyroid blood flow is also decreased following superior cervical ganglionectomy during the period corresponding to noradrenergic nerve terminal degeneration (Cardinali *et al.*, 1982).

Exactly how these effects relate to the overall functioning of the thyroid is, however, not clear. It has long been known that exophthalmos is a complication of hyperthyroidism and, initially, this was mistaken as the proptosis caused by sympathetic stimulation (see Soderberg, 1959 for review). This led to the assumption that sympathetic nerves have a goitrogenic effect. However, it has now been suggested that the cervical sympathetic nerves normally exert a negative influence on thyroid function (Pisarev *et al.*, 1981). Recent experiments in rats show that superior cervical ganglionectomy of one week duration enhances the thyroid growth which occurs in the remaining thyroid lobe after hemithyroidectomy. On the other hand, blood flow, as estimated from the uptake of a tracer dose of ^{86}Rb, is decreased significantly after this denervation procedure (Pisarev *et al.*, 1981). Therefore, any progoitrogenic effect of superior cervical ganglionectomy in this instance would not appear to be due to an increase in blood flow. In contrast to reports of decreased thyroid blood flow at certain times following removal of the SCG, acute (one-half hour) or chronic (two weeks) extirpation of this ganglion has no overall effect on thyroid blood flow in normal rats (Hedge, Huffman and Connors, 1986; Michalkiewicz, Huffman and Hedge, 1990).

Intraarterial or intravenous administration of adrenaline or noradrenaline (NA) causes vasoconstriction which is often followed by vasodilatation. The degree of vasoconstriction is proportional to the log of the dose of the catecholamine injected, but varies with initial circulatory state within the thyroid. Thus, the most pronounced vasoconstriction is elicited in animals with a high resting blood flow, whereas in animals with low resting blood flow, there is hardly any constriction even with a five times higher dose of adrenaline. However, the vasoconstrictor effect of NA is five to ten times weaker than that of adrenaline (Soderberg, 1958a). Similar effects have been observed by other investigators (Ahn, Athans and Rosenberg, 1969). In another study, it has been shown that small intraarterial doses of NA may cause thyroidal vasodilatation, whereas adrenaline at all doses causes vasoconstriction. For instance, when infused intravenously at a large dose of 0.1 μg/min, NA causes thyroidal vasoconstriction but, when infused at a smaller dose of 0.01 μg/min, it causes thyroidal vasodilatation. On the other hand, adrenaline in all doses ranging from 0.01 to 0.1 μg/min causes thyroidal vasoconstriction (Mowbray and Peart, 1960).

The presence of α and β adrenoceptors on thyroid follicular cells has already been shown by *in vivo* and *in vitro* studies (Dumont *et al.*, 1981; Toccafondi *et al.*, 1983). However, there is very little information available in the literature about the presence of adrenoceptors on thyroid blood vessels and their relation to thyroid blood flow. Since thyroid blood vessels are responsive to both adrenaline and NA, it may be logically presumed that, like many other vascular beds, thyroid blood vessels also contain both α and β adrenoceptors.

Cholinergic mechanisms

Changes in the parasympathetic neural input can also affect thyroid vasomotor tone. Stimulation of the vagus (Soderberg, 1958a; Ishii, Shizume and Okinaka, 1968) or more specifically, the superior laryngeal nerve (Soderberg, 1958a; Ito *et al.*, 1987) is almost always accompanied by an acute increase in thyroid blood flow. While such effects on thyroid blood flow appear to be sustained during the period of stimulation, this vasodilatory activity abates shortly after stimulus cessation. A counterbalancing effect from sympathetic nerves is suggested by the observation that the vasodilatation elicited by vagal stimulation is enhanced following resection of cranial sympathetic ganglia (Ishii, Shizume and Okinaka, 1968). In contrast to reports of enhanced thyroid blood flow during superior laryngeal nerve stimulation, acute (one half hour) or chronic (two weeks) transection of this nerve has no apparent effect on thyroid vasomotor tone in normal rats (Michalkiewicz, Huffman and Hedge, 1990). This finding could suggest that there is a functional compensation of remaining autonomic pathways to the thyroid during this time or the expression of local blood flow regulatory mechanisms. Alternatively, the superior laryngeal nerve may play no role in the control of thyroid blood flow under basal conditions and may only exert an important influence during conditions when this gland is challenged (i.e., during goitrogenic stimulation).

The contribution of the inferior laryngeal (recurrent) nerve to the regulation of thyroid vasomotor tone is less clear. In general, stimulation or transection of this nerve has no effect on thyroid blood flow (Soderberg, 1958a; Michalkiewicz, Huffman and Hedge, 1990).

Acetylcholine (ACh) is a likely candidate as one of the neurotransmitters contributing to the vasodilatory response to vagal or superior laryngeal nerve stimulation. Infusions of ACh increase thyroid blood flow and this effect can be blocked by atropine (Soderberg, 1958a; Huffman *et al.*, 1991). The suggestion that muscarinic cholinergic mechanisms mediate the vascular response to superior laryngeal nerve stimulation under some conditions is supported by the observation that atropine can block thyroidal vasodilatation elicited by low frequency-stimulation of this nerve (Ito *et al.*, 1987). However, atropine does not abolish the increases in thyroid blood flow seen at higher frequencies of stimulation and other influences (i.e., peptidergic) appear to contribute significantly to these responses (see later section).

Nonadrenergic, noncholinergic mechanisms

In addition to evidence that the classical neurotransmitters, NA and ACh, play some role in the modulation of thyroid vasomotor tone, it is increasingly likely that nonadrenergic, noncholinergic neural mechanisms also contribute to the regulation of the thyroidal circulation. The potential for neuropeptides and other putative neurotransmitters to influence the thyroid circulation is evidenced by observations that the administration of such substances may be associated with changes in thyroid blood flow (Table 15.2). Unravelling the role that each of these vasoactive substances plays in the neural regulation of the thyroid vasculature under normal and pathological states is the next challenge.

VIP and homologues: The first indication that VIP might participate in the neural regulation of the thyroid circulation came from immunohistochemical studies showing

TABLE 15.2

Effects of neurotransmitters, vasoactive substances or neuropeptides on
thyroid blood flow or vascular conductance

Neurotransmitter, vasoactive substance, or neuropeptide	Species	Route	Effect	Reference[c]
Adrenaline	rabbit, cat	iv or ia[a]	↓ [b]	Soderberg, 1958a
	dog	ia	↓	Mowbray and Peart, 1960
	human	iv	↓	Mowbray and Peart, 1960
		iv	↓	Ahn, Athans, and Rosenberg, 1969
Noradrenaline	human	iv	↑	Mowbray and Peart, 1960
	dog	ia	↓ high dose; ↑ low dose	Mowbray and Peart, 1960
Acetylcholine	rabbit, cat	iv	↑	Soderberg, 1958a
	rat	iv or topical	↑	Huffman et al., 1991
Serotonin	rabbit, cat	ia	↑	Soderberg, 1958a
	rat	iv	↑	Melander et al., 1975b
Histamine	rat	iv	↑	Melander et al., 1975b
	rat	topical	↔	Huffman et al., unpub. obs.
2-chloroadenosine	rat	topical	↔	Huffman et al., unpub. obs.
VIP and/or homologues	rabbit	iv	↑	Nilsson and Bill, 1984
	rat	iv or topical	↑	Huffman and Hedge, 1986a
		iv	↑ (VIP>PHI>secretin) > GRF	Huffman, Connors and Hedge, 1988
	rat	ia	↑	Ito et al., 1987
NPY	rat	iv	↓	Hedge, Huffman and Connors, 1987
Substance P	rat	iv	↔	Huffman and Hedge, 1986b
CGRP	rat	iv	↔	Huffman et al., unpub. obs.

[a] iv = intravenous; ia = intraarterial; topical = applied with cotton pads directed to the thyroid gland.
[b] ↓ = decrease; ↑ = increase; ↔ = no change.
[c] Note: see Soderberg, 1958a and Kapitola, 1973 for references to literature prior to 1958.

a substantial number of VIP-containing nerve fibres in close association with blood vessels in the thyroid gland (see later section). Subsequent to this observation, the administration of exogenous VIP was shown to cause prompt and striking increases in thyroid blood flow (Figure 15.4; Nilsson and Bill, 1984; Huffman and Hedge, 1986a; Ito et al., 1987). This effect of VIP is dose-dependent (Huffman and Hedge, 1986a) and is not modified by anaesthesia (Bouder, Huffman and Hedge, 1988). Furthermore, VIP appears to act directly at the thyroidal vasculature since the effect is seen with localized topical or close intraarterial administration, and occurs in the absence of observable effects on thyroidal follicular function (Huffman and Hedge, 1986a; Ito et al., 1987; Huffman et al., 1988). The mechanism whereby VIP induces thyroidal vasodilatation has not been explored. In other vascular beds, the vasodilator action of VIP appears to be closely associated with the arterial accumulation of both cGMP and cAMP and may be mediated by prostaglandins (Wei, Kontos and Said, 1980; Ignarro et al., 1987). Since VIP can markedly increase thyroid

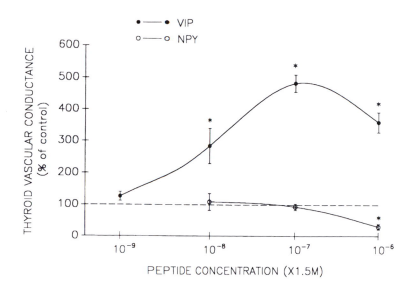

Figure 15.4   Vascular conductance in the thyroid glands of rats infused with VIP (closed circles) or NPY (open circles) at the doses indicated. Results are presented as a percent of control values from saline-infused rats. * represents $p < 0.05$ versus saline-infused. Adapted from Hedge, Huffman and Connors, 1987 and Huffman, Connors and Hedge, 1988.

cAMP levels (Ahren *et al.*, 1980; Toccafondi, Brandi and Melander, 1984), it seems likely that this second messenger may participate in VIP-induced vasodilatation in the thyroid gland. Whether the vasodilator effect of VIP on the thyroid is dependent upon an intact endothelium is not known; both endothelium-dependent and -independent mechanisms have been postulated for this peptide in different vascular beds (Duckles and Said, 1982; Davies and Williams, 1984).

The participation of endogenous VIP in the neural control of the thyroid circulation is suggested by the observation that atropine pretreatment does not abolish the increases in thyroid blood flow seen during high frequency parasympathetic stimulation, and furthermore, that there is an increase in thyroidal VIP outflow under such conditions (Ito *et al.*, 1987). Thus, as in other vascular beds (e.g., the salivary gland), VIP appears to be a prime candidate for the mediation of some nonadrenergic, noncholinergic neural effects. The role which VIP may play under basal conditions or conditions during which thyroid blood flow is altered is less clear. The administration of each of three putative antagonists of VIP was without effect on basal thyroid blood flow; however, in this same study, it was also found that these compounds were unable to block the vasodilator effect of exogenous VIP (Michalkiewicz, Huffman and Hedge, 1987; unpublished observations). Such results suggest that these particular pharmacologigal substances cannot be used to evaluate the role of endogenous VIP in the modulation of thyroid vascular tone. The neutralization of VIP with antibodies is another approach which has been attempted. Upon systemic administration of a specific VIP antiserum, systemic mean arterial blood pressure increased and prolactin levels decreased. Such responses are consistent with effective neutralization of endogenous VIP activity. However, under these conditions, basal thyroid blood flow was not changed, suggesting that the contribution of VIP to the maintenance of vascular tone under normal conditions is minimal (Michalkiewicz, Huffman and Hedge, 1987).

In order to further evaluate the role of VIP in the regulation of thyroid blood flow, thyroidal VIP content has been measured under conditions associated with changes in thyroid blood flow. The observation that a high iodine diet is associated both with decreases in thyroid blood flow and VIP content is consistent with the hypothesis that a reduction in VIP effects at the thyroid vasculature may, in part, account for the reduced thyroid blood flow under these conditions (Michalkiewicz et al., 1989a). However, VIP content is not changed under hypothyroid conditions (e.g., following propylthiouracil or low iodine diet treatment or after hemithyroidectomy) which are associated with marked increases in thyroid blood flow (Michalkiewicz et al., 1987; Connors, Huffman and Hedge, 1988; Michalkiewicz et al., 1989a, 1989b). Conversely, treatment with thyroxine results in decreases in thyroid blood flow, with no change in VIP content (Michalkiewicz et al., 1987; Connors, Huffman and Hedge, 1988). These results suggest that the underlying mechanisms whereby thyroid blood flow may be changed in response to various challenges may be quite complex. In addition, observations regarding changes, or lack of changes, in VIP economy in the thyroid need also to be interpreted along with data regarding the effectiveness of VIP on the thyroidal vasculature under these conditions. For instance, changes in VIP receptor number or vascular responsiveness to VIP during hypo- or hyperthyroid conditions will need to be addressed before the role of VIP in the regulation of thyroid blood flow will be fully understood.

VIP shares sequence homology with a number of other peptides i.e., PHI, helodermin, secretin, growth hormone releasing hormone (GRF), and gastric inhibitory peptide. In general, the vasodilator potency of these peptides at the thyroid corresponds to the degree of structural homology with VIP (Huffman, Connors and Hedge, 1988). This observation is consistent with an action of these peptides at the same vascular receptor, or perhaps at different receptors, but with a common mechanism beyond the receptor site. Since one of these homologues (i.e., PHI) is found in the thyroid gland in conjunction with VIP-containing nerve fibres, its involvement in the neural regulation of thyroid blood flow warrants further attention.

Other neuropeptides: In addition to VIP and its structural homologue, PHI, a host of other neuropeptides has been localized to nerve fibres within the thyroid gland (see later section). The occurrence of these peptides in nerves which are in close proximity to blood vessels suggest that they may participate in the regulation of thyroid blood flow.

NPY, as in other vascular beds, is a vasoconstrictor agent in the thyroid (Figure 15.4; Hedge, Huffman and Connors, 1987). Although the mechanism of this thyroidal effect has not been explored, NPY has been described as having three primary sites of action in other organ systems (Wahlestedt et al., 1990). These sites of action are: a direct post-junctional vasoconstrictor effect; an indirect post-junctional effect to enhance NA-induced vasoconstriction; and a pre-junctional effect to inhibit the stimulated release of NA. The vasoconstriction elicited by NPY in the thyroid gland is most likely by one of the first two mechanisms described, or a combination of these. However, further experiments utilizing appropriate pharmacological tools and measurements of endogenous NPY levels under conditions of altered thyroid blood flow will be necessary in order to determine the importance of NPY in the modulation of thyroid vasomotor tone.

Other peptides which occur in nerve fibres in close association with the thyroidal vasculature include substance P, CGRP, galanin and neurokinin A. Substance P and CGRP have no apparent effect on thyroid blood flow when tested under conditions during which VIP and NPY have pronounced effects (Huffman and Hedge, 1986b; unpublished observations). These peptides have, however, been implicated as having a sensory role in other systems (Pernow, 1983; Jansen et al., 1990), and a similar situation may exist in the thyroid gland (see below). To date, the possible modulation of thyroid vasomotor tone by galanin or neurokinin A has not been addressed.

Interestingly, cholecystokinin is a peptide which occurs preferentially in fibres that innervate thyroid follicular cells (Ahren et al., 1983). An "indirect" neural control of the thyroid circulation by this peptide is possible through its potential influence on the metabolic activity of thyroid follicular cells. Although acute infusions of cholecystokinin do not alter thyroid blood flow (Huffman et al., 1990), this peptide could play a role in the regulation of functional changes in the thyroid after goitrogen treatment (i.e., growth of the gland and the associated hyperaemia).

Other putative neurotransmitters: In certain blood vessels, it is becoming increasingly clear that purinergic compounds function to modulate vascular tone (Burnstock, 1987). Adenosine 5'-triphosphate (ATP) can coexist with NA or ACh in nerve terminals, and a role for ATP as an excitatory co-transmitter with NA in the circulatory control of a variety of blood vessels has been proposed. In these instances, ATP appears to interact with P_{2X}-purinoceptors on vascular smooth muscle cells. In addition to a neural vasoconstrictor action, purines such as ATP and adenosine can have potent vasodilator actions on vascular preparations. These effects appear to be mediated via P_{2Y}-purinoceptors on endothelial cells or P_1-purinoceptors on vascular smooth muscle cells. The extent to which purines may be involved in the regulation of thyroid vascular tone has not been extensively studied, however, we have found that the topical application of adenosine to the thyroid is without effect on thyroid blood flow under normal conditions (unpublished observations). Whether purinergic neurotransmission plays a role in the circulatory control of the thyroid is an unanswered question. Similarly, nothing is known about the participation of GABA in the regulation of thyroidal vascular tone.

Interactions between neurotransmitters, neuropeptides, other vasoactive substances, and humoral factors

Interactions between neurotransmitters and neuropeptides: The extensive co-localization of neurotransmitters and neuropeptides, or different neuropeptides within fibres which innervate the vasculature of the thyroid gland (see later section) suggests that these substances may interact in the regulation of thyroid blood flow. This area has not been explored to a great extent, but it is likely that a complex interplay exists in the modulation of thyroid vasomotor tone.

An important source of VIP in the thyroid is the superior laryngeal nerve (Michalkiewicz, Huffman and Hedge, 1990). This is part of the parasympathetic nervous input to the gland and, as described earlier, stimulation of this nerve increases thyroid blood flow. The participation of both ACh and VIP in the mediation of this response is likely since atropine can partly, but not completely, abolish this effect and VIP outflow is increased at high frequencies (Ito et al., 1987). The observation that the effect of VIP on thyroid vascular conductance is actually enhanced following muscarinic blockade suggests that an antagonism between the actions of endogenous ACh and VIP may exist in the modulation of thyroid vascular tone (Huffman et al., 1991). This apparent situation in the thyroid differs from what has been described in the salivary gland, where a synergism between ACh and VIP on both vasodilatory and secretory responses has been described (Lundberg, 1981).

As discussed earlier, an important action of NPY in other vascular beds is an enhancement of NA-induced vasoconstriction. Given the coexistence of NPY with NA in nerve fibres in the thyroid gland, this is a potentially important mechanism for the regulation of thyroid blood flow which has not been addressed to date. The observation that a variety of peptides coexist in the thyroid, and have been shown to interact in the regulation of thyroid follicular cell activity (Grunditz et al., 1984), suggests that complementary interactions for these peptides may exist in the modulation of thyroid vasomotor tone.

Interactions between neurotransmitters and other vasoactive substances: As alluded to previously, it is possible that the neural regulation of the thyroid vasculature may be "indirect" via an effect on follicular function, and thus a consequence of altered metabolic activity of the gland. Other possible mechanisms whereby nerves may influence thyroid blood flow include the modulation of release of vasoactive substances from mast cells or parafollicular (C) cells within the thyroid.

Although the suggestion that nerves may influence the release of vasoactive mast cell products is purely speculative at this time, significant nerve/mast cell associations can occur in the body (Bienenstock et al., 1987). Histamine and serotonin released from mast cells within the thyroid can markedly increase thyroid blood flow (Melander et al., 1975b) and one postulated mechanism for TSH-induced increases in thyroid blood flow is through the mobilization of these amines (Clayton and Szego, 1967; Melander et al., 1975a). In our preliminary experiments, topical treatment of the thyroid with histamine had no effect on thyroid blood flow in normal, untreated rats (unpublished observations). However, the previously described effect of histamine or serotonin to increase thyroid blood flow was observed in T_4-pretreated rats or mice. It is very likely that the status of the thyroid gland (i.e., iodine economy) influences gland responsiveness. Furthermore, the involvement of a neurally-mediated mast cell response in thyroid autoimmune disease states (e.g., Graves disease) which are associated with changes in thyroid blood flow should be considered.

In addition to possible effects at mast cells, nerves might also influence thyroid blood flow via the release of vasoactive substances from parafollicular (C) cells. Although this has not been demonstrated, neurotransmitters can influence C cell activity and C cells can form or store vasoactive substances (Melander et al., 1975a; Cardinali et al., 1986).

Interactions between neurotransmitters and thyrotropin: Thyrotropin (TSH), secreted by the pituitary gland, stimulates virtually all functional processes of thyroid epithelial cells and hypophysectomy is associated with decreases in thyroid blood flow which can be restored to normal with the administration of exogenous TSH (Csernay, Laszlo and Kovacs,

1968; Connors, Huffman and Hedge, 1988). However, it has been shown that increases in circulating TSH levels *per se* are not always accompanied by increases in thyroid blood flow (Kapitola, Schreiberova and Jahoda, 1967; Connors *et al.*, 1991). Thus, it appears that TSH-associated elevations in thyroid blood flow are dependent upon the functional state of this gland and are most dramatically seen when intrathyroidal iodine economy is compromised. Therefore, the possibility exists that TSH through a direct action, or via changes in follicular cell function, may affect neurotransmitter actions on thyroid blood vessels and that this mechanism could, in part, underlie the differential effect of TSH on thyroid blood flow under varying thyroid states. Although this issue has not been addressed extensively to date, such TSH-dependent changes in thyroid blood flow do not appear to be associated with changes in the concentration of intrathyroidal VIP (Michalkiewicz *et al.*, 1987).

In addition to the possibility that TSH-mediated effects at the thyroid may affect neurotransmitter release or action at this gland, neurally-mediated changes in thyroidal vasomotor tone could influence the delivery rate of TSH to the thyroid and thereby affect thyroid function. However, the finding of an enhanced goitrogenic response to TSH in superior cervical ganglionectomized rats with decreased thyroid blood flow does not support this concept (Pisarev *et al.*, 1981).

Thus, while significant interactions between TSH and nerves in the control of thyroid follicular function have been described (see Ahren, 1986 and Melander, 1986 for reviews), there is limited information available to date regarding the interrelationship between nerves and TSH in the control of thyroid blood flow.

Interactions between neurotransmitters and iodine: Thyroid gland function can be strikingly influenced by iodine availability (Nagataki and Ingbar, 1986). One such adjustment that occurs in response to a decreasing iodine supply is a marked increase in thyroid blood flow (Michalkiewicz *et al.*, 1989a). Conversely, increasing the iodine supply by the provision of a high iodine diet is accompanied by decreases in thyroid blood flow (Michalkiewicz *et al.*, 1989a). Since these changes can occur in the absence of alterations in circulating TSH levels, other mechanisms must be invoked to explain the striking effects of iodine on thyroid blood flow. As noted earlier (see previous section), ingestion of a high iodine diet is accompanied by decreases in VIP content. Assuming that VIP synthesis and release are also decreased under these conditions, this may indicate that a neural link exists between such high iodine diet effects on thyroid blood flow. It is also possible that plasma iodide may alter the thyroid blood flow response to TSH (i.e., alter the sensitivity of thyroid blood flow to TSH) as has been hypothesized for other thyroidal autoregulatory processes (Field, 1986). Neural elements may play a significant role in this adjustment, however, as indicated in the previous section, further studies will be necessary to define the interactions which may exist between humoral factors, such as iodide or TSH, and neurotransmitters in the regulation of thyroid blood flow.

AFFERENT AUTONOMIC CONTROL AND CENTRAL INTEGRATION

The participation of the central nervous system in the control of thyroid function is best described by the classical hypothalamo-pituitary-thyroid axis in which thyrotropin-releasing hormone is an important hormonal factor acting to regulate thyroid function. However, some evidence supports the existence of a reflex pathway by which nerves transmit information from the thyroid to the central nervous system and from the central nervous system to the thyroid.

Hemithyroidectomy is a condition in which a compensatory increase in thyroid blood flow is seen in the contralateral lobe (Michalkiewicz et al., 1989b). Hemithyroidectomy is also associated with increases in hypothalamic thyrotropin-releasing hormone content (Gerendai et al., 1985). Since thyrotropin-releasing hormone, given intracerebroventricularly, can result in increases in thyroid blood flow via the activation of vagal pathways (Tonoue and Nomoto, 1979), a possible reflex may be envisioned whereby the condition of "subtotal thyroidectomy" is relayed to the CNS by the remaining thyroid sensory nerves which contain Substance P and CGRP. In the CNS, thyrotropin-releasing hormone-containing neurons would be activated, leading to an increase in superior laryngeal nerve activity and increased thyroid blood flow. It is already known that the increase in TSH which accompanies hemithyroidectomy can not fully account for the increases in thyroid blood flow seen in this condition (Michalkiewicz et al., 1991), and neural involvement in this phenomenon has been suggested. A test of the model proposed above would be to administer capsaicin (i.e., deplete Substance P/CGRP from nerve endings) and then perform hemithyroidectomy. An attenuation of the compensatory increase in thyroid blood flow under these conditions would provide support for this hypothesis.

FUNCTIONAL SIGNIFICANCE OF THE NEURAL CONTROL OF THE THYROID CIRCULATION

It is evident from the review of the literature presented that nerves and associated neurotransmitters can act to influence the thyroid circulation. Exactly how neural control of the thyroid vasculature may be linked with thyroid function during physiological and pathological states is, however, still not well understood. Soderberg (1958a, 1958b) concluded from his extensive studies that the rate of thyroidal iodine uptake was generally proportional to the blood flow through this gland, whereas the secretion of thyroid hormones and vasomotor activity were not well correlated. Data from other laboratories support this finding (Brown-Grant and Gibson, 1956; Ahn, Athans and Rosenberg, 1969). The idea that thyroidal iodide trapping would be dependent upon thyroid blood flow was initially proposed on purely theoretical grounds by Riggs in 1952. Since the thyroid is normally trapping most of the iodide it receives, it can not be expected to make major adjustments in absolute uptake by modulating only the trap activity; once extraction efficiency is maximal, iodide supply will be flow-limited, and thus could increase only if blood flow increases. Therefore, it is likely that the neural regulation of thyroid vasomotor tone is important in modulating thyroidal iodine uptake and thus assuring that a sufficient supply of iodine is available for thyroid hormone synthesis. This may be especially important under conditions of relative iodine deficiency and this concept is supported by the observation that iodine uptake can be enhanced by VIP treatment in rats receiving a low-iodine, but not a normal, diet (Pietrzyk et al., 1992).

It is also tempting to speculate that the delivery rate of TSH to the thyroid gland may be dependent upon neurally mediated changes in thyroid blood flow. Thus, nerves may indirectly exert control over the rate of hormone output through changes in the responsiveness to TSH. Such a phenomenon has been proposed for both the thyroid (Soderberg, 1958b) and other endocrine glands (Porter and Klaiber, 1965; Urquhart and Li, 1969; Niswender *et al.*, 1976). While this is an attractive proposal, doses of VIP which markedly enhance thyroid blood flow do not alter TSH-stimulated thyroid hormone release in the rat (Huffman *et al.*, 1988), and there is currently little experimental evidence to indicate a link between the rate of delivery of tropic hormone and thyroidal responsiveness. Instead, the available literature is most consistent with a neural modulation of TSH responsiveness via a direct interaction between neurotransmitters and TSH at thyroidal follicular cells (see Ahren, 1986; Melander, 1986 for reviews).

A third manner in which changes in thyroid blood flow may be linked to alterations in thyroid activity could be in the redistribution of blood flow within the gland. A functional heterogeneity in growth, iodine metabolism and thyroglobulin synthesis exists within follicular epithelial cells (Studer, Peter and Gerber, 1989) and neurally-mediated changes in blood flow may contribute to these differences. Such changes, as described here or above, could be exerted through short-term alterations in vascular tone or long-term structural (i.e., angiogenic) influences.

In conclusion, while theoretical considerations and some experimental results suggest that neural influences on the thyroid circulation may have an important effect on thyroid function by influencing iodine uptake, TSH-responsiveness, and/or heterogeneity of activity, there is a dearth of information causally linking neurally-mediated changes in thyroid vasomotor tone to changes in thyroid activity. The future design and execution of such experiments will greatly clarify the functional significance of the neural control of the thyroid circulation.

ACKNOWLEDGEMENTS

Studies performed in the authors' laboratory were supported by NIH grants DK35037 and DK07312 and NSF grant DCB-8904470.

REFERENCES

Ahn, C.S., Athans, J.C. and Rosenberg, I.N. (1969). Effects of epinephrine and of alteration in glandular blood flow upon thyroid function: studies using thyroid vein cannulation in dogs. *Endocrinology*, **84**, 501–507.

Ahren, B. (1986). Thyroid neuroendocrinology: neural regulation of thyroid hormone secretion. *Endocrine Reviews*, **7**, 149–155.

Ahren, B., Alumets, J., Ericsson, M., Fahrenkrug, J., Fahrenkrug, L., Håkanson, R., et al. (1980). VIP occurs in intrathyroidal nerves and stimulates thyroid hormone secretion. *Nature*, **287**, 343–345.

Ahren, B., Grunditz, T., Ekman, R., Håkanson, R., Sundler, F. and Uddman, R. (1983). Neuropeptides in the thyroid gland: distribution of substance P and gastrin/cholecystokinin and their effects on the secretion of iodothyronine and calcitonin. *Endocrinology*, **113**, 379–383.

Amenta, F., Caporuscio, D., Ferrante, F., Porcelli, F. and Zomparelli, M. (1978). Cholinergic nerves in the thyroid gland. *Cell and Tissue Research*, **195**, 367–370.

Bienenstock, J., Tomioka, M., Matsuda, H., Stead, K. I., Quinonez, G., Simon, G.T., et al. (1987). The role of mast cells in inflammatory processes: evidence for nerve/mast cell interactions. *International Archives of Allergy and Applied Immunology*, **82**, 238–243.

Bouder, T.G., Huffman, L.J. and Hedge, G.A. (1988). Effects of vasoactive intestinal peptide on vascular conductance are unaffected by anaesthesia. *American Journal of Physiology*, **255**, R968–R973.

Brown-Grant, K. and Gibson, J.G. (1956). The effect of exogenous and endogenous adrenaline on the uptake of radio-iodine by the thyroid gland of the rabbit. *Journal of Physiology*, **131**, 85–101.

Burnstock, G. (1987). Present status of purinergic neurotransmission — implications for vascular control. In *Neuronal Messengers in Vascular Function*, edited by A. Nobin, C. Owman and B. Arneklo-Nobin, pp. 327–340. New York: Elsevier Science Publishers.

Cannon, W.B. and Cattell, M. (1916). Studies on the conditions of activity in endocrine glands. II. The secretory innervation of the thyroid gland. *American Journal of Physiology*, **41**, 58–73.

Cardinali, D.P., Pisarev, M.A., Barontini, M., Juvenal, G.J., Boado, R.J. and Vacas, M.I. (1982). Efferent neuroendocrine pathways of sympathetic superior cervical ganglia. *Neuroendocrinology*, **35**, 248–254.

Cardinali, D.P., Sartorio, G.C., Ladizesky, M.G., Guillen, C.E. and Soto, R.J. (1986). Changes in calcitonin release during sympathetic nerve degeneration after superior cervical ganglionectomy of rats. *Neuroendocrinology*, **43**, 498–503.

Clayton, J.A. and Szego, C.M. (1967). Depletion of rat thyroid serotonin accompanied by increased blood flow as an acute response to thyroid-stimulating hormone. *Endocrinology*, **80**, 689–698.

Connors, J.M., Huffman, L.J. and Hedge, G.A. (1988). Effects of thyrotropin on the vascular conductance of the thyroid gland. *Endocrinology*, **122**, 921–929.

Connors, J.M., Huffman, L.J., Michalkiewicz, M., Chang, B.S.H., Dey, R.D. and Hedge, G.A. (1991). Thyroid vascular conductance: differential effects of elevated plasma TSH induced by treatment with thioamides or TSH-releasing hormone. *Endocrinology*, **129**, 117–125.

Csernay, L., Laszlo, F.A. and Kovacs, K. (1968). The effect of hypophysectomy on adrenal, thyroid and testicular blood flow in the rat. *Acta Physiologica Academiae Scientiarum Hungaricae*, **33**, 291–295.

Davies, J.M. and Williams, K.I. (1984). Endothelial-dependent relaxant effects of vasoactive intestinal polypeptide and arachidonic acid in rat aortic strips. *Prostaglandins*, **27**, 195–202.

Duckles, S.P. and Said, S.I. (1982). Vasoactive intestinal peptide as a neurotransmitter in the cerebral circulation. *European Journal of Pharmacology*, **78**, 371–374.

Dumont, J.E., Takeuchi, A., Lamy, F., Gervy-Decoster, C., Cochaux, P., Roger, P., et al. (1981). Thyroid control: an example of complex cell regulation network. *Advances in Cyclic Nucleotide Research*, **14**, 479–489.

Field, J.B. (1986). Mechanism of action of thyrotropin. In *The Thyroid*, edited by S.H. Ingbar and L.E. Braverman, pp. 288–318. Philadelphia: J.B. Lippincott.

Folkman, J. and Klagsbrun, M. (1987). Angiogenic factors. *Science*, **235**, 442–447.

Fujita, H. (1975). Fine structure of the thyroid gland. *International Review of Cytology*, **40**, 197–280.

Fujita, H. and Murakami, T. (1974). Scanning electron microscopy on the distribution of the minute blood vessels in the thyroid gland of the dog, rat, and rhesus monkey. *Archivum Histologicum Japonicum*, **36**, 181–188.

Gerendai, I., Nemeskeri, A., Faivre-Bauman, A., Grouselle, D. and Tixier-Vidal, A. (1985). Effect of unilateral or bilateral thyroidectomy on TRH content of hypothalamus halves. *Journal of Endocrinological Investigation*, **8**, 321–323.

Goodman, A. and Rone, J.D. (1987). Thyroid angiogenesis: endotheliotropic chemoattractant activity from rat thyroid cells in culture. *Endocrinology*, **121**, 2131–2140.

Green, S.T. (1987). Intrathyroidal autonomic nerves can directly influence hormone release from rat thyroid follicles: a study *in vitro* employing electrical field stimulation and intracellular microelectrodes. *Clinical Science*, **72**, 233–238.

Greil, W., Rafferzeder, M., Bechtner, G. and Gartner, R. (1989). Release of an endothelial cell growth factor from cultured porcine thyroid follicles. *Molecular Endocrinology*, **3**, 858–867.

Grunditz, T., Håkanson, R., Rerup, C., Sundler, F. and Uddman, R. (1984). Neuropeptide Y in the thyroid gland: neuronal localization and enhancement of stimulated thyroid hormone secretion. *Endocrinology*, **115**, 1537–1542.

Grunditz, T., Ekman, R., Håkanson, R., Rerup, C., Sundler, F. and Uddman, R. (1986a). Calcitonin gene-related peptide in thyroid nerve fibres and C cells: effects on thyroid hormone secretion and response to hypercalcemia. *Endocrinology*, **119**, 2313–2324.

Grunditz, T., Håkanson, R., Hedge, G., Rerup, C., Sundler, F. and Uddman, R. (1986b). Peptide histidine isoleucine amide stimulates thyroid hormone secretion and coexists with vasoactive intestinal polypeptide in intrathyroid nerve fibres from laryngeal ganglia. *Endocrinology*, **118**, 783–790.

Grunditz, T., Håkanson, R., Sundler, F. and Uddman R. (1987). Neurokinin A and galanin in the thyroid gland: neuronal localization. *Endocrinology*, **121**, 575–585.

Grunditz T., Ekman, R., Håkanson, R., Sundler, F. and Uddman, R. (1988a). Neuropeptide Y and vasoactive intestinal peptide coexist in rat thyroid nerve fibres emanating from the thyroid ganglion. *Regulatory Peptides*, **23**, 193–208.

Grunditz, T., Håkanson, R., Sundler, F. and Uddman R. (1988b). Neuronal pathways to the rat thyroid revealed by retrograde tracing and immunocytochemistry. *Neuroscience*, **24**, 321–335.

Hansen, J. and Skaaring, P. (1973). Scanning electron microscopy of normal rat thyroid. *Anatomischer Anzeiger*, **134**, 177–185.

Hedge, G.A., Huffman, L.J., Grunditz, T. and Sundler, F. (1984). Immunocytochemical studies of the peptidergic innervation of the thyroid gland in the Brattleboro rat. *Endocrinology*, **115**, 2071–2076.

Hedge, G.A., Huffman, L.J. and Connors, J.M. (1986). Effects of neuropeptides and TSH on thyroid blood flow and hormone secretion. In *Frontiers in Thyroidology*, edited by G. Medeiros Nero and E. Gaitan, pp. 335–338. New York: Plenum Publishing Corporation.

Hedge, G.A., Huffman, L.J. and Connors, J.M. (1987). Functional significance of peptidergic thyroid nerves. In *Integrative Neuroendocrinology: Molecular, Cellular and Clinical Aspects*, edited by S.M. McCann and R.I. Weiner, pp. 115–126. Basel: Karger.

Herveg, J.P. and Wollman, S.H. (1977). Changes in the volume of epithelium, capsule and blood vessels during the development of thyroid hyperplasia in rats. *Annales d' endocrinologie*, **38**, 46A.

Holmgren, H. and Naumann, B. (1949). A study of the nerves of the thyroid gland and their relationship to glandular function. *Acta Endocrinologica*, **3**, 215–235.

Huffman, L. and Hedge, G.A. (1986a). Effects of vasoactive intestinal peptide on thyroid blood flow and circulating thyroid hormone levels in the rat. *Endocrinology*, **118**, 550–557.

Huffman, L. and Hedge, G.A. (1986b). Neuropeptide control of thyroid blood flow and hormone secretion in the rat. *Life Sciences*, **39**, 2143–2150.

Huffman, L.J., Connors, J.M. and Hedge, G.A. (1988). VIP and its homologues increase vascular conductance in certain endocrine and exocrine glands. *American Journal of Physiology*, **254**, E435–E442.

Huffman, L.J., Connors, J.M., White, B.H. and Hedge, G.A. (1988). Vasoactive intestinal peptide treatment that increases thyroid blood flow fails to alter plasma T_3 or T_4 levels in the rat. *Neuroendocrinology*, **47**, 567–574.

Huffman, L., Michalkiewicz, M., Pietrzyk, Z. and Hedge, G.A. (1990). Helodermin, but not cholecystokinin, somatostatin, or thyrotropin releasing hormone, acutely increases thyroid blood flow in the rat. *Regulatory Peptides*, **31**, 101–114.

Huffman, L.J., Michalkiewicz, M., Connors, J.M., Pietrzyk, Z. and Hedge, G.A. (1991). Muscarinic modulation of the vasodilatory effects of vasoactive intestinal peptide at the rat thyroid gland. *Neuroendocrinology*, **53**, 69–74.

Hultgardh-Nilsson, A., Nilsson, J., Jonzon, B. and Dalsgaard, C.-J. (1988). Growth-inhibitory properties of vasoactive intestinal polypeptide. *Regulatory Peptides*, **22**, 267–274.

Ignarro, L.J., Byrns, R.E., Buga, G.M. and Woods, K.S. (1987). Mechanisms of endothelium-dependent vascular smooth muscle relaxation elicited by bradykinin and VIP. *American Journal of Physiology*, **253**, H1074–H1082.

Imada, M., Kurosumi, M. and Fujita, H. (1986a). Three-dimensional imaging of blood vessels in thyroids from normal and levothyroxine sodium-treated rats. *Archivum Histologicum Japonicum*, **49**, 359–367.

Imada, M., Kurosumi, M. and Fujita, H. (1986b). Three-dimensional aspects of blood vessels in thyroids from normal, low iodine diet-treated, TSH-treated, and PTU-treated rats. *Cell and Tissue Research*, **245**, 291–296.

Ishii, J., Shizume, K. and Okinaka, S. (1968). Effect of stimulation of the vagus nerve on the thyroidal release of ^{131}I-labeled hormones. *Endocrinology*, **82**, 7–16.

Ito, H., Matsuda, K., Sato, A. and Tohgi, H. (1987). Cholinergic and VIPergic vasodilator actions of parasympathetic nerves on the thyroid blood flow in rats. *Japanese Journal of Physiology*, **37**, 1005–1017.

Jansen, I., Alafaci, C., Uddman, R. and Edvinsson, L. (1990). Evidence that calcitonin gene-related peptide contributes to the capsaicin-induced relaxation of guinea pig cerebral arteries. *Regulatory Peptides*, **31**, 167–178.

Johanson, V., Ofverholm, T. and Ericson, L.E. (1987). A method for selective infusion in the thyroid artery of the rat and mouse. *Acta Endocrinologica*, **119**, 37–42.

Kapitola, J. (1973). Contemporary notions on the blood flow through the thyroid gland. *Endocrinologia Experimentalis*, **7**, 147–158.

Kapitola, J., Schreiberova, O. and Jahoda, I. (1967). Interrelations between the thyroid function and blood flow in rats. *Endocrinologia Experimentalis*, **1**, 165–171.

Laurberg, P. (1976). T_4 and T_3 release from the perfused canine thyroid isolated *in situ*. *Acta Endocrinologica*, **83**, 105–113.

Lewinski, A. (1981). Inhibitory effect of intrathyroidal injections of 6-hydroxydopamine on the compensatory thyroid hyperplasia in rats. *Neuroendocrinology Letters*, **3**, 341–346.

Lundberg, J.M. (1981). Evidence for coexistence of vasoactive intestinal polypeptide (VIP) and acetylcholine in neurons of cat exocrine glands. *Acta Physiologica Scandinavica Supplementum*, **496**, 1–57.

Melander, A. (1986). Autonomic nervous control: adrenergic, cholinergic, and peptidergic regulation. In *The Thyroid*, edited by S.H. Ingbar and L.E. Braverman, pp. 331–338. Philadelphia: J.B. Lippincott.

Melander, A. and Sundler, F. (1979). Presence and influence of cholinergic nerves in the mouse thyroid. *Endocrinology*, **105**, 7–9.

Melander, A., Sundler, F. and Westgren, U. (1973). Intrathyroidal amines and the synthesis of thyroid hormone. *Endocrinology*, **93**, 193–200.

Melander, A., Ericson, L.E. and Ljunggren J.G. (1974). Sympathetic innervation of the normal human thyroid. *Journal of Clinical Endocrinology and Metabolism*, **39**, 713–718.

Melander, A., Ericson, L.E., Sundler, F. and Ingbar, S.I. (1974). Sympathetic innervation of the mouse thyroid and its significance in thyroid hormone secretion. *Endocrinology*, **94**, 959–966.

Melander, A., Ericson, L.E., Sundler, F. and Westgren, U. (1975a). Intrathyroidal amines in the regulation of thyroid activity. *Reviews of Physiology, Biochemistry and Pharmacology*, **73**, 39–71.

Melander, A., Sundler, F. and Westgren, U. (1975). Sympathetic innervation of the thyroid: variation with species and age. *Endocrinology*, **96**, 102–106.

Melander, A., Westgren, U., Sundler, F. and Ericson, L.E. (1975b). Influence of histamine- and 5-hydroxytrypt-amine-containing thyroid mast cells on thyroid blood flow and permeability in the rat. *Endocrinology*, **97**, 1130–1137.

Michalkiewicz, M., Huffman, L.J., Connors, J.M. and Hedge, G.A. (1987). Measurement of thyroidal VIP content by RIA under hyper- and hypothyroid conditions. *17th Annual Meeting, Society for Neuroscience*, 1311.

Michalkiewicz, M., Huffman, L.J. and Hedge, G.A. (1987). Effects of vasoactive intestinal peptide (VIP) antagonists or antiserum on thyroid blood flow (TBF) and plasma T_3/T_4 levels in the rat. *Federation Proceedings*, **46**, 842.

Michalkiewicz, M., Huffman, L.J., Connors, J.M. and Hedge, G.A. (1989a). Alterations in thyroid blood flow induced by varying levels of iodine intake in the rat. *Endocrinology*, **125**, 54–60.

Michalkiewicz, M., Connors, J.M., Huffman, L.J. and Hedge, G.A. (1989b). Increases in thyroid gland blood flow after hemithyroidectomy in the rat. *Endocrinology*, **124**, 1118–1123.

Michalkiewicz, M., Huffman, L.J. and Hedge, G.A. (1990). Effects of thyroid denervation on thyroid blood flow and VIP content. *20th Annual Meeting, Society for Neuroscience*, 188.

Michalkiewicz, M., Connors, J.M., Huffman, L.J., Pietrzyk, Z. and Hedge, G.A. (1991). Compensatory changes in thyroid blood flow are only partially mediated by thyrotropin. *American Journal of Physiology*, **260**, E608–E612.

Molne, J., Jortso, E., Smeds, S. and Ericson, L.E. (1987). Vascularization of normal human thyroid tissue transplanted to nude mice. *Experimental Cell Biology*, **55**, 104–114.

Mowbray, J.F. and Peart, W.S. (1960). Effects of noradrenaline and adrenaline on the thyroid. *Journal of Physiology*, **151**, 261–271.

Nagataki, S. and Ingbar, S.H. (1986). Autoregulation: effects of iodine. In *The Thyroid*, edited by S.H. Ingbar and L.E. Braverman, pp. 319–338. Philadelphia: J.B. Lippincott.

Nilsson, J., von Euler, A.M. and Dalsgaard, C.-J. (1985). Stimulation of connective tissue cell growth by substance P and substance K. *Nature*, **315**, 61–63.

Nilsson, S.F.E. and Bill, A. (1984). Vasoactive intestinal polypeptide (VIP): effects in the eye and on regional blood flows. *Acta Physiologica Scandinavica*, **121**, 385–392.

Niswender, G.D., Reimers, T.J., Diekman, M.A. and Nett, T.M. (1976). Blood flow: a mediator of ovarian function. *Biology of Reproduction*, **14**, 64–81.

Nonidez, J.F. (1931a). Innervation of the thyroid gland. I. The presence of ganglia in the thyroid of the dog. *Archives of Neurology and Psychiatry*, **25**, 1175–1190.

Nonidez, J.F. (1931b). Innervation of the thyroid gland. II. Origin and course of the thyroid nerves in the dog. *American Journal of Anatomy*, **48**, 299–329.

Nonidez, J.F. (1935). Innervation of the thyroid gland. III. Distribution and termination of the nerve fibres in the dog. *American Journal of Anatomy*, **57**, 135–169.

Pernow, B. (1983). Substance P. *Pharmacological Reviews*, **35**, 85–141.

Pietrzyk, Z., Michalkiewicz, M., Huffman, L.J. and Hedge, G.A. (1992). Vasoactive intestinal peptide (VIP) enhances thyroidal iodide uptake during dietary iodide deficiency. *Endocrine Research*, **18**, 213–228.

Pisarev, M.A., Cardinali, D.P., Juvenal, GJ., Vacas, M.I., Barontini, M. and Boado, R.J. (1981). Role of the sympathetic nervous system in the control of the goitrogenic response in the rat. *Endocrinology*, **109**, 2202–2207.

Porter, J.C. and Klaiber, M.S. (1965). Corticosterone secretion in rats as a function of ACTH input and adrenal blood flow. *American Journal of Physiology*, **209**, 811–814.

Riggs, D.S. (1952). Quantitative aspects of iodine metabolism in man. *Pharmacological Reviews*, **4**, 284–370.

Romeo, H.E., Solveyro, C.G., Vacas, M.I., Rosenstein, R.E., Barontini, M. and Cardinali, D.P. (1986). Origins of the sympathetic projections to rat thyroid and parathyroid glands. *Journal of the Autonomic Nervous System*, **17**, 63–70.

Shinaberger, J.H. and Bruner H.D. (1956). Blood flow in the thyroid gland in the dog. *Federation Proceedings*, **15**, 483.

Sloan, L.W. (1971). Surgical anatomy of the thyroid. In *The Thyroid*, edited by S.C. Werner and S.H. Ingbar, pp. 323–334. New York: Harper & Row.

Smeds, S. and Wollman, S.H. (1983). ^{3}H-Thymidine labeling of endothelial cells in thyroid arteries, veins, and lymphatics during thyroid stimulation. *Laboratory Investigation*, **48**, 285–291.

Soderberg, U. (1958a). Short term reactions in the thyroid gland revealed by continuous measurement of blood flow, rate of uptake of radioactive iodine and rate of release of labelled hormones. *Acta Physiologica Scandinavica*, **42**, Supplementum 147, 1–112.

Soderberg, U. (1958b). The relation between activity and blood flow in the thyroid gland. *Experientia*, **14**, 229–231.

Soderberg, U. (1959). Temporal characteristics of thyroid activity. *Physiological Reviews*, **39**, 777–810.

Studer, H., Peter, H.J. and Gerber, H. (1989). Natural heterogeneity of thyroid cells: the basis for understanding thyroid function and nodular goiter growth. *Endocrine Reviews*, **10**, 125–135.

Thomas, O.L. (1945). The vascular bed in normal and thiourea activated thyroid glands of the rat. *Anatomical Record*, **93**, 23–45.

Tice, L.W. and Creveling, C.R. (1975). Electron microscopic identification of adrenergic nerve endings on thyroid epithelial cells. *Endocrinology*, **97**, 1123–1129.

Toccafondi, R.S., Brandi, M.L., Rotella, C.M. and Zonefrati, R. (1983). Studies of catecholamine effect on cAMP in human cultured thyroid cells: their interaction with thyrotropin receptor. *Acta Endocrinologica*, **102**, 62–67.

Toccafondi, R.S., Brandi, M.L. and Melander, A. (1984). Vasoactive intestinal peptide stimulation of human thyroid cell function. *Journal of Clinical Endocrinology and Metabolism*, **58**, 157–160.

Tonoue, T. and Nomoto, T. (1979). Central nervous system mediated stimulation by thyrotropin-releasing hormone of microcirculation in thyroid gland of rats. *Endocrinologica Japonica*, **26**, 749–752.

Tzinas, S., Droulias, C., Harlaftis, N., Akin, J.T., Jr., Gray, S.W. and Skandalakis, J.E. (1976). Vascular patterns of the thyroid gland. *American Surgeon*, **42**, 639–644.

Uchiyama, Y., Murakami, G. and Ohno, Y. (1985). The fine structure of nerve endings on rat thyroid follicular cells. *Cell and Tissue Research*, **242**, 457–460.

Urquhart, J. and Li, C.C. (1969). Dynamic testing and modeling of adrenocortical secretory function. *Annals of the New York Academy of Sciences*, **156**, 756–778.

Van Sande, J., Dumont, J.E., Melander, A. and Sundler, F. (1980). Presence and influence of cholinergic nerves in the human thyroid. *Journal of Clinical Endocrinology and Metabolism*, **51**, 500–502.

Wahlestedt, C., Grundemar, L., Håkanson, R., Heilig, M., Shen, G.H., Zukowska-Grojec, Z., *et al.* (1990). Neuropeptide Y receptor subtypes, Y1 and Y2. *Annals of the New York Academy of Sciences*, **611**, 7–26.

Watts, C.F. (1915). Changes in iodine content of the thyroid gland following changes in the blood flow through the gland. *American Journal of Physiology*, **38**, 356–368.

Wei, E.P., Kontos, H.A. and Said, S.I. (1980). Mechanism of action of vasoactive intestinal polypeptide on cerebral arterioles. *American Journal of Physiology*, **239**, H765–H768.

Wollman, S.H., Herveg, J.P., Zeligs, J.D. and Ericson, L.E. (1978). Blood capillary enlargement during the development of thyroid hyperplasia in the rat. *Endocrinology*, **103**, 2306–2314.

Index